CW01455913

Daniel A. Paesani (Editor)

# Bruxism: Theory and Practice

# Bruxism: Theory and Practice

*Editor:*
*Daniel A. Paesani*

*Contributors:*
Monica Andersen, Taro Arima,
Lene Baad-Hansen, Marta M. Barreiro,
Gunnar E. Carlsson, Fernando Cifuentes,
Sergio Fuster, Jorge Mario Galante,
Carlos Gianoni, Fernando Goldberg,
Hans L. Hamburger, Faramarz Jadidi,
Anders Johansson, Ann-Katrin Johansson,
Takafumi Kato, Marcelo Kreiner,
Stephanos Kyrkanides, Frank Lobbezoo,
Ricardo L. Macchi, Daniele Manfredini,
Arturo E. Manns Freese, Machiel Naeije,
Luca Guarda Nardini, Ridwaan Omar,
Claudia Restrepo, Xiomara Restrepo-J.,
Andres R. Sanchez, Guillermo Schinini,
Teresa Cristina Barros Schütz,
José T. T. de Siqueira, Peter Svensson,
Ross H. Tallents, Sergio Tufik

QUINTESSENCE PUBLISHING

London, Berlin, Chicago, Tokyo, Barcelona,
Beijing, Istanbul, Milan, Moscow, New Delhi,
Paris, Prague, São Paulo, Seoul, and Warsaw

*This book is dedicated to the memory of*
*Rosalia Cuddé and Graciela Slutzky*

British Library Cataloguing in Publication Data
Paesani, Daniel A.
Bruxism : theory and practice.
1. Bruxism. 2. Bruxism--Diagnosis. 3. Bruxism--Complications.
4. Bruxism--Treatment.
I. Title
617.6-dc22
ISBN-13: 9781850971917



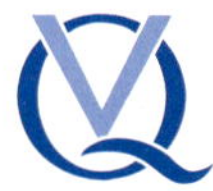

**Quintessence Publishing Co. Ltd**
Quintessence House, Grafton Road
New Malden, Surrey KT3 3AB
United Kingdom
www.quintpub.co.uk

Production: Juliane Richter, Quintessenz Verlags-GmbH, Berlin
Printing: Bosch-Druck GmbH, Ergolding



ISBN: 978-1-85097-191-7
Printed in Germany

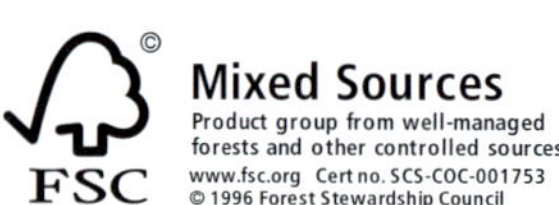

# Foreword

For years the dental profession has been intrigued, fascinated, and sometimes even obsessed with the phenomenon we call bruxism. It has been underdiagnosed, overdiagnosed, and even misdiagnosed. Some have described it as the most destructive process affecting the masticatory structures, while others refer to it as a benign routine activity. Some suggest it is rare, while others say it is very common. Some say it is a major contributor to temporomandibular disorders, while others say it is not even related.

The etiology of bruxism has been hotly debated for years. Some believe it is a peripherally generated activity associated with tooth contacts, while others believe it is a central brainstem-driven process. There is a long list of suggested causes of bruxism such as eccentric tooth contacts, dental malocclusion, emotional stress, anxiety, sleep disturbances, genetic factors, medications, alcohol consumption, breathing disorders, allergies, mental disorders, and even pin worms. Bruxism is even mentioned in the Holy Bible as the "gnashing of teeth" associated with anger and frustration.

The dental profession has learned that studying bruxism is difficult and controversial. Most patients are unaware of their bruxing activity and therefore deny it. Bed partners are sometimes more reliable reporters. We dentists seem to inform all our patients that they brux; they just don't know it. We most probably do this because we see the evidence of tooth wear, yet timing may be a serious issue. For instance, significant tooth wear in a 40-year-old patient may present as a dental problem; yet this wear might have occurred 20 years earlier and bruxism is no longer a contributing factor.

Clinicians have also developed a wide variety of treatments for bruxism, many with no scientific evidence. Dental treatments have ranged from selectively adjusting the occlusion to prosthetic or orthodontic therapies. We have developed a wide variety of occlusal appliances, most with limited to no supportive data. We have suggested non-dental therapies such as medications, biofeedback, stress reduction, and acupuncture. We have even used negative-feedback devices including electric shocks, loud noises, and taste aversion. It is obvious that we need to understand and document the most effective method to manage bruxism.

It is quite evident that the profession needs a comprehensive review of this complex phenomenon known as bruxism. Dr. Daniel Paesani recognized this need and has put together the most thorough body of information ever created by the profession. He has assembled some of our finest experts from around the world to contribute their knowledge and insights to this text. His comprehensive list of chapters has left no stone unturned. This text is the most complete overview of bruxism the profession has ever had opportunity to review.

There are several reasons why I am very pleased to have been asked to write the foreword to this textbook. First, this text represents the first comprehensive attempt to review bruxism, and the profession needs to be enlightened and informed about this important subject. I am also very pleased because I have known Daniel Paesani for almost 30 years and I know and appreciate his dedication to the field. Dr. Paesani was one of my very first international residents in our Orofacial Pain Center and he came from Rosario, Argentina to Lexington, Kentucky with much passion for the field and personal sacrifice. I have always admired his dedication and work ethic, and this text is a product of just that. I believe it will serve our profession well.

Jeffrey P. Okeson, DMD
*Chair, Department of Oral Health Science*
Director, Orofacial Pain Program
University of Kentucky College of Dentistry
Lexington, Kentucky, USA

# Preface and Acknowledgments

Over my 12 years as Professor of Masticatory System Physiology in the School of Odontology of the Universidad del Salvador/AOA (Buenos Aires, Argentina), the biggest problem we have had to face has been the lack of scientific compilations on bruxism, which are needed for students to take bruxism as an object of study.

At first, we used to request students to visit the Medline web page – the most important biomedical-literature database worldwide – and perform searches, but before long we realized that was not the right track. The students faced the difficulty of having to select which pieces of information to use from the thousands of publications retrieved by search engines. Of course, since these were first-degree students, they were not yet sufficiently qualified to differentiate concepts that had been validated by scientific method from concepts based simply on mysticism and dogma. We, the professors, would spend long hours assisting them with these issues, and we would use the scarce, precious time available to us to select and compile the study material rather than to teach.

This experience made me wonder why – researchers and published books being so many and bruxism being such an important entity in the odontological field – not a single volume existed devoted exclusively to bruxism. When I found no answer to this question, I started to think about taking on the responsibility to compile information with the aim of publishing a volume exclusively devoted to bruxism and its treatment.

After preparing an extensive list of chapters, and with the purpose of addressing all the topics related to bruxism, I invited a group of colleagues whose brilliant professional careers, experience, and dedication to the subject would *a priori* guarantee their addressing the specific topics with scientific and scholarly rigor. The premise was that each paragraph, each idea, each suggestion should be based on scientific evidence, so that the work, apart from being useful to college professors and students, is an interesting book for general practitioners, one that provides answers to the many questions arising in everyday dental practice. Also, specialists in craniomandibular disorders will benefit from the in-depth analysis of the subjects and the extensive, up-to-date bibliographies contained herein, which provide a quick, well-organized way to access the evidence they need in their professional practice and as a tool for planning future research. So, the volume is divided into three sections.

- The first section comprises eight chapters dealing with bruxism knowledge and guidelines for diagnosis, sleep physiology, main etiological theories, influence of peripheral and emotional factors, movement disorders, and bruxism in children.
- The second section comprises nine chapters and is devoted to the effects of bruxism on the masticatory system components. Some of the topics are: the noxious action of bruxism on dental pulp, periodontal ligament, temporomandibular joints, muscles, and its relation-

ship with pain. Some bruxism effects that are currently controversial are discussed, for which purpose a wide review of the literature on the subject is provided. Special emphasis has been placed on tooth wear and on the differential diagnosis of bruxism's several causes. One chapter has been specifically devoted to dental erosion, and another chapter to endogenous erosion mechanisms, since general practitioners often mistake tooth wear caused by endogenous erosion for tooth wear caused by bruxism.

- The third section comprises eight chapters and deals with various aspects related to the treatment of bruxism. The pharmacological effects of certain central-action drugs and some peripheral-action drugs, such as botulinum toxin, are described. The text also deals with the treatment of bruxism involving dental implants and appliances constructed with dental materials particularly recommended for bruxers. Topics related to dental occlusion are discussed with the aim of facilitating understanding of the concepts needed to enter the fascinating world of complex oral rehabilitation. One chapter deals with techniques used for the reconstruction of teeth affected by significant wear.

The volume also includes a review of the scientific evidence on the treatment of bruxism, especially bruxism splints. The different procedures used for protecting the masticatory system against the effects of bruxism are described and illustrated by means of case reports.

***Acknowledgments***

I would like to express my gratitude to:

- the contributing authors, whose valuable expertise and thorough dedication ensured the excellent coverage of a wide range of topics related to bruxism
- Professors Jeffrey Okeson, Ross Tallents, Per-Lennart Westesson, and Annika Isberg for introducing me to the marvelous world of science
- Quintessence Publishing for believing in this book and accepting it for publication
- professional translators Ángela Giottonini (Chapters 1, 15, and 21) and María Mirela Perusia (Chapters 2, 9–14, 20, 23, and 25) for their brilliant translations of the original Spanish text into English
- Valeria Castillo for proofreading the original Spanish text
- the staff of the library of the Asociación Odontológica Argentina (Dental Association of Argentina) for their valuable help in obtaining the innumerable bibliographical references I have used
- my assistants Liliana Rivalta, Gabriela Allo, and Patricia Peloso for their endless patience and dedication and their invaluable help in the management of the numerous patients and in the process of obtaining the clinical photographs
- my family, Triana, Guido, Julia, Pedro, Susana, and Candela, who, in all their love, gave up sharing many irretrievable days with me.

Daniel Angel Paesani
*Editor*

# List of all contributors

### *Editor*

**Daniel A. Paesani, DDS**
Professor of Stomatognathic Physiology
School of Dentistry
University of Salvador/AOA
Buenos Aires, Argentina

### *Contributors*

**Monica Andersen, PhD**
Associate Professor
Department of Psychobiology
School of Medicine
Universidade Federal de São Paulo
(UNIFESP)
São Paulo, Brazil

**Taro Arima, DDS, PhD**
Assistant Professor
Department of Oral Rehabilitation
Graduate School of Dental Medicine
University of Hokkaido
Sapporo, Japan

**Lene Baad-Hansen, DDS, PhD**
Associate Professor
Department of Clinical Oral Physiology
School of Dentistry
Aarhus University
Aarhus, Denmark

**Marta M. Barreiro, DDS, Dr Dent**
Professor of Dental Materials
School of Dentistry
University of Buenos Aires
Buenos Aires, Argentina

**Gunnar E. Carlsson, LDS, Odont Dr/ PhD, Dr Odont hc, Dr Dent hc, FDSRCS**
Professor Emeritus
Department of Prosthetic Dentistry/
Dental Materials Science
Specialist in Prosthodontics and TMD/
Orofacial Pain
Institute of Odontology
The Sahlgrenska Academy
University of Gothenburg
Göteborg, Sweden

**Fernando Cifuentes, DDS**
Assistance Professor
Department of Stomatognatic Physiology
School of Dentistry
University of Salvador/AOA
Buenos Aires, Argentina

**Sergio Fuster, MD**
Gastroenterology Specialist
Private Practice, Rosario, Argentina

**Jorge Mario Galante, DDS**
Associate Professor
School of Dentistry
University of Buenos Aires
Buenos Aires, Argentina

**Carlos Gianoni, MD**
Gastroenterology Specialist
Private Practice
Rosario, Argentina

**Fernando Goldberg, DDS, PhD**
Professor
Department of Endodontics
School of Dentistry
University of Salvador/AOA
Buenos Aires, Argentina

**Hans L. Hamburger, MD, PhD**
Neurologist
Department of Clinical Neurophysiology
Amsterdam Center for Sleep-Wake Studies
Slotervaart Hospital
Amsterdam, The Netherlands

**Faramarz Jadidi**
PhD student
Department of Clinical Oral Physiology
School of Dentistry, Aarhus University
Aarhus, Denmark

**Anders Johansson, DDS, Odont Dr/PhD**
Professor
Department of Clinical Dentistry - Prosthodontics
Specialist in Prosthodontics and TMD/
Orofacial Pain
Faculty of Medicine and Dentistry
University of Bergen
Bergen, Norway

**Ann-Katrin Johansson, DDS, Odont Lic/MSc, Odont Dr/PhD**
Associate Professor and Head of Cariology
Department of Clinical Dentistry - Cariology
Specialist in Pediatric Dentistry
Faculty of Dentistry, University of Bergen
Bergen, Norway

**Takafumi Kato, DDS, PhD**
Associate Professor
Institute for Oral Science
Graduate School of Oral Medicine
Matsumoto Dental University
Chief
Dental Sleep Medicine Clinic
Matsumoto Dental University Hospital
Matsumoto, Japan

**Marcelo Kreiner, DDS**
Professor and Chairman
Department of General and Oral Physiology
School of Dentistry
Universidad de la República
Montevideo, Uruguay

**Stephanos Kyrkanides, DDS, MS, PhD**
Professor and Chairman
Department of Orthodontics
and Pediatric Dentistry
School of Dental Medicine
Stony Brook University
Stony Brook
New York, NY, USA

**Frank Lobbezoo, DDS, PhD**
Professor
Department of Oral Function
Academic Centre for Dentistry Amsterdam
(ACTA), Amsterdam, The Netherlands

**Ricardo L. Macchi, DDS, MS, Dr Dent**
Professor Emeritus of Dental Materials
School of Dentistry
University of Buenos Aires
Buenos Aires, Argentina

**Daniele Manfredini, DDS**
Visiting Professor
TMD Clinic
Department of Maxillofacial Surgery
University of Padova, Padova, Italy

**Arturo E. Manns Freese, DDS, PhD**
Professor of Oral Physiology and Occlusion
School of Dentistry, University of the Andes
Santiago, Chile

**Machiel Naeije, PhD**
Professor and Chair
Department of Oral Function
Academic Centre for Dentistry Amsterdam (ACTA), Amsterdam, The Netherlands

**Luca Guarda Nardini, MD, DDS**
Director
TMD Clinic, Department of Maxillofacial Surgery
University of Padova, Padova, Italy

**Ridwaan Omar, BSc, BDS, LDSRCS, MSc, FRACDS, FDSRCSEd**
Professor and Head of Prosthodontics
Vice Dean for Academic & Clinical Affairs
Department of Restorative Sciences
Faculty of Dentistry, Kuwait University
Kuwait

**Claudia Restrepo, DDS**
Pediatric Dentist
Teacher, Postgraduate Program of Pediatric Dentistry and Preventive Orthodontics
Director of the CES-LPH Research Group
CES University, Medellin, Colombia

**Xiomara Restrepo-J., DDS**
General Practice Resident
Department of General Dentistry
Eastman Institute for Oral Health
Rochester, NY, USA

**Andres R. Sanchez, DDS, MS**
Private Practice, Eden Prairie, MN, USA
Former Assistant Professor in Periodontics
Marquette University School of Dentistry
Milwaukee, WI, USA

**Guillermo Schinini, DDS**
Clinical Assistant Professor
Department of Periodontology
Maimonides University
Private Practice
Rosario, Argentina

**Teresa Cristina Barros Schütz, DDS, PhD**
Researcher
Department of Psychobiology
School of Medicine
Universidade Federal de São Paulo (UNIFESP)
São Paulo, Brazil

**José T. T. de Siqueira, DDS, PhD**
Head of Orofacial Pain Team
Dentistry Division
Hospital das Clínicas, School of Medicine
Universidade de São Paulo (USP)
Researcher
Department of Psychobiology
School of Medicine
Universidade Federal de São Paulo (UNIFESP)
São Paulo, Brazil

**Peter Svensson, DDS, PhD, Dr Odont**
Professor
Department of Clinical Oral Physiology
School of Dentistry, Aarhus University
Aarhus, Denmark

**Ross H. Tallents, DDS**
Professor of Dentistry
Department of Orthodontics and Prosthodontics
Eastman Institute for Oral Health
Rochester, NY, USA

**Sergio Tufik, MD, PhD**
Professor
Department of Psychobiology
School of Medicine
Universidade Federal de São Paulo (UNIFESP)
São Paulo, Brazil

# Contents

# Part 1

# Overview of the problem

# Chapter 1

# Introduction to Bruxism

*Daniel A. Paesani*

## Introduction

In the glossary of terms of the American Academy of Orofacial Pain, bruxism is defined as a "total parafunctional daily or nightly activity that includes grinding, gnashing, or clenching of the teeth. It takes place in the absence of subjective consciousness and it can be diagnosed by the presence of tooth wear facets which have not resulted from the chewing function".[1]

In order to understand the remoteness of the act of "gnashing the teeth", we can cite the following passages from the Bible:

Psalm 35:16 "Like profane mockers at a feast, they gnash at me with their teeth"

Psalm 112:10 "The sinner shall see and be angry, he shall gnash his teeth and consume away"

Job 16:9 "he grinds his teeth at me"

Matthew 8:12 "But the children of the kingdom shall be cast out into outer darkness: there shall be weeping and gnashing of teeth"

At the beginning of the twentieth century, Karolyi used the term "traumatic neuralgia" to refer to the grinding of the teeth and described it as the cause of a periodontal condition by then called *pyorrhea*.[2] The term "bruxism" comes from the Greek expression *brychein odontas* that means grinding the teeth. In French, *bruxomanie* was used for the first time by Marie and Pietkiewicz in 1907.[3] Then, Frohman was responsible for the first publication in the odontological literature when he referred to "bruxomania" as a pure psychological state.[4]

## The Importance of Bruxism in Daily Care

Bruxism may be considered a normal habit; but under certain circumstances, such as an increase in the frequency of episodes and the strength of masseter contractions, it may turn into a phenomenon with pathological consequences.[5] Bruxism may dramatically change the result and the duration of the delicate and careful treatments performed by clinicians. Whereas a soft form of bruxism hardly ever affects oral structures, a hard manifestation may cause frustrating problems for both the patient and the professional. A simple plastic obturation, an endodontic treatment, a crown, or fixed dental prosthesis may be destroyed faster than usual due to bruxism.

When the most evident effect of bruxism is wear of dentition, the patient is the only one to blame; but if there is quick wear of a treatment done by a clinician, a conflict between the patient and the professional can arise. It is likely that practitioners have always experienced this. Quite often, the powerful effect of bruxism is underestimated and every dental specialization is likely to be affected, to a certain degree, by this devastating habit.

For these reasons, it is advisable to put into practice early instruction on bruxism, and if possible as a specialized subject. Unfortunately, in many dental schools, bruxism teaching is limited to partial classes in different subjects. It is often confusing to read the discussions and contradictions of this concept. In the following chapters, the aim is to clarify the current concept of bruxism, its effects, diagnosis, and treatment, and future investigations, to try to put an end to the controversies.

## Oral Habits

The masticatory system is very complex and accomplishes specific vital functions such as mastication, swallowing, and speaking. The rest of the activities are considered "non-functional", and for this reason they are called *parafunctions*. Some people call them self-destructive oral habits because they produce a type of aggression towards the body – including bruxism. The following is a list of the so-called parafunctions:

- long-lasting teeth clenching
- teeth grinding
- sustained contraction of the muscles of mastication (without dental contact)
- biting the lip, cheeks, or tongue
- lingual thrust
- nail biting
- cuticle biting
- biting different objects
- alteration in jaw posture (such as keeping a protruded jaw position).

## Classification of Bruxism according to the Type and Timing of Activity

Bruxism can be experienced by the patient while awake or asleep. In the past it was classified as day or nightly bruxism; but following the suggestion made by the American Academy of Sleeping Disorders,[6] and due to the fact that some people sleep during the day and may also grind, it is more accurate to refer to *sleep and awake bruxism*. Bruxism involves teeth grinding as well as a continuous clenching, or both at the same time.

Sleep bruxism involves the development of a rhythmic jaw muscle activity, which can be divided into three types:[7]

- *phasic:* corresponds to at least three muscle contraction bursts of 0.25 to 2.0 seconds of duration separated by two inter-burst intervals[8]
- *tonic:* corresponds to a muscle contraction burst that lasts more than 2.0 seconds[8]
- *mixed:* a combination of phasic and tonic episodes separated by a 30-second interval.[9]

During sleep, teeth grinding caused by a certain muscle contraction, also called "eccentric or phasic bruxism", is more common. This kind of bruxism is accompanied by a very characteristic sound that can be rather annoying for bed partners. People who grind their teeth during sleep can only be aware of this disturbing behaviour when somebody who has heard the grinding sound tells them or, on very few occasions, when the grinding sound is so loud that it interrupts the person's sleep. This kind of bruxism generally causes a specific kind of tooth wear called attrition that manifests as "wear facets".

Other people have a silent type of bruxism, that is, they constantly clench their teeth without any movements. This type of bruxism – known as "centric or tonic" – is less frequent. Finally, the combination of the phasic and tonic types of bruxism is called "mixed" bruxism.

Studies on bruxers carried out by Lavigne and co-workers[9] in laboratories using polysomnography have revealed the following distribution of the different types of bruxism:

- 52.5% phasic
- 11.4% tonic
- 36.1% mixed.

During wakefulness, the most common type of bruxism involves teeth clenching. This type of bruxism has not been studied in depth. Some patients say that they are surprised to find out that they brux involuntarily when they are performing a task that demands concentration or when they are emotionally stressed.

On the other hand, some people grind their teeth while awake. This parafunction is generally mild and so does not produce the typical grinding sound, with the exception of those people who suffer from neurological conditions or a brain lesion.[10]

Some people brux both during wakefulness (clenching) and while sleeping (grinding). Another type of bruxism – called "secondary or pharmacologic bruxism" – has been discovered in patients with psychiatric conditions as a side-effect of neuroleptic and antidepressant medication. This topic is dealt with in Chapter 18.

## Etiology

The etiology of bruxism is a controversial subject. Karolyi's mystical approach,[2] which postulated occlusion interferences as the alleged cause, has fallen out of favor over the years. At present, even though the etiology of bruxism is an unsolved question, there seems to be an agreement on establishing a difference between awake and sleep bruxism and on the fact that they are associated with different etiological factors.

Awake bruxism is considered a tic and has been related to daily stress.[11] In contrast, sleep bruxism originates in the central nervous system (CNS) and is associated with lightening of the sleep, or so-called micro-arousal.[12,13] Bruxism etiology is dealt with comprehensively in Chapter 4.

## Genetics

Since the first epidemiological study of the prevalence of bruxism in the population in general, a statistically significant correlation has been established between sleep bruxers and the number of blood relatives who also suffer from bruxism.[14] Three hypotheses have been postulated: (1) an inherited factor, (2) the same "emotional environment" shared by relatives, and (3) an increased degree of consciousness of the habit. A similar correlation was found in another study, but the author states that the determination of genetic factors is confusing owing to the overlapping presence of environmental factors.[15] Between 21% and 50% of patients who develop sleep bruxism have a direct relative who also suffers from the same condition.[16,17]

Dooland and co-workers[18] carried out a study on a group of monozygotic twins and another group of bizygotic twins. Based on the belief that wear facets on canines would be the consequence of gnashing habits, the authors compared the maxillary primary canine wear facets present in both groups and found that all individuals showed signs of wear. They concluded that bruxism is a universal phenomenon in children.

Two studies support the idea of the inherited nature of sleep bruxism by stating that bruxism prevalence is more frequent in monozygotic siblings than in bizygotic ones.[19,20] However, another study carried out on twins showed no genetic correlation for sleep bruxism.[21]

Diverse opinions remain regarding genetic factors. The roles of genetic and family environmental factors should be clarified by future controlled investigations.

*Table 1-1*

**Prevalence of bruxism (%) from cross-sectional epidemiologic studies in the general population.**

| Author | Method | Gender | Age | Wk Cl | Slp Gr | Cl+Gr |
|---|---|---|---|---|---|---|
| Egermark-Eriksson et al[24] | Q | F+M | 7<br>11<br>15 | 9<br>11<br>11 | 20<br>10<br>11 | –<br>–<br>– |
| Nilner[64] | PI | F+M | 7–14<br>15–18 | 20<br>13 | 16<br>7 | –<br>– |
| Könönen et al[65] | PI | F<br>M | 10–16 | 16<br>6 | 10<br>18 | –<br>– |
| Ingervall et al[30] | Q | M | 21–54 | 44.7 | 12.8 | – |
| Reding et al[14] | Q | F+M | 3–17<br>16–36 | –<br>– | 15.1<br>5.1 | –<br>– |
| Molin et al[66] | Q | M | 18–25 | 10 | 4 | – |
| Glaros[15] | Q | F<br>M | 19 | 7<br>10 | 5<br>3 | 3<br>3 |
| Matsuka et al[67] | Q | F+M | 20–70 | 30 | 34 | – |
| Rieder et al[37] | Q | F<br>M | 13–86 | 37.1<br>29.2 | 13.7<br>20.2 | –<br>– |
| Winocur et al[28] | Q | F | 15–16 | 18 | 4.7 | – |
| Glass et al[68] | TI | F+M | ≥18 | 17.9 | 14.5 | – |
| Pow et al[69] | TI | F+M | ≥18 | – | – | 24.6 |
| Goulet et al[70] | TI | F+M | ≥18 | 20 | 6 | – |
| Ohayon et al[71] | TI | F+M | ≥15 | – | 8.2 | – |
| Swanljung and Rantanen[36] | PI | F<br>M | 18–64 | 2.7 | 9<br>15 | –<br>– |
| Ciancaglini et al[57] | PI | F+M | 18–75 | – | – | 31.4 |
| Gross et al[72] | PI | F+M | 3–89 | 19.2 | 12.1 | – |
| Choy and Smith[73] | Q | F<br>M | x~65 | 36.5<br>28 | –<br>– | –<br>– |

contd.

*Table 1-1*

| Author | Method | Gender | Age | Wk Cl | Slp Gr | Cl+Gr |
|---|---|---|---|---|---|---|
| Gavish et al[29] | Q | F | 15–16 | 22 | 12.7 | – |
| Agerberg and Carlsson[74] | Q | F+M | 15–74 | 20 | 10 | – |
| De Vis et al[75] | Q | F+M | 3–6 | – | 7.7 | – |
| Widmalm et al[76] | PI | F+M | 4–6 | – | 20 | – |
| Ng et al[77] | PI | F+M | x~6.4 | – | 8.5 | – |
| Ng et al[78] | TI | F+M | 6–12 | – | 20.5 | – |
| Chuanjedong et al[56] | Q | F+M | >15 | – | – | 17.8 |
| Lavigne and Montplaisir[54] | PI | F+M | >18 | – | 8 | – |
| Cheifetz et al[27] | Q | F+M | <17 | – | 38 | – |
| Demir et al[79] | Q | F+M | 7–19 | – | 12.6 | – |
| Ow et al[80] | PI+Q | F+M | 55–91 | 3.9 | 3.6 | – |
| Duckro et al[81] | TI | F+M | ≥21 | 10.8 | 12.8 | – |
| Agerberg and Bergenholtz[82] | PI | F | 25 | 26.1 | 15.6 | – |
| | | M | | 19.3 | 17.3 | – |
| | | F | 35 | 28.1 | 11.3 | – |
| | | M | | 16.8 | 15.3 | – |
| | | F | 50 | 28.3 | 7.1 | – |
| | | M | | 19.4 | 8.4 | – |
| | | F | 65 | 24.6 | 3.1 | – |
| | | M | | 18.7 | 6.4 | – |
| Mercado and Faulkner[58] | PI | F | 54–89 | – | – | 36.6 |
| | | M | 47–88 | – | – | 25 |
| Norheim and Dahl[83] | Q | F | 20–69 | – | 4 | – |
| | | M | | – | 7 | – |
| Jensen et al[38] | Q | F | 25–64 | 28.9 | 18.9 | – |
| | | M | | 15.8 | 12 | – |

Q = questionnaire; PI = personal interview; TI = telephone interview; Wk Cl = wake clenching; Slp Gr = sleep grinding; Cl+Gr = clenching + grinding; x = mean

*Table 1-2*

**Prevalence of bruxism (%) in patients with temporomandibular disorders (TMD).**

| Author | Method | Population | Gender | Age | Wk Cl | Slp Gr | Cl+Gr |
|---|---|---|---|---|---|---|---|
| Agerberg and Helkimo[84] | Q | TMD | F+M | 11–84 | – | – | 37 |
| Droukas et al[85] | Q | TMD | F+M | 16–40 | 46 | 38 | – |
| Gelb and Bernstein[86] | Q | TMD | F+M | 10–80 | – | – | 58 |
| Pergamalian et al[52] | Q+PI | TMD | F+M | 18–60 | – | – | 79.7 |
| Butler et al[87] | Q | TMD | F+M | 16–73 | 48 | 21 | – |
| Cacchiotti et al[88] | Q | TMD<br>Controls | F+M | 19–40<br>22–39 | 33<br>44 | 36<br>32 | –<br>– |
| Suvinen et al[89] | Q | TMD<br>Controls | F+M | 38.4<br>33.4 | –<br>– | –<br>– | 62.5<br>23 |
| Agerberg and Carlsson[90] | Q | Controls<br>TMD | F+M | 15–74 | 20<br>52 | 10<br>17 | –<br>– |
| Marbach et al[40] | Q | TMD<br>Controls | F+M | 38<br>39.9 | –<br>– | –<br>– | 27<br>28 |
| Manfredini et al[91] | Q | TMD<br>Controls | F+M | 34.7<br>33.6 | –<br>– | –<br>– | 58<br>44.1 |
| Koidis et al[92] | Q | TMD | F<br>M | 16–70 | 65<br>59 | 18<br>26 | –<br>– |

Q = questionnaire; PI = personal interview; Wk Cl = wake clenching;
Slp Gr = sleep grinding; Cl+Gr = clenching + grinding

*Table 1-3*

**Prevalence of bruxism (%) from longitudinal studies.**

| Author | Method | Gender | Age | Wk Cl | Slp Gr | Cl+Gr |
|---|---|---|---|---|---|---|
| Laberge et al[93] | Q | F+M | 3–10 | – | 19.2 | – |
| | | | 11 | – | 13.8 | – |
| | | | 12 | – | 11.2 | – |
| | | | 13 | – | 9.3 | – |
| Holm and Arvidsson[94] Holm[95–97] | PI | F+M | 3 | – | 24 | – |
| | | | 4 | – | 28 | – |
| | | | 5 | – | 32 | – |
| | | | 8 | – | 21 | – |
| Onizawa and Yoshida[98] | Q | F+M | 18 | – | – | 13.5 |
| | | | 25 | – | – | 28.7 |
| Heikinheimo et al[99] | Q | F | 12 | – | – | 40.4 |
| | | | 15 | – | – | 36.9 |
| | | M | 12 | – | – | 31.3 |
| | | | 15 | – | – | 29.9 |
| Könönen and Nyström[100] | PI | F+M | 14 | 9 | 14 | – |
| | | | 15 | 5 | 9 | – |
| | | | 18 | 10 | 11 | – |
| Magnusson et al[101] | Q | F+M | 7 | – | – | 26 |
| | | | 11 | – | – | 27 |
| | | | 11 | – | – | 19 |
| | | | 15 | – | – | 29 |
| Magnusson et al[102] | Q | F+M | 15 | 12 | 10 | – |
| | | | 20 | 21 | 14 | – |
| Magnusson et al[103] | Q | F+M | 7 | 12 | 19 | – |
| | | | 17 | 34 | 24 | – |
| | | | 11 | 11 | 14 | – |
| | | | 21 | 48 | 28 | – |
| | | | 15 | 11 | 15 | – |
| | | | 25 | 45 | 38 | – |
| Magnusson et al[104] | Q | F+M | 15 | 11 | 15 | – |
| | | | 20 | 21 | 14 | – |
| | | | 25 | 45 | 38 | – |
| | | | 35 | 46 | 33 | – |
| Pilley et al[105] | Q+PI | F+M | 12 | 24 | 19.7 | – |
| | | | 15 | 41 | 21 | – |

Q = questionnaire; PI = personal interview; Wk Cl = wake clenching;
Slp Gr = sleep grinding; Cl+Gr = clenching + grinding

*Table 1-4*

**Prevalence of bruxism (%) from cross-sectional studies where dental wear was included.**

| Author | Method | Population | Gender | Age | Wk Cl | Slp Gr | Cl+Gr | DW |
|---|---|---|---|---|---|---|---|---|
| Lindqvist[39] | Q+CE | Students | F+M | 10–13 | 1 | 15 | – | 47 |
| Lindqvist[19] | ME+CE | Twins | F+M | 10–14 | – | – | – | 54 |
| Nilner and Lassing[44] | PI+CE | Students | F+M | 7–14 | 20 | 16 | – | 100 |
| Seligman et al[22] | Q+ME | Students | F+M | 19–40 | 21 | – | 23 | 91.5 |
| Dooland et al[18] | ME+CE | Twins | F+M | 8 | – | – | – | 100 |

Q = questionnaire; CE = clinical examination; ME = model examination; PI = personal interview; Wk Cl = wake clenching; Slp Gr = sleep grinding; Cl+Gr = clenching + grinding; DW = dental wear

## Epidemiology

In the general population it is very difficult to accurately determine the prevalence of bruxism. Tables 1-1 to 1-5 present the results of various epidemiologic studies.

No significant differences regarding sex have been found, and epidemiologic studies have reported great variability of bruxism prevalence – the reported percentages range from 6% to 91%.[14,22] These wide differences can be attributed to:

- the methodology applied for diagnosis
- characteristics of the studied population
- types of bruxism.

### *The Methodology Applied for Diagnosis*

Bruxism measurement is an extremely complicated process, so differences among the methodologies used for identifying bruxism have a great influence on the prevalences reported. The simplest and most economical methodologies (questionnaires, models, electromyography) are usually inaccurate, whereas more accurate methods (sleep studies) are more complex and expensive.

*Questionnaires*

Questionnaires are widely used in epidemiologic surveys because they are a rapid and inexpensive instrument to gather information. Other available methods are personal and telephone interviews that, unlike questionnaires, guarantee a more accurate answer from the interviewee thanks to the direct contact.

The accuracy of questionnaires for recording self-evaluation of habits has been thrown into doubt.[23] For example, the questionnaire response can be influenced by the patient's age – the older the person is, the more intellectually mature and the more aware of habits he or she will be. Moreover, when the same questionnaire is used more than once in a longitudinal study (see Table 1-3), patients can pay more attention to their actions and can find it easier to spot initially unconscious habits or behaviors. This can relatively increase bruxism prevalence results. It is also believed that questionnaires underestimate bruxism prevalence because some people may completely ignore their bruxing habit.[24]

Some patients start to think they are bruxers after their dentist has diagnosed it (based on pres-

*Table 1-5*

**Prevalence of dental wear (%) obtained from clinical examination and/or model examination.**

| Author | Method | Gender | Age | Dental wear |
|---|---|---|---|---|
| Fareed et al[106] | ME | F+M | 19–25 | 100 |
| Abdullah et al[107] | ME | F+M | 17–24 | 100 |
| Warren et al[108] | ME | F+M | 5 | 100 |
| Pintado et al[109] | ME | F+M | 22–30 | 50 |
| Milosevic and Lo[110] | CE | F+M | 14–77 | 100 |
| Casanova-Rosado et al[111] | CE | F+M | 14–19 | 33.3 |
| Silness et al[112] | ME | F+M | 21–28 | 98 |
| Ogunyinka et al[113] | CE | F+M | 12–18 | 8.52 |
| Egermark-Eriksson et al[114] | CE | F+M | 20 | 86 |
| Kampe et al[115] | CE+ME | F+M | 17–22 | 93 |
| Hugoson et al[53] | CE | F+M | 3<br>5<br>10<br>15<br>20 | 37<br>81<br>22<br>49<br>65 |
| Hugoson et al[49] | CE | F+M | 20<br>30<br>40<br>50<br>60<br>70<br>80 | 65<br>80<br>68<br>82<br>86<br>74<br>77 |

CE = clinical examination; ME = model examination

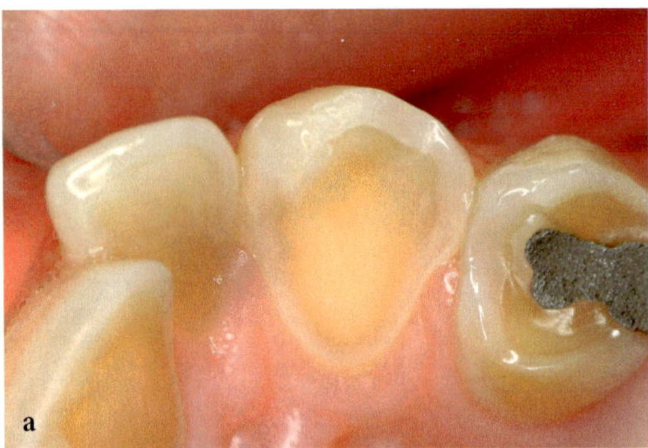

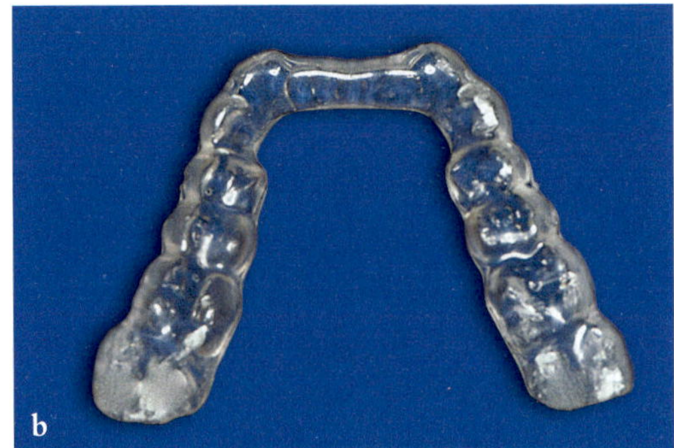

Fig 1-1 **(a)** Tooth wear in a patient referred for "bruxism treatment". In fact, the diagnosis confirmed that the lesions were caused by gastroesophageal reflux. **(b)** Splint worn by a patient for two years to protect his teeth against "bruxism". The absence of marks on the splint shows that tooth wear in this patient cannot be ascribed to bruxism.

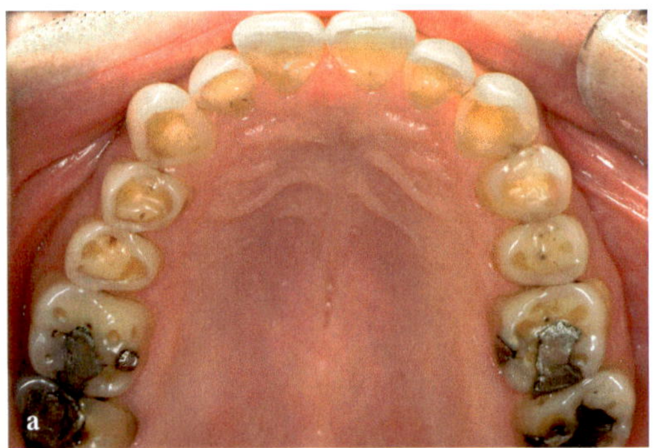

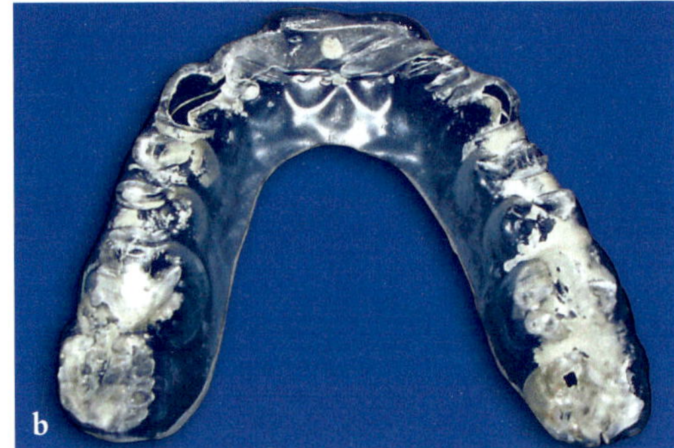

Fig 1-2 **(a)** Generalized tooth wear in a patient with gastroesophageal reflux. Note the typical cupping lesions or volcano-shaped lesions and amalgam restorations in high relief, which are characteristic of erosion by acid. **(b)** Bruxism splint belonging to the same patient after three years of use. The significant wear confirms sleep bruxism. The evidence demonstrates that tooth wear in this patient results from the combined action of bruxism and erosion.

ence of excessive wear) and has made night guards for them. Very frequently these mouth guards do not show any signs of bruxism after some time (Fig 1-1), while research has proved that real bruxers *do* leave antagonist teeth marks on splints (Fig 1-2).[25,26]

A wholly different scenario arises when a third person confirms that the patient produces grinding sounds while sleeping. These witnesses can easily perceive the sound because they are roommates or bed partners – unless they are used to the noise, or do not hear it because teeth grinding can sometimes be performed silently. So, except for some situations, patients who grind their teeth and sleep alone are completely unaware of their condition.

In the case of young bruxers, their parents are the ones who frequently testify that they can hear their children grinding. A questionnaire filled in by 5- and 6-year-old children's parents showed a prevalence of 15%; nevertheless, 15.5% of children presented clinical evidence of the habit which was not detected by their parents.[17] An increase in bruxism prevalence of 1.7 times was the result of a study in which the parents of children and adolescents were asked whether they heard their children grinding when the bedroom door was left open.[27] Moreover, it must be taken into account that the younger the children are, the more the parents keep an eye on their children's sleep.[14]

Table 1-1 presents a cross-sectional compilation of epidemiologic works that used questionnaires and personal or telephone interviews to identify sleep bruxism, awake bruxism, or a combination of both types. If we analyze two pieces of research carried out on similar groups of 15- to 16-year-old teenagers, in the same country and using the same questionnaire, we can easily understand how difficult it is to compare epidemiologic studies. One of the studies reported 4.7% nightly grinding whereas the other study reported 12.7%; that is, three times more.[28,29] This difference was ascribed to sociocultural differences between the groups.[28]

Some questionnaires establish a difference between bruxism as a permanent habit and another type of bruxism performed only on certain occasions.[30] These two types of bruxism classified according to the chronologic sequence of the habit make the results even more inaccurate. Even though it has been proved that bruxism is not constant over time,[31] we are far from knowing whether there is a real, spontaneous, and definite remission of the habit. In fact, the presence of bruxism at an early age indicates that the habit will continue into adulthood.[32] Since awake clenching is related to fluctuating factors such as stress and emotional alterations, it is reasonable to think that this kind of bruxism has the same irregularity.[15,33–35] Thus, this irregularity of the habit represents the normal fluctuation in teeth clenching as a response to the different day-to-day stresses experienced by a patient. It is hard to decide whether to take into account those people who say they "sometimes" brux, or the bruxers who "always" do it, because the results are generally inconsistent. Those who say that they are "always" clenching their teeth are 4.6% of the population whereas the number rises to 40.1% if those who "sometimes" clench are included.[30] Since we are trying to get information about clenching prevalence, perhaps the correct thing to do is to add both results, leading to 44.7%. However, if we compare this result with another study result (also performed in Scandinavia) in which the awake clenching percentage was 2.7%, we find that the difference in prevalence is 20 times.[36] It is worthwhile mentioning that a population of military men was exclusively studied in the former study, while a general sample of both sexes was studied in the second one. Nevertheless, it is not easy to explain such different results because, in contrast, the prevalence of awake clenching in females is larger.[37,38]

The validity of answers given to a questionnaire can be corroborated by means of personal questioning; for example: "How do you know you grind your teeth when you are sleeping? Has anybody told you?" Clinical accuracy of grinding sounds during sleep (heard by a third person) had 78% sensitivity and 94% specificity when it was compared with polysomnography.[9]

### *Tooth wear facets*

Some studies determine bruxism magnitude in relation to tooth wear by means of directly observing the patient's mouth or by using cast models. As can be seen in Table 1-4, some of these studies found non-physiologic dentition wear that suggests a bruxism prevalence of approximately 50% in the population.[19,39] These numbers are much larger than those obtained by the same patients' answers to a questionnaire, which show that only 30% of the patients presenting with tooth wear know they grind their teeth while sleeping.[39] A similar situation arises if we analyze Seligman and collaborators' work: out of 91.5% of the population that presented dentition wear, only 23% acknowledged in the questionnaire being aware of their sleep grinding habit.[22] From these analyses, it can be said that questionnaires underestimate bruxism, or else, dentition wear overestimates the real presence of the habit.

The clinical specificity and reliability of tooth wear as an indicator of bruxism has been questioned,[40] and a longitudinal epidemiologic study showed that only 3% of tooth wear is attributable to bruxism.[41] Other studies that have compared tooth wear magnitude with the masseter muscle electromyographical (EMG) level have not found a significant relationship between them.[42,43] Similar results were found when comparing bruxism awareness by means of personal questioning or questionnaires and by means of tooth wear.[22,39,44] As discussed in a more comprehensive manner in Chapter 9, tooth wear can be triggered by many individual or combined factors. Tooth wear is highly prevalent in the population,[22,44] so bruxism is one of the least relevant factors and could represent only an association.

### *Studied Population Characteristics*

When analyzing the epidemiology of bruxism, special care should be taken with regard to the population characteristics because these have a significant effect on prevalence.

#### *Age*

Some pediatric practitioners state that bruxism is a very frequent but self-limiting childhood condition that does not progress into adulthood bruxism.[45] It is seen as the result of occlusal interferences, the product of the eruption of permanent teeth during mixed dentition, and thus as a physiologic process to dental occlusion maturity.[46] Contrary to this belief, it has been shown by means of longitudinal examinations of patients who brux from an early age that the habit persists into adulthood.[16,32] To set alongside this, there is a lot of evidence that shows how bruxism frequency fluctuates in time.[8,47,48] However, it seems quite unlikely that a spontaneous remission of the habit occurs. This has been suggested by Hublin and coworkers who reported that only 15% of the adults who do not brux during sleep did brux in their childhood.[20]

The relationship between age and bruxism depends on the methodology used to detect this habit. Tooth wear is irreversible, so attrition increases progressively. That is why some studies associate tooth wear with age.[46,49–52] Physiologic and pathologic variations of the human dentition should be taken into account when dealing with epidemiology. For example, Table 1-5 shows how wear increases in children aged 3 to 5 years (primary dentition), while at the age of 10 it decreases (mixed dentition) and then it goes up again at the age of 20. These fluctuations in amount of wear are influenced by primary dentition exfoliation which has been adding wear since eruption. When permanent teeth erupt, wear signs will be seen again with the passing of time.[53] Additionally, the more advanced the age, the higher the probability of tooth loss because of caries, periodontal disease, fracture, etc., and this will be reflected in the wear amount to be quantified.

Age is an important factor to bear in mind when carrying out sleep bruxism studies because bruxism has been reported to decrease with age.[54] In another study, a significant reduction in episodes of bruxism with age was found in subjects who were over 60 years old.[55]

#### *Patients with temporomandibular disorders versus the general population*

According to studies which generally employed questionnaires, bruxism prevalence is much higher when people with a temporomandibular disorder (TMD) are included in the studied population. This is apparent in Table 1-2. The relationship between bruxism and TMD is highly complex, so a whole chapter has been devoted to it (Chapter 16).

Generally, TMD patients classify themselves as bruxers under the influence of those clinicians who view a direct relationship between TMD and bruxism. A study of this class of patient concluded that most of them repeat their former dentists' explanations to explain the origin of pain. So, in order to avoid sample bias, it is recommended to carefully investigate the origin of the patients' statements about bruxism.[40] In this regard, when studying TMD patients, Pergamalian and coworkers did not find any correlation between tooth wear amounts and self-reported bruxism levels.[52] Moreover, no significant relationship could be found between tooth wear degree and bruxism level registered with EMG.[42]

### *The Type of Bruxism*

Bruxism is a condition that includes teeth grinding and clenching, and these two different habits (or a combination) can be performed while sleeping or awake. Although clenching is more common when people are not sleeping, and grinding generally takes place during sleep, there are individual exceptions. So to establish accurate epidemiologic numbers, it is necessary to make a distinction between sleep and awake bruxism because they are not always simultaneously present in the same patient and consequently respective prevalence amounts will also be different.[37]

One study showed a bruxism prevalence of 17.8% but it did not specify whether the investigation focused on sleep or awake bruxism or on a combination of both.[56] Other research which considered both bruxism habits – that is, clenching and grinding – did not clarify whether they were referring to sleep or awake bruxism in the questionnaires, so the reported conclusion may include the addition of both types of bruxism.[57,58] Generally, in a great number of studies, awake bruxism prevalence is double that of sleep bruxism.

## Bruxism Variability

Some evidence suggests that bruxism is not a constant habit. Although awake bruxism has not been extensively studied, patients' anecdotal evidence seems to indicate an important chronologic habit fluctuation. On countless occasions, patients say that they clench their teeth more frequently when they are under acute stress. These statements could be completely subjective, but they deserve to be taken into account owing to the fact that they are commonly encountered in dental practice worldwide. This constitutes another unsolved issue about bruxism, but particularly about awake bruxism.

Logically, there are reasons for this lack of scientific information since it is not simple to measure human bruxism objectively when people are naturally performing their many daily activities. Nonetheless, some subjective measurements obtained by questionnaires and psychometric testing have showed a direct relationship between emotional stress and awake bruxism.[15,33–35] This assumption was confirmed by Glaros and Rao when they provided evidence that confirmed awake bruxers (clenchers) respond to stress situations differently to non-bruxers.[59]

It has been shown that confirmed bruxers do not systematically perform this parafunctional activity whenever they sleep.[8,47,48] Different investigations conducted using portable EMG during several sleeping nights also pointed out a great variability in the recorded electromyographic levels.[60–62]

Bruxism variability has also been illustrated in sleep laboratories, although the observations were made on the same person on repeated occasions.[63] All this research has established that bruxism levels vary significantly over time, ranging from intense periods of bruxism to periods with almost no bruxism activity. For this reason – and to avoid both underestimating and overestimating bruxism presence – some authors have suggested performing measurements over many different nights.[31,61]

## References


1. Okeson JP. Orofacial Pain: Guidelines for Assessment, Diagnosis, and Management. Chicago: Quintessence, 1996.
2. Karolyi M. Beobachtungen über Pyorrhea Alveolaris. Oesterreichischungarische Vierteljahrsschrift für Zahnheilkunde 1901;17:279–283.
3. Marie MM, Pietkiewicz M. La bruxomanie. Revue Stomatol 1907;14:107–116.

4. Frohmann BS. The application of psychotherapy to dental problems. Dent Cosmos 1931;73:1117–1122.
5. Sjöholm T, Lehtinen II, Helenius H. Masseter muscle activity in diagnosed sleep bruxists compared with non-symptomatic controls. J Sleep Res 1995;4:48–55.
6. Thorpy MJ. Diagnostic Classification Steering Committee. International Classification of Sleep Disorders: Diagnostic and Coding Manual. Rochester, MN: American Sleep Disorders Association and Allen Press, 1990.
7. Velly Miguel AM, Montplaisir J, Rompre PH, Lund JP, Lavigne GJ. Bruxism and other orofacial movements during sleep. J Craniomandib Disord 1992;6:71–81.
8. Reding GR, Zepelin H, Robinson JE, Zimmerman SO, Smith VH. Nocturnal teeth-grinding: all-night psychophysiologic studies. J Dent Res 1968;47:786–797.
9. Lavigne GJ, Rompre PH, Montplaisir JY. Sleep bruxism: validity of clinical research diagnosis criteria in a controlled polysomnographic study. J Dent Res 1996;75: 546–552.
10. Perlstein MA, Barnett HE. Nature and recognition of cerebral palsy in infancy. J Am Dent Assoc 1952;148:1389–1397.
11. Molin C, Levi L. A psycho-odontologic investigation of patients with bruxism. Acta Odontol Scand 1966;24: 373–391.
12. Macaluso GM, Guerra P, Di Giovanni G, Boselli M, Parrino L, Terzano MG. Sleep bruxism is a disorder related to periodic arousals during sleep. J Dent Res 1998;77: 565–573.
13. Kato T, Rompre P, Montplaisir JY, Sessle BJ, Lavigne GJ. Sleep bruxism: an oromotor activity secondary to micro-arousal. J Dent Res 2001;80:1940–1944.
14. Reding GR, Rubright WC, Zimmerman SO. Incidence of bruxism. J Dent Res 1966;45:1198–1204.
15. Glaros AG. Incidence of diurnal and nocturnal bruxism. J Prosthet Dent 1981;45:545–549.
16. Abe K, Shimakawa M. Genetic and developmental aspects of sleeptalking and teethgrinding. Acta Paedopsychiatr 1966;33:339–344.
17. Kuch EV, Till MJ, Messer LB. Bruxing and nonbruxing children: a comparison of their personality traits. Pediatr Dent 1979;1:182–187.
18. Dooland KV, Townsend GC, Kaidonis JA. Prevalence and side preference for tooth grinding in twins. Aust Dent J 2006;51:219–224.
19. Lindqvist B. Bruxism in twins. Acta Odontol Scand 1974; 32:177–187.
20. Hublin K, Kaprio J, Partinen M, Koskenvuo M. Sleep bruxism based on self-report in a nationwide twin cohort. J Sleep Res 1998;7:61–67.
21. Michalowicz BS, Pihlstrom BL, Hodges JS, Bouchard TJ. No heritability of temporomandibular joint signs and symptoms. J Dent Res 2000;79:1573–1578.
22. Seligman DA, Pullinger AG, Solberg WK. The prevalence of dental attrition and its association with factors of age, gender, occlusion, and TMJ symptomatology. J Dent Res 1988;67:1323–1333.
23. Lipinski D, Nelson RO. The reactivity and unreliability of self-recording. J Consult Clin Psychol 1974;42:118–123.
24. Egermark-Eriksson I, Carlsson GE, Ingervall B. Prevalence of mandibular dysfunction and orofacial parafunction in 7-, 11-, and 15-year old Swedish children. Eur J Orthod 1981;3: 163–172.
25. Holmgren K, Sheikholeslam A, RiiseC. Effect of a full-arch maxillary occlusal splint on parafunctional activity during sleep in patients with nocturnal bruxism and signs and symptoms of craniomandibular disorders. J Prosthet Dent 1993;69:293–297.
26. Chung S, Kim Y, Kim H. Prevalence and patterns of nocturnal bruxofacets on stabilization splints in temporomandibular disorder patients. J Craniomandibular Pract 2000;18: 92–97.
27. Cheifetz AT, Osganian SK, Allred EN, Needleman HL. Prevalence of bruxism and associated correlates in children as reported by parents. J Dent Child 2005;72:67–73.
28. Winocur E, Gavish A, Finkelshtein T, Halachmi M, Gazit E. Oral habits among adolescent girls and their association with symptoms of temporomandibular disorders. J Oral Rehabil 2001;28:624–629.
29. Gavish A, Halachmi M, Winocur E, Gazit E. Oral habits and their association with signs and symptoms of temporomandibular disorders in adolescent girls. J Oral Rehabil 2000;27:22–32.
30. Ingervall B, Mohlin B, Thilander B. Prevalence of symptoms of functional disturbances of the masticatory system in Swedish men. J Oral Rehabil 1980;7:185–197.
31. Lavigne GJ, Guitard F, Rompre PH, Montplaisir JY. Variability in sleep bruxism activity over time. J Sleep Res 2001;10:237–244.
32. Carlsson GE, Egermark I, Magnusson T. Predictors of bruxism, other oral parafunctions, and tooth wear over a 20-year follow-up period. J Orofac Pain 2003;17:50–57.
33. Olkinuora M. A factor analytic study of psychosocial background in bruxism. Proc Finn Dent Soc 1972;68: 184–199.
34. Olkinuora M. A psychosomatic study of bruxism with emphasis on mental strain and familiar predisposition factors. Proc Finn Dent Soc 1972;68:110–123.
35. Olkinuora M. Psychosocial aspects in a series of bruxists compared with a group of non-bruxists. Proc Finn Dent Soc 1972;68:200–208.
36. Swanljung O, Rantanen T. Functional disorders of the masticatory system in Southwest Finland. Community Dent Oral Epidemiol 1979;7:177–182.
37. Rieder CE, Martinoff JT, Wilcox SA. The prevalence of mandibular dysfunction. Part I: Sex and age distribution of related signs and symptoms. J Prosthet Dent 1983;50: 81–88.
38. Jensen R, Rasmussen BK, Lous I, Olesen J. Prevalence of oromandibular dysfunction in a general population. J Orofac Pain 1993;7:175–182.
39. Lindqvist B. Bruxism in children. Odontol Revy 1971; 22:413–424.

40. Marbach JJ, Raphael KG, Dohrenwend BP, Lennon MC. The validity of tooth grinding measures: etiology of pain dysfunction syndrome revisited. J Am Dent Assoc 1990; 120:327–333.
41. Ekfeldt A, Hugoson A, Bergendal T, Helkimo M. An individual tooth wear index and an analysis of factors correlated to incisal and occlusal wear in an adult Swedish population. Acta Odontol Scand 1990;48:343–349.
42. Dettmar DM, Shaw RM, Tilley AJ. Tooth wear and bruxism: a sleep laboratory investigation. Aust Dent J 1987;32:421–426.
43. Pierce C, Close J, Krause A. Relation between wear faceting and EMG-measured bruxing activity. J Dent Res 1996;75:1588 (abstract).
44. Nilner M, Lassing SA.Prevalence of functional disturbances and diseases of the stomatognathic system in 7–14 year olds. Swed Dent J 1981;5:173–187.
45. Kieser JA, Groeneveld HT. Relationship between juvenile bruxing and craniomandibular dysfunction. J Oral Rehabil 1998;25:662–665.
46. Nyström M, Kononem M, Alaluusua S, Ebalahti M, Vartiovaara J. Development of horizontal tooth wear in maxillary anterior teeth from 5 to 18 years of age. J Dent Res 1990;69:1765–1770.
47. Rugh JD, Harlan J. Nocturnal bruxism and temporomandibular disorders. In: Jankovic J, Tolosa E (eds). Advances in Neurology. New York: Raven Press, 1988: 329–341.
48. Rugh JD, Ohrbach R. Occlusal parafunction. In: Mohl ND, Zarb GA, Carlsson GE, Rugh JD (eds). A Textbook of Occlusion. Chicago: Quintessence, 1988:249–261.
49. Hugoson A, Bergendal T, Ekfeldt A, Helkimo M. Prevalence and severity of incisal and occlusal tooth wear in an adult Swedish population. Acta Odontol Scand 1988;46: 255–265.
50. Lambrechts P, Braem M, Vuyistede-Wauters M, Vanherle G. Quantitative in-vivo wear of human enamel. J Dent Res 1989;68:1752–1754.
51. Smith BG, Robb ND. The prevalence of tooth wear in 1007 dental patients. J Oral Rehabil 1996;23:232–239.
52. Pergamalian A, Rudy TE, Zaki HS, Greco CM. The association between wear facets, bruxism, and severity of facial pain in patients with temporomandibular disorders. J Prosthet Dent 2003;90:194–200.
53. Hugoson A, Ekfeldt A, koch G, Hallonsten A. Incisal and occlusal tooth wear in children and adolescents in a Swedish population. Acta Odontol Scand 1996;54:263–270.
54. Lavigne GJ, Montplaisir JY. Restless legs syndrome and sleep bruxism: prevalence and association among Canadians. Sleep 1994;17:739–743.
55. Okeson JP, Phillips BA, Berry DTR, Cook Y, Paesani D, Galante J. Nocturnal bruxing events in healthy geriatric subjects. J Oral Rehabil 1990;17:411–417.
56. Chuanjedong P, Kedjarune-leggat U, Kerpton D, Chongsuvivat-Wong V, Benjakul P. Associated factors of tooth wear in southern Thailand. J Oral Rehabil 2002;29:997–1002.
57. Ciancaglini R, Gherlone EF, Radaelli G. The relationship of bruxism with craniofacial pain and symptoms from the masticatory system in the adult population. J Oral Rehabil 2001;28:842–848.
58. Mercado MDF, Faulkner KDB. The prevalence of craniomandibular disorders in completely edentulous denture-wearing subjects. J Oral Rehabil 1991;18:231–242.
59. Glaros AG, Rao SM. Electromyographic correlates of experimentally induced stress in diurnal bruxists and normals. J Dent Res 1979;58:1872–1878.
60. Rugh JD, Solberg WK. Electromyographic studies of bruxist behavior before and during treatment. J Calif Dent Assoc. 1975;3:56–59.
61. Ikeda T, Nishgawa K, Kondo K, Takeuchi H, Clark GT. Criteria for the detection of sleep-associated bruxism in humans. J Orofac Pain 1996;10:270–282.
62. Funch DP, Gale EN. Factors associated with nocturnal bruxism and its treatment. J Behav Med 1980;3:385–397.
63. Dal Fabbro C, De Lourdes Ventura M, Tufik S. A linear study of a man with sleep bruxism for 30 consecutive nights-correlation reports. J Sleep Res 1997;26:547.
64. Nilner M. Functional disturbances and diseases in the stomatognathic system among 7- to 18-year-olds. J Craniomandibular Pract 1985;3:358–367.
65. Könönen M, Nyström M, Kleemola-Kujala E et al. Signs and symptoms of craneomandibular disorders in a series of Finnish children. Acta Odontol Scand 1987;45:109–114.
66. Molin C, Carlsson GE, Friling B, Hedegård B. Frequency of symptoms of mandibular dysfunction in young Swedish men. J Oral Rehabil 1976;3:9–18.
67. Matsuka Y, Yatani H, Kuboki T, Yamashita A. Temporomandibular disorders in the adult population of Okayama city, Japan. J Craniomandibular Pract 1996;14:158–162.
68. Glass EG, McGlynn FD, Glaros AG, Melton K, Romans K. Prevalence of temporomandibular disorder symptoms in a major metropolitan area. Cranio 1993;11:217–220.
69. Pow EHN, Leung KCM, McMillan AS. Prevalence of symptoms associated with temporomandibular disorders in Hong Kong Chinese. J Orofac Pain 2001;15:228–234.
70. Goulet JP, Lund JP, Montplaisir JY, Lavigne GJ. Daily clenching, nocturnal bruxing, and stress and their association with TMD symptoms. J Orofac Pain 1993;7: 120–127.
71. Ohayon MM, Li KK, Guilleminault C. Risk factors for sleep bruxism in the general population. Chest 2001; 119:53–61.
72. Gross AJ, Rivera-Morales WC, Gale EN. A prevalence study of symptoms associated with TM disorders. J Craniomandib Disord 1988;2:191–195.
73. Choy E, Smith DE. The prevalence of temporomandibular joint disturbances in complete denture patients. J Oral Rehabil 1980;7:331–352.
74. Agerberg G, Carlsson GE. Functional disorders of the masticatory system. I: Distribution of symptoms according to age and sex as judged from investigation by questionnaire. Acta Odontol Scand 1972;30:597–613.

75. De Vis H, De Boever JA, van Cauwenberghe P. Epidemiologic survey of functional conditions of the masticatory system in Belgian children aged 3–6 years. Community Dent Oral Epidemiol 1984;12:203–207.
76. Widmalm SE, Christiansen RL, Gunn SM, Hawley LM. Prevalence of signs and symptoms of craniomandibular disorders and orofacial parafunction in 4–6-year-old African-American and Caucasian children. J Oral Rehabil 1995;22: 87–93.
77. Ng DK, Kwok KL, Poon G, Chau KW. Habitual snoring and sleep bruxism in a pediatric outpatient population in Hong Kong. Singapore Med J 2002;43:554–556.
78. Ng DK, Kwok KL, Cheung JM et al. Prevalence of sleep problems in Hong Kong primary school children: a community-based telephone survey. Chest 2005;128: 1315–1323.
79. Demir A, Uysal T, Guray E, Basciftci FA. The relationship between bruxism and occlusal factors among seven- to 19-year-old Turkish children. Angle Orthod 2004;74: 672–676.
80. Ow RKK, Loh T, Neo J, Khoo J. Symptoms of craniomandibular disorder among elderly people. J Oral Rehabil 1995;22:413–419.
81. Duckro PN, Tait RC, Margolis RB, Deshields TL. Prevalence of temporomandibular symptoms in a large United States metropolitan area. J Craniomandibular Pract 1990;8: 131–138.
82. Agerberg G, Bergenholtz A. Craniomandibular disorders in adult populations of West Bothnia, Sweden. Acta Odontol Scand 1989;47:129–140.
83. Norheim PW, Dahl BL. Some self-reported symptoms of temporomandibular joint dysfunction in a population in Northern Norway. J Oral Rehabil 1978;5:63–68.
84. Agerberg G, Helkimo M. Symptomatology of patients referred for mandibular dysfunction: evaluation with the aid of a questionnaire. J Craniomandibular Pract 1987;5: 157–163.
85. Droukas B, Lindee C, Carlsson GE. Occlusion and mandibular dysfunction: a clinical study of patients referred for functional disturbances of the masticatory system. J Prosthet Dent 1985;53:402–406.
86. Gelb H, Bernstein I. Clinical evaluation of two hundred patients with temporomandibular joint syndrome. J Prosthet Dent 1983;49:234–243.
87. Butler JH, Folke LE, Bandt CL. A descriptive survey of signs and symptoms associated with the myofascial pain-dysfunction syndrome. J Am Dent Assoc 1975;90: 635–639.
88. Cacchiotti DA, Bianchi P, McNeill C. Signs and symptoms in samples with and without temporomandibular disorders. J Craniomandib Disord 1991;5:167–172.
89. Suvinen TI, Reade PC, Sunden B, Gerschman JA, Koukounas E. Temporomandibular disorders. 1: a comparison of symptoms profiles in Australian and Finnish patients. J Orofac Pain 1997;11:58–66.
90. Agerberg G, Carlsson GE. Symptoms of functional disturbances of the masticatory system. Acta Odontol Scand 1975;33:183–190.
91. Manfredini D, Cantini E, Romagnoli M, Bosco M. Prevalence of bruxism in patients with different research diagnostic criteria for temporomandibular disorders (RDC/ TMD) diagnoses. Cranio 2003;21:279–285.
92. Koidis PT, Zarifi A, Grigoriadou E, Garefis P. Effect of age and sex on craniomandibular disorders. J Prosthet Dent 1993;69:93–101.
93. Laberge L, Tremblay RE, Vitaro F, Montplaisir JY. Development of parasomnias from childhood to early adolescence. Pediatrics 2000;106:67–74.
94. Holm AK, Arvidsson S. Oral health in preschool Swedish children. Odontol Revy 1974;25:81–98.
95. Holm AK. Oral health in 4-year-old Swedish children. Community Dent Oral Epidemiol 1975;3:25–33.
96. Holm AK. Oral health in 5-year-old Swedish children. Community Dent Oral Epidemiol 1975;3:184–189.
97. Holm AK. Dental health in a group of Swedish 8-year-olds followed since the age of 3. Community Dent Oral Epidemiol 1978;6:71–77.
98. Onizawa K, Yoshida H. Longitudinal changes of symptoms of temporomandibular disorders in Japanese young adults. J Orofac Pain 1996;10:151–156.
99. Heikinheimo K, Salmi K, Myllärniemi S, Kirveskari P. Symptoms of craniomandibular disorder in a sample of Finnish adolescents at the ages of 12 and 15. Eur J Orthod 1989;11:325–331.
100. Könönen M, Nyström M. A longitudinal study of craniomandibular disorders in Finnish adolescents. J Orofac Pain 1993;7:329–336.
101. Magnusson T, Egermark-Eriksson I, Carlsson GE. Four-year longitudinal study of mandibular dysfunction in children. Community Dent Oral Epidemiol 1985;13: 117–120.
102. Magnusson T, Egermark-Eriksson I, Carlsson GE. Five-year longitudinal study of signs and symptoms of mandibular dysfunction in adolescents. J Craniomandibular Pract 1986;4:338–344.
103. Magnusson T, Carlsson GE, Egermark I. Changes in subjective symptoms of craniomandibular disorders in children and adolescents during a 10-year period. J Orofac Pain 1993;7:76–82.
104. Magnusson T, Egermark I, Carlsson GE. A longitudinal epidemiologic study of signs and symptoms of temporomandibular disorders from 15 to 35 years of age. J Orofac Pain 2000;14:310–319.
105. Pilley JR, Mohlin B, Shaw WC, Kingdon A. A survey of craniomandibular disorders in 800 15-year-olds: a follow-up study of children with malocclusion. Eur J Orthod 1992;152–161.
106. Fareed K, Johansson A, Omar R. Prevalence and severity of occlusal wear in a young Saudi population. Acta Odontol Scand 1990;48:279–285.

107. Abdullah A, Sherfudhin H, Omar R, Johansson A. Prevalence of occlusal tooth wear and its relationship to lateral and protrusive contact schemes in a young adult Indian population. Acta Odontol Scand 1994;52:191–197.
108. Warren JJ, Yonezu T, Bishara SE. Tooth wear patterns in the deciduous dentition. Am J Orthod Dentofacial Orthop 2002;122:614–618.
109. Pintado MR, Anderson GC, DeLong R, Douglas WH. Variation in tooth wear in young adults over a two-year period. J Prosthet Dent 1997;77:313–320.
110. Milosevic A, Lo MS. Tooth wear in three ethnic groups in Sabah (Northern Borneo). Int Dent J 1996;46: 572–578.
111. Casanova-Rosado JF, Medina-Solis CE, Vallejos-Sanchez AA et al. Dental attrition and associated factors in adolescents 14 to 19 years of age: a pilot study. Int J Prosthodont 2005;18:516–518.
112. Silness J, Berge M, Johannessen G. A 2-year follow-up study of incisal tooth wear in dental students. Acta Odontol Scand 1995;53:331–333.
113. Ogunyinka A, Dosumu OO, Otuyemi OD. The pattern of toothwear amongst 12–18-year-old students in a Nigerian population. J Oral Rehab 2001;28:601–605.
114. Egermark-Eriksson I, Carlsson GE, Magnusson T. A long-term epidemiologic study of the relationship between occlusal factors and mandibular dysfunction in children and adolescents. J Dent Res 1987;66:67–71.
115. Kampe T, Hannerz H, Ström P. Facet pattern in intact and restored dentition of young adults: a comparative study. Acta Odontol Scand 1984;42:225–233.

Chapter 2

# Diagnosis of Bruxism

*Daniel A. Paesani*

## Introduction

Diagnosis is the process of identifying a medical condition. Early diagnosis of bruxism is extremely important for both the clinician and the patient. The condition should be identified by the clinician on seeing a patient for the first time. This will then allow the professional to devise a specific treatment plan according to the patient's activity (grinding or clenching), the degree of bruxism (mild, moderate, or severe), and the time when it happens (in sleep, during wakefulness, or both). In the case of severe bruxers, unless the necessary precautions are taken, just wearing a self-cure acrylic-resin 3-unit provisional bridge in the mouth for some time may not result in the expected outcome. Early identification of patients with such a profile will allow the dentist to prevent undesirable situations. This applies to simple plastic restoration of molars, complex occlusal rehabilitation, and orthodontic treatments. Bruxism will defy any method of odontological treatment. Determining the time at which bruxism starts and the kind of bruxism a patient develops will also be helpful in sparing unnecessary treatments. What would be the use of prescribing a night guard to a patient who clenches only during daytime?

Early diagnosis also allows patients to be aware of their habit in case a treatment proves not to be effective. (By no means should this be understood as an abdication of responsibility on the part of the clinician.) This prevents unpleasant conflicts that may affect the clinician–patient relationship and may cause a lawsuit to be filed.

Accurately diagnosing bruxism is important also for researchers, who need to identify and measure it. In order to do this, it is necessary to use technology that is usually not available to the practitioner. The tools for identifying and assessing bruxism are:

- *clinical diagnosis:* symptoms (questionnaires and personal interview); and signs (observation, and mouth, model, and photographic examination to quantify tooth wear)

Table 2-1

**Questionnaire for detection of bruxism.**

| | *Yes* | *No* | *Don't know* |
|---|---|---|---|
| Do you grind your teeth when you sleep? | | | |
| Has anybody heard you grind your teeth while you sleep? | | | |
| On waking up, do you usually find that you are clenching your teeth? | | | |
| When you wake up, do you usually have jaw pain or jaw fatigue? | | | |
| When you wake up, do you usually have the feeling that your teeth are loose? | | | |
| When you wake up, do you usually have sore teeth and/or sore gums? | | | |
| When you wake up, do you usually have a headache in the temples? | | | |
| When you wake up, do you usually have a jaw lock? | | | |
| Have you ever found that you were clenching your teeth in the daytime? | | | |
| Have you ever found that you were grinding your teeth in the daytime? | | | |

- *complementary methods:* use of intraoral devices for tooth wear quantification (splints; Bruxcore®, Boston, MA, USA) and bite force detectors; masseter electromyography (EMG, ambulatory EMG, disposable EMG devices such as BiteStrip®); and sleep polysomnography.

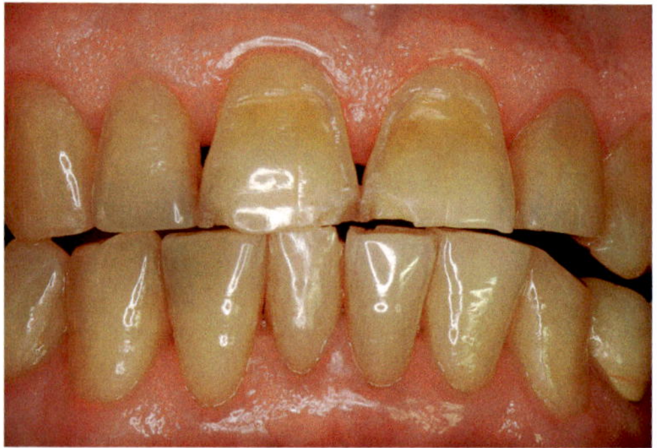

Fig 2-1 Enamel fracture in both central incisors, as a result of bruxism in the protrusive direction. Note also the abrasive wear of vestibular enamel, caused by hard tooth brushing.

## Clinical Diagnosis

### *Symptoms*

A rapid way of collecting information is to request the patient to answer a questionnaire. It is the most widely available method to be used in everyday practice. Chapter 1 has already discussed the advantages and disadvantages of this method in the diagnosis of bruxism symptoms.

Questionnaires are very useful for obtaining a great amount of information in a short time. A good questionnaire should include a wide range of questions concerning the patient's general health status, diseases, medication, etc. Of course, as the main subject of this book is bruxism, we will just be dealing with the questions that specifically refer to it.

Table 2-1 shows sample questions that can be added to the general questionnaire usually used during the patient's first appointment; such a general questionnaire is simply about a collection of symptoms that can be attributed to bruxism. It is advisable to include "Don't know" among the

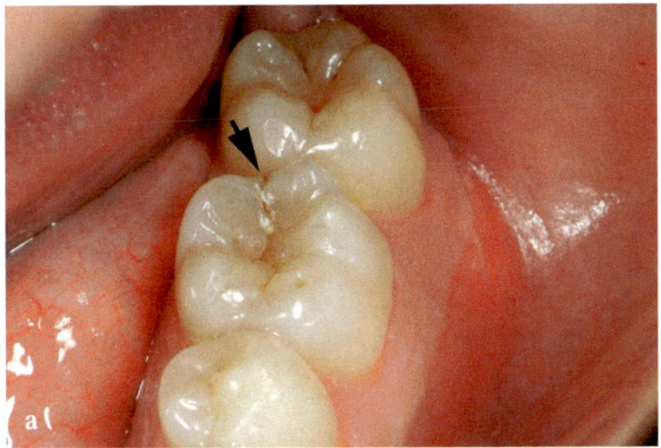


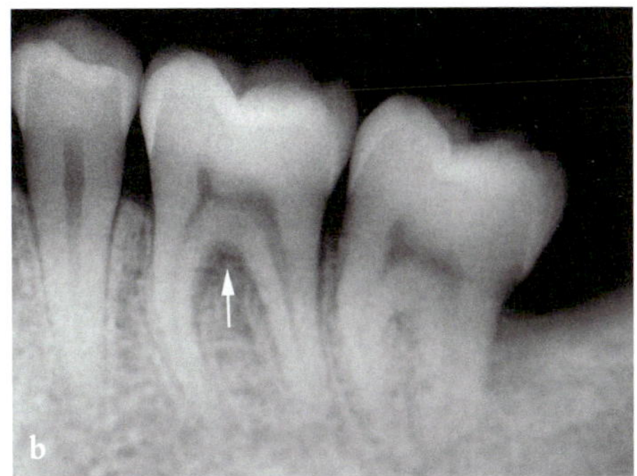


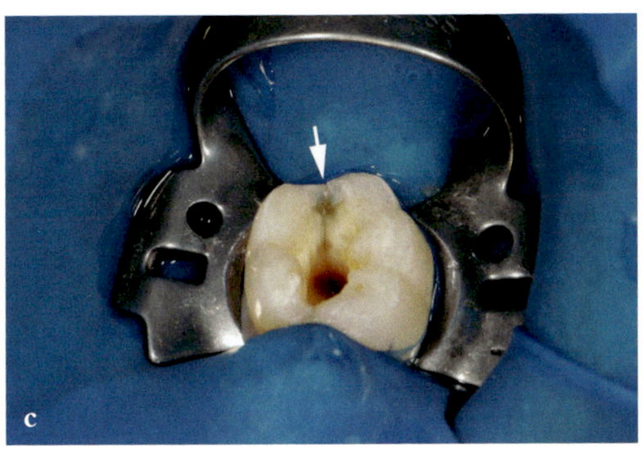


Fig 2-2 **(a)** Fracture line in a mandibular molar (arrow) caused by bruxism of the clenching type. **(b)** No fracture is evident in the periapical radiograph, although a reactive area in the interradicular space can be seen (arrow). **(c)** Opening of the molar reveals that the fracture has reached the pulp chamber (arrow).

possible choices; this will prevent false-positive and false-negative answers from patients who are not sure of how to respond. At the first appointment, during history taking, it is recommended that the clinician quickly asks the patient the same questions from the questionnaire again in order to confirm the accuracy of the patient's answers.

### *Signs*

In the clinical examination, some signs may be present to suggest bruxism. The character of these signs (and symptoms) is "relative", since they alone are not sufficient evidence of bruxism; although frequently mentioned in the literature, the fact is that they have not yet been validated by scientific method. Future controlled investigations will have to determine the corresponding sensitivity and specificity values for each of them. So far, only the clinical validity of tooth-grinding sounds during sleep (witness statements based on two episodes per week) has been studied. When checked against polysomnography, they showed a sensitivity of 78% and a specificity of 98%.[1]

#### *Tooth wear*

Although this has a strong association with bruxism, it is not a specific sign since there are many causes of tooth wear. Grinding causes the teeth to deteriorate in a specific way (attrition). Tooth wear can be studied by direct visual inspection of the mouth, by examining plaster models of the patient's teeth, and by taking a look at intraoral pictures. This subject is discussed in detail in Chapter 9.

#### *Fractures*

There may be fractures in natural teeth, prostheses, dental implants, and dental restorations (Figs 2-1 to 2-11).

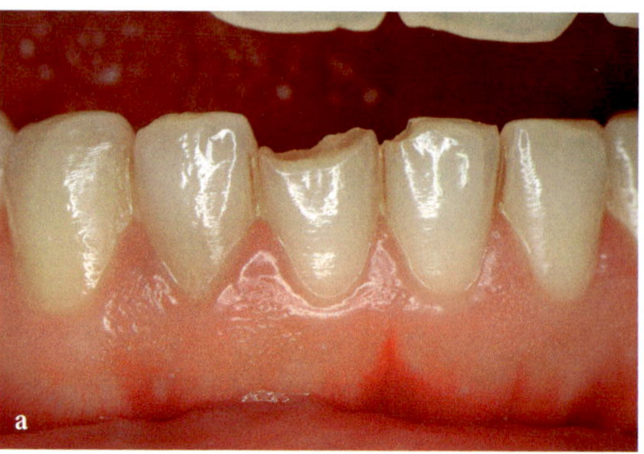


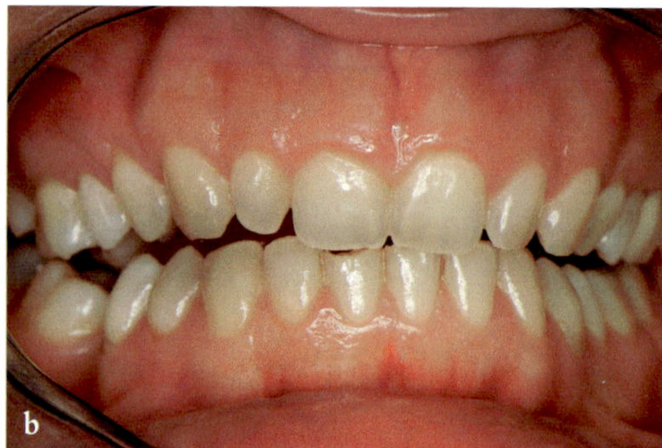


Fig 2-3 **(a)** Fracture of the mandibular central incisors caused by protrusive bruxism. **(b)** Bruxism pattern reproduction.

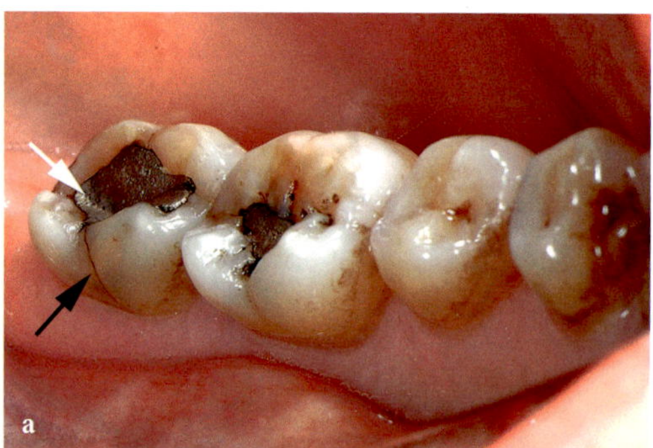


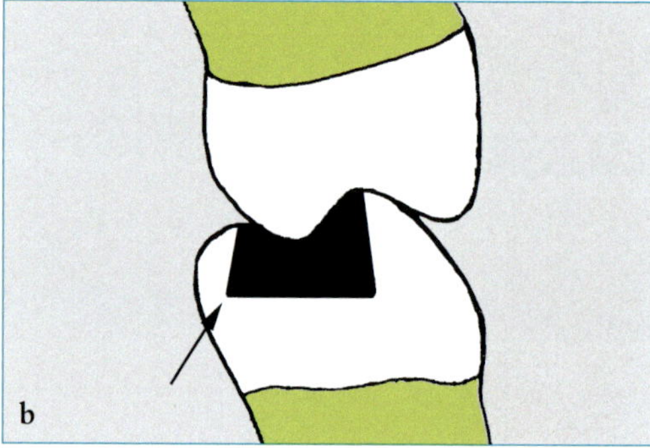


Fig 2-4 **(a)** Fracture line (black arrow) affecting the distolingual cusp of a mandibular second molar. Note the attrition (white arrow) caused by a closely fitting antagonist cusp over an amalgam restoration and enamel distal marginal ridge. This clencher had significant hypertrophy of both masseters. **(b)** Area weakened by the carving of the cavity (arrow), which predisposes it to fracture.

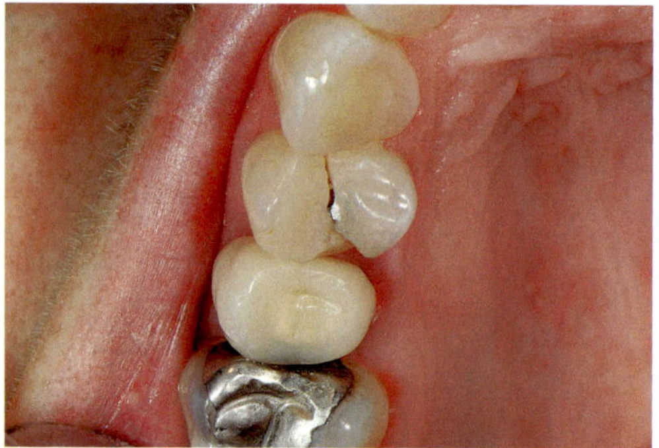

Fig 2-5 Vertical fracture of a maxillary premolar.

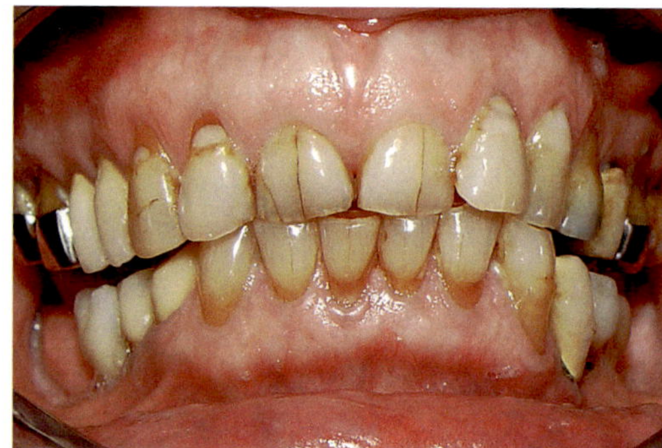

Fig 2-6 Maxillary incisor vestibular enamel fracture in a woman with intense eccentric bruxism.

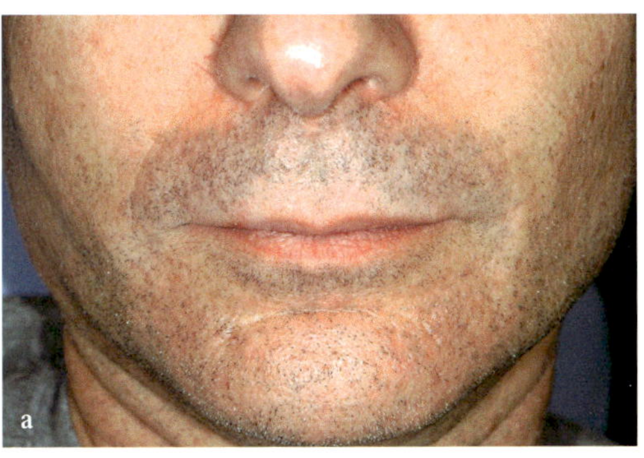


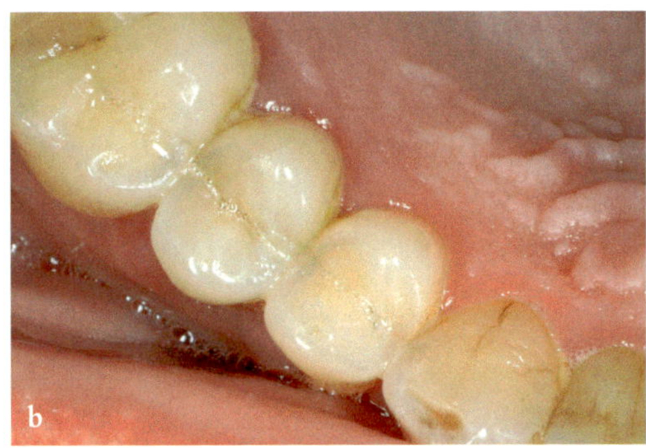


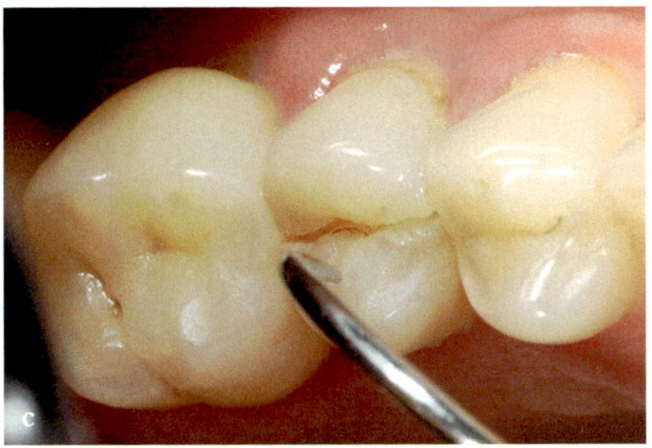


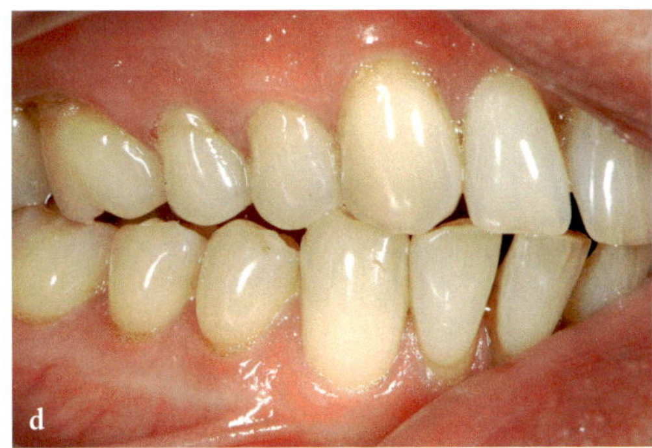


Fig 2-7 **(a)** Clencher showing signs of masseter hypertrophy. **(b)** The second premolar is fractured, though there is no clinical evidence of it. The patient complained of acute pain but was unable to identify its source. **(c)** The fracture was detected with the aid of an explorer. **(d)** Canine protection indicates that the fracture could not have been caused by grinding. **(e)** No signs of fracture are evident in the periapical radiograph, although both the second premolar and the two molars show periodontal widening resulting from sustained tooth clenching.

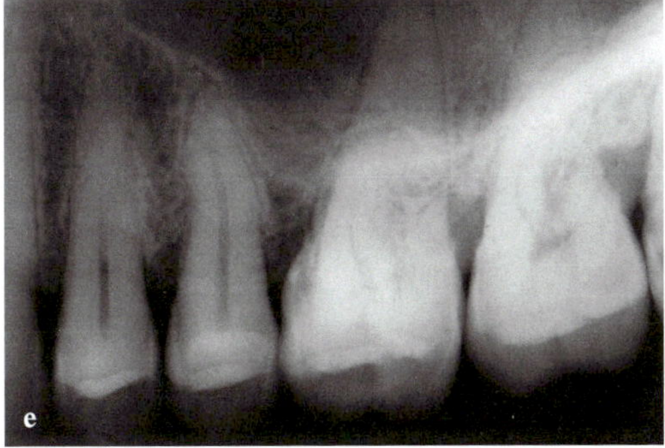

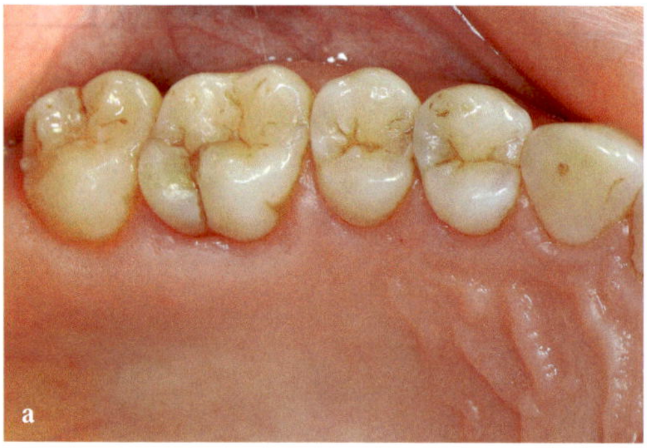

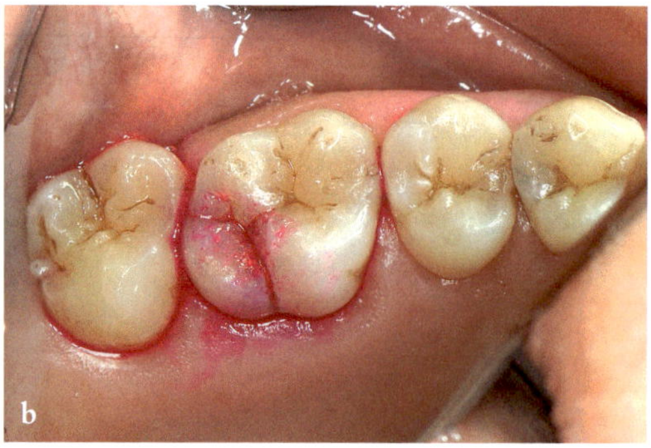

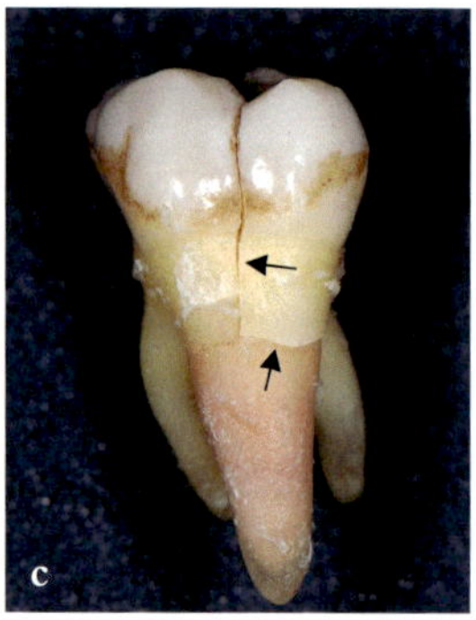

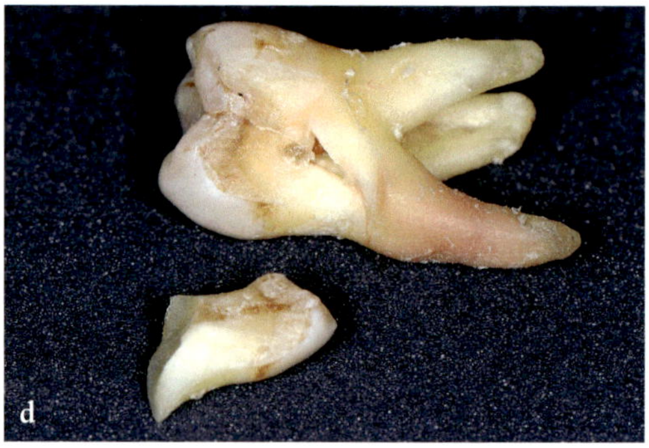

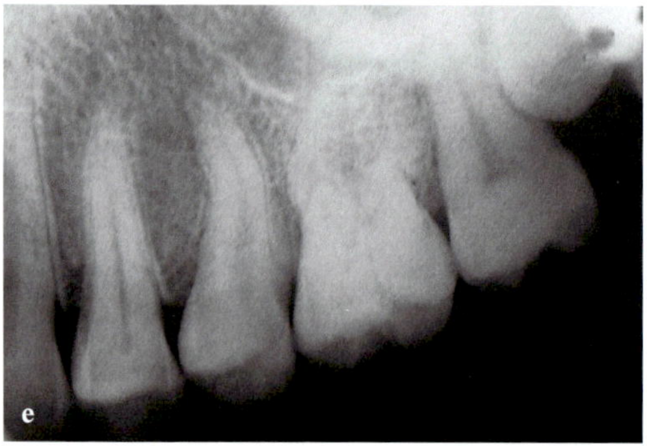

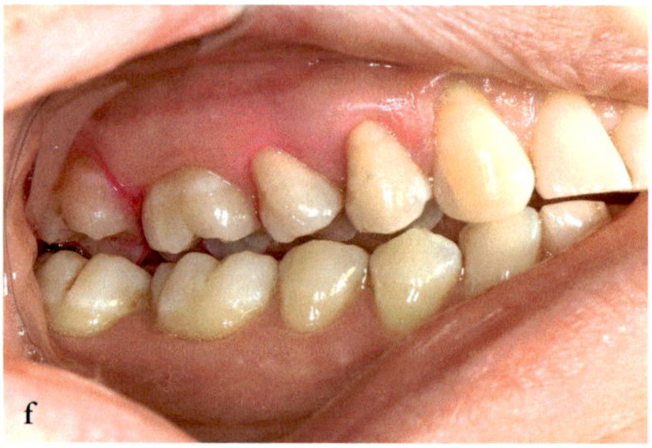

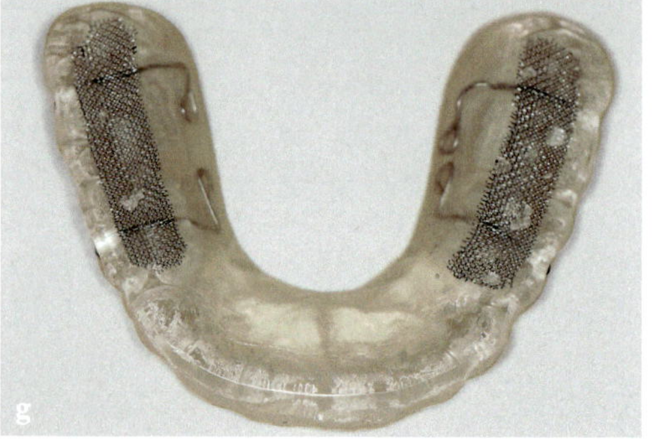

Fig 2-8 **(a)** The first molar shows a fracture that is not seen clinically. **(b)** The fracture of the distopalatal cusp can be detected with the aid of a caries detector. **(c)** Fracture lines (arrows). **(d)** Note how the fracture affects the pulp chamber. **(e)** Fracture of the molar is not seen in the periapical radiograph. **(f)** Canine protection is present during lateral movement. **(g)** This female patient wears a night guard, the surface of which shows signs of clenching. She acknowledged that she clenches hard during the daytime, so it is likely that the fracture occurred while she was in a state of consciousness.

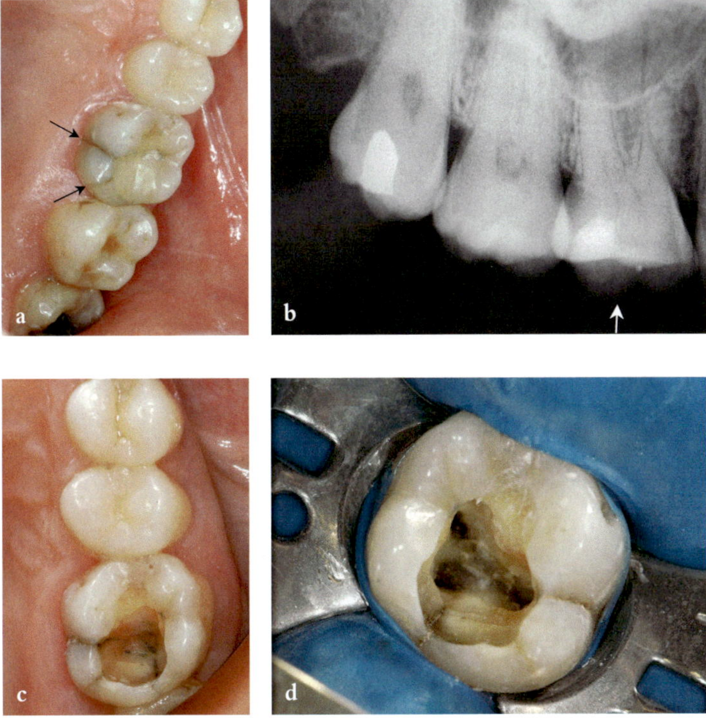

**Fig 2-9** **(a)** Two fractures (arrows) in the maxillary first molar of a female clencher. The composite restoration shows signs of clenching. The patient was on carbamazepine at a dose of 600 mg/day as treatment for intense pain ascribed to potential trigeminal neuralgia diagnosed by a neurologist. **(b)** Periapical radiograph showing significant decrease in the size of the first molar's pulp chamber (arrow). **(c)** After restoration removal, the two fracture lines can be seen involving the pulp chamber roof. The molar was vital, so anesthesia was used during the procedure. **(d)** On opening the pulp chamber, penetration of the distal fracture into the chamber could be observed. There was scarce pulp tissue, and no bleeding occurred during its removal. The pain remitted completely, and the patient was able to stop taking carbamazepine.

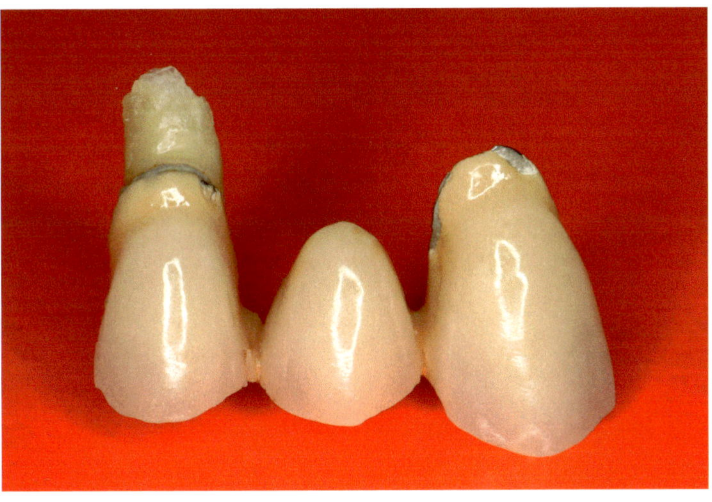

**Fig 2-10** A fixed prosthesis fracture.

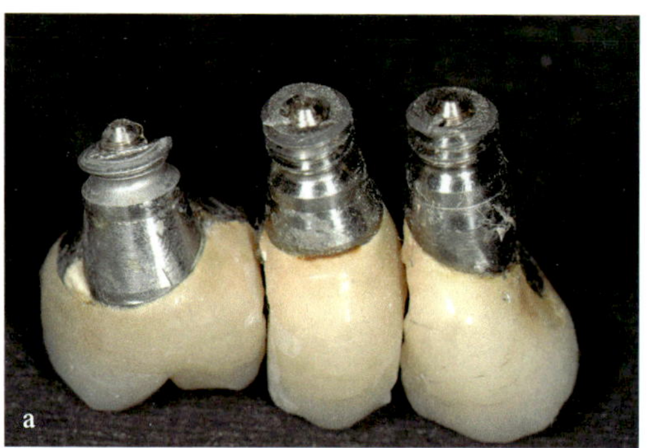


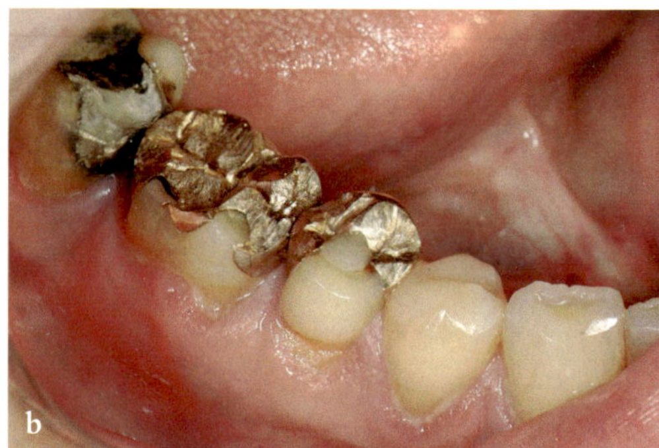


**Fig 2-11** **(a)** Fracture of three implants. **(b)** Antagonists showing attrition caused by eccentric bruxism.

*Tooth mobility*

This can be caused by the widening of the periodontal ligament due to trauma, with no periodontal disease involved (Figs 2-12 and 2-13).

*Pulp necrosis*

There may be death of pulp tissue caused by the continuous occlusal trauma (Figs 2-14 and 2-15).

*Traumatic ulcers*

Traumatic ulcers of the oral mucosa can be caused by continuous clenching and grinding over removable prostheses supported by the oral mucosa.

*Masticatory muscle hypertrophy*

The presence of excessively developed masseter and temporalis muscles during voluntary contraction is another sign of constant clenching (Fig 2-16).

*Linea alba*

A hyperkeratinized white line in the cheek mucosa is another sign that has been ascribed to bruxism.[2–4] As shown in Fig 2-17, this line is located inside the cheek, parallel to the occlusal plane and matching the occlusal plane. Whenever present, it is always bilateral.[3–5] Some authors claim that the formation of the buccal mucosa ridging, or "linea alba", is not related to bruxism in any way.[6] Others ascribe it to the cheek pressure exerted during deglutition.[5]

*Tongue indentations*

This refers to the impressions made by the teeth on the circumferential edge of the tongue (Fig 2-18). They result from the force that the tongue exerts against the dental arches simultaneously with clenching. Some authors[7–9] consider them to be a clinical sign of bruxism, but others disagree.[6,10]

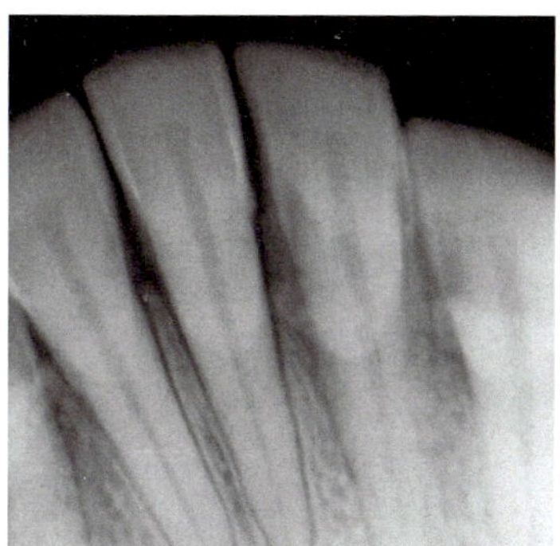

Fig 2-12 Periodontal widening caused by bruxism.

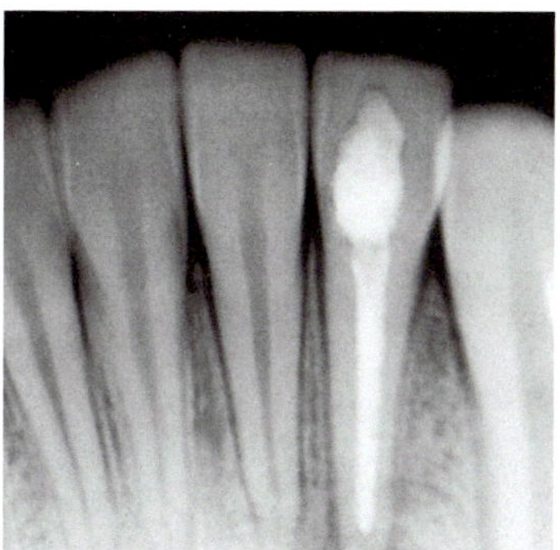

Fig 2-13 Intense bruxing in this patient caused not only periodontal widening but also pulp necrosis in a mandibular lateral incisor. Root canal treatment was required.

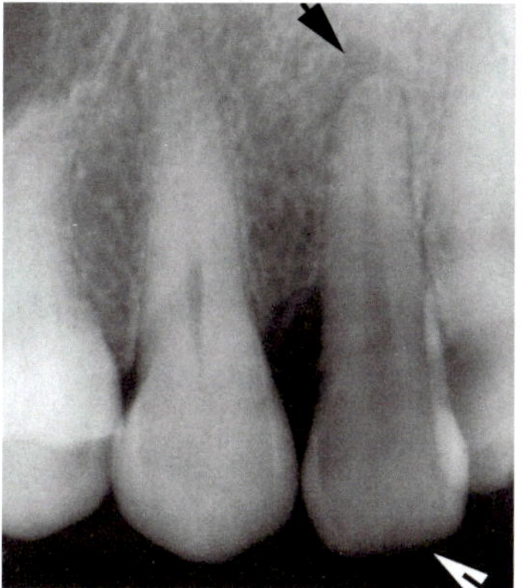

Fig 2-14 Canine pulpal necrosis. Attrition (white arrow) caused by bruxism and an apical radiolucency (black arrow) can be seen.

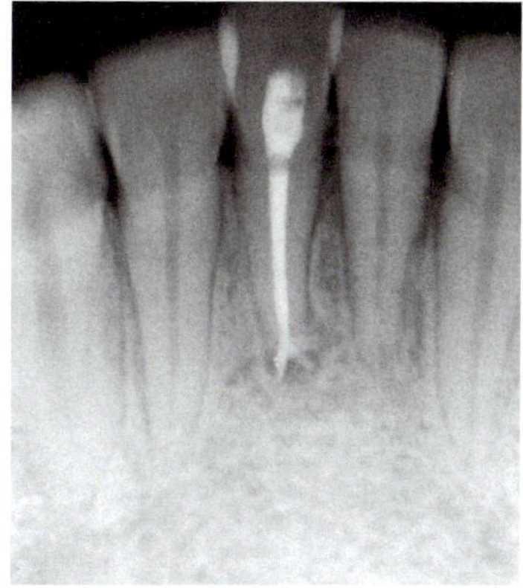

Fig 2-15 A mandibular central incisor that was treated endodontically because of pulpal necrosis due to bruxism.

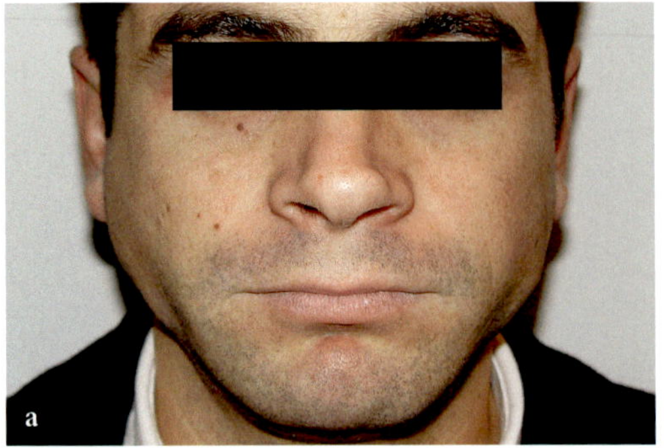


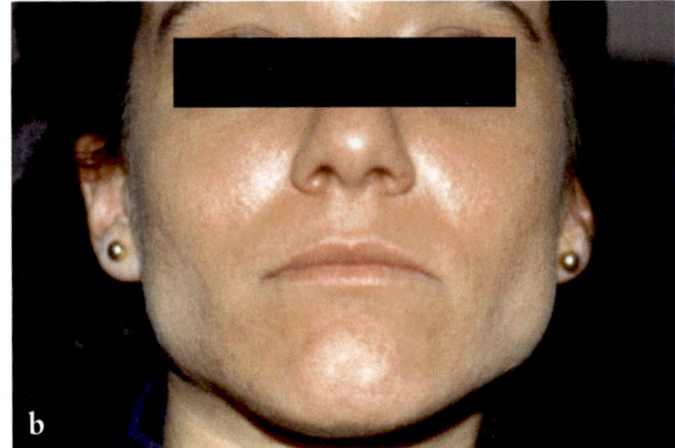


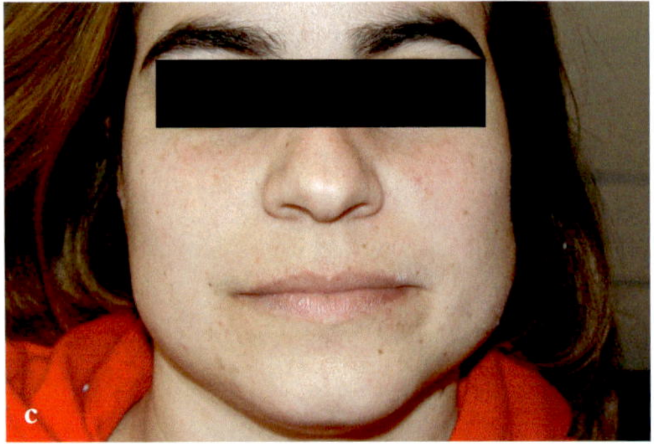


Fig 2-16 **(a–c)** Three patients with masseter hypertrophy.

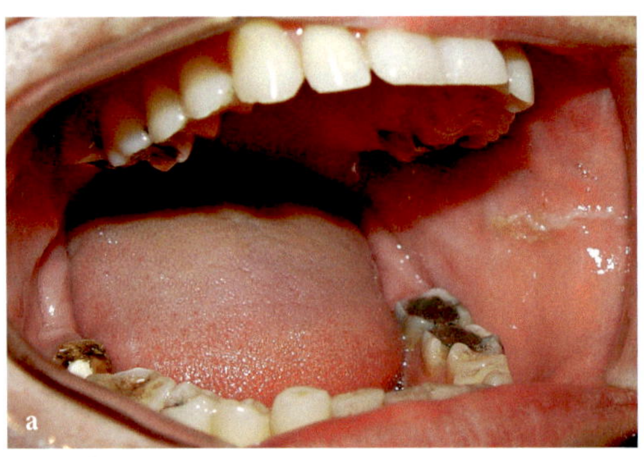


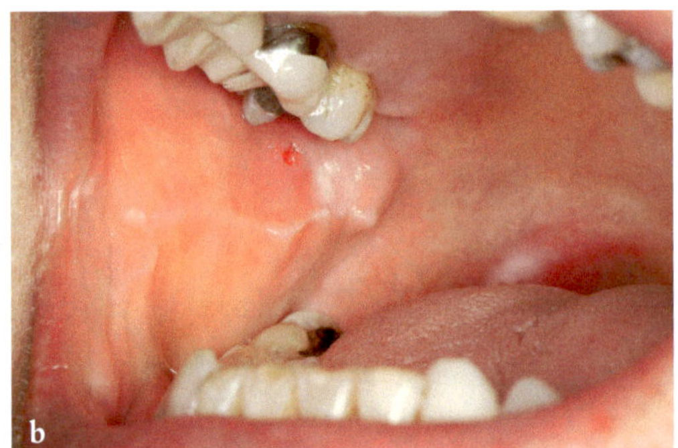


Fig 2-17 **(a and b)** Buccal mucosa ridging, or linea alba.

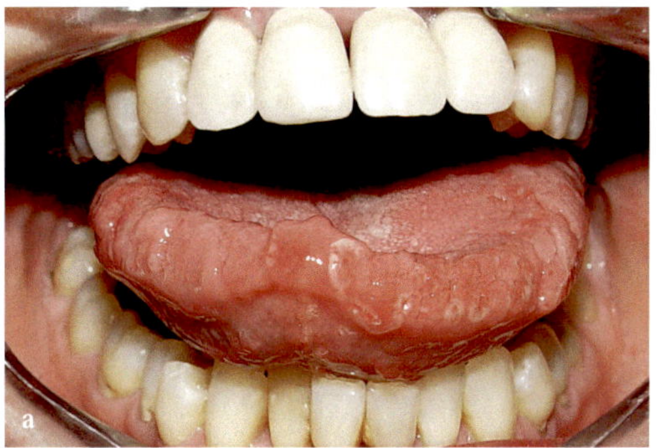

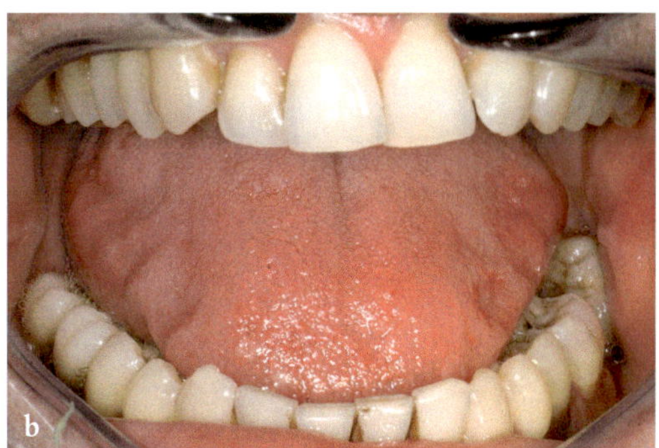

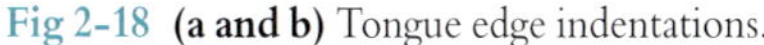

Fig 2-18 **(a and b)** Tongue edge indentations.

## Complementary Methods for Diagnosis

The interpretation of clinical signs and symptoms provides clinicians with valuable information that can be used to diagnose bruxism. Nevertheless, in the research field these data are not sufficient because they do not enable accurate quantification of the activity. Thus, it is necessary to use complementary quantification methods to corroborate etiology theories, assess response to treatments, etc. Complementary methods for bruxism research include intraoral devices, portable EMG devices, and polysomnography.

### *Intraoral Devices*

Some researchers have proposed the use of intraoral devices to measure bruxism in an objective way. There are two approaches: those that help assess bruxism through the interpretation of superficial bite plate wear, and those that measure the bite force through sensors embedded in the bite plates.

#### *Bite plate wear quantification*

Clinicians who regularly treat bruxers will often observe impressions made by bruxism on the sleep-time devices used by these patients (Fig 2-19). This has led to research based on the interpretation of splint wear caused by bruxism.

#### *Bruxofacets in splints*

A group of researchers reported on cases of bruxers who used night guards.[11] They found that all of them bruxed over the splints. Sixty-one percent of the patients showed repetition of the wear pattern in the control visits every 2 weeks; the remaining 39% also showed wear repetition but after longer periods. Wear facets always occured in the same place and with the same direction and movement patterns. Seventy-one percent of them were caused by bilateral grinding, 13% by unilateral grinding, 13% by sustained clenching and a minimum of lateral movements, while 3% of the facets were in the protrusive direction. The study confirms that sleep bruxism is mostly of the grinding kind, and that the wear pattern is constant and repeats over time. Bruxism fluctuations were checked also; in 39% of patients, wear was not produced according to a constant chronological pattern. These results were later confirmed in a similar paper.[12] Subsequently, other researchers introduced a splint digitalization system for three-dimensional measurement of wear.[13] They were able to report on wear features more accurately; on comparing wear produced on each side of the splint, and anterior and posterior wear, they found it to be unsymmetrical. Unfortunately, no studies seem to have evaluated the accuracy of these methods for measuring bruxism.

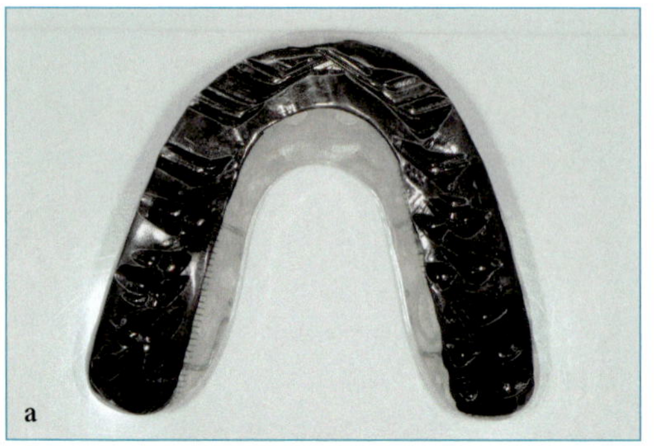


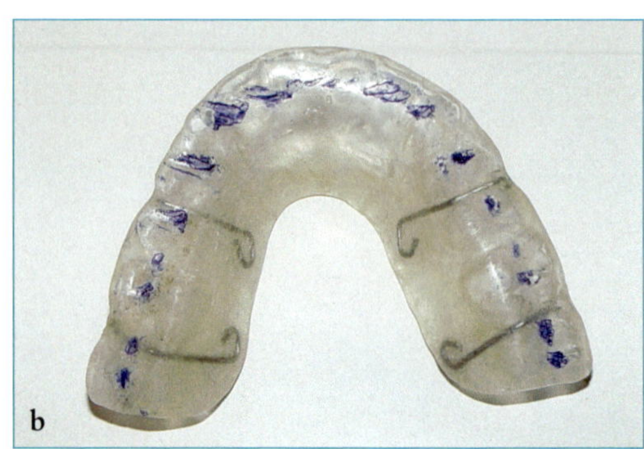


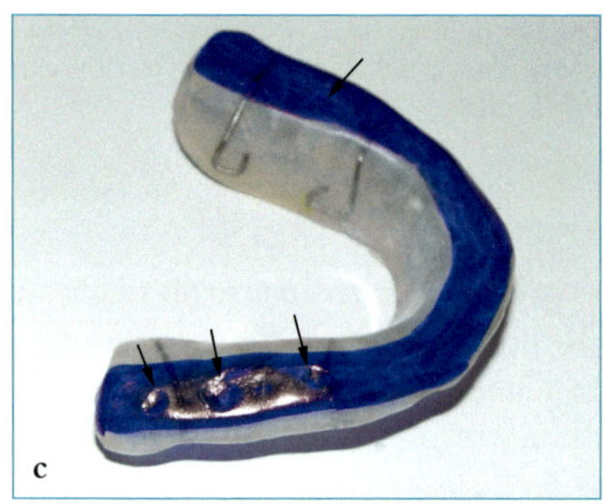


Fig 2-19 **(a)** A splint belonging to a patient showing phasic bruxism during sleep. Note the impressions left by the antagonist cusps on the splint surface during lateral movement. **(b)** This bite plate reflects a unilateral, rightward, grinding type of bruxism pattern. **(c)** This splint shows clearly the impressions left by bruxism of the clenching type (tonic).

*Bruxcore*

Another suggested quantification method uses Bruxcore. This system measures the volume of wear caused by bruxism.[14,15] It consists of a 0.51 mm-thick polyvinyl chloride sheet with four colored layers (two red and two white layers arranged alternately) and a medium-shaded grid with 0.14 mm-diameter microdots printed on its surface. The plate contains 2,228 microdots per square centimeter. It can be made very easily by thermoforming it and vacuum-stamping it over a model of the patient's dental arch, and then cutting it in a similar way to a splint. The wear area can be objectively measured by counting the number of missing microdots, whereas the number of worn-through layers accounts for wear depth. Then, both parameters are combined and a number is obtained which represents the bruxism index. In short, Bruxcore can be said to be a splint made of a material comprising several layers of different colors which allows one to measure bruxism by counting the number of microdots that wear away (Fig 2-20).

Recently, a computerized system for wear analysis has been presented which improves objectivity by resorting to an algorithm for measuring the abrasion area in pixels.[16] The validity of this system, though, has been called into question, since Bruxcore alone can alter the oral environment and therefore modify the parafunctional activity.[17]

*Bite force detectors*

Teams of researchers have created systems for detecting the forces generated by sleep bruxism.[18,19]

*Intra-splint force detector*

This innovative system uses a 100 μm-thick piezoelectric film that is embedded 1 mm below the splint occlusal surface and is extremely sensitive to splint deformation caused by bruxism. A threshold is set, and every time it is exceeded the information

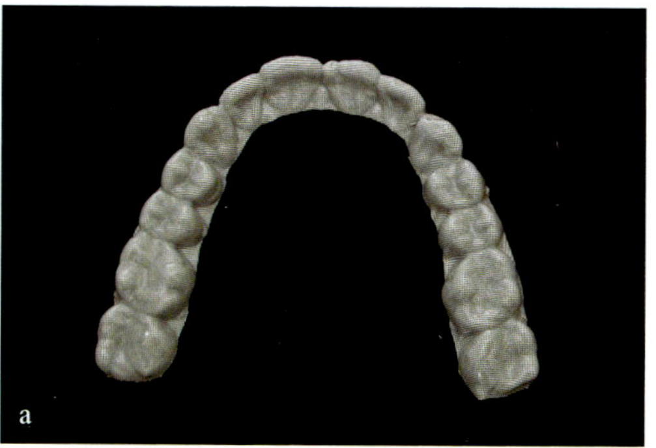


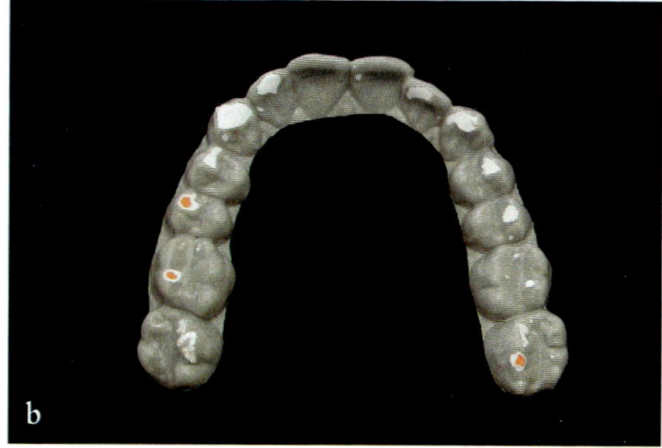


Fig 2-20 **(a)** Bite plate made with a Bruxcore sheet. The patient wore it for five consecutive nights, but no signs of parafunctional activity can be observed. **(b)** Bruxcore plate worn for five consecutive nights by another bruxer; bruxism impressions may be observed over the surface of the device. (Both pictures courtesy of Dr Michelle A. Ommerborn, Department of Operative and Preventive Dentistry and Endodontics, Heinrich-Heine-University, Düsseldorf, Germany.)

is sent through a wire to an amplifier-detector and then to a computer programmed to record and store data in 1-second resolution text files.[20] To date, only one paper has been published on this subject; it reports on the case of just one patient who was simultaneously studied with the piezoelectric detector and polysomnography for a whole night in a sleep laboratory (described later). The researchers used masseter EMG as the "gold standard" and reported a sensitivity of 0.89; the correlation ratio between the events registered by the piezoelectric detector and those registered by the EMG was 0.80.[19]

As reported by the system developers, the advantage of piezoelectric detectors over portable EMG devices is that they do not require the use of surface electrodes (position reproducibility; sounds generated by poor adherence to the skin) which often leads to misreading; in contrast, piezoelectric detectors work in a much simpler way, because just splint placement and turning on of the device are required.

*Force measurement by intraoral splints*

Nishigawa and co-workers developed a system that measures bruxism by means of strain gauge sensors embedded in acrylic splints.[18] Two sensors are placed in the upper splint, one to the right and the other to the left, in the molar area. In the lower splint, two transducers are placed as antagonists. Every time the patient clenches his or her teeth the transducers record vertical bite force. The study of a group of 10 patients evaluated over three nights revealed that sleep bruxism bite forces can exceed the amplitude of daytime maximum voluntary bite force. In the series, the average bite force was 42.3 kgf. One subject was reported to have a bite force of 81.2 kgf – he exceeded his maximum daytime voluntary bite force by 111.6%. The average event duration was 7.1 ± 5.3 seconds, and the number of bruxism episodes was 3.6 per hour.

Nevertheless, as is the case with Bruxcore, the use of splints alters the oral environment and, consequently, bruxism values, and this may be confusing. This subject will be discussed in detail in Chapter 25, where we analyze the effect of the splints on bruxism.

### *Masseter Electromyography Records*

Bruxism can be assessed in an ambulatory way through EMG recording of the masseter activity. The possibility of recording bruxism without affecting the nature of the oral environment allows more accurate assessment.

*Portable EMG devices*

The many advantages of portable EMG devices include their relatively low cost and the possibility of studying subjects in their own homes, without the need for them to go to a research center every day. This makes it easier to study a large number of subjects time and again, and over long periods. The pitfall, though, is that it is impossible to maintain strict control over the study, in terms of electrode position reproducibility, prior thorough cleaning of the skin, potential electrical artifacts generated by badly adhered electrodes, etc. Also, other rhythmic activities of the masticatory muscles (e.g., deglutition, facial gesticulation, jaw movements without tooth contact) may be misrecorded as bruxism episodes. The fact that these non-bruxing activities may be included in the records is misleading for researchers.

Muscle activities without tooth contact have been reported in both non-bruxers and bruxers.[10,21–23] A study by Lavigne and co-workers,[24] conducted in a sleep laboratory, found that 60% of normal individuals will show rhythmic muscle activities (of the masticatory muscles) without tooth contact, the frequency of such activities being three times as low in control subjects as it is in bruxers. The authors recommend the use in sleep studies of a microphone connected to a recorder, so that real tooth-grinding episodes can be distinguished from rhythmic movements without tooth contact.

Several portable EMG models have been used in bruxism research. The first portable EMG device was developed in the 1970s and had only one channel which recorded cumulative masseter activity; this was then divided by the amount of time the activity was monitored for and converted into EMG units expressed in microvolts.[25] Portable EMG devices allow sensitivity to be varied, so that only muscle activity that exceeds the set threshold value is recorded. This prevents the recording of other minor muscle activities which are not consistent with tooth grinding or tooth clenching. Several values have been used in research; thresholds have been set to 20 μV, 30 μV, and 100 μV.

A plethora of literature has been published on the use of portable EMG devices.[26–28] Some authors attempted to use them to demonstrate that bruxism has a strong association with emotional factors.[29] Their work was later called into question due to methodology errors generally involving a low number of participants in the study population and lack of a control group.

Some of these devices have an alarm which triggers whenever there is a muscle contraction that exceeds the set threshold. This allows the patient to wake up and interrupt the bruxism event. This is known as "biofeedback"; it is also helpful in training patients how to relax facial and masticatory muscles.[30,31]

In 1982, by adding a pulse identification system, Zaharkin improved the equipment which Solberg and Rugh had used for the first time in 1972. The audible signals recorded by a recorder would then be transformed into a polygraph chart which could be analyzed by a laboratory technician. These modifications enabled the EMG devices to quantify bruxism activity, and the recording of the frequency and duration of bruxism events made it possible to distinguish between clenching and grinding episodes.

Some years later, research carried out using another improved portable EMG device was reported.[32] The system included a clock that allowed chronological recording of bruxism episodes within periods of 15 minutes. The effects of a true splint were compared with the effects of a placebo splint and it was found that both splints reduced the frequency of bruxism.

A significant number of publications have reported on research using several portable EMG device models. This has allowed study of the relationships between bruxism and dental occlusion, emotional status, the different days of the week, the efficiency of selective grinding, etc.[26,28,29,31,33,34] Unfortunately, the lack of standardization among

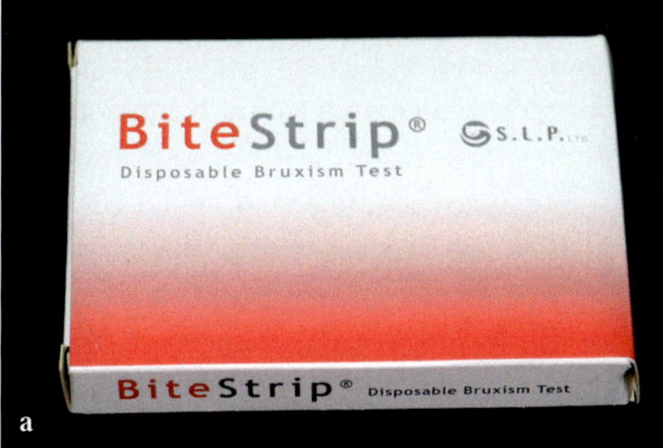


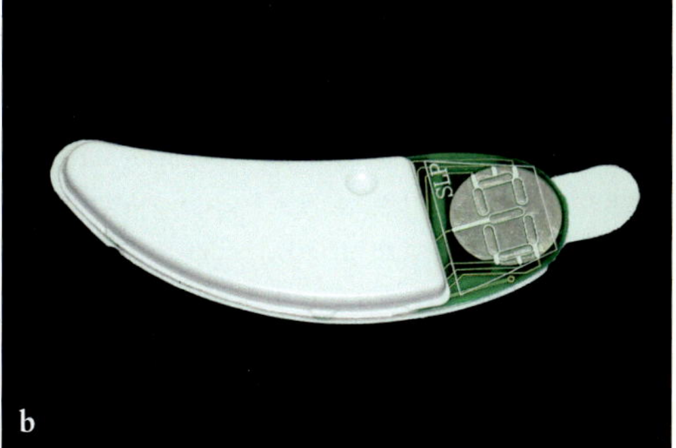


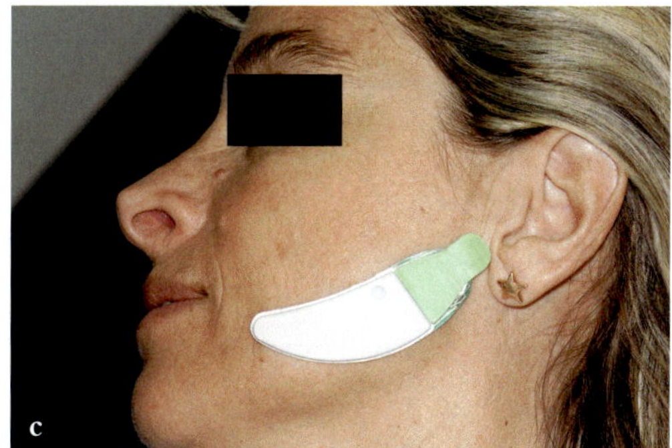


Fig 2-21 **(a–c)** BiteStrip miniature EMG device.

the equipment used makes valid comparison of the publications difficult.[35]

A device that has some advantages over the earlier devices has recently been launched to the market.[36,37] It has various channels that allow the simultaneous assessment of four muscles (two temporalis muscles and two masseters) and includes a novel amplification technology that filters the signal and avoids the recording of electrical noise and other artifacts generated by body movements in sleep. The information is recorded on a memory card and then downloaded to a computer and analyzed with specially developed software, which allows detection of the different bruxism events and the duration of each episode.

*Disposable miniature EMG device: BiteStrip®*

A tiny disposable device that records sleep bruxism activity has recently been launched to the market. BiteStrip (S.L.P., Israel) is a miniature electronic system measuring 7 cm by 2 cm and weighing 4 g. It has two electrodes that stick to the skin over the masseter muscle area and record masseter contractile activities. The device comprises an EMG amplifier and a central processing unit (CPU) with software for real-time analysis of bruxism intensity and the number of bruxism episodes. It is powered by a lithium battery, and the results are shown on a chemical display for further analysis. The patient's maximum voluntary contraction (MVC) before starting the test is recorded and used as the threshold. Activities above 30% of MVC are considered to be bruxism events. BiteStrip records every EMG peak for a period of up to 6 hours (Fig 2-21a–c).

The BiteStrip system was simultaneously compared with EMG during a polysomnography performed in five suspected bruxers.[38] After analysis of the participants' records, a sensitivity of 63% and a specificity of 73% using a threshold value of >40% of MVC were reported. Thus, the system proved to be a cost-effective tool for subjects with mild to severe bruxism.

### Polysomnography

See Chapter 3 for a thorough understanding of the studies of sleep bruxism.

#### *Research*

Polysomnography (PSG) conducted in a sleep laboratory is the most accurate method for studying bruxism. It records biologic signals such as EMG, electroencephalogram (EEG), electro-oculogram (EOG), and electrocardiogram (ECG), as well as audio and video signals. Interactions between bruxism and sleep physiology are currently known thanks to studies based on this method.

In a brief abstract published in 1961, Takahama was the first to report on a bruxism study conducted in a sleep lab.[39] Correlation with EEG findings revealed that bruxism occurred predominantly during the light sleep stage and was preceded by pulse, breathing, and cortical activity alterations. This suggested a relationship between sleep bruxism and activity of the autonomic nervous system.

Later, in 1964, some more thorough research was conducted by Reding and co-workers.[40] They studied 12 bruxers and 4 control subjects using polysomnography. They found that bruxism occurred mainly during the rapid eye movement (REM) stage and within 2 minutes after the beginning of the non-REM I and non-REM II stages. Three years later, though, after redefining the episodes, they rectified their previous work by reporting that bruxism occurs in all sleep stages, though predominantly in the non-REM II stage.[41] It has also been demonstrated that each bruxism episode is preceded by a quickening of the pulse rate.[21,42–44]

During sleep, other activities occur, including myoclonic contractions, coughing, moaning, face rubbing, deglutition, snoring, and normal opening and closing movements of the mouth. All these activities alternate with tooth-grinding episodes; thus, it is essential to distinguish the former from the latter.[45]

For this reason, polysomnography is complemented by monitoring of the subject by means of an infrared video camera focused on the head and neck, and a microphone is also placed over the head. This allows thorough control of the study and accurate identification of the true tooth-grinding episodes, so as to distinguish them from other misleading activities (Fig 2-22).

Sleep studies also led to the discovery of rhythmic masticatory muscle activity (RMMA), which has been associated with subjects with bruxing habits.[46,47] However, this kind of muscle activity has also been seen in normal subjects who do not grind their teeth, and in subjects who suffer from somnambulism and nightmares. Some authors have defined RMMA as "masticatory automatism".[48]

RMMA is seen in 60% of normal individuals. It is not associated with sleep disorders, since it occurs mostly in subjects with a normal sleep architecture. However, comparison between groups of non-bruxers and groups of bruxers showed that the latter experience more RMMA episodes, more peaks per episode, and higher-amplitude peaks.[24] Sixty percent of RMMAs are related to deglutition, in both bruxers and non-bruxers.[49]

Sleep organization is similar in bruxers and non-bruxers who have RMMA without tooth grinding. With regard to stage efficiency, duration and distribution, both groups have a normal sleep architecture; that is why bruxers do not usually complain of sleep alterations.[10] Several studies agree that most bruxism episodes occur in the light sleep stage – in the non-REM II stage.[10,21,23,50,51]

A relationship between an abrupt temporary lightening of the sleep (micro-arousal) prior to bruxism episodes was first reported by Reding and

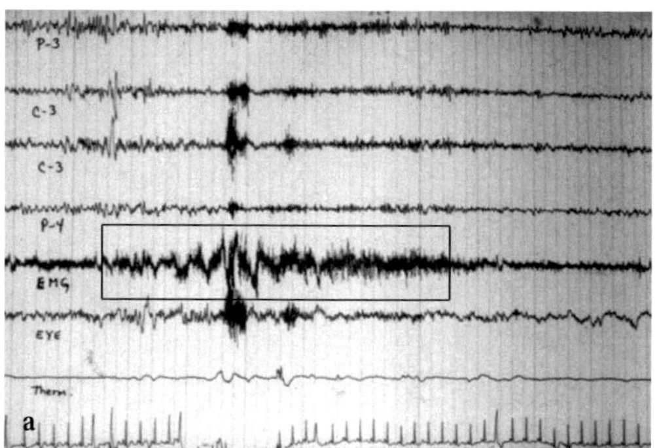

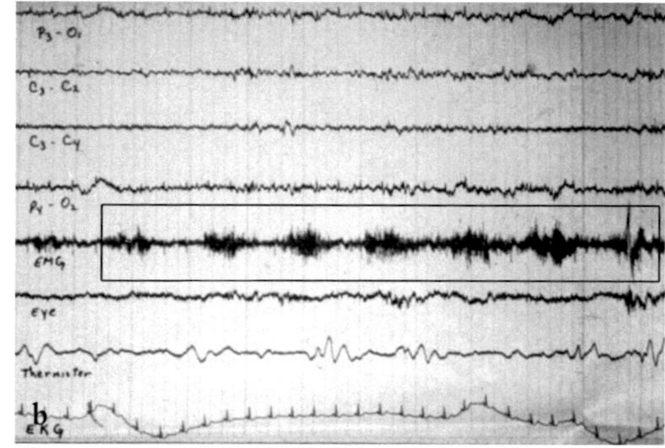

Fig 2-22 **(a)** Polysomnography. The box shows right-masseter EMG activity during a sustained tooth-clenching episode of 12 seconds. **(b)** The box shows seven tooth-grinding episodes recorded over the right-masseter EMG channel. Each episode averages 2 seconds, and the inactivity spaces in between represent left-masseter activity.

co-workers in 1968, in a study of a group of bruxers and control subjects with polysomnography.[21] Later, in an uncontrolled study, it was possible to experimentally induce bruxism episodes in sleepers by provoking micro-arousals through sensory stimuli. The authors concluded that, apparently, bruxism was an arousal reaction.[52]

Micro-arousals are commonly seen in normal non-bruxers in a similar number per hour, regardless of the subjects showing RMMA or not. In contrast, micro-arousals are 67% more frequent in subjects who grind their teeth during sleep than in normal subjects, though these values are not above those in normal subjects reported by other studies.[53,54] Thus, and as Satoh and Harada suggest,[52] bruxism is apparently an arousal reaction[24] and not an arousal pathology.[46] Recently, micro-arousals were experimentally induced in a controlled study, and, as in the experiment by Satoh and Harada, RMMA episodes were evoked. This RMMA was more frequent in bruxers than in normal subjects. Bruxers showed tooth grinding in 71% of evoked RMMAs. These findings contribute to the hypothesis that bruxism is an exaggerated kind of motor activity associated with micro-arousals.[55]

*Sleep bruxism identification criteria*

For polysomnography interpretation, EMG thresholds must be set so as to determine whether the muscle activity found is consistent or not with bruxism episodes. This is not easy, because a threshold too high may cause many bruxism episodes to be ignored, while a threshold too low may lead to mistaking non-bruxing episodes for bruxing episodes. A well-devised research project should also include a control population (non-bruxers).

The criterion by which to assign each subject to the correct study population can present a challenge. The American Sleep Disorders Association (ASDA) suggested that clinical diagnosis of sleep bruxism should be based mainly on tooth-grinding or tooth-clenching reports plus the presence of at least some of the following clinical findings: sounds associated with bruxism, tooth wear, and sore muscles on waking.[56] Scientific proof of the validity of these criteria is still required. In 1996, Lavigne and co-workers compared a population of bruxers with a control population (non-bruxers) in a controlled study.[1] They demonstrated the accuracy of the inclusion criteria suggested by ASDA. The clinical validity of the patients, after laboratory confirmation of the grinding sounds reported by them in the clinical evaluation, showed a sensitivity of 78% and a specificity of 94%. Tooth wear was seen in 16 out of the 18 bruxers studied. These results show that it will be possible for studies that choose to select subjects by using the above-mentioned criteria to include very homogeneous study populations. Besides, this information is very important for general practitioners who, in addition to clinical examination, will be able to accurately identify sleep bruxers by using a simple questionnaire.

Only 6 out of 18 bruxers reported experiencing morning pain or morning fatigue in the questionnaire answered by both bruxers and control subjects. During the clinical interrogation, though, none of them reported experiencing this problem. Significantly, 16 out of 18 bruxers showed masseter hypertrophy – not listed by ASDA as an inclusion criterion. Also, the authors suggest the following cutoff values for identifying bruxism episodes with polysomnograpy:

- more than 4 bruxism episodes per hour of sleep
- more than 6 bruxism peaks per episode and/or 25 bruxism peaks per hour of sleep
- at least 2 events with tooth-grinding sounds.

The individuals from the control population never reached these cutoff values. Bruxers showed three times the number of bruxism episodes per night and per hour of sleep; they also showed more bruxism peaks per episode. In both groups, 80% of the episodes occurred in the non-REM I and II stages. Sleep variables in both groups were similar, which confirms that bruxers do not suffer from sleep architecture disorders, as other authors suggested.[57,58] The results of this study have confirmed the validity of the cutoff values suggested by the authors, which allow one to distinguish bruxism episodes from other rhythmic muscle activities occurring during sleep.

## References


1. Lavigne GJ, Rompre PH, Montplaisir JY. Sleep bruxism: validity of clinical research diagnosis criteria in a controlled polysomnographic study. J Dent Res 1996; 75:546–552.
2. Crispian S, Stephen RF, Stephen RP. Oral Diseases, ed 2. Singapore: Toppan Printing Co., 1996:217.
3 Gary CC, John FN. Principles of Oral Diagnosis. Montana, USA: Mosby Yearbook, 1993:64.
4. Malcom AL. Oral Medicine, ed 9. Philadelphia: Lippincott, 1994:56.
5. Takagi I, Sakurai K. Investigation of the factors related to the formation of the buccal mucosa ridging. J Oral Rehabil 2003;30:565–572.
6. Piquero K, Ando T, Sakurai K. Buccal mucosa ridging and tongue indentation: incidence and associated factors. Bull Tokyo Dent Coll 1999;40:71–78.
7. Sapiro SM. Tongue indentations as an indicator of clenching. Clin Prev Dent 1992;14:21–24.
8. Long JH. A device to prevent jaw clenching. J Prosthet Dent 1998;79:353–354.
9. Kampe T, Tagdac T, Bader G, Edman G, Karlsson S. Reported symptoms and clinical findings in a group of subjects with longstanding bruxing behavior. J Oral Rehabil 1997;24:581–587.
10. Yanagisawa K, Takagi I, Sakurai K. Influence of tongue pressure and width on tongue indentation formation. J Oral Rehabil 2007;34:827–834.
11. Holmgren K, Sheikholeslam A, Riise C. Effect of a full-arch maxillary occlusal splint on parafunctional activity during sleep in patients with nocturnal bruxism and signs and symptoms of craniomandibular disorders. J Prosthet Dent 1993;69:293–297.
12. Chung S, Kim Y, Kim H. Prevalence and patterns of nocturnal bruxofacets on stabilization splints in temporomandibular disorder patients. J Craniomandibular Pract 2000;18:92–97.
13. Korioth TWP, Bohlig KC, Anderson GC. Digital assessment of occlusal wear patterns on occlusal stabilization splints: a pilot study. J Prosthet Dent 1998;80:209–213.
14. Forgione AG. A simple but effective method of quantifying bruxism behavior. J Dent Res 1974;53:127.
15. Heller RF, Forgione AG. An evaluation of bruxism control: massed negative practice and automated relaxation training. J Dent Res 1975;54:1120–1123.
16. Ommerborn MA, Giraki M, Schneider C et al. A new analyzing method for quantification of abrasion on the Bruxcore device for sleep bruxism. J Orofac Pain 2005; 19:223–238.

17. Pierce CJ, Gale EN. Methodological considerations concerning the use of Bruxcore plates to evaluate nocturnal bruxism. J Dent Res 1989;68:1110–1114.
18. Nishigawa K, Bando E, Nakano M. Quantitative study of bite force during sleep associated bruxism. J Oral Rehabil 2001;28:485–491.
19. Baba K, Clark GT, Watanabe T, Ohyama T. Bruxism force detection by a piezoelectric film-based recording device in sleeping humans. J Orofac Pain 2003;17:58–64.
20. Takeuchi H, Ikeda T, Clark GT. A piezoelectric film-based intrasplint detection method for bruxism. J Prosthet Dent 2001;86:195–202.
21. Reding GR, Zepelin H, Robinson JE, Zimmerman SO, Smith VH. Nocturnal teeth-grinding: all-night psychophysiologic studies. J Dent Res 1968;47:786–797.
22. Sjoholm T, Lehtinen I, Helenius H. Masseter muscle activity in diagnosed sleep bruxists compared with non-symptomatic controls. J Sleep Res 1995;4:48–55.
23. Macaluso GM, Guerra P, Di Giovanni G et al. Sleep bruxism is a disorder related to periodic arousals during sleep. J Dent Res 1998;77:565–573.
24. Lavigne GJ, Rompre PH, Poirier G et al. Rhythmic masticatory muscle activity during sleep in humans. J Dent Res 2001;80:443–448.
25. Solberg WK, Rugh JD. The use of bio-feedback devices in the treatment of bruxism. J South Calif Dent Assoc 1972;40:852–853.
26. Clark GT, Beemsterboer PL, Solberg WK, Rugh JD. Nocturnal electromyographic evaluation of myofascial pain dysfunction in patients undergoing oclusal splint therapy. J Am Dent Assoc 1979;99:607–611.
27. Clark GT, Rugh JD, Handelman SL. Nocturnal masseter muscle activity and urinary catecholamine levels in bruxers. J Dent Res 1980;59:1571–1576.
28. Rugh JD, Barghi N, Drago CJ. Experimental occlusal discrepancies and nocturnal bruxism. J Prosthet Dent 1984;51:548–553.
29. Rugh JD, Solberg WK. Electromyographic studies of bruxist behavior before and during treatment. J Calif Dent Assoc 1975;3:56–59.
30. Rugh JD, Johnson RW. Temporal analysis of nocturnal bruxism during EMG feedback. J Periodontol 1981;52: 263–265.
31. Pierce CJ, Gale EN. A comparison of different treatments for nocturnal bruxism. J Dent Res 1988;67:597–601.
32. Cassisi JE, McGlynn FD, Mahan PE. Occlusal splint effects on nocturnal bruxing: an emerging paradigm and some early results. Cranio 1987;5:64–68.
33. Solberg WK, Clark GT, Rugh JD. Nocturnal electromyographic evaluation of bruxism patients undergoing short term splint therapy. J Oral Rehabil 1975;2:215–223.
34. Rugh JD, Graham GS, Smith JC, Ohrbach RK. Effects of canine versus molar occlusal splint guidance on nocturnal bruxism and craniomandibular symptomatology. J Craniomandib Disord 1989;3:203–210.
35. Rugh JD, Schwitzgebel RL. Methods and designs variability in commercial electromyographic biofeedback devices. Behav Res Methods Instrum Comput 1977;9: 281–285.
36. Hiyama S, Ono T, Ishiwata Y, Kato Y, Kuroda T. First night effect of an interocclusal appliance on nocturnal masticatory muscle activity. J Oral Rehabil 2003;30: 139–145.
37. Harada T, Ichiki R, Tsukiyama Y, Koyano K. The effect of oral splint devices on sleep bruxism: a 6-week observation with an ambulatory electromyographic recording device. J Oral Rehabil 2006;33:482–488.
38. Minakuchi H, Clark GT, Haberman PB, Maekawa K, Kuboki T. The sensitivity and specificity of miniature bruxism detection device. J Orofac Pain 2006;20:92 (abstract).
39. Takahama Y. Bruxism. J Dent Res 1961;40:227 (abstract).
40. Reding GR, Rubright WC, Rechtschaffen A, Daniels RS. Sleep pattern of tooth-grinding: its relationship to dreaming. Science 1964;145:725–726.
41. Reding GR, Zepelin H, Robinson JE, Smith VH, Zimmerman SO. Sleep pattern of bruxism: a revision. Psychophysiology 1967;4:396 (abstract).
42. Okura k, Nakano M, Bando E et al. Analysis of biological signals during sleep associated bruxism. J Jpn Soc Stomatognath Funct 1996;3:83–93.
43. Huynh N, Kato T, Rompre PH et al. Sleep bruxism is associated to micro arousals and an increase in cardiac sympathetic activity. J Sleep Res 2006;15:339–346.
44. Kato T, Rompre P, Montplaisir JY, Sessle BJ, Lavigne GJ. Sleep bruxism: an oromotor activity secondary to micro-arousal. J Dent Res 2001;80:1940–1944.
45. Velly Miguel AM, Montplaisir J, Rompre PH, Lund JP, Lavigne GJ. Bruxism and other orofacial movements during sleep. J Craniomandib Disord 1992;6:71–81.
46. Thorpy MJ. International Classification of Sleep Disorders: Diagnostic and Coding Manual. Rochester, MN: Allen Press, 1997.
47. Lavigne GJ, Manzini C. Sleep bruxism and concomitant motor activity. In: Kryger MH, Roth T, Dement WC (eds). Principles and Practice of Sleep Medicine. Philadelphia: Elsevier Saunders, 2000:773–785.
48. Halasz P, Ujszaszi J. Chewing automatism in sleep connected with micro-arousals: an indicator of propensity to confusional awakenings? In: Koella WP, Obal F, Schulz OF, Visser P (eds). Sleep '86. Stuttgart: Gustav Fisher Verlag, 1988:235–239.
49. Miyawaki S, Lavigne GJ, Pierre M, Guitard F, Montplaisir JY, Kato T. Association between sleep bruxism, swallowing-related laryngeal movement, and sleep position. Sleep 2003;26:461–465.
50. Okeson JP, Phillips BA, Berry DTR, Baldwin RM. Nocturnal bruxing events: a report of normative data and cardiovascular response. J Oral Rehabil 1994;21:623–630.

51. Bader GG, Kampe T, Tagdae T, Karlsson S, Blomqvist M. Descriptive physiological data on a sleep bruxism population. Sleep 1997;20:982–990.
52. Satoh T, Harada Y. Tooth-grinding during sleep as an arousal reaction. Experientia 1971;27:785–786.
53. Mathur R, Douglas NJ. Frequency of EEG arousals from nocturnal sleep in normal subjects. Sleep 1995;18:330–333.
54. Boselli M, Parrino L, Smerieri A, Terzano MG. Effect of age on EEG arousals in normal sleep. Sleep 1998;21: 351–357.
55. Kato T, Montplaisir JY, Guitard F, Sessle BJ, Lund JP, Lavigne GJ. Evidence that experimentally induced sleep bruxism is a consequence of transient arousal. J Dent Res 2003;82:284–288.
56. Thorpy MJ for Diagnostic Classification Steering Committee. International Classification of Sleep Disorders: Diagnostic and Coding Manual. Rochester, MN: American Sleep Disorders Association and Allen Press, 1990.
57. Dettmar DM, Shaw RM, Tilley AJ. Tooth wear and bruxism: a sleep laboratory investigation. Aust Dent J 1987;32: 421–426.
58. Pierce C, Close J, Krause A. Relation between wear faceting and EMG-measured bruxing activity. J Dent Res 1996;75:1588.

Chapter 3

# Sleep Physiology and Bruxism

*José T. T. de Siqueira, Teresa Cristina Barros Schütz, Monica Andersen, and Sergio Tufik*

## Introduction

From time immemorial, teeth grinding during sleep, as common as it is, has been the subject of popular imagination. Only in recent decades, however, has this disorder been examined scientifically, and despite numerous studies on the subject, doubts as to its pathophysiological and clinical nature still linger.

Fortunately, studies in the fields of sleep medicine and sleep biology have yielded a body of literature that has improved the comprehension of sleep and its disturbances, its importance in the body's homeostasis,[1] as well as how sleep is associated with the curious act of teeth grinding. From the investigation of dental occlusion, researchers went on to examine orofacial movements such as mastication, which led to pinpointing the role of the central nervous system (CNS) in the rhythmic activity of mastication muscles and sleep bruxism.[2,3]

Clinically, bruxism causes concern in parents, patients, and dentists alike as this is a disorder that causes complications that directly affect the masticatory system. Epidemiologic studies show that some sleep disturbances – such as obstructive sleep apnea, snoring, and leg movements – are risk factors for bruxism.[4] Also, there is the possibility that bruxism is a manifestation of either a neurologic or psychiatric condition, or an effect of medication or drugs,[5] creating a context in which precise diagnosis is required once the risk factors have been singled out. As a result, clinicians are increasingly sought for the treatment of oral problems associated with sleep disorders.[6] That is when such professionals face yet another challenge, which is to understand the pathophysiology of bruxism in the context of the physiology of sleep.[7] Therefore, it is of utmost importance to know how a sleep laboratory conducts research and what parameters are used in the assessment of a polysomnograph (PSG) that includes the monitoring of mastication muscles.

## Basic Facts of Sleep Physiology and Pathophysiology

Sleep differs from other states of consciousness in that it is fully reversible, a state that has evoked fascination and interest – making it the subject of folklore and tradition, as ancient documents can attest. Sleep accounts for nearly one-third of our lives and is essential for the maintenance of our health and indispensable for the soundness of our minds and emotions. Its influence can clearly be noted after a single bad night of sleep. The daily amount of sleep falls as one becomes older and continues to fall with advanced age. Babies sleep for 16 hours, adults for 8 hours, and the elderly for even less. It is interesting to note that it is at advanced ages that sleep resumes its polyphasic patterns, as observed in newborns.

The concept of sleep held at the beginning of the 20th century – as being passive and uniform – was reformulated from 1929 after the discovery of human electroscillograms by Berger. The oscillations he observed were cortex potentials and were dubbed electroencephalograms (EEG: a specific name for the recordings made by means of electrodes located over the scalp); and then, in 1937, Loomis and co-workers[8,9] described interactive oscillations of the human EEG recorded over periods of several hours. They described the phases of sleep, from the most superficial to the deepest stages that were later called synchronized sleep or "non-REM". In 1953, Aserinsky and Kleitman[10] described the cyclic occurrence of fast ocular movements during sleep and associated them with increased frequency of cortical activity, similar to what happened in the awake state despite the presence of muscle atonia (the reason why it was called desynchronized sleep). But it was in 1957 that Dement and Kleitman[11] demonstrated that ocular activity took place simultaneously with the desynchronized phase of sleep and was associated with the content of dreams in humans – and so they called it "rapid eye movement" (REM) sleep. The technique to assess sleep was first described in 1968 by Rechtschaffen and Kales,[12] based on the results of the EEG, electro-oculogram (EOG), and electromyogram (EMG). In 2007, the American Academy of Sleep Medicine published a manual for the scoring of sleep and associated events to provide more comprehensive standardized specifications and scoring rules for characterizing natural sleep as performed in PSG.[13] Indeed, the parameters became the standard reference in the assessment of sleep for researchers and sleep physicians. Such electroencephalographic standards – as well as the durations of the different sleep stages – change throughout life, as children and adults have different sleep needs (for a review, see, e.g., Tufik[7]).

### *Phases of Sleep*

Sleep has two distinct and alternating phases: sleep without fast ocular movements (non-REM or NREM) and sleep with rapid eye movements (REM). Each possesses its own, distinct neural mechanism, electrophysiologic indicators, and behavior. NREM sleep (synchronized sleep; quiet, slow sleep; or slow-wave sleep) is so called because its electroencephalographic characteristics show an inhibitory–excitory electrical rhythm potential that is generated by thalamic and cortical neurons that form high-amplitude, low-voltage synchronized waves, or slow delta waves.[14] NREM sleep can be observed distributed in the first half of the night especially. NREM sleep includes three stages: N1, N2, and N3.[13] During REM sleep, neurons in the brain stem, located in the pontine tegmentum and known as REM sleep-on cells, are particularly active.[14] At present, sleep is considered an active and complex state and the alternating REM–NREM constitutes the architecture of sleep.[15]

### *Sleep: From Newborn to Old Age*

Newborns may sleep from 16 to 20 hours a day, alternating sleep and awake in cycles of 3–4 hours in what is called "polyphasic sleep". A newborn's EEG is less organized than an adult's; 50% of the total sleep time is REM sleep, evidence that this phase is critical in the initial development of the brain. Between the ages of 3 and 4 years, children spend about 3–4 hours in REM sleep, 3 hours in deep NREM, and fewer than 5 hours in light NREM sleep each night.

The consolidation of nocturnal sleep occurs at around 3 months of age (but with significant individual variations) and with the presence of at least two daytime sleep episodes, one in the morning and one in the afternoon. These disappear in adulthood. When the child reaches prepuberty at close to 10 years of age (with individual variations), the amount of REM sleep falls by approximately 2 hours per night, similar to that of a healthy adult.[16] The recommended polysomnographic parameters for children and adolescents from 1 to 15 years of age are the following:[17] stage N1 4.1% (±4.1%); stage N2 48.9% (±9.7%); stage N3 25.2% (±9.1%); REM sleep 17.4% (±5.7%); and awakening rate 5.3% (±3.5%). Obstructive sleep apnea of up to 1 episode per hour of sleep, central apnea index 0.9, basal saturation of oxyhemoglobin >92%, and maximum desaturation 89% are the standards expected for children.[17]

The amount of deep NREM sleep falls during adolescence, at between 11 and 17 years of age. However, the need for total sleep time increases, indicating that puberty is associated with a higher need for sleep due to behavioral alterations that include an altered sleep–wake cycle. Adolescents go to bed and wake up later than pre-pubertal youngsters.[18–21] This pattern of behavior has been attributed to an altered psychosocial environment and, more recently, to the circadian modifications during puberty. Also, adolescents have delayed secretion of melatonin when compared to children in a more precocious stage of development.[18,22,23] Polysomnographically, in mature adolescents, an increase in stage N2 and reduction in stage N3 is observed when compared to pre-pubertal adolescents or children.[24–26]

Mature adolescents may present a decrease in sensibility to extended periods of wakefulness and experience less pressure to go to bed than pre-pubertal adolescents and children.[27] But after 14 to 18 hours of vigil, sleep latency becomes significantly lower in mature adolescents compared to pre-pubertal individuals, regardless of the circadian cycle.[25] In contrast, the physiologic mechanisms involved in the decrease of sensibility to sleep loss during puberty are not completely known and it is believed that they may be associated with accelerated changes in brain development occurring during adolescence.[28] A recent study proposes that the high tolerance to prolonged awake periods observed in mature adolescents may be in preparation for the adult lifestyle, and for the shortening of sleep periods that is common in adults.[29]

Adults aged between 20 and 30 years have relatively stable sleep and normally spend 25% of the time in stage N3. The total sleep time lasts on average 7.5 hours per night, of which about 75% accounts for deep NREM sleep and 25% for REM sleep.

Sleep patterns begin to change at 40–45 years of age in men and at 50–55 years in women. There is reduction of quality of sleep as age advances, be it subjective or objective. Epidemiologic studies show that women report more sleep complaints than men at all ages, including adulthood and old age.[30–32] After middle age, the amount of deep NREM sleep gradually reduces. Indeed, adults between 50 and 60 years may spend only 10% or less of the total sleep time in NREM stages of sleep. As one becomes older, there is an increase in the number of awakenings during sleep. Most individuals over 65 have long awakenings that last close to 30 minutes, and they tend to remain awake in bed for 15–20% of the time. Elderly individuals over 70 sleep under 7 hours each night, and most of their sleep is superficial and often interrupted.

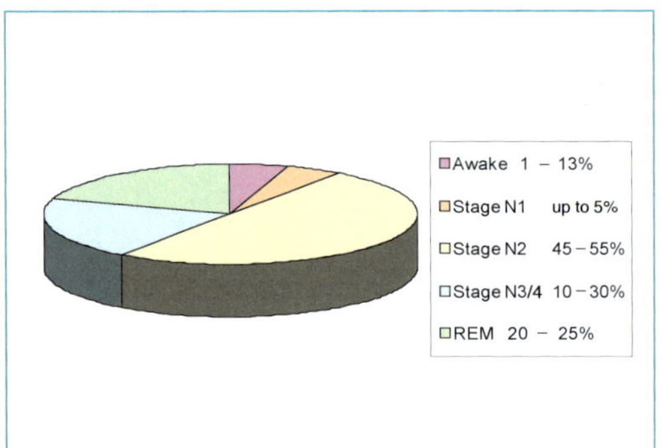


Fig 3-1 The awake state represents 1–13% of the total sleep time and takes place prior to the onset of sleep, and in the brief awakenings that number between 5 and 15 episodes per hour that generally occur in stage shifts. Awakenings are accompanied by subtle body movements and in the morning arousal.

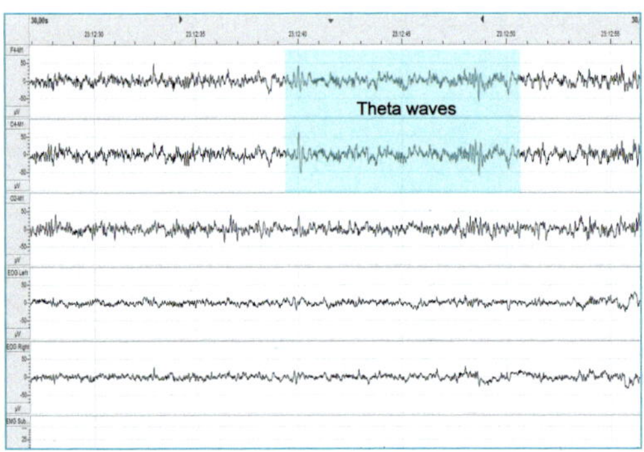


Fig 3-2 Stage N1 of the NREM sleep represents the transition between wakefulness and sleep, characterized by the theta wave (4–7 Hz).

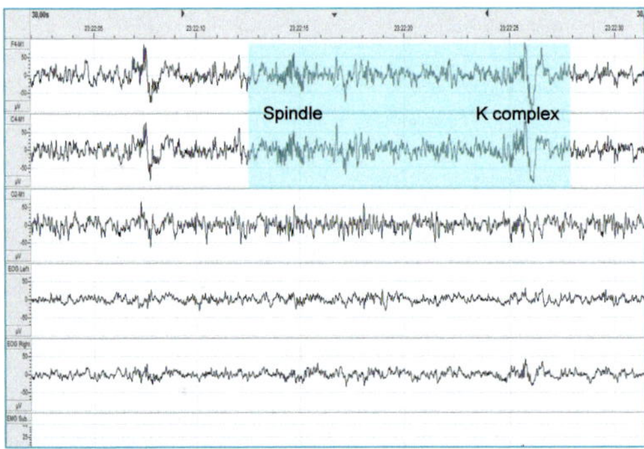


Fig 3-3 Stage N2 of the NREM sleep. K-complex waves can be observed, which are biphasic waves of high amplitude, with a duration of 0.5 seconds, and with an acute negative phase and a slower positive phase.

## Sleep Architecture

It is in the awake state that the countless number of human activities occur. In PSG recordings, wakefulness is part of the sleep architecture, and is one of the stages of the hypnogram (for a review, see Pinto and Silva[33]). Wakefulness represents 1–13% of the total sleep time and takes place prior to the onset of sleep (Fig 3-1). Beta waves are observed in the attentive awake state when an individual carries out tasks. When a person is relaxed and with eyes closed, wakefulness becomes characterized by occipital alpha waves (waves at 8 to 13 Hz, whose amplitude is greater in the occipital portion of the skull). Such waves occur spontaneously as one closes the eyes.

### *NREM Sleep*

Stage N1 (Fig 3-2) represents the transition from wakefulness to sleep. During this stage, 50% of individuals state they are conscious and are able to repeat actions that occur in their surroundings. The appearance of low-voltage and -frequency (4–7 Hz) theta waves is characteristic of stage N1. Eye movements are slow and intermittent, and the EMG features reduction of muscular tone. Stage N1 may occupy up to 5% of the total sleep time. There is a gradual increase of voltage in the EEG as the individual progresses from stage N1 to the following stages. Stage N2 is characterized by the presence of sleep spindles (sigma waves that have high amplitude and frequency at 12–14 Hz and lasting at least 0.5 seconds, especially in the central region of the skull), and of K complexes, which are biphasic waves of high amplitude with a duration of 0.5 seconds, and with an acute negative phase and a slower positive phase (Fig 3-3). Synchrony of electrical activity within the brain occurs in this phase, which reflects a decrease in the level of activity of cortical neurons in addition to a nearly complete cessation of eye movements. Stage N2 may last 5–15 minutes and occurs through the night, occupying 45–55% of the total sleep time.

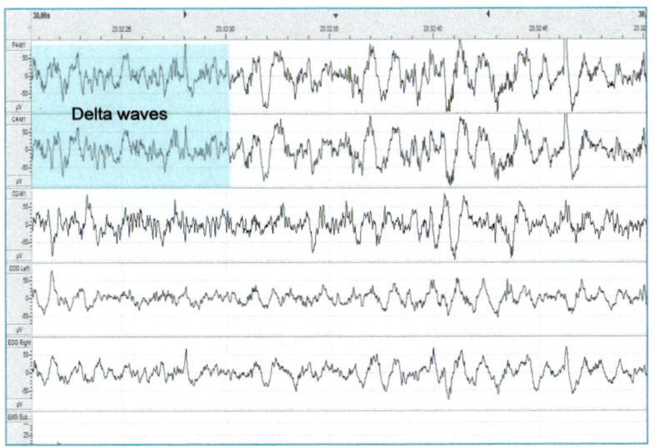


Fig 3-4 Stage N3 of the NREM sleep is characterized by delta waves of high amplitude (over 75 μV) and low frequency (1–2 Hz), which constitute at least 20% of the EEG recording.

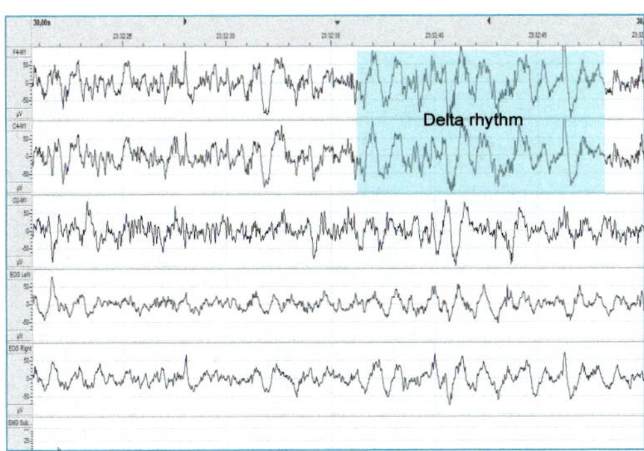


Fig 3-5 Stage N3 of the NREM sleep. We observed a high incidence of delta waves related to the deep sleep.

Sleep stage N3 (Figs 3-4 and 3-5) is characterized by delta waves of high amplitude (over 75 μV) and low frequency (1– 2 Hz), which constitute at least 20% of the EEG recording as depicted in Figures 3-4 and 3-5. In this stage, eye movements are rare and muscular tone reduces progressively. Stage N3 is the most profound sleep, is commonly called "slow-wave sleep", and takes up 10–30% of the total sleep time. NREM sleep consists of stages 1–4, and is concentrated in the first half of the night.

## *REM Sleep*

The EEG of REM sleep shows desynchronized cortical activity resulting from activation of the mesencephalic reticular formation, and features theta waves with low voltage and mixed frequency. At some point in the recording these waves form the saw tooth waves from the frontal and central region (Fig 3-6). The presence of these waves helps in the reconnaissance of REM sleep. Thus, the REM sleep is similar to the waking state, because, despite being a state of deep sleep, it is similar to the waking EEG, but with the absence of muscle tone. For instance, individuals present loss of tone in the skeletal muscles of the limbs, lips, tongue, head, as well as eardrum muscles, but eye oscillations remain unaltered.

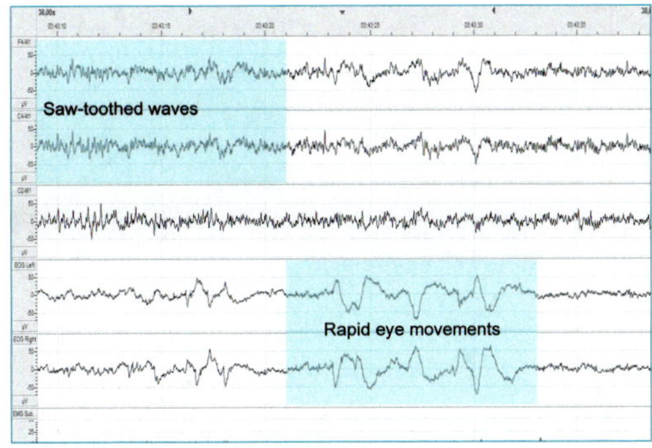


Fig 3-6 REM sleep. In this phase, the theta waves in some moments of recording form the sawtooth waves from the frontal and central region. Rapid eye movements characterize this sleep stage.

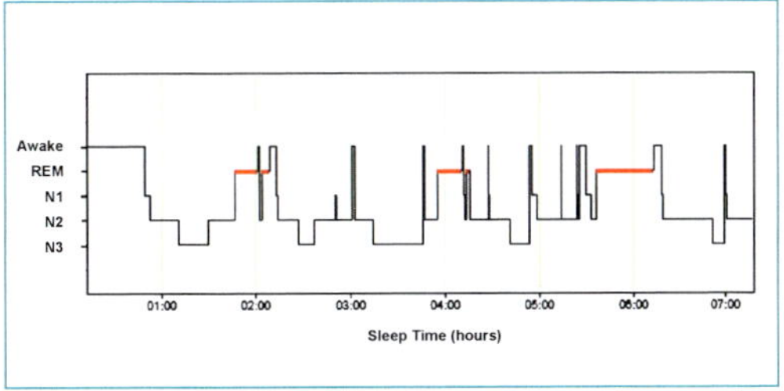


Fig 3-7 The general sleep architecture can be observed in this hypnogram, wherein an overview of the sleep period can be appreciated. The NREM sleep is mainly observed distributed in the first half of the night.

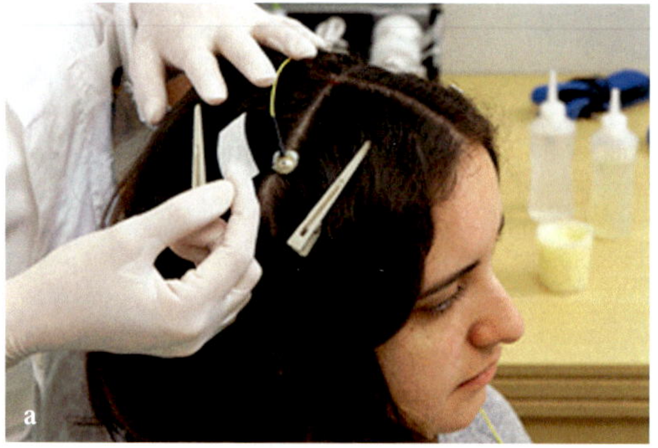

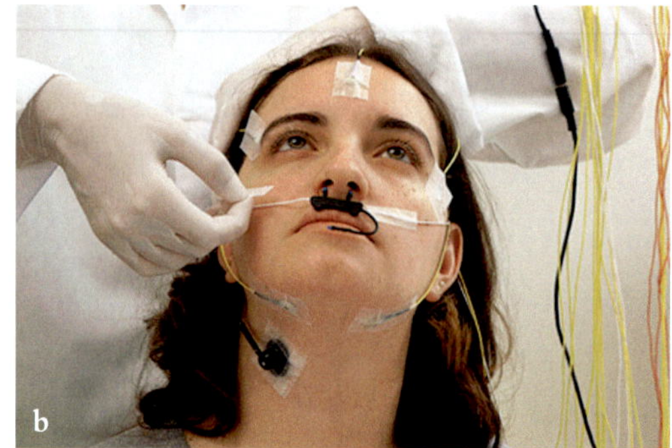

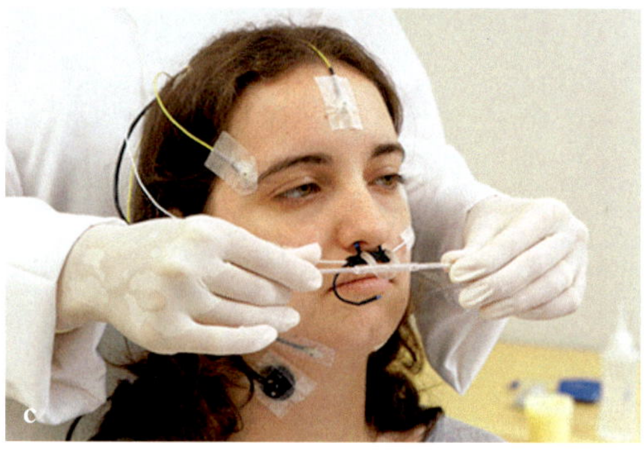

Fig 3-8 **(a–c)** A patient is prepared for the recording in accordance with the technique described by Rechtschaffen and Kales in 1968.

The presence of dreams is the main characteristic of REM sleep and rapid eye movements occur at irregular intervals; this pattern of sleep corresponds to 20–25% of the total sleep time.

REM sleep presents distinct characteristics with *phasic events* (rapid eye movements, muscular or distal myoclonal twitching, fast sudden movement of the limbs and lips, and ponto-geniculo-occipital waves) and *tonic events* (loss of skeletal muscular tone, desynchronized cortical EEG, and cardiorespiratory fluctuations). REM sleep is concentrated in the second half of the night, especially in the last third of the period (Fig 3-7). During the sleeping period, 4–6 cycles normally take place, each lasting 90–100 minutes, and each of those cycles is composed of NREM and REM sleep phases. Upon falling asleep we shift to stages N1, N2, and N3, and subsequently return to stage N2 prior to the first episode of REM sleep, as depicted in Figure 3-7. The period between the onset of sleep until the end of the first REM stage constitutes a sleep cycle.

The methodology and interpretation of the different EEG patterns was established in 2007 by the American Academy of Sleep Medicine[13] and the chronological sequence of the stages was called "sleep architecture". The representation of the sleep architecture of an entire night is done through hypnograms (Fig 3-7).

Sleep prepares us to be in an effective state of wakefulness. Both NREM and REM are essential for a healthy life, but the precise function of each of these states is not yet elucidated. It is assumed that NREM is associated with the release of hormones, while the increase in brain blood flow and memory consolidation seems to involve REM sleep. The fact is that the total period of sleep should be enough for such needs.

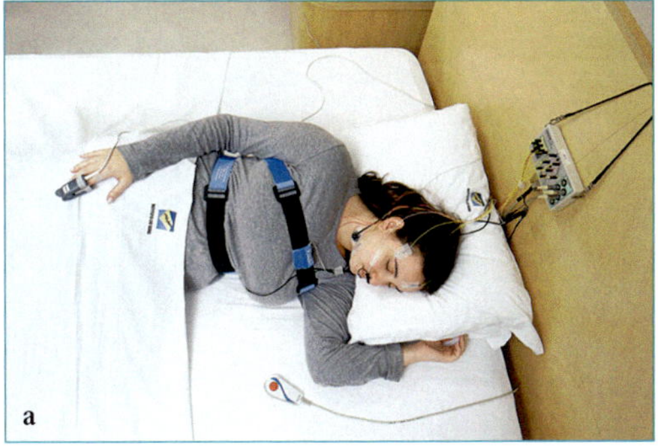

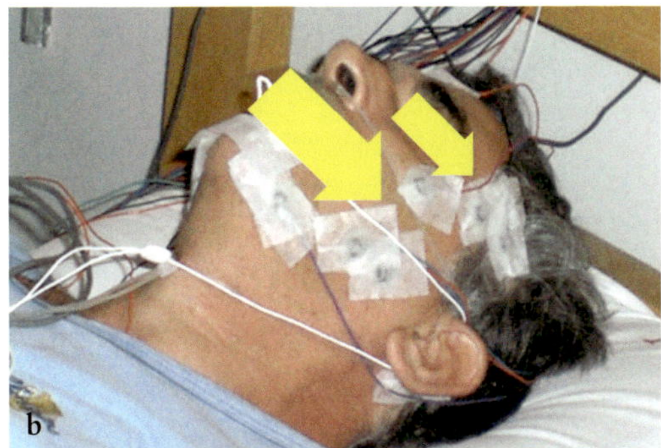

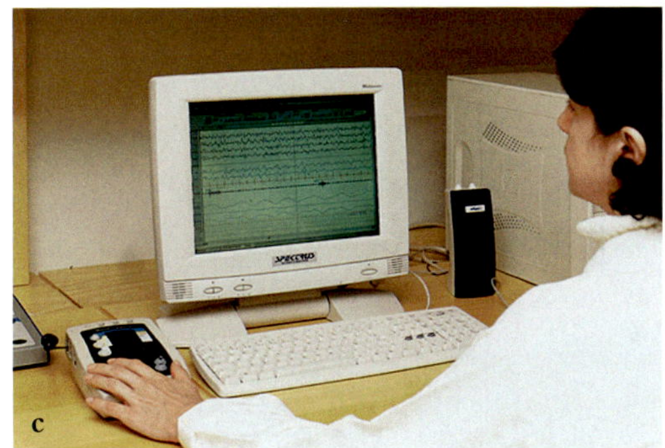

Fig 3-9 A patient ready to make a PSG. **(a)** Note the placement of electrodes to register the general characteristics of sleep. **(b)** The patient has electrodes over masticatory muscles, masseter and temporal (arrows). **(c)** The patient is monitored throughout the night.

## The Sleep Laboratory

A PSG recording should be performed in a dark, sound-attenuated, and temperature-controlled room,[12] and for the purpose of research it is recommended that two consecutive nights in a sleep laboratory be recorded.[34] The first night is used for adaptation to the environment and to allow time to rule out other sleep disorders, whereas the second is used to collect the data. The patient is prepared for the recording (Fig 3-8) in accordance with the technique previously described[13] and is monitored throughout the night, as depicted in Figure 3-9.

A PSG recording includes EEG derivations, bilateral EOG, EMG of chin and anterior tibialis muscles, electrocardiogram (ECG), airflow parameters, respiratory effort of chest and abdomen, oxygen saturation, and body position. Additional EMG of bilateral masseter electrodes may be placed at the discretion of the investigator or clinician.[13]

Prior to the sleep recordings, each patient performs a series of tasks to allow signal recognition and calibration of the EMG: swallowing, coughing, and maximum voluntary contraction.

Assessment of the PSG is done directly from the computer screen and readings are done in 30-second pages, called "epochs". Data can be stored and printed for later use.

## Understanding Bruxism in a PSG

As described by Sjöholm and colleagues,[35] the rhythmic masticatory muscles activity (RMMA) is monitored by means of EMG of the masseter and/or of the temporal muscles. The former is more commonly used for the purpose of investigation of sleep. RMMA may occur in up to 60% of individuals who have no history of bruxism, and in those who do RMMA is three times more frequent than in individuals with no history of tooth-grinding

*Table 3-1*

**International Classification of Sleep Disorders, 2005.**

| | | |
|---|---|---|
| A | The patient reports, or is aware of, tooth-grinding sounds or tooth clenching during sleep. | |
| B | One or more of the following is present: | |
| | (i) | abnormal wear of the teeth |
| | (ii) | jaw discomfort, fatigue, or pain and jaw lock upon awakening |
| | (iii) | masseter muscle hypertrophy upon voluntary forceful clenching. |
| C | The jaw muscle activity is not better explained by another current sleep disorder, medical or neurological sleep medication use, or substance use disorder. | |

sounds.[36,37] At present, diagnosis of sleep bruxism (SB) is made when certain requisites are met, namely intensity, frequency, and type of mandible movement that occurred during sleep and that were duly recorded in a PSG.[38,39] It is known that SB does not occur evenly, and oscillations in intensity and frequency can reach 20% in 30 sleep nights of a given individual[40] and up to 25% in groups of patients who have a history of SB and who have been observed for several years.[38,39] Thus, SB varies in frequency and intensity and may be classified as light, moderate, or severe according to the number of nights SB occurs throughout a week.[39] EMG recordings of RMMA may be carried out by means of portable devices where the person regularly sleeps or, better, at a sleep lab where there are the means to assess a host of other sleep parameters along with orofacial movements.[41–43]

The most meaningful and pioneering work on PSG and bruxism was conducted in the 1960s and 1970s. Reding and colleagues[44] assessed the sleep of 40 volunteers; in this study the sound of teeth grinding, whether or not associated with RMMA, was adopted as the criterion for bruxism. The predominance of stage N2 was observed in bruxism spells, despite the fact these occurred in all sleep phases, and episodes were accompanied by an increase in heart rate. No alteration in the sleep architecture was observed. Satoh and Harada[45] compared bruxism with the H-reflex that occurs in the calf of the leg, in the gastrocnemius muscle, and observed that such reflex was abolished during the bruxism episodes. This led those researchers to conclude that activity within the spinal motor system during bruxism was similar to that during body movement. Later, the same researchers assessed the sleep of 15 individuals with a history of bruxism and observed that the episodes of bruxism occurred mainly during rapid-wave sleep, often preceded by complex K-waves and followed by alpha waves.[46] Also, the episodes preceded sympathetic activity (vasoconstriction at the fingertips and tachycardia), and the episodes could be caused by awakening stimuli. Finally, they were similar to spontaneous episodes. The researchers concluded that bruxism is triggered by sleep becoming abruptly superficial, which seemed like part of an awakening reaction. Several other studies have helped to consolidate this information.[47–51]

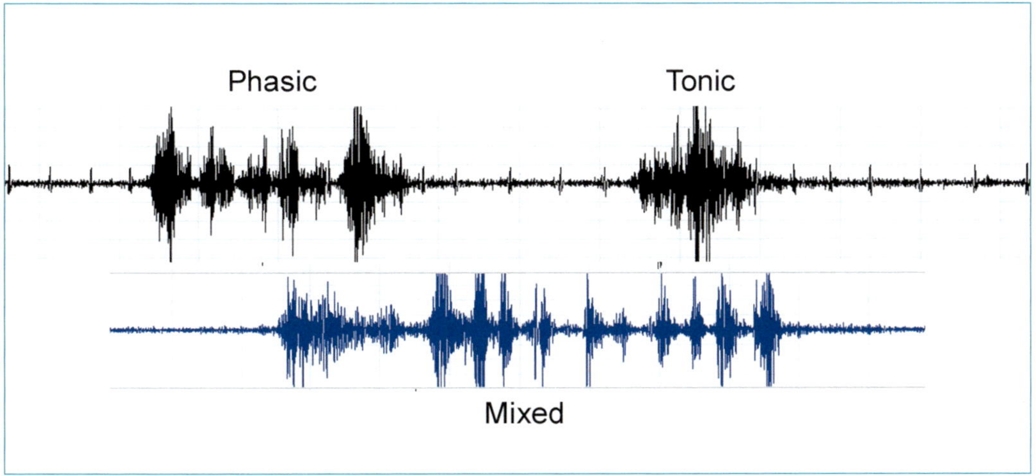


Fig 3-10 Bruxism episodes. A phasic episode corresponds to at least three EMG bursts of 0.25–2.0 seconds, separated by two interburst intervals. A tonic episode corresponds to an EMG burst lasting over 2.0 seconds.

Recently, Lavigne and colleagues have proposed a new hypothesis for RMMA/SB.[3] They have proposed that an episodic and transitory activation of the ascending awakening system serves to activate the mastication muscles due to a possible excitation or suppression of an inhibitory factor that may exist in the motor neurons of the trigemini or in the interneurons of the CPG (central pattern generator) within the trigeminal reticular formation.

Other orofacial movement during sleep (e.g., mandibular myoclonus) may occur in 10% of the patients who have SB[1] and can be distinguished from SB provided the recommended criteria are adopted[38] – considering respiratory disturbances, abnormal swallowing, night terrors, confused awakenings, daily dyskinesia, and epilepsy, among others.[52,53] At any rate, SB is established only when RMMA meets certain previously established criteria,[38] as we shall see below.

### *Sleep Bruxism Criteria*

According to the International Classification of Sleep Disorders,[1] the criteria for the diagnosis of SB are as shown in Table 3-1.

The criteria for assessment of RMMA and sleep bruxism that are currently used in research were validated by Lavigne and co-workers[38,39] from pre-existing data in the literature.[44,54–56] These criteria presented 72% sensitivity and 94% specificity and require validation in large population samples.[38,39] According to Lavigne and co-workers, RMMA may be done in the masseter muscle as well as in the temporal muscle, but it is the former that is most used for this purpose (see Fig 3-9). An infrared camera and microphone are used to monitor orofacial movement and sounds produced by teeth grinding. During the calibration of the recording the patient is asked to strongly press the maxilla to maximum voluntary contraction (MVC). The recording allows for the detection of the amplitude of the EMG potential. The criteria for assessment of RMMA and SB are:

- The amplitude of the EMG for the recording of the RMMA is defined as being 10–20% of the MVC.
- Bruxism episodes may be of three kinds: phasic (grinding), tonic (clenching), or mixed (both). A phasic episode corresponds to at least three EMG bursts of 0.25–2.0 seconds

duration, separated by two interburst intervals, while a tonic episode corresponds to an EMG burst lasting over 2.0 seconds (Fig 3-10).
- In order to confirm moderate and severe sleep bruxism, one must present:[38,39] (a) more than 4 episodes per hour; (b) more than 6 bursts per episode and/or 25 bursts per hour of sleep; and (c) at least 2 episodes with dental noise during sleep.
- Patients with low sleep bruxism (2–4 episodes/h) have an increased risk of reporting facial pain or headache on awakening.[57]

Quite similar to the criteria described by Lavigne and colleagues,[38,39] the American Academy of Sleep Medicine Manual[13] recommended other rules for scoring bruxism in the PSG recording (note: these criteria require further validation because the use of the chin to represent bruxism episodes remains controversial):

1) Bruxism may consist of brief (phasic) or sustained (tonic) elevations of chin EMG activity that are at least twice the amplitude of background EMG.
2) Brief elevations of chin EMG activity are scored as bruxism if they are 0.25–2 seconds in duration and if at least three such elevations occur in a regular sequence.
3) Sustained elevations of chin EMG activity are scored as bruxism if the duration is more than 2 seconds.
4) A period of at least 3 seconds of stable background chin EMG must occur before a new episode of bruxism can be scored.
5) Bruxism can be scored reliably by audio in combination with PSG by a minimum of 2 audible tooth grinding episodes/night of PSG in the absence of epilepsy.

## Conclusion

Sleep bruxism affects a significant portion of the population, but its etiology remains uncertain and so far there is no consensus on treatment. Although its clinical manifestations are well known, they are, ironically, accompanied by conditions of high prevalence in the general population – namely toothache, pain caused by temporomandibular disorders, other forms of orofacial pain, and headache – and therefore require accurate diagnosis. Moreover, its association with other sleep disorders – such as obstructive sleep apnea and restless leg syndrome – is relevant in that these abnormalities are risk factors that affect general health.

Diagnosing sleep bruxism by means of well-defined criteria is essential not only in the determination of its true clinical significance, but also to establish how it affects the associated clinical conditions. Comprehension of such mechanisms will enable the creation of therapeutic strategies for SB specifically, or for the consequences it gives rise to, as both treatments are not necessarily the same.

The clinician, on hearing a complaint from a patient, should be able to make the diagnosis based on scientific data in order to reduce the risk of iatrogenic sequelae and to minimize deterioration in the patient's quality of life.

## Acknowledgment

We are grateful to Dr. Rogério Santos-Silva for his technical comments on a final revision of this text.

## References


1. American Academy of Sleep Medicine. The International Classification of Sleep Disorders. Diagnostic and Coding Manual, ed 2. Westchester, IL: American Academy of Sleep Medicine, 2005.
2. Rugh JD, Barghi N, Drago CJ. Experimental occlusal discrepancies and nocturnal bruxism. J Prosthet Dent 1984;51:548–553.
3. Lavigne GJ, Huynh N, Kato T et al. Genesis of sleep bruxism: motor and autonomic–cardiac interactions. Arch Oral Biol 2007;52:381–384.
4. Ohayon MM, Li KK, Guilleminault C. Risk factors for sleep bruxism in the general population. Chest 2001;119: 53–61.
5. Kato T, Sessle BJ, Lavigne GJ, Rompré PH, Montplaisir JY. Sleep bruxism: an oromotor activity secondary to micro-arousal. J Dent Res 2001;80:1940–1944.
6. Lavigne GL, Lobbezoo F. Sleep disorders and the dental patient: an overview. Oral Surg Oral Med Oral Pathol Oral Radiol Endod 1999; 88:257–272.
7. Tufik S. Medicina e Biologia do Sono. São Paulo: Manoli, 2008.
8. Berger H. On the electroencephalogram of man: third report. Electroencephalogr Clin Neurophysiol 1969a; Suppl 28:95.
9. Berger H. On the electroencephalogram of man: eighth report. Electroencephalogr Clin Neurophysiol 1969b; Suppl 28:209.
10. Aserinsky E, Kleitman N. Regularly occurring periods of eye motility, and concomitant phenomena, during sleep. Science 1953;118:273–274.
11. Dement W, Kleitman N. Cyclic variations in EEG during sleep and their relation to eye movements, body motility, and dreaming. Electroencephalogr Clin Neurophysiol 1957;9:673–690.
12. Rechtschaffen A, Kales A. Manual of Standardized Terminology, Techniques and Scoring System for Sleep Stages of Human Subjects. Los Angeles, CA: Brain Information Service, 1968.
13. Iber C, Ancoli-Israel S, Chesson Jr A, Quan S. The AASM Manual for the Scoring of Sleep and Associated Events: Rules, Terminology and Technical Specifications. Westchester, IL: American Academy of Sleep Medicine, 2007.
14. Steriade M. Basic mechanisms of sleep generation. Neurology 1992;42(7):9–17.
15. Hobson JA. Sleep and dreaming. J Neurosci 1990;10(2): 371–382.
16. Coble PA, Reynolds CF, Kupper DJ, Houck P. Electroencephalographic sleep of healthy children. II: Findings using automated delta and REM sleep measurement methods. Sleep 1987;10:551–562.
17. Uliel S, Tauman R, Greenfeld M, Sivan Y. Normal polysomnographic respiratory values in children and adolescents. Chest 2004;125:872–878.
18. Carskadon MA, Vieira C, Acebo C. Association between puberty and delayed phase preference. Sleep 1993;16: 258–262.
19. Wolfson AR, Carskadon MA. Sleep schedules and daytime functioning in adolescents. Child Dev 1998;69: 875–887.
20. Laberge L, Trembly RE, Vitaro F, Montplaisir J. Development of parassomnias from childhood to early adolescence. Pediatrics 2000;106:67–74.
21. Gau SF, Soong WT. The transition of sleep-wake patterns in early adolescence. Sleep 2003;26:449–454.
22. Carskadon MA, Acebo C, Richardson GS, Tate BA, Seifer R. An approach to studying circadian rhythms of adolescent humans. J Biol Rhythms 1997;12:278–289.
23. Carskadon MA, Acebo C, Jenni OG. Regulation of adolescent sleep: implications for behavior. Ann N Y Acad Sci 2004;1021:276–291.
24. Jenni OG, Carskadon MA. Spectral analysis of the sleep electroencephalogram during adolescence. Sleep 2004; 27:774–783.
25. Jenni OG, Achermann P, Carskadon MA. Homeostatic sleep regulation in adolescents. Sleep 2005;28:1446–1454.
26. Jenni OG, Van Reem E, Carskadon MA. Regional differences of the sleep electroencephalogram in adolescents. J Sleep Res 2005;14:141–147.
27. Taylor DJ, Jenni OG, Acebo C, Carskadon MA. Sleep tendency during extended wakefulness: insights into adolescent sleep regulation and behavior. J Sleep Res 2005;14: 239–244.
28. Spear LP. The adolescent brain and age-related behavioral manifestations. Neurosci Biobehav Rev 2000;24:417–463.
29. Jenni OG, O'Connor BB. Children's sleep: an interplay between culture and biology. Pediatrics 2005;115(Suppl 1): 204–216.
30. Groeger JA, Zijlstra FR, Dijk DJ. Sleep quantity, sleep difficulties and their perceived consequences in a representative sample of some 2000 British adults. J Sleep Res 2004;13:359–371.
31. Ursin R, Bjorvatn B, Holsten F. Sleep duration, subjective sleep need, and sleep habits of 40- to 45-year-olds in the Hordaland Health Study. Sleep 2005;28:1260–1269.
32. Silva A, Andersen ML, De Mello MT et al. Gender differences in polysomnographic findings and sleep complaints in a clinical population. Braz J Med Biol Res 2008; 41:1067–1075.
33. Pinto LR, Silva RS. Polissonografia normal e nos principais distúrbios de sono. In: Tufik S (ed) Medicina e Biologia do Sono. São Paulo: Manoli, 2008:161–180.
34. Thorpy MJ. Parasomnias. In: International Classification of Sleep Disorders: Diagnostic and Coding Manual (ASDA). Rochester: Allen Press, 1990:142–185.

35. Sjöholm TT, Lehtinem I, Helenius H. Masseter muscle activity in diagnosed sleep bruxists compared with non-symptomatic controls. J Sleep Res 1995;4(1):48–55.
36. Gastaut H, Batini C, Broughton R, Fressy J, Tassinari CA. Étude électroencéphalographique des phénomènes épisodiques non épileptiques au cours du sommeil. In: Le sommeil de nuit normal et pathologique. Paris: Masson, 1965.
37. Lavigne GJ, Rompré PH, Poirier HH, Kato T, Montplaisir JY. Rhythmic muscle activity during sleep in humans. J Dent Res 2001;80:443–448.
38. Lavigne GJ, Rompré PH, Montplaisir JY. Sleep bruxism: validity of clinical research diagnostic criteria in a controlled polysomnographic study. J Dent Res 1996;75: 546–552.
39. Lavigne GJ, Rompré PH, Guitard F, Montplaisir JY. Variability in sleep bruxism activity over time. J Sleep Res 2001;10:237–244.
40. Dal'fabbro C, de Siqueira JTT, Tufik S. Long term PSG in a bruxism patient: the role of daily anxiety. Sleep Med 2009;10:813.
41. Rugh JD, SolbergWK. Electromyographic studies of bruxist behavior before and during treatment. J Calif Dent Assoc 1975;3:56–59.
42. Gallo LM, Salis PH, Gross SS, Palla S. Nocturnal masseter EMG activity of healthy subjects in a natural environment. J Dent Res 1999;78:1436–1444.
43. Van Selms MKA, Lobbezoo F, Wicks DJ, Hamburger HL, Naeije M. Craniomandibular pain, oral parafunctions, and psychological stress in a longitudinal case study. J Oral Rehabil 2004;31:738–745.
44. Reding GR, Zepelin H, Robinson JE, Zimmerman SO, Smith VH. Nocturnal teeth-grinding: all-night physicophysiologic studies. J Dent Res 1968;45:1198–1204.
45. Satoh T, Harada Y. Depression of H-reflex during tooth grinding in sleep. Physiol Behav 1972;9(5):893–894.
46. Satoh T, Harada Y. Electrophysiological study of tooth grinding during sleep. Electroencephalogr Clin Neurophysiol 1973;35:267–275.
47. Okura K, Makano M, Bando E et al. Analysis of biological signals during sleep-associated bruxism. J Jpn Soc Stomatognath Funct 1996;3:83–93.
48. Macaluso GM, Guerra P, Di Giovanni G et al. Sleep bruxism is a disorder related to periodic arousals during sleep. J Dent Res 1998;77:565–573.
49. Kato T, Sessle BJ, Lavigne GJ, Rompré PH, Montplaisir JY. Sleep bruxism: an oromotor activity secondary to micro-arousal. J Dent Res 2001;80:1940–1944.
50. Kato T, Montplaisir JY, Guitard F, Sessle BJ, Lund JP, Lavigne GJ. Evidence that experimentally-induced sleep bruxism is a consequence of transient arousal. J Dent Res 2003;82:284–288.
51. Huynh N, Kato T, Rompré PH et al. Sleep bruxism is associated to micro-arousals and an increase in cardiac sympathetic activity. J Sleep Res 2006;3:339–346.
52. Velly-Miguel AM, Montplaisir J, Rompré PH, Lund JP, Lavigne GJ. Bruxism and other orofacial movements during sleep. J Craniomandib Disord 1992;6:71–81.
53. Kato T, Montplaisir JY, Blanchet PJ, Lund JP, Lavigne GJ. Idiopathic myoclonus in the oromandibular region during sleep: a possible source of confusion in sleep bruxism diagnosis. Mov Disord 1999;14(5):865–871.
54. Rugh JD, Harlam J. Nocturnal bruxism and temporomandibular disorders. In: Janckovic J, Tolosa E (eds). Advances in Neurology. New York: Raven Press, 1988: 329–341.
55. Ware JC, Rugh JD. Destructive bruxism: sleep stage relationship. Sleep 1988;11(2):172–181.
56. Okeson JP, Phillips BA, Berry DT et al. Nocturnal bruxing events in healthy geriatric subjects. J Oral Rehabil 1990;17:411–418.
57. Rompré PH, Daily-Landry D, Guitard F, Montplaisir JY, Lavigne GJ. Identification of a sleep bruxism subgroup with a higher risk of pain. J Dent Res 2007;86:837–42.

# Chapter 4

# Etiology of Bruxism

*Frank Lobbezoo, Hans L. Hamburger, and Machiel Naeije*

## Introduction

Bruxism is a stereotyped oral movement disorder that is characterized by daytime and/or sleep-related teeth grinding and/or clenching.[1,2] The disorder has a prevalence in the general adult population of about 10% and is usually regarded as one of the possible causative factors for, *inter alia*, temporomandibular pain and tooth wear in the form of attrition.[3] These possible musculoskeletal and dental consequences of bruxism illustrate the clinical importance of this disorder.

In the past decades, bruxism has been studied extensively, and many research papers and review articles have been published. To illustrate this, a Medline search was performed in September 2006, using the National Library of Medicine's (NLM) Medical Subject Headings (MeSH) Database and PubMed. The search term "Bruxism" [MeSH Terms] OR bruxism [Text Word] yielded 1,910 papers, 215 of which were reviews. When using the truncated search term bruxi*, thereby turning off automatic term mapping and the automatic explosion of MeSH terms, 1,930 papers were found, 219 of them being reviews. A pure MeSH search on this subject (i.e., "bruxism" [MeSH]) resulted in 1,717 papers, including 182 reviews. About 20% of the papers, found with any of these three search strategies, were published during the past five years; the remaining papers appeared between 1966 and 2001. This shows that there is a growing interest in bruxism, illustrated by the scatter plot in Fig 4-1.

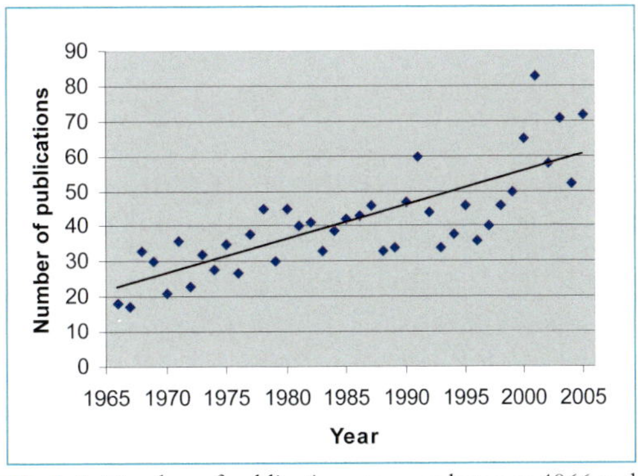


Fig 4-1 Number of publications per year between 1966 and 2005 in which bruxism was used as a MeSH term.

This chapter is based on Lobbezoo and Naeije[13] and Lobbezoo et al.[14]

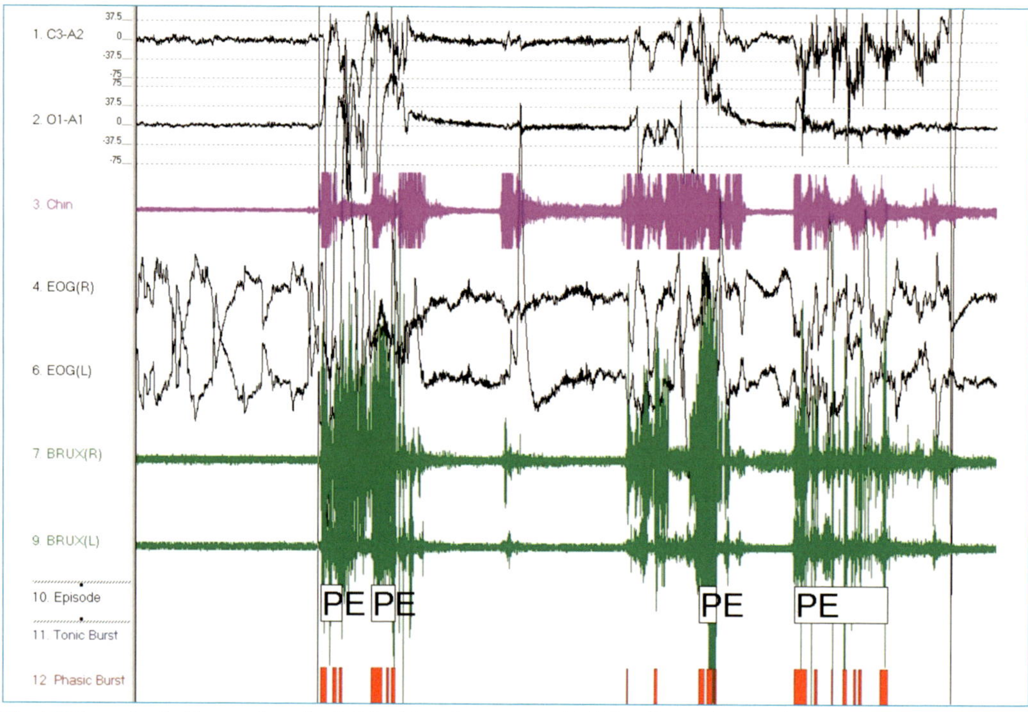


Fig 4-2 Example of a 30-second epoch of a full-night polysomnographic ("sleep") recording. A selection of the 16 channels used is indicated on the left side. Channels 1 and 2 are electroencephalographic signals; channel 3 is a submental electromyographic recording; channels 4 and 6 are the electro-oculographic recordings from the right and left sides; and channels 7 and 9 are the electromyographic signals of both masseter muscles. Below these masseter signals, the results of the automatic sleep bruxism detection is shown, PE indicating the significant presence of so-called phasic episodes (i.e., at least three bursts, repetitive at a frequency of approximately 1 Hz and with burst durations between 0.25 and 2.0 seconds.

Despite this growing interest, bruxism remains difficult to grasp and controversial.[4] For example, there is still no agreement regarding the definition and diagnosis of bruxism.[5] As a consequence, the available articles on the etiology of bruxism are difficult to compare and therefore hard to interpret unequivocally. The interpretation of the literature is further hampered by the fact that the effects of factors such as gender and race on the prevalence of the disorder are not yet clarified.[6] This makes the generalization of certain findings difficult. Moreover, insight into study design has improved considerably during the past decade. For instance, control subjects are frequently absent in previous studies, and regularly the phenomenon of interest, bruxism, was quantified with indirect measures.

Notwithstanding these difficulties, many etiological theories to explain bruxism have been formulated over the years. Although these theories are hard to confirm or refute owing to the controversial character of the disorder, most suggest a multifactorial etiology.[5,7–9] Basically, three groups of etiologic factors can be distinguished: a group of peripheral (morphologic) factors, and two groups of central factors, psychologic and pathophysiologic. Below, these groups will be reviewed and their relative contributions to the etiology of bruxism will be discussed.

Some authors stress the importance of discriminating between sleep-related bruxism and bruxism during wakefulness, because they might have different etiologies.[10–12] In this review, bruxism will be considered as the combination of all parafunctional clenching and grinding activities, exerted both during sleep and while awake, because as yet both phenomena are not or only inadequately distinguished in most related articles. However, most data regarding the etiology of bruxism come from studies of sleep-related bruxism, because this type is better suited for a reliable diagnosis in a scientific research setting owing to the application of full-night, multi-channel sleep recordings (polysomnography; see Lavigne and Manzini[5]). Figure 4-2 shows an example of a polysomnographic recording that was automatically scored for the presence of sleep-related bruxism events.

The purpose of this chapter – a combined and adapted version of the reviews by Lobbezoo and Naeije[13] and Lobbezoo and co-workers[14] – is to review the literature on the etiology of bruxism to try to establish which group of etiologic factors can be considered most implicated in the disorder. Insight into the etiology is also clinically important, because it enables the clinician to choose a treatment that might influence or even eliminate one or more of the factors that perpetuate the disorder.

## Categories

As mentioned above, the factors that may play a role in the etiology of bruxism can be divided into three categories: morphologic, pathophysiologic, and psychosocial. Of the most recent papers (i.e., those that were published during the past 5 years), relatively few deal with morphologic factors (~10%), while only slightly more papers have the role of psychosocial factors in the etiology of bruxism as their main focus (~20%). The vast majority of the selected papers (~70%) deal with possible etiologic factors that can be classified among the pathophysiologic ones. These percentages corroborate the commonly observed trend in bruxism research, away from a main focus on occlusion and towards a more biomedical/ biopsychosocial point of view (see, e.g., the reviews by Kato and co-workers,[15–17] De Laat and Macaluso,[18] Lavigne and co-workers,[19] and Lobbezoo and co-workers[3]). In the following sections, the possible role of morphological (occlusal) factors will be discussed first, followed by that of various psychosocial factors. Finally, several pathophysiologic factors will be described in relation to their purported role in the etiology of bruxism.

## Morphologic Factors

Within the group of morphologic factors, anomalies in dental occlusion and articulation as well as in the (bony) anatomy of the orofacial region can be distinguished. Seen in the historical perspective reviewed below, these factors were formerly considered the most important initiating and perpetuating etiologic factors for bruxism. More recently, the role of occlusal–anatomic factors is believed to be much smaller, if at all present. This shift is illustrated by the fact that the term "occlusal disturbance" is more and more being replaced by the term "occlusal characteristic". A disturbance usually indicates that something needs to be corrected, while a characteristic only suggests that something more or less noteworthy is present without there being a need for any corrections whatsoever. Nowadays, there is growing agreement on the insight that it is not really important how someone's occlusion looks, but it does matter how one "copes" with a certain type of occlusion. It is the dental professional's task to prevent the creation of "occlusal neurotics", which might easily occur when occlusal adjustment procedures are discussed with the patient.[20]

### *Occlusion and Articulation*

A frequently cited study regarding bruxism is the classical one by Ramfjord[10] in which the clinical phenomenon "bruxism" was studied with electromyographic (EMG) techniques. Although Ramfjord also saw a role for "neurotic tensions" in the etiology of bruxism, he held certain occlusal characteristics mainly responsible for the initiation of the disorder. Especially discrepancies between retruded contact position and intercuspal position, and also the presence of mediotrusive (balancing-side) contacts during articulation, were thought to be involved in the etiology. Ramfjord reported that occlusal adjustments (grinding procedures) always led to a disappearance of bruxism. The presence or absence of bruxism was determined during a 45–60-minute EMG protocol, during which the patient performed a couple of movement tasks. It is, however, doubtful whether these tasks were indicative of bruxism, because no direct measures of actual parafunctional activities were performed. Ramfjord supported his results with his own (unpublished) observations in rhesus monkeys, which only stopped their bruxism activities when they completed the elimination of the overfilled part of a restoration in the first molar. Bruxism would thus be an instrument with which an individual tries to eliminate occlusal interferences. The interferences were believed to cause a reflexly mediated excitation of the jaw-closing muscles through the stimulation of periodontal mechanoreceptors.

Although in Ramfjord's EMG study no controls were included, and although the use of indirect measures for bruxism renders the results impossible to interpret according to more recent insights into study design, the conclusions of this study have had a major impact on clinical dentistry for many decades. There is still research going on into the role of occlusion and articulation in the etiology of bruxism (see below), although these factors are already being put aside by the outcomes of better controlled studies. For example, Rugh and co-workers[21] studied the influences of artificial occlusal interferences, incorporated in crowns in the molar region, on masticatory muscle activity (MMA) during sleep. MMA was quantified by means of EMG recordings from the sleeping patient. In contrast with the findings of Ramfjord, artificial interferences caused a significant decrease in sleep-related MMA in 90% of the cases. This result sheds some serious doubt on the role of occlusion in the etiology of bruxism. The other side of the medal is that artificial interferences cannot directly be compared with natural ones, the latter possibly being the effect of bruxism rather than its cause.

In better controlled studies, the elimination of interferences in occlusion and articulation was shown to have no influence on bruxism activities.[22,23] Moreover, not every bruxer has occlusal interferences and not every person with such interferences is a bruxer.[24] Nevertheless, several occlusal factors (e.g., large and/or inverse overjets and overbites) are still being suggested in relation to self-reported bruxism in a study with children.[25] Griffin[26] even states that, for effective management of bruxism, the establishment of harmony between maximum intercuspation and centric relation is required. However, most studies on this subject now agree that there is no (or hardly any) relationship between self-reported and/or clinically established bruxism on the one hand and occlusal factors on the other, neither in adult samples[27–29] nor in child samples.[30] Importantly, Manfredini and co-workers[31] state, on the basis of a review of the literature, that there is still a lack of methodologically sound studies to definitively refute the importance of occlusal factors in the etiology of bruxism.

Therefore, the conclusion is justified that even though occlusal schemes are relevant for the distribution of the forces that go with bruxism activities,[12] there is no scientific proof for a role of occlusion and articulation in the etiology of bruxism.[32] Future research on this subject should include more objective techniques to establish the presence or absence of bruxism (e.g., electromyography or polysomnography), using the proper design for studies to cause-and-effect relationships; that is, prospective, longitudinal trials.

### *Orofacial Anatomy*

Two studies have examined the possible relationship between bruxism and the anatomy of the orofacial region. Miller and co-workers[33] found a more pronounced asymmetry in condylar height in bruxers as compared with non-bruxers; Young and co-workers[34] observed larger bizygomatic and cranial widths in bruxers. In neither of these studies, however, was the presence or absence of bruxism confirmed polysomnographically, as assessed by self-report and a clinical examination, and this hampers the interpretation of their results. The absence of a polysomnographic confirmation of the (non-)bruxer status also hampers the interpretation of the study by Menapace and co-workers,[35] although these authors found no differences in the dentofacial morphology between bruxers and non-bruxers. In another study, which primarily focused on tooth wear in relation to the morphology of the craniofacial structures,[36] a more rectangular form of the maxillary dental arch was found in patients with severe dental attrition than in control subjects. In addition, these authors found that patients with severe attrition had a more rectangular facial morphology than controls, in combination with an anteriorly rotated mandible, a small anterior facial height, and a large bimaxillary interincisal angle. Again, unfortunately, the researchers did not use polysomnography to classify their patients.

So far, only one controlled study on the relationship between bruxism and morphologic factors has been performed with the use of polysomnography to confirm or refute the presence of bruxism.[37] In that study, Lobbezoo and co-workers compared 26 occlusal variables and 25 cephalometric variables between bruxers and non-bruxers and found no differences between the groups. As for the interferences in dental occlusion and articulation, we therefore conclude that there is no proof for a role of factors related to the anatomy of the orofacial skeleton in the etiology of bruxism.

## Psychosocial Factors

Rosales and co-workers[38] evoked emotional stress in rats by letting them observe other rats that underwent electrical foot shocks in a neighboring cage. Compared to rats that did not observe the foot-shocked rats, the "observing" rats had high levels of brux-like masseter muscle activity. Although it is unknown whether this brux-like behavior in rats is in any way related to bruxism in man, Slavicek and Sato[39] consider such behavior in experimental animals as an emergency exit during periods of psychic overloading. The findings and suggestions of these animal studies are in line with many observations in humans that suggest a causal relationship between psychosocial factors such as stress on the one hand and bruxism on the other. As mentioned before, Ramfjord[10] saw a role for "neurotic tensions" in the etiology of bruxism. Besides in this classical study, stress and personality have been implicated in the etiology of bruxism for many years. However, the exact contribution of these (and other) psychosocial factors to this etiology remains the subject of debate.

A major problem is the fact that psychosocial factors are difficult to make operational. The combination of such factors with an equivocally defined disorder such as bruxism obviously yields a difficult area of research. Nevertheless, a large number of studies have been performed on possible interactions between psychosocial factors and bruxism, mostly using questionnaires.

### *Questionnaire Studies*

A controlled questionnaire study by Olkinuora[40] demonstrated that bruxers can be considered emotionally out of balance and that they tend to develop more psychosomatic disorders. Their personalities would be characterized by perfectionism and an increased tendency towards anger and aggression. These findings were later confirmed by Kampe and co-workers,[41] who also demonstrated increased anxiety in a group of bruxers. Further, bruxers differ from healthy controls in the presence of increased levels of hostility,[42] as well as in the presence of depression and stress sensitivity.[27,31] The use of a specific questionnaire for the amount of psychologic disturbance, the Minnesota Multiphasic Personality Inventory (MMPI), however, indicated that bruxers do not differ from non-bruxers within a population of patients with facial pain.[43]

Interestingly, an increased amount of aggression and somatization can already be found in bruxing 5- and 6-year-olds.[44] Bruxing children are apparently more anxious than non-bruxers,[45] while 50-year-old bruxers more frequently report, *inter alia*, being single and having a higher educational level.[46]

A series of papers about the presence of bruxism and psychosocial factors among the employees of the Finnish Broadcasting Company describes that self-reports of bruxism may reveal, *inter alia*, ongoing stress in normal work life[47] and dissatisfaction with one's work shift schedule.[48] Therefore, Ahlberg and co-workers[49] state that factors such as perceived stress should be taken into account when treating bruxism-related temporomandibular pain. A multinational, large-scale population study of sleep bruxism revealed "highly stressful life" as a significant risk factor.[50] Likewise, in a longitudinal case study by van Selms and co-workers,[51] it was demonstrated that daytime clenching could significantly be explained by experienced stress.

### *Electromyography and Polysomnography*

Only rarely, electromyography or polysomnography has been used in study of the role of psychosocial factors in the etiology of bruxism. A unique "electromyography case" was described by Rugh and Robbins.[52] During a 6-month period, they continuously recorded the masticatory electromyographic activity of a young woman. In times of increased stress due to, for example, exams and fights with her partner, she developed an increase in her sleep-related masticatory muscle activity. Although interesting, it is still a case, and this relationship is less obvious in groups of bruxers (see below).

An important study on the possible relationship between stress and bruxism is that by Pierce and co-workers.[53] These authors investigated in 100 bruxers the amount of self-reported stress in relation to electromyographically recorded bruxism during the night before the stress report (anticipatory stress) and the night following the report (experienced stress). A total of 15 nights was recorded. For both anticipatory stress and experienced stress, significant (positive) correlations with bruxism were found in eight individuals only. For the entire sample, no association between stress and bruxism could be demonstrated. Also, Watanabe and co-workers[54] and van Selms and co-workers[51] failed to demonstrate a relationship between experienced and anticipated stress on the one hand and sleep-related bruxism on the other. Similarly, Goulet and co-workers[55] found only a weak correlation between self-reported stress and bruxism. Finally, in a controlled polysomnographic study of vigilance and reaction time, an increased level of anxiety was found in sleep bruxers.[56] Anxiety was the only psychosocial outcome variable to reach statistical significance in this study.

Taken the findings of all these studies together, the body of evidence for a possible causal relationship between bruxism and various psychosocial factors is growing, though not yet conclusive. It appears that this relationship differs between individuals and is probably smaller than previously assumed. Clearly, there is a need for more, well-designed, controlled studies on this subject, in which the *susceptibility* of an individual to psychosocial factors should be taken into account.[57]

## Pathophysiologic Factors

More and more, pathophysiologic factors are suggested to be involved in the precipitation of bruxism.[5,9] For example, bruxism has been linked to sleep disturbances, an altered brain chemistry, the use of certain medications and illicit drugs, smoking, the consumption of alcohol, and certain traumas and diseases. In this review, genetic factors are included among the pathophysiologic factors as well.

### *Sleep-related Factors*

Since bruxism often occurs during sleep, the physiology of sleep has been studied extensively in the search for possible causes of the disorder. While Nagels and co-workers[58] report a significantly lower percentage of slow-wave sleep in bruxers than in healthy controls, other authors report macrostructural sleep quality and architecture to be normal in bruxism patients.[54,59] Interestingly, and in contrast to one's expectations, experimental deprivation of slow-wave sleep (this sleep stage being the one during which the least bruxism activity reportedly occurs) did not significantly influence sleep bruxism.[60] In contrast to these macrostructural sleep studies, in a study of sleep microstructure, the sleep of bruxers was found to be characterized by a low incidence of K-complexes and K-alphas in the EEG.[59] This illustrates the importance of including microstructural analyses of sleep in future studies of sleep bruxism.

The so-called "arousal response" has been the subject of many studies (e.g., Wrubble and co-workers[61]). An arousal response is a sudden change in the depth of sleep, during which the individual either arrives in a lighter sleep stage or actually wakes up.[62] Such a response is accompanied by gross body movements (e.g., turning), the appearance of K-complexes in the EEG, an increased heart rate, respiratory changes, peripheral vasoconstrictions, and increased muscle activities. Macaluso and co-workers[63] showed that, in 86% of cases, bruxism episodes were associated with an arousal response. Besides the above-mentioned characteristics of an arousal response, involuntary leg movements were present in association with about 80% of the bruxism episodes. These observations suggest that bruxism is part of an arousal response indeed.

Several recent papers corroborate this suggestion. Kato and co-workers,[64] using a case–control design, found evidence for the suggestion that sleep bruxism is an oromotor manifestation secondary to the microstructural sleep event "micro-arousal" (i.e., an abrupt change in the frequency of cortical EEG that is occasionally associated with motor activity). Similarly, experimentally induced micro-arousals were followed by masticatory motor events in all sleep bruxers in another study by Kato and co-workers.[65] Based on a review of the literature, Kato and co-workers[17] suggest a sequence of events from autonomic (cardiac) changes and brain cortical activation (sleep arousal) to the genesis of sleep-related masticatory muscle activities (bruxism). Interestingly, associations have also been observed between bruxism activities on the one hand and a supine sleeping position, gastroesophageal reflux, episodes of decreased esophageal pH, and swallowing on the other.[66–69] The exact temporal relationship of these factors to bruxism is, as yet, unknown. Future studies should therefore aim at unraveling an all-embracing sequence of events.

In relation to sleep quality and architecture, bruxism and habitual snoring were found to be closely related.[70] Ohayon and co-workers[50] even report an increased risk of reported sleep bruxism in the presence of loud snoring and obstructive sleep apnea syndrome (OSAS). According to Sjoholm and co-workers,[71] these relationships are due to the disturbed sleep of habitual snorers and OSAS patients. However, whether these relationships indicate a true physiologic association is still unknown.

### *Neurochemical Factors*

From a recent series of papers, it can be derived that certain disturbances in the central neurotransmitter system may be involved in the etiology of bruxism.[72–74] From these papers, it can be hypothesized that the balance between the direct and indirect pathways of the basal ganglia, a group of five subcortical nuclei that are involved in the coordination of movements, is disturbed in bruxers. The direct output pathway goes directly from the striatum (one of the five basal ganglia) to the thalamus, from where afferent signals project to the cerebral cortex. The indirect pathway, on the other hand, passes by several other nuclei before the thalamus is reached. If there is an imbalance between both pathways, movement disorders are the result, as in Parkinson's disease.[75] The cause of such an imbalance can be found in the so-called "nigrostriatal projection", a feedback loop within the complex of nuclei that constitute the basal ganglia. The imbalance goes with disturbances in the dopamine-mediated transmission of action potentials. In case of actual nigrostiatal degeneration, Parkinson's disease emerges due to a lack of endogenous dopamine, which can be influenced by pharmacologic therapy (e.g., dopamine precursors, dopamine agonists). In cases of bruxism, there may be an imbalance between both output pathways as well, however without signs of degeneration of the nigrostriatal feedback loop. The acute short-term use of L-dopa (a dopamine precursor of bromocriptine, a D2 receptor agonist[73,74]) and of pergolide (a D1/D2 receptor agonist[76]) inhibits bruxism activity in controlled polysomnographic studies. However, it should be noted that the chronic long-term use of L-dopa by patients with Parkinson's disease is known to cause bruxism.[77]

Similarly, the chronic use of neuroleptics by psychiatric patients gives rise to bruxism during wakefulness.[78] Also, medications that exert an indirect influence on the dopaminergic system, like selective serotonine reuptake inhibitors (SSRIs), may cause bruxism after long-term use.[79–82] This is corroborated by the observation by Amir and co-workers[83] that the beta-blocker propranolol relieved bruxism secondary to antipsychotic drug exposure in two cases. It appears that there may be two types of bruxism: an idiopathic type that can be suppressed by a short-term treatment with dopamine agonists, and an iatrogenic type that is caused by the long-term application of several dopaminergic medicines. The only study so far that complicates this view is a recent one by Lavigne and co-workers,[84] in which bruxism could not be influenced by the acute use of bromocriptine. A possible explanation for this deviant finding may be the fact that bromocriptine was combined with domperidone to suppress peripheral side-effects.

Bruxism was found more frequently in heavy drug addicts.[85] Furthermore, two case reports describe severe bruxism in relation to an addiction to amphetamine, which can be explained through amphetamine's disturbing influence on the dopaminergic system.[86,87] In line with these reports, the amphetamine-like medications that are used in the management of attention deficit hyperactivity disorder (ADHD), such as methylphenidate, have bruxism as a possible side-effect, as shown in a case–control study by Malki and co-workers.[88] Also, the amphetamine-like substance XTC reportedly has excessive tooth wear and bruxism as side-effects.[89,90] Based on a study with rats, Arrue and co-workers[91] give a possible explanation for this side-effect of XTC – the XTC-induced reduction of the jaw-opening reflex.

Nicotine stimulates central dopaminergic activities, which might explain the finding that smokers of cigarettes report bruxism almost two times more than non-smokers[49,92,93] and that smokers show about five times more bruxism episodes per night than non-smokers.[92] According to Ohayon and co-workers,[50] smokers are at higher risk than non-smokers of reporting sleep bruxism, as are drinkers of caffeine and alcohol. Hartmann[57] found that alcohol could lead to bruxism; more than four units per day would then be necessary. This observation also fits well into the view that bruxism is mainly a centrally mediated disorder.

In an attempt to establish a link between the role of occlusal disharmonies and that of alterations in central dopaminergic neurotransmission in experimentally induced bruxism in the rat, Gomez and co-workers[94] and Areso and co-workers[95] found that an acrylic cap on the mandibular central incisors, which was worn for a prolonged period of time, resulted in an imbalance in dopa accumulation between the hemispheres in the basal ganglia. However, Lobbezoo and co-workers[37] were not able to demonstrate a similar phenomenon in humans: no significant correlations were found between morphologic factors and asymmetries in striatal D2 receptor expression in a group of patients with polysomnographically confirmed sleep-related bruxism. It should be stated, however, that it is difficult to compare artificial occlusal interferences in experimentally bruxing rats with "natural" ones in patients with sleep-related bruxism.

In short, all of the above-summarized papers suggest that disturbances in the central dopaminergic system can be linked to bruxism. However, as stated by Winocur and co-workers,[96] more controlled, evidence-based research on this underexplored subject is needed. Further, it should be noted that information about dopaminergic substances in relation to the etiology of bruxism is more readily available than that about other neurochemicals. Thus, although it may seem from the available evidence that mainly the dopaminergic system plays a role in the etiology of bruxism, the lack of focus on other substances in the literature – as well as the presence of many possible interactions between dopamine and other neurochemicals – indicates the need for more research.

### *Heredity*

Many clinicians have the impression that bruxism runs in families. Hublin and co-workers[97] demonstrated in a large-scale questionnaire study with about 4,000 twin pairs that the contribution of heredity to bruxism varies from 39% to 64%. Bruxism was also shown to share a common genetic background with sleep-talking, another parasomnia.[98] Hublin and Kaprio[99] therefore take the stand that genetic effects have a significant role in the origin of bruxism, although the exact mechanisms of transmission are still unknown. Many recent publications thus favor the role of genetics in the etiology of bruxism. In contrast, however, Michalowicz and co-workers[100] concluded, on the basis of a combined questionnaire and clinical study with almost 250 pairs of twins, that there is no such role. Hence, whether or not bruxism is, to a greater or lesser extent, genetically determined still remains unclear.

### *Trauma and Diseases*

As reviewed extensively by Lavigne and Montplaisir in 1995,[101] bruxism has been related to a host of traumas and diseases. Recently, brain damage was described as a possible cause for bruxism in the case series and case report by Millwood and Fiske[102] and Pidcock and co-workers,[103] respectively. Further, certain diseases of mainly neurologic and psychiatric nature have been linked to the etiology of bruxism: basal ganglia infarction,[104] cerebral palsy,[105,106] Down syndrome,[107] epilepsy,[108] Huntington's disease,[109,110] Leigh's disease,[111] meningococcal septicemia,[112] multiple system atrophy,[113] Parkinson's disease,[114] post-traumatic stress disorder,[115,116] and Rett syndrome.[117] With the exception of the study by Rodrigues dos Santos and co-workers on cerebral palsy,[105] which had a case–control design, all other references in the afore-given list of diseases in relation to the etiology of bruxism are case series or case reports. This indicates that a lot of well-designed research still needs to be performed to further evaluate the nature of the relationships that were found between bruxism on the one hand and trauma and diseases on the other.

On the basis of the above overview, it can be concluded that bruxism can be associated with several pathophysiologic factors.

## Conclusion

From epidemiologic studies, we know that rhythmic, sleep-related masticatory muscle activities occur in almost 60% of the adult population.[8] The percentage of people that actually fulfill the cut-off criteria for a sleep bruxism diagnosis is considerably smaller.[118] Hence, rhythmic masticatory muscle activities may be considered normal sleep-related motor behavior. Possibly, one or more of the factors described in the above overview contribute to an increase in frequency, duration, and intensity of these muscle activities, thus enabling a diagnosis of sleep-related bruxism. This hypothesis was formulated in 1995 by Lavigne and Montplaisir and is known as the bruxism generator model.[101]

This model fits nicely with the proposed multifactorial etiology of bruxism. Based on the evidence reviewed above, it seems that bruxism has a multifactorial etiology indeed. There is strong evidence that the role of occlusal characteristics and other morphological factors is small, if at all present. There is convincing evidence, however, that (sleep-related) bruxism is part of an arousal response. Disturbances in the central dopaminergic system are implicated in the etiology of bruxism as well. Further, there is a role for factors such as smoking, alcohol, heredity, trauma, and diseases, while the proposed role of stress and other psychosocial factors is probably smaller than hitherto assumed. In short: bruxism is mainly centrally mediated, not peripherally.

There is still a need for well-designed studies. Evidence-based information about these subjects would be welcomed in the dental clinic, where the causes and consequences of bruxism still frustrate (and fascinate) practitioners.

## References

1. American Academy of Sleep Medicine. International Classification of Sleep Disorders: Diagnostic and Coding Manual. Chicago, IL: AASM, 2001.
2. Okeson JP. Orofacial Pain: Guidelines for Assessment, Diagnosis, and Management. Chicago, IL: Quintessence, 1996.
3. Lobbezoo F, van der Zaag J, Visscher CM, Naeije M. Oral kinesiology: a new postgraduate programme in the Netherlands. J Oral Rehabil 2004;31:192–198.
4. Lavigne GJ, Goulet JP, Zuconni M, Morisson F, Lobbezoo F. Sleep disorders and the dental patient. Oral Surg Oral Med Oral Pathol Oral Radiol Endod 1999;88: 257–272.
5. Lavigne GJ, Manzini C. Bruxism. In: Kryger MH, Roth T, Dement WC (eds). Principles and Practice of Sleep Medicine. Philadelphia, PA: WB Saunders 2000:773–785.
6. Lavigne GJ, Lobbezoo F, Montplaisir JY. The genesis of rhythmic masticatory muscle activity and bruxism during sleep. In: Morimoto T, Matsuya T, Takada K (eds). Brain and Oral Functions. Amsterdam: Elsevier Science, 1995: 249–255.
7. Attanasio R. An overview of bruxism and its management. Dent Clin North Am 1997;41:229–241.
8. Lobbezoo F, Lavigne GJ. Do bruxism and temporomandibular disorders have a cause-and-effect relationship? J Orofac Pain 1997;11:15–23.
9. Bader G, Lavigne GJ. Sleep bruxism: an overview of an oromandibular sleep movement disorder. Sleep Med Rev 2000;4:27–43.
10. Ramfjord SP. Bruxism, a clinical and electromyographic study. J Am Dent Assoc 1961;62:21–44.
11. Glaros A. Incidence of diurnal and nocturnal bruxism. J Prosthet Dent 1981;45:545–549.
12. Rugh JD, Harlan J. Nocturnal bruxism and temporomandibular disorders. Adv Neurol 1988;49:329–341.
13. Lobbezoo F, Naeije M. Bruxism is mainly regulated centrally, not peripherally. J Oral Rehabil 2001;28: 1085–1091.
14. Lobbezoo F, Zaag J van der, Naeije M. Bruxism: its multiple causes and its effects on dental implants. An updated review. J Oral Rehabil 2006;33:293–300.
15. Kato T, Thie NM, Montplaisir JY, Lavigne GJ. Bruxism and orofacial movements during sleep. Dent Clin North Am 2001;45:657–684.
16. Kato T, Dal-Fabbro C, Lavigne GJ. Current knowledge on awake and sleep bruxism: overview. Alpha Omegan 2003;96:24–32.
17. Kato T, Thie NM, Huynh N, Miyawaki S, Lavigne GJ. Topical review: sleep bruxism and the role of peripheral sensory influences. J Orofac Pain 2003;17:191–213.
18. De Laat A, Macaluso GM. Sleep bruxism as a motor disorder. Mov Disord 2002;17(Suppl 2):S67–S69.
19. Lavigne GJ, Kato T, Kolta A, Sessle BJ. Neurobiological mechanisms involved in sleep bruxism. Crit Rev Oral Biol Med 2003;14:30–46.
20. Greene CS, Mohl ND, McNeill C, Clark GT, Truelove EL. Temporomandibular disorders and science: a response to the critics. J Prosthet Dent 1998;80:214–215.
21. Rugh JD, Barghi N, Drago CJ. Experimental occlusal discrepancies and nocturnal bruxism. J Prosthet Dent 1984;51:548–553.

22. Kardachi BJR, Bailey JO, Ash MM. A comparison of biofeedback and occlusal adjustment on bruxism. J Periodontol 1978;49:367.
23. Bailey JO, Rugh JD. Effect of occlusal adjustment on bruxism as monitored by nocturnal EMG recordings. J Dent Res 1980;59:317.
24. Greene CS, Marbach JJ. Epidemiologic studies of mandibular dysfunction: a critical review. J Prosthet Dent 1982;48:184–190.
25. Sari S, Sonmez H. The relationship between occlusal factors and bruxism in permanent and mixed dentition in Turkish children. J Clin Pediatr Dent 2001;25:191–194.
26. Griffin KM. Mandibular adaptive reposturing: the etiology of a common and multifaceted autodestructive syndrome. Gen Dent 2003;51:62–67.
27. Manfredini D, Landi N, Romagnoli M, Bosco M. Psychic and occlusal factors in bruxers. Aust Dent J 2004;49: 84–89.
28. Manfredini D, Landi N, Tognini F, Montagnani G, Bosco M. Occlusal features are not a reliable predictor of bruxism. Minerva Stomatol 2004;53:231–239.
29. Demir A, Uysal T, Guray E, Basciftci FA. The relationship between bruxism and occlusal factors among seven- to 19-year-old Turkish children. Angle Orthod 2004;74: 672–676.
30. Cheng HJ, Chen YQ, Yu CH, Shen YQ. The influence of occlusion on the incidence of bruxism in 779 children in Shanghai. Shanghai Kou Qiang Yi Xue 2004;13:98–99.
31. Manfredini D, Cantini E, Romagnoli M, Bosco M. Prevalence of bruxism in patients with different research diagnostic criteria for temporomandibular disorders (RDC/ TMD) diagnoses. Cranio 2003;21:279–285.
32. Clark GT, Adler RC. A critical evaluation of occlusal therapy: occlusal adjustment procedures. J Am Dent Assoc 1985;110:743–750.
33. Miller VJ, Yoeli Z, Barnea E, Zeltser C. The effect of parafunction on condylar asymmetry in patients with temporomandibular disorders. J Oral Rehabil 1998;25:721–724.
34. Young DV, Rinchuse DJ, Pierce CJ, Zullo T. The craniofacial morphology of bruxers versus nonbruxers. Angle Orthod 1999;69:14–18.
35. Menapace SE, Rinchuse DJ, Zullo T, Pierce CJ, Shnorhokian H. The dentofacial morphology of bruxers versus non-bruxers. Angle Orthod 1994;64:244–245.
36. Waltimo A, Nyström M, Könönen M. Bite force and dentofacial morphology in men with severe dental attrition. Scand J Dent Res 1994;102:92–96.
37. Lobbezoo F, Rompré PH, Soucy JP et al. Lack of associations between occlusal-cephalometric measures, side imbalance in striatal D2 receptor binding, and sleep-related oromotor activities. J Orofac Pain 2001;15:340–346.
38. Rosales VP, Ikeda K, Hizaki K et al. Emotional stress and brux-like activity of the masseter muscle in rats. Eur J Orthod 2002;24:107–117.
39. Slavicek R, Sato S. Bruxism: a function of the masticatory organ to cope with stress. Wien Med Wochenschr 2004; 154:584–589.
40. Olkinuora M. Psychosocial aspects in a series of bruxists compared with a group of non-bruxists. Proc Finn Dent Soc 1972;68:200–208.
41. Kampe T, Edman G, Bader G, Tagdae T, Karlsson S. Personality traits in a group of subjects with long-standing bruxing behaviour. J Oral Rehabil 1997;24:588–593.
42. Molina OF, dos Santos J. Hostility in TMD/bruxism patients and controls: a clinical comparison study and preliminary results. Cranio 2002;20:282–288.
43. Harness DM, Peltier B. Comparison of MMPI scores with self-report of sleep disturbance and bruxism in the facial pain population. Cranio 1992;10:70–74.
44. Kuch EV, Till MJ, Messer LB. Bruxing and non-bruxing children: a comparison of their personality traits. Pediatr Dent 1979;1:182–187.
45. Monaco A, Ciammella NM, Marci MC, Pirro R, Giannoni M. The anxiety in bruxer child: a case–control study. Minerva Stomatol 2002;51:247–250.
46. Johansson A, Unell L, Carlsson G et al. Associations between social and general health factors and symptoms related to temporomandibular disorders and bruxism in a population of 50-year-old subjects. Acta Odontol Scand 2004;62:231–237.
47. Ahlberg J, Rantala M, Savolainen A et al. Reported bruxism and stress experience. Community Dent Oral Epidemiol 2002;30:405–408.
48. Ahlberg K, Ahlberg J, Kononen M et al. Reported bruxism and stress experience in media personnel with or without irregular shift work. Acta Odontol Scand 2003;61: 315–318.
49. Ahlberg J, Savolainen A, Rantala M, Lindholm H, Kononen M. Reported bruxism and biopsychosocial symptoms: a longitudinal study. Community Dent Oral Epidemiol 2004;32:307–311.
50. Ohayon MM, Li KK, Guilleminault C. Risk factors for sleep bruxism in the general population. Chest 2001;119: 53–61.
51. van Selms MKA, Lobbezoo F, Wicks DJ, Hamburger HL, Naeije M. Craniomandibular pain, oral parafunctions, and psychological stress in a longitudinal case study. J Oral Rehabil 2004;31:738–745.
52. Rugh JD, Robbins JW. Oral habit disorders. In: Ingersoll BD (ed). Behavioral Aspects in Dentistry. New York, NY: Appleton-Century-Crofts, 1982:179–202.
53. Pierce CJ, Chrisman K, Bennett ME, Close JM. Stress, anticipatory stress, and psychologic measures related to sleep bruxism. J Orofac Pain 1995;9:51–56.
54. Watanabe T, Ichikawa K, Clark GT. Bruxism levels and daily behaviors: 3 weeks of measurement and correlation. J Orofac Pain 2003;17:65–73.
55. Goulet JP, Lund JP, Montplaisir JY, Lavigne GJ. Daily clenching, nocturnal bruxism, and stress and their association with TMD symptoms. J Orofac Pain 1993;7:120.
56. Major M, Rompré PH, Guitard F et al. A controlled daytime challenge of motor performance and vigilance in sleep bruxers. J Dent Res 1999;78:1754–1762.

57. Hartmann E. Bruxism. In: Kryger MH, Roth T, Dement WC (eds). Principles and Practice of Sleep Medicine. Philadelphia, PA: WB Saunders, 1994:598–601.
58. Nagels G, Okkerse W, Braem M et al. Decreased amount of slow wave sleep in nocturnal bruxism is not improved by dental splint therapy. Acta Neurol Belg 2001;101:152–159.
59. Lavigne GJ, Rompre PH, Guitard F et al. Lower number of K-complexes and K-alphas in sleep bruxism: a controlled quantitative study. Clin Neurophysiol 2002;113: 686–693.
60. Arima T, Svensson P, Rasmussen C et al. The relationship between selective sleep deprivation, nocturnal jaw-muscle activity and pain in healthy men. J Oral Rehabil 2001;28: 140–148.
61. Wrubble MK, Lumley MA, McGlynn FD. Sleep-related bruxism and sleep variables: a critical review. J Craniomandib Disord 1989;3:152–158.
62. Thorpy MJ. Glossary of terms used in sleep disorders medicine. In: Thorpy MJ (ed). Handbook of Sleep Disorders. New York, NY: Marcel Dekker, 1990:779–795.
63. Macaluso GM, Guerra P, Di Giovanni G et al. Sleep bruxism is a disorder related to periodic arousals during sleep. J Dent Res 1998;77:565–573.
64. Kato T, Rompre P, Montplaisir JY, Sessle BJ, Lavigne GJ. Sleep bruxism: an oromotor activity secondary to micro-arousal. J Dent Res 2001;80:1940–1944.
65. Kato T, Montplaisir JY, Guitard F et al. Evidence that experimentally induced sleep bruxism is a consequence of transient arousal. J Dent Res 2003;82:284–288.
66. Thie NM, Kato T, Bader G, Montplaisir JY, Lavigne GJ. The significance of saliva during sleep and the relevance of oromotor movements. Sleep Med Rev 2002;6:213–227.
67. Miyawaki S, Tanimoto Y, Araki Y et al. Association between nocturnal bruxism and gastroesophageal reflux. Sleep 2003;26:888–892.
68. Miyawaki S, Lavigne GJ, Pierre M et al. Association between sleep bruxism, swallowing-related laryngeal movement, and sleep positions. Sleep 2003;26:461–465.
69. Miyawaki S, Tanimoto Y, Araki Y et al. Relationships among nocturnal jaw muscle activities, decreased esophageal pH, and sleep positions. Am J Orthod Dentofacial Orthop 2004;126:615–619.
70. Ng DK, Kwok KL, Poon G, Chau KW. Habitual snoring and sleep bruxism in a paediatric outpatient population in Hong Kong. Singapore Med J 2002;43:554–556.
71. Sjoholm TT, Lowe AA, Miyamoto K, Fleetham JA, Ryan CF. Sleep bruxism in patients with sleep-disordered breathing. Arch Oral Biol 2000;45:889–896.
72. Lobbezoo F, Soucy JP, Montplaisir JY, Lavigne GJ. Striatal D2 receptor binding in sleep bruxism: a controlled study with iodine-123-iodobenzamide and single photon emission computed tomography. J Dent Res 1996;75: 1804–1810.
73. Lobbezoo F, Lavigne GJ, Tanguay R, Montplaisir JY. The effect of the catecholamine precursor L-dopa on sleep bruxism: a controlled clinical trial. Mov Disord 1997;12: 73–78.
74. Lobbezoo F, Soucy JP, Hartman NG, Montplaisir JY, Lavigne GJ. Effects of the dopamine D2 receptor agonist bromocriptine on sleep bruxism: report of two single-patient clinical trials. J Dent Res 1997;76:1611–1615.
75. Strange PG. Dopamine receptors in the basal ganglia: relevance to Parkinson's disease. Mov Disord 1993;8:263–270.
76. Zaag J van der, Lobbezoo F, Avoort PGGL van der et al. Effects of pergolide on severe sleep bruxism in a patient experiencing oral implant failure. J Oral Rehabil 2007;34: 317–322.
77. Magee KR. Bruxism related to levodopa therapy. J Am Med Assoc 1970;214:147.
78. Micheli F, Pardal MF, Gatto M et al. Bruxism secondary to chronic antidopaminergic drug exposure. Clin Neuropharmacol 1993;16:315–323.
79. Jaffee MS, Bostwick JM. Buspirone as an antidote to venlafaxine-induced bruxism. Psychosomatics 2000;41: 535–536.
80. Lobbezoo F, van Denderen RJ, Verheij JG, Naeije M. Reports of SSRI-associated bruxism in the family physician's office. J Orofac Pain 2001;15:340–346.
81. Wise M. Citalopram-induced bruxism. Br J Psychiatry 2001;178:182.
82. Miyaoka T, Yasukawa R, Mihara T et al. Successful electroconvulsive therapy in major depression with fluvoxamine-induced bruxism. J ECT 2003;19:170–172.
83. Amir I, Hermesh H, Gavish A. Bruxism secondary to antipsychotic drug exposure: a positive response to propranolol. Clin Neuropharmacol, 1997;20:86–89.
84. Lavigne GJ, Soucy JP, Lobbezoo F et al. Double Blind, crossover, placebo-controlled trial with bromocriptine in patients with sleep bruxism. Clin Neuropharmacol 2001; 24:145–149.
85. Winocur E, Gavish A, Volfin G, Halachmi M, Gazit E. Oral motor parafunctions among heavy drug addicts and their effects on signs and symptoms of temporomandibular disorders. J Orofac Pain 2001;15:56–63.
86. Ashcroft GW, Eccleston D, Waddell JL. Recognition of amphetamine addicts. BMJ 1965;5426:57.
87. See SJ, Tan EK. Severe amphethamine-induced bruxism: treatment with botulinum toxin. Acta Neurol Scand 2003;107:161–163.
88. Malki GA, Zawawi KH, Melis M, Hughes CV. Prevalence of bruxism in children receiving treatment for attention deficit hyperactivity disorder: a pilot study. J Clin Pediatr Dent 2004;29:63–67.
89. Milosevic A, Agrawal N, Redfearn PJ, Mair LH. The occurrence of toothwear in users of Ecstasy (3,4-methylene-dioxymethamphetamine). Community Dent Oral Epidemiol 1999;27:283–287.
90. McGrath C, Chan B. Oral health sensations associated with illicit drug abuse. Br Dent J 2005;198:159–162.
91. Arrue A, Gomez FM, Giralt MT. Effects of 3,4-methylenedioxymethamphetamine (Ecstasy) on the jaw-opening reflex and on the alpha-adrenoceptors which regulate this reflex in the anesthetized rat. Eur J Oral Sci 2004;112:127–133.

92. Lavigne GJ, Lobbezoo F, Rompré PH, Nielsen TA, Montplaisir JY. Cigarette smoking as a risk or exacerbating factor for restless legs syndrome and sleep bruxism. Sleep 1997;20:290–293.
93. Madrid S, Vranesh JG, Hicks RA. Cigarette smoking and bruxism. Percept Mot Skills 1998;87:898.
94. Gomez FM, Areso MP, Giralt MT, Sainz B, Garcia-Vallejo P. Effects of dopaminergic drugs, occlusal disharmonies and chronic stress on non-functional masticatory activity in the rat assessed by incisal attrition. J Dent Res 1998;77:1454–1464.
95. Areso MP, Giralt MT, Sainz B et al. Occlusal disharmonies modulate central catecholaminergic activity in the rat. J Dent Res 1999;78:1204–1213.
96. Winocur E, Gavish A, Voikovitch M, Emodi-Perlman A, Eli I. Drugs and bruxism: a critical review. J Orofac Pain 2003;17:99–111.
97. Hublin C, Kaprio J, Partinen M, Koskenvuo M. Sleep bruxism based on self-report in a nationwide twin cohort. J Sleep Res 1998;7:61–67.
98. Hublin C, Kaprio J, Partinen M, Koskenvu M. Parasomnias: co-occurrence and genetics. Psychiatr Genet 2001; 11:65–70.
99. Hublin C, Kaprio J. Genetic aspects and genetic epidemiology of parasomnias. Sleep Med Rev 2003;7:413–421.
100. Michalowicz BS, Pihlstrom BL, Hodges JS, Bouchard TJ. No heritability of temporomandibular joint signs and symptoms. J Dent Res 2000;79:1573–1578.
101. Lavigne GJ, Montplaisir JY. Bruxism: Epidemiology, diagnosis, pathophysiology, and pharmacology. Adv Pain Res Ther 1995;21:387–404.
102. Millwood J, Fiske J. Lip-biting in patients with profound neuro-disability. Dent Update 2001;28:105–108.
103. Pidcock FS, Wise JM, Christensen JR. Treatment of severe post-traumatic bruxism with botulinum toxin-A: case report. J Oral Maxillofac Surg 2002;60:115–117.
104. Tan EK, Chan LL, Chang HM. Severe bruxism following basal ganglia infarcts: insights into pathophysiology. J Neurol Sci 2004;217:229–232.
105. Rodrigues dos Santos MT, Masiero D, Novo NF, Simionato MR. Oral conditions in children with cerebral palsy. J Dent Child (Chic) 2003;70:40–46.
106. Manzano FS, Granero LM, Masiero D, dos Maria TB. Treatment of muscle spasticity in patients with cerebral palsy using BTX-A: a pilot study. Spec Care Dentist 2004;24:235–239.
107. Boyd D, Quick A, Murray C. The Down syndrome patient in dental practice. II: clinical considerations. N Z Dent J 2004;100:4–9.
108. Meletti S, Cantalupo G, Volpi L et al. Rhythmic teeth grinding induced by temporal lobe seizures. Neurology 2004;62:2306–2309.
109. Louis ED, Tampone E. Bruxism in Huntington's disease. Mov Disord 2001;16:785–786.
110. Nash MC, Ferrell RB, Lombardo MA, Williams RB. Treatment of bruxism in Huntington's disease with botulinum toxin. J Neuropsychiatry Clin Neurosci 2004;16: 381–382.
111. Diab M. Self-inflicted orodental injury in a child with Leigh disease. Int J Paediatr Dent 2004;14:73–77.
112. Coyne BM, Montague T. Teeth grinding, tongue and lip biting in a 24-month-old boy with meningococcal septicaemia: report of a case. Int J Paediatr Dent 2002;12: 277–280.
113. Wali GM. Asymmetrical awake bruxism associated with multiple system atrophy. Mov Disord 2004;19:352–355.
114. Srivastava T, Ahuja M, Srivastava M, Trivedi A. Bruxism as presenting feature of Parkinson's disease. J Assoc Physicians India 2002;50:457.
115. Patients with PTSD risk damaging teeth [news]. J Dent Hyg 2001;75:115.
116. Wright EF, Thompson RL, Paunovich ED. Post-traumatic stress disorder: considerations for dentistry. Quintessence Int 2004;35:206–210.
117. Magalhaes MH, Kawamura JY, Araujo LC. General and oral characteristics in Rett syndrome. Spec Care Dentist 2002;22:147–150.
118. Lavigne GJ, Rompré PH, Montplaisir JY. Sleep bruxism: validity of clinical research diagnostic criteria in a controlled polysomnographic study. J Dent Res 1996;75: 546–552.

Chapter 5

# Role of Peripheral Sensory Factors in Bruxism: A Physiologic Interpretation for Clinical Dentistry

*Takafumi Kato*

## Introduction

Bruxism has been defined as an oral parafunctional activity that includes clenching, bracing, gnashing, and grinding of the teeth while asleep or awake (see Chapter 1).[1] Bruxism is considered to be a clinically relevant problem in dentistry because it can be associated with tooth wear, failure of dental prostheses and implants, and orofacial pain. Although a definitive understanding of pathophysiology and the management strategies have yet to be established, it has long been thought in clinical dentistry that local or peripheral factors play an important role in the pathophysiology. Thus, the interest of most practitioners has focused on the relationship between the maxillary and mandibular dentition (e.g., occlusion).

However, more recent literature does not strongly support the validity of occlusal disharmony (or malocclusion) as a primary cause of bruxism (see also Chapter 4).[2–11] For example, epidemiologic or observational studies have reported both negative and positive correlations between reports of tooth grinding and clenching, and the presence of occlusal interferences. Furthermore, the nature of these studies is limited: diagnosis was based mainly on a clinical interpretation (e.g., tooth wear) and on subjective reports (e.g., self-awareness), and most were cross-sectional studies. Even though a positive correlation was found between the presence of bruxism and occlusal observations, the results can only demonstrate an association between these variables; it is difficult to link these clinical data to physiologic mechanisms.

This chapter will present current physiologic knowledge about bruxism in order to promote a better understanding of peripheral factors in bruxism in clinical dentistry. It will review basic information concerning peripheral sensory influences on jaw motor activities. Then jaw posture and tooth contacts will be presented in association with muscle activity, followed by several putative peripheral factors related to bruxism. To finish, the physiologic role of the oral splint in the management of bruxism is discussed.

Table 5-1

**Behavioral and physiologic differences between wakefulness and sleep.**

| | Wakefulness | Sleep |
|---|---|---|
| *Behavior* | | |
| Alertness | Alert and conscious | Unconscious but reversible |
| Posture | Elect, sitting, standing | Recumbent |
| Mobility/movements | Normal | Reduced or absent |
| Response to stimuli | Normal | Reduced |
| Eye | Open | Closed |
| *Physiology* | | |
| Motor | Normal | Reduced activity in NREM<br>Nearly absent in REM |
| Sensory | Normal | Reduced but selective |
| Respiratory | Normal | Slow and steady in NREM<br>Irregular in REM |
| Cardiovascular | Normal | Reduced but changeable, e.g., heart rate is low in NREM but high in REM |
| Autonomic | Normal | Changeable, related to sleep cycles, e.g., sympathetic activity is low in NREM and high in REM |

Bruxism is classified as being: (1) either primary (idiopathic) or secondary (related to neurologic, psychiatric, sleep, movement disorders or of an iatrogenic type associated with drug use); and (2) occurring during either sleep or wakefulness.[12–14] In this chapter, discussion will be limited to *primary bruxism*, since medical conditions related to secondary bruxism are often associated with an alteration of the sensorimotor system (see Chapter 1).[15,16] In addition, wakefulness and sleep are characterized by different conscious, behavioral, and physiologic states that can be associated with different kinds of sensorimotor integration (see Chapter 3).[11,17] In the clinical literature, bruxism during wakefulness is thought to be characterized by tooth clenching (habit).[12,16] In contrast, 90% of sleep bruxism is associated with rhythmic masticatory muscle activity (RMMA) with or without tooth grinding.[13,18,19] Therefore bruxism occurring during wakefulness and sleep will be discussed separately here. Because of the availability of physiologic information, the majority of this chapter will be devoted to sleep bruxism.

## Basic Knowledge of Orofacial Sensorimotor Systems

Sleep and wakefulness are very different behavioral and physiologic conditions (Table 5-1). For example, wakefulness is characterized by conscious vigilance to sensory stimuli and various behaviors, while sleep is characterized by unconsciousness and behavioral quiescence. The difference between the two conditions should be recognized in any discussion of the role of peripheral factors in bruxism.

### *Sleep Architecture*

Since sleep architecture has been reviewed in another chapter (Chapter 3), only the fundamental information will be summarized here (Fig 5-1).

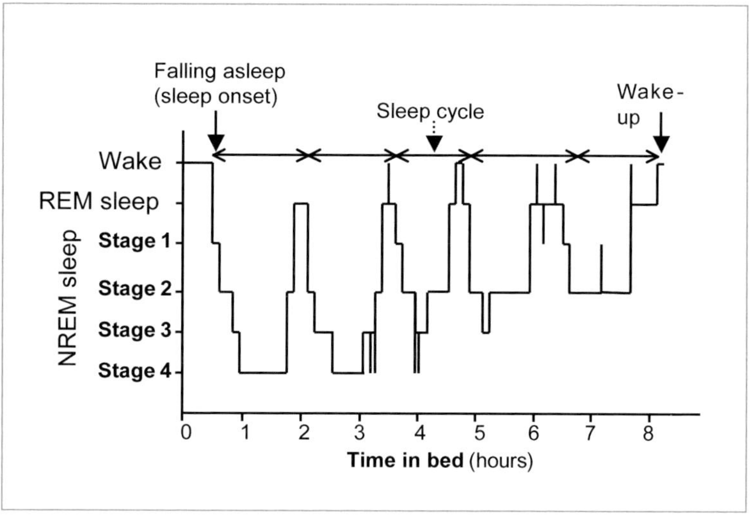


Fig 5-1 Sleep architecture.

Sleep usually lasts 7–9 hours in adults.[17] In mammals, sleep macrostructure is divided into nonrapid eye movement (NREM) and rapid eye movement (REM) sleep. In humans, NREM sleep is further classified into four stages, from light (stages 1 and 2) to deep (stages 3 and 4). Each stage is characterized by brain activity, autonomic activity, and motor activity.[20] After a normal subject falls into NREM sleep stage 1 (sleep onset), sleep progresses to stage 2 and to stages 3 and 4, and returns light NREM sleep before reaching REM sleep. This "sleep cycle" is repeated every 90–120 minutes.

A sleep stage is not a simple and stable state. Various transient and phasic physiologic events occur within any given sleep stage.[20,21] These events include K-complexes and sleep spindles in sleep stage 2, or transient arousal events (not full awakenings). As will be discussed later, transient arousals without full awakening (or consciousness), such as micro-arousals, occur frequently during sleep in association with brief cortical, autonomic–cardiac and even jaw motor activations. Micro-arousals occur at a frequency of 10–15 times per hour of sleep and tend to occur at the end of a NREM period.[22] A more intense arousal activity, awakening, is less frequent (3–4 times per hour of sleep) and is often associated with body movement and sleep stage shift (e.g., from a deeper to a lighter stage). Cyclic alternating patterns (CAP) are clusters of phasic and arousal activities that are repeated every 20–60 seconds.[22] These phasic events can be triggered or modified by peripheral sensory stimuli (e.g., sound and touch) or by endogenous stimuli (e.g., a change in blood pressure)[23,24] because they represent conditions of sleep (instability or stability) that regulate the sleep process.[24] As will be discussed later, the occurrence of sleep bruxism is very much correlated with the above sleep processes.

### *Orofacial Sensory Afferents and Reflexes*

Clinicians have long associated peripheral factors (e.g., occlusal interferences) with the genesis of bruxism (e.g., initiation of jaw-closing activity as seen on electromyography (EMG)). The following basic summary of trigeminal sensory physiology outlines how peripheral sensory inputs reflect on the motor system and how the peripheral sensory system differs between wakefulness and sleep (Fig 5-2).

| Tissues | Sensory types | Location of primary afferent | Activity | | |
|---|---|---|---|---|---|
| | | | aefuness | Seep | |
| | | | | NREM | REM |
| Skin/mucosa | Touch<br>Thermal<br>Nociception | TG<br>TG<br>TG | ↑by contacts between skin/ mucosa /food during chewing | ↓ | ↑or↓ |
| Teeth | Nociception | TG | | ↓ | ↓ |
| Periodontium | Stretch<br>Nociception | TG&MesV<br>TG | ↑ by tooth contact during chewing/biting | unknown<br>unknown | unknown<br>unknown |
| Jaw muscles | Stretch<br>Muscle<br>Tendon<br>Nociception | MesV<br>TG<br>TG | ↑ by jaw opening<br>↑ during chewing/biting | unknown<br>unknown | unknown<br>unknown |
| TMJ | Pressure<br>Stretch<br>Nociception | TG<br>TG | ↑ by jaw movement | unknown<br>unknown | unknown<br>unknown |

**Fig 5-2** Orofacial sensory inputs and their modulation during wakefulness and sleep.

*Skin and mucosal receptor afferents*

Sensory inputs from facial/perioral skin and oral mucosa (lip, tongue, palate, and gingiva) include tactile (touch), thermal (cold, heat) and nociceptive (e.g., pain) information. These afferents provide sensory information for coordinating jaw, lip, and tongue movements during mastication, swallowing, and speaking.[25] Tactile information is generated from mechanoreceptors in the cutaneous or mucosal tissues when the receptor is deformed by strain or pressure in the skin and mucosa of the cheek, tongue, or lips.[25] Tactile information from orofacial structures usually activates jaw-closing muscles while noxious stimulation inhibits jaw-closing muscles.[25,26] We have little knowledge of the skin and mucosal sensory afferent activities during sleep. In some animal studies, sensory information from trigeminal nerves is suppressed in NREM sleep compared with REM sleep.[23]

*Periodontal afferents*

Mechanoreceptors in the periodontal ligament respond to forces applied to the teeth (e.g., contact between teeth and food during chewing, and tonic clenching). Rapidly adapting receptors respond abruptly to the force while slowly adapting receptors can be activated as the force applied to the teeth gradually increases.[25,27] The rapidly adapting receptors have higher force thresholds compared with slowly adapting receptors. When excessive or unexpected force is applied to teeth during chewing, sensory inputs from the former receptors are more likely to inhibit jaw-closing muscles and activate jaw-opening muscles.[26,28,29] Sensory inputs from the latter receptors are more likely to facilitate jaw-closing muscle activity when biting force is necessary for chewing hard food.[30,31] Unfortunately, no evidence is available to speculate that these modulations occur during sleep.

Subjects with an awareness of tooth grinding during sleep did not differ in perioral and tooth tactile sensitivity.[32] However, in a recent study, subjects with higher masseter EMG activity during sleep exhibited a lower interocclusal tactile threshold (e.g., ability to detect a thinner object) compared with those without.[33] The clinical significance of this difference needs further investigation.

*Muscle afferents*

Muscle sensory afferents are classified into several groups according to fiber diameter.[31] The larger afferents (groups Ia and II) innervate the intrafusal fibers in muscle spindles. Note that muscle spindles are located mainly in jaw-closing muscles (masseter) while there are very few in the jaw-opening digastric muscle. These afferents are mainly responsive to the velocity and length of muscle stretch. These afferent activities facilitate jaw-closing muscle activity while chewing hard food.[34,35] Group Ib afferents convey information about muscle tension detected by Golgi tendon organs. They become excited by muscle stretch and by jaw muscle contraction during chewing.[31] The smaller afferents (groups III and IV) carry mechanical or nociceptive information. The activation of nociceptive afferents reduces jaw-closing muscle activity during chewing.[36] Several studies have reported a decrease of oromotor episodes during sleep in sleep bruxism (SB) patients with jaw muscle pain.[37-39] In a large-sample polysomnographic study, SB patients with low levels of SB activity were more at risk of reporting pain compared with those with high SB activity.[40] During wakefulness, however, some studies reported that orofacial pain patients can exhibit increased parafunctional jaw muscle activity.[41] The discrepancy between sleep and waking conditions needs to be clarified for a better understanding of the relationship between pain and jaw motor activity/behavior and to improve the clinical management strategies of orofacial pain patients.

There are no studies recording jaw muscle afferents during sleep. The activity of limb muscle spindle afferents is suppressed during NREM sleep and is decreased further in REM sleep.[42] A transient facilitation of the afferent activity during sleep can be observed in association with arousal-related activation.[42,43]

*Temporomandibular joint (TMJ) afferents*

The TMJ afferents innervate the joint capsule and are sensitive to mechanical and nociceptive stimuli.[31] Only a few studies have investigated the role of TMJ afferents on jaw motor control.[44,45] No study has been done during sleep.

*Table 5-2*

**Jaw reflexes during sleep compared with wakefulness.**

| | NREM sleep | REM sleep |
|---|---|---|
| Excitability of jaw motoneurons | ⇩ | ⇩ ⇩ ⇩ |
| Jaw-opening reflex (disynaptic reflex) | ⇩ or ⇨ | ⇩ ⇩ |
| Jaw-closing reflex (monosynaptic reflex) | ⇩ or ⇨ | ⇩ ⇩ |

## *Trigeminal Reflexes (Table 5-2)*

*Jaw-opening reflex (JOR)*

The JOR is a rapid di-synaptic reflex following the activation of mechanoreceptors or nociceptive receptors in the orofacial skin, mucosal, and periodontal ligaments.[30,31] In JOR, jaw-closing muscle activity is inhibited while jaw-opening muscle activity is not facilitated clearly in humans compared with animals.[30,31] The activity of the JOR is modulated during chewing in animals.[30,31] The JOR, triggered by non-painful stimulation (e.g., low threshold afferents), is inhibited during the closing phase but not during the opening phase. By contrast, when the JOR is induced by stimulation of high-threshold mechanoreceptors (e.g., probably nociceptive or harmful stimuli), the reflex is facilitated during the closing phase and inhibited during the opening phase. The latter reflex modulation is useful to protect orofacial structures from damage, for example when one bites unexpectedly on a cherry stone.

In animal studies, the JOR is induced by the electrical stimulation of the alveolar nerve. The JOR was not found to decrease during NREM sleep while it was strongly reduced in REM sleep in animals.[46,47] However, the JOR seems to be facilitated during transient arousal. In these studies, the types of sensory afferents triggering the JOR were not differentiated.

*Jaw-closing reflex (JCR)*

The JCR is a monosynaptic reflex that can be triggered by a mechanical chin tap that stretches muscle receptors abruptly and excites muscle spindle afferents in the trigeminal nerve (H-reflex).[30,31] The JCR is facilitated during the jaw-closing phase of chewing and during tooth-clenching tasks.[48–50] In animals, a monosynaptic reflex like the JCR can be induced by electrical stimulation of muscle spindle afferents. The amplitude of the JCR did not significantly decrease from wakefulness to NREM sleep, and was markedly suppressed during REM sleep.[47,51] However, there are controversial findings indicating that the amplitude of the JCR is facilitated or suppressed in relation to rapid eye movement episodes during REM sleep.[47,51]

### *Comment*

Regardless of wakefulness or sleep, it is clear that sensory information is generated by the deformation of sensory receptors in orofacial tissues as a consequence of orofacial motor activity and movements. This implies that sensory influence may have a modulatory role for oromotor activities such as bruxism. Compared to wakefulness, orofacial sensory information and reflex activity are decreased during sleep without jaw movement. However, it is not known how sensory and reflex activities interact with jaw motor activity during bruxism. The lack of this information prevents us from correctly understanding the physiologic relevance of occlusal therapy in clinical management (e.g., using a splint).

## Which Event Comes First: Tooth Contact or Jaw Muscle Activity?

This is an important question to consider when discussing the relevance of peripheral occlusal factors in the genesis of bruxism. This section will review jaw posture and tooth contacts in association with jaw motor activity, during wakefulness and sleep.

### *Jaw Posture, Motor Events, and Tooth Contacts during Wakefulness*

When we sit upright, our maxillary and mandibular teeth are separated by a distance of 3–5 mm when the jaw is in its resting position (habitual mandibular position).[52] The habitual mandibular position is maintained by the visco-elasticity of muscles and perioral soft tissues, and by postural jaw muscle tone. It is known that jaw-closing muscle tone is not at a minimum at the so-called "resting mandibular position".[52] Thus, residual activity of the jaw muscles exists while there is no tooth contact (Fig 5-3).

When the jaw is functioning, such as chewing and swallowing, tooth contacts between maxillary and mandibular dentitions, or contacts between food and teeth occur very frequently (2–3 times per second while chewing) in association with masticatory muscle activations.[53,54] During the periods when the jaw is not functioning, jaw-closing muscles can be activated in association with non-functional oromotor activities.[55,56] This jaw-closing muscle activity could increase the chance for maxillary and mandibular teeth to contact each other.[57,58] Either during stressful or non-stressful conditions, masseter muscle activity is higher in subjects with an awareness of tooth clenching during wakefulness than in those without, suggesting that subjects with an awareness of tooth clenching might show an increased number of tooth contacts.[59–62] A recent controlled study reports that habitual jaw-closing muscle activity during a non-eating waking period decreases when occlusal interference with gold foil (2 x 8 x 0.25 mm) is created to disturb the intercuspal position in normal subjects.[56] The decrease is more apparent for muscle bursts with high activity. These suggest that subtle occlusal disturbances can modify jaw muscle activity during non-eating waking periods. However, it remains to be determined whether decreased masseter muscle activity during wakefulness in response to occlusal interference could be associated with avoiding unpleasant sensations or with reflex activity.

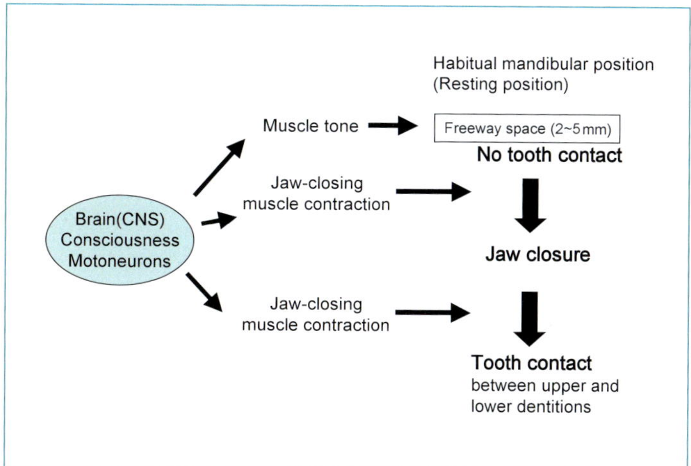


Fig 5-3 Physiologic process of tooth contact during wakefulness.

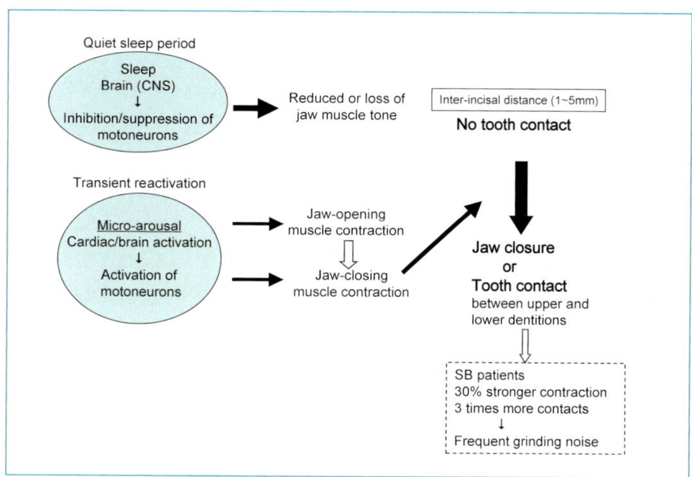


Fig 5-4 Physiologic process of tooth contact during sleep.

In conclusion, tooth contacts can occur during wakefulness as a result of increased jaw-closing muscle activity (Fig 5-3). People aware of tooth clenching can exhibit a higher number of tooth contacts than those without. The physiologic mechanisms of these observations and sensory influences on spontaneous tooth clenching activity are not well understood in terms of cognitive awakeness or reflex modulation.

### *Jaw Posture, Motor Events, and Tooth Contacts during Sleep*

During sleep, masticatory muscle tone is usually lower in REM sleep than in NREM sleep owing to the different motor controls in the central nervous system.[63] As has been observed in skeletal muscles, masticatory muscle tone decreases from wakefulness to sleep.[64,65] Because of a decrease in jaw muscle tone, the jaw is usually open 1–5 mm for approximately 90% of total sleeping time (see

Fig 5-4).[66] The magnitude of jaw opening is associated with a decrease in muscle tone; jaw opening magnitude is significantly greater during REM sleep than in NREM sleep. In addition, the jaw can be located further back during sleep, especially in a supine position – a condition that contributes to a narrowing of the airway during sleep.[67] The maxillary and mandibular teeth are unlikely to contact each other during the majority of the sleep period.

Nonetheless, tooth contacts can occur occasionally during sleep. Several studies have directly measured tooth contacts during sleep using intraoral sensors although no recordings were made for sleep variables.[53,68,69,70] In normal subjects, tooth contacts were found to be associated with swallowing and body movements during sleep, since jaw-closing muscles are activated following a transient arousal in these events.[66] In addition, tooth contacts occurred in clusters every 90–120 minutes during the night.[68,70,71] Interestingly, recent polysomnographic studies have revealed that SB occurs in clusters in association with sleep cycles[72,73] (see next section and Fig 5-5). The above observations suggest that tooth contacts, or periodontal inputs, are not necessary for the jaw muscle to be activated during sleep (Fig 5-4). This idea is also supported indirectly by the clinical observation that edentulous subjects can exhibit either rhythmic or tonic masseter muscle activity even when they sleep without wearing dentures.[74,75]

One study reported that the frequency and duration of tooth contacts was significantly higher in SB patients with temporomandibular disorder (TMD) compared with normal subjects and patients with TMD[76] (Table 5-3). Using polysomnographic recording with audio–video, the incidence of tooth grinding-related noise has been found to be more frequent in SB patients than in normal subjects.[77,78] The increased number of tooth contacts during sleep in SB patients can be assumed from the results of several studies recording masseter muscle EMG activity during sleep (see Fig 5-3). Jaw motor episodes have been observed more frequently in SB patients (between 3.5 and 6.8 episodes per hour of sleep) than in normal subjects (0.3–1.9 episodes) and the total duration of these episodes per hour of sleep is longer in SB patients (0.4–1.65 minutes) compared to normal subjects (0.12–0.9 minutes).[19,78,80] In addition, SB patients show approximately 40% higher EMG burst amplitudes during sleep than normal subjects.[19,80] Although different methods and criteria have been used to record SB and tooth contacts, and to score SB episodes, it can be summarized that SB patients exhibit episodes of intense jaw-closing muscle activity 2–5 times more often and for a longer duration than normal subjects (Table 5-3). These findings suggest that SB is an exaggerated form of transient motor (muscle) activity during sleep. Thus the exaggerated jaw motor episodes in SB patients can be associated with the frequent occurrence of tooth contacts and tooth grinding noises.

### *From Physiological Sequence to Tooth Contact during Sleep*

Sleep bruxism is a transient motor event with a duration ranging, on average, from 5 to 15 seconds.[19,74,77–82] In SB patients aware of frequent tooth grinding, more than 80% of these episodes are characterized by RMMA.[19,77,80] These patients exhibit approximately three times more RMMA episodes compared to normal subjects (Table 5-3).

Young and healthy SB patients usually exhibit normal sleep macrostructure as well as microstructures, and do not complain of sleep disturbance.[11] In these patients, 60–80% of SB episodes occur in stages 1 and 2 of NREM sleep. Very few SB episodes occur in stages 3 and 4 of NREM sleep (<5%) and in REM sleep (<10 %).[19,72,77,82,] In addition, within the sleep cycle, SB occurs in clusters during NREM periods where the sleep stage is getting lighter from deep NREM to REM sleep (see arrowheads in Fig 5-5).[72] This period is characterized by increased activity in terms of micro-arousals and CAP[22,73] (Fig 5-5).

*Table 5-3*

**Comparison of jaw motor events and tooth contacts in sleep bruxism patients (SBp) and normal subjects.[a]**

| Authors | | Frequency[c] | Ratio (frequency)[b] | Duration[d] | Ratio (duration)[b] |
|---|---|---|---|---|---|
| *Jaw motor events* | | | | | |
| Nishigawa et al (2001) | Normal | 3.5 (0.3–11.5) | | 0.4 min (0.02–1.4) | |
| | SB | 3.5 (0.5–7.5) | 1.0 | 0.4 min (0.03–0.9) | 1.0 |
| Kydd & Daly (1985) | Normal | – | | 0.4 min (0.4–0.6) | |
| | SBp | – | – | 1.4 min (0.4–2.0) | 3.5 |
| Sjöholm et al (1995) | Normal | 1.9 | | 0.9 min (0.3–1.4) | |
| | SBp | 4.8 | 2.5 | 1.65 min (1.0–3.2) | 1.8 |
| Lavigne et al (2001) | Normal | 1.8 (0.1–12.6) | | – | |
| | SBp | 5.8 (1.2–15.2) | 3.2 | – | |
| Miyawaki et al (2003) | Normal | 0.5 | | 0.12 min (0.05–0.25) | |
| | SBp | 6.8 | 13.6 | 1.15 min (0.68–1.9) | 9.6 |
| *Tooth contact/grinding noise* | | | | | |
| Reding et al[e] (1968) | Normal | 0 | | 0 | |
| | SBp | 5.8 | – | 0.34 min | – |
| Trenouth[f] (1979) | Normal | 45 | | 0.68 min | |
| | SBp | 165 | 3.6 | 4.8 min | 7.0 |
| Lavigne et al[e] (1996) | Normal | 0 | | – | |
| | SBp | 0.97 | – | – | – |
| Lavigne et al[e] (2001) | Normal | 0 | | – | |
| | SBp | 1.9 | – | – | – |
| Miyawaki et al[e] (2003) | Normal | 0.1 (0–0.3) | | 0.03 min (0–0.07) | |
| | SBp | 3.4 (0.1–10) | 34 | 0.62 min (0.01–1.54) | 20.3 |

[a]Only the studies comparing SB patients and controls are presented. See Kato et al[11] for other studies.
[b]Ratios were calculated by dividing the number of SB patients by that of normal subjects.
[c,d]Frequency and duration (mean [range] were presented as times per hour of sleep and minutes per hour of sleep, respectively.
[e]Episodes with tooth grinding noise were counted.
[f]Tooth contacts were directly measured.

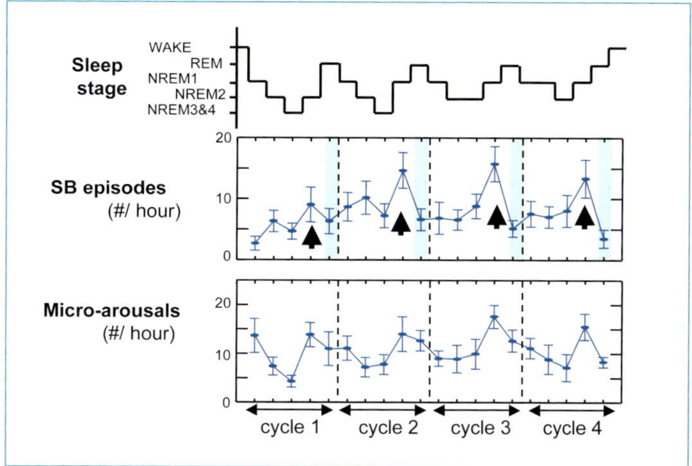


Fig 5-5 Sleep architecture and the occurrence of sleep bruxism and micro-arousals.

Polysomnographic studies have reported a time relation between the genesis of SB and transient arousal events such as transient brain electroencephalographic (EEG) activation, increases in heart rate, and frequent sleep stage shifts.[19,73,77,80,82–84] In most of these studies, changes in brain EEG activity (e.g., alpha activity) and an increase in heart rate are observed before jaw-closing muscle activity related to RMMA episodes. Subsequently, the following physiological sequence was demonstrated in relation to the genesis of SB episodes:[19,72,85] (1) an increase in sympathetic activity 4 minutes before, (2) an increase in brain EEG activity 4 seconds before, (3) an increase in heart rate one cardiac cycle (approximately 1 second) before, and (4) an increase in suprahyoid muscle activity (jaw-opening muscle) 0.8 seconds before the onset of masseter muscle activation.

The above studies suggest that tooth contacts can occur as a last event in a sequence of arousal–jaw motor activation during sleep, not as an initial event generating each sleep bruxism episode (Fig 5-4). The exaggerated number of jaw muscle episodes can be associated with increased jaw motor responsiveness to micro-arousals in SB patients.

### *Comment*

The mandible opens at a resting mandibular position during wakefulness. Teeth in the maxilla and the mandible can contact when jaw–closing muscles are activated in association with functional and non-functional oromotor activities. It is clear that, during sleep, arousal is followed by an increase in jaw muscle activity and jaw closure: brain and cardiac activation clearly precede SB episodes. Thus, tooth contact is a consequence of jaw motor activation rather than a cause. Occlusal and intraoral peripheral factors are not direct triggering factors for bruxism. Alternatively, bruxism jaw muscle EMG events and tooth contact occur more frequently in patients than in normal subjects. Increased activity of jaw-closing muscles and an increased number of tooth contacts can be associated with increased mechanical loads on teeth, muscle, joint, and dental prostheses in patients with bruxism.

## Sensory Stimuli and Sleep Bruxism

Peripheral sensory inputs can influence jaw motor activity during wakefulness. However, there is little information on orofacial sensory stimuli and bruxism during wakefulness. As previously discussed, sleep bruxism is subject to sleep regulation and secondary to micro-arousal. Interestingly, several studies have reported that SB activity could be modified by applying sensory stimulation during sleep. These findings are not surprising since it is known that all sensory inputs from orofacial and other body tissues can influence sleep architecture.[23]

### *Sensory Stimuli Associated with the Genesis of SB*

In a biofeedback experiment, sensory stimuli were applied at the onset of a SB episode in order to prevent SB. Each stimulus was triggered when masticatory EMG activity and/or biting force exceeded a predefined non-sleep threshold (Fig 5-6). When using loud stimuli, the duration but not the frequency of SB episodes was found to decrease.[86–90] Similarly, when non-noxious electrical stimulation to the lip was applied at the time of tooth contact, the duration of SB episodes was decreased rather than the number of episodes.[91] Another study showed that electrical stimulation of forehead skin has a decreasing effect on SB episodes.[92] In a few case studies, a vibratory stimulus or an unpleasant taste stimulus applied into the mouth reduced SB activity and the effects lasted over several months.[93,94]

Thus, jaw-closing muscle activity during sleep can be disturbed by sensory stimuli given to either the orofacial or the non-orofacial region. In order to determine the precise roles of sensory stimulation in these paradigms, it will be necessary to

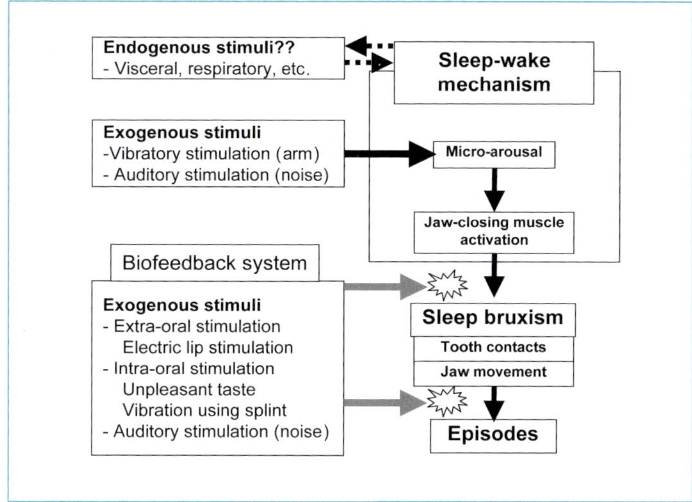


Fig 5-6 Summary of sensory influences on sleep bruxism.

make further investigation of the mechanisms involved in relation to sleep architecture (e.g., sleep stages, micro-arousal), trigeminal nerve excitability (e.g., reflex) and cognitive function (e.g., awareness of stimuli).[15,64]

In contrast to previous studies, a few studies have reported that SB can be induced by applying sensory stimulation during quiet periods of sleep. An increase in masseter EMG activity was observed following a loud noise (>60 dB) or a vibration applied to the arm.[95,96] Tooth grinding episodes during sleep occasionally follow experimental arousals (approximately 8% of vibration, noise, and light) in SB patients.[83,95] Moreover, the probability of experimentally induced SB episodes was seven times more frequent in SB patients than in normal subjects.[95] Tooth grinding episodes were induced in SB patients only.[95] These suggest that SB–tooth grinding is more easily induced by sensory stimulation when it triggers micro-arousal (i.e., RMMA in SB patients is more responsive to micro-arousals compared to normal subjects) (see Fig 5-6). This further supports the idea that arousal activity is a prerequisite to inducing jaw motor activity during sleep.

### *Oroesopharyngeal Functions and Sleep Bruxism*

Many orofacial motor activities occur during sleep. These include swallowing, grimacing, talking, sighing, and coughing.[97] The occurrence of these motor activities is also associated with micro-arousals.

During sleep, swallowing occurs in association with arousals at a frequency of 5–10 times per hour – a rate that is 5–10 times lower during wakefulness.[78] The decreased rate of swallowing during sleep may be associated with decreased salivary flow.[98] Several studies have reported that chemical acid stimulation of vagal sensory afferents in the esophagus triggers arousals and swallowing during sleep.[99] Transient arousals and swallowing occur more frequently during sleep in patients with gastroesophageal reflux (GER).[100,101] However, healthy subjects exhibit swallowing in the absence of reflux events during sleep.[102,103] Thus, the role of swallowing in combination with salivation is thought to be a mechanism protecting oroesopharyngeal structures from acid reflux during sleep.[99] Interestingly, close to 60% of SB episodes occurred concomitantly with swallowing.[78] A recent study showed that in SB patients

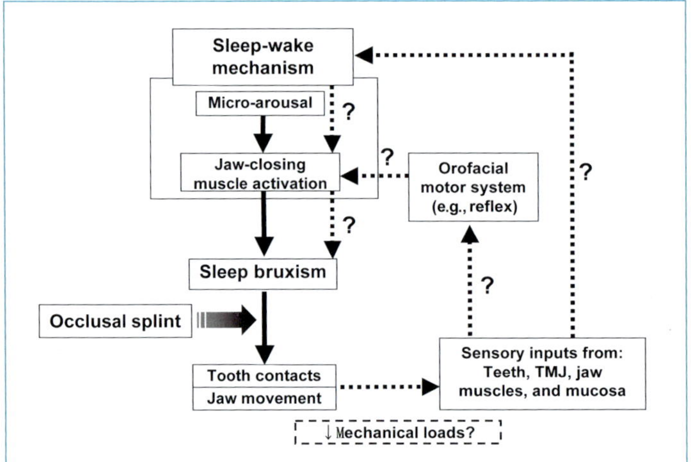


Fig 5-7 Putative actions of an occlusal splint on sleep bruxism.

without clinical signs and symptoms of GER the occurrence of SB is associated with a decrease in esophageal pH during sleep, while another did not demonstrate this.[104,105] It has been noted that visceral fluctuations are regulated by the autonomic nervous system that fluctuates in association with sleep processes.[99] It remains to be determined how factors such as swallowing, esophageal pH, micro-arousals, and salivation interact in the genesis of sleep bruxism.

Respiratory disturbance during sleep is another physiologic issue associated with mandibular position. As mentioned earlier, during sleep, especially in a supine position, the decrease in jaw muscle tone results in retrusion, the opening of the mandible, and tongue collapse.[66,67] The changes in mandibular and tongue position are associated with airway narrowing in normal subjects or with airway obstruction in patients with obstructive sleep apnea syndrome (OSAS).[106] Thus, in dental management of OSAS, a bimaxillary oral appliance is used to increase or maintain the airway space by moving the mandible into an advanced position.[107] It is important to note that several craniofacial morphologies resulting in airway narrowing, such as macroglossia and microngathia, are thought to be a risk for OSAS; these factors can underlie genetic or ethnic differences in the occurrence of OSAS.[106,108] Physiologic studies have reported that respiratory events such as apnea or hypopnea are often terminated with jaw-closing muscle activation.[109] In this condition, apnea and hypopnea events result in micro-arousal and awakening, which often leads to tonic, rather than rhythmic, muscle contractions in jaw-opening and jaw-closing muscles. Jaw muscle activation at the termination of respiratory events is necessary to restore airway patency.[65] Several physiologic studies have reported that RMMA or tooth grinding are not associated with the termination of apnea.[110,111] However, SB seems more prevalent in patients with snoring or OSAS.[112] The putative association between SB, mandibular position, and respiratory modulation needs further investigation.[10]

### *Comment*

The above findings suggest that sleep bruxism can be influenced by orofacial sensory stimuli or other sensory stimuli (e.g., sound, vibration). When stimuli are given after SB initiation, ongoing SB can be interrupted. Moreover, SB episodes can be triggered by sensory-induced micro-arousals. We may therefore surmise that there is an interaction between sensory input, jaw muscle activity, and sleep mechanisms in the genesis of sleep bruxism.

The influence of visceral sensory stimuli on sleep arousal and oromotor activity has been well documented in the literature. However, the concomitant occurrence of SB and swallowing in relation to visceral sensory stimuli and salivation still needs to be investigated. The association between respiratory events and SB raises other morphologic issues in the pathophysiology of sleep bruxism. Thus, putative peripheral factors contributing to sleep bruxism may not be limited to teeth in the oral cavity but could also involve oroesopharyngeal structures. These notions provide us with another paradigm for further understanding the effect of the occlusal splint on sleep bruxism. This paradigm will be discussed in the next section.

## Can the Peripheral Sensory System Explain the Role of an Oral Splint in SB Management?

### *Influences of the Occlusal Splint on SB Activity*

One common strategy used by clinicians to manage bruxism is the use of an oral device.[74,113] Patients are usually instructed to use these devices during sleep. Therefore, this management strategy is aimed at sleep bruxism rather than bruxism during wakefulness. In this context, there are many studies recording jaw-closing muscle activity during sleep when patients use an oral device. When average masseter EMG activity during the night was assessed using a portable EMG recording system, EMG activity was not only reduced in most patients but also increased or did not change in some patients.[114–117] The decreasing influence did not continue when the splint was withdrawn.[114,116] However, specific influences on SB genesis were difficult to assess because the frequency, intensity, and duration of the SB episodes was not evaluated. In several studies, SB episodes were selected based on an EMG threshold using automatic software, or the episodes were discriminated from other non-specific orofacial activities (e.g., swallowing) using a combination of analytic software and audio–video recording. These studies again showed that the effects of an oral splint on the frequency, intensity, and duration of SB episodes varied between or within studies (20–50% variability).[79,90,118–121]

There are several studies comparing the effects of different oral devices on sleep bruxism. The average masseter EMG activity during sleep did not differ between the splints with canine guidance or group-function guidance.[115] Using a crossover design (reversing the order of application of the devices), a few studies compared the effects of an occlusal splint and a palatal splint not covering maxillary teeth. One study reported no change but the others reported a decrease in SB activity for both devices.[119,120] More importantly, these three studies reported that no difference in the effects on SB activity was found between the two devices. In a 6-week follow-up study, the decreasing effects lasted for only 2 weeks after insertion of an occlusal and horseshoe-shaped palatal splint.[121]

In another study, an oral splint covering the incisors significantly reduced the frequency and intensity of SB, whereas a normal occlusal splint had no effect.[122] When subjects wore palatal splints of different thicknesses for several nights, SB decreased with the use of the splint that completely filled the palatal space.[123] Finally, the effect on SB was compared between an occlusal splint and a mandibular advancement device (e.g., slightly [<40% of maximal advancement] and moderately [>40%] advanced jaw position).[124] Sleep bruxism activity was significantly less using the mandibular advancement device with moderate advancement than when an occlusal splint was used.

### *Can We Explain how an Oral Splint Works for Bruxism?*

Despite the evidence of the studies mentioned above, it is very difficult to draw a clear conclusion about how oral devices act on SB genesis or activity. There are several reasons for this. First, the studies use different methodologies to record SB (portable EMG recording or polysomnographic recordings) and different methods to assess SB activity (e.g., automatic detection, visual scoring and a calculation of average nightly activity). Second, the diagnosis of SB patients (e.g., clinical exams, polysomnographic recording) is not standardized. Third, some studies did not use a control condition (e.g., a crossover study design or a comparison between two devices). Fourth, the design of the oral devices differed between studies.

As has been discussed in the previous sections, SB is not triggered directly by tooth contact. Occlusal devices that do not cover the teeth (e.g., palatal splints) have similar effects on SB compared to normal occlusal splints. Moreover, in several studies, in which the effects of occlusal adjustment and experimental occlusal interferences on SB activity were tested, SB activity did not change very much.[125,126] Thus, occlusal devices do not seem to work for the genesis of SB by removing occlusal interferences.[113] Accordingly an oral splint can be used to protect teeth or orofacial tissues from mechanical impacts or consequences generated after tooth contact[8,12,113,127,128] (Fig 5-7).

Several studies have reported that the patterns of jaw muscle contractions (e.g., in closer and opener muscles) and jaw movements related to SB are unique compared to awake chewing.[64,129–132] During SB, jaw-closing and jaw-opening muscles often show co-contraction and jaw-closing muscles on the reciprocal side seem more activated. These findings suggest that the mechanical loads placed on the orofacial structures as well as reflex modulation can differ between chewing during wakefulness and tooth grinding during sleep.[133] Unfortunately, there is little scientific evidence available to define "appropriate" tooth contact patterns (e.g., either static or functional) and to appropriately control mechanical loads and orofacial consequences in SB patients (see Fig 5-7).

As discussed in the previous section, nonspecific stimulation can interrupt SB in the biofeedback system. One putative interpretation for the role of an oral splint is that, when patients wear an oral device during sleep, tooth and mucosal contacts on oral devices (cheek, lip, tongue, and palate) may generate unusual sensory information that warns sleeping patients not to grind their teeth strongly.[98,113] In a few studies where splint therapy reduced SB activity, sleep and EEG parameters (e.g., micro-arousals) were not altered.[119,134] In scientific studies, relevant sensory information (e.g., pain, noise, alarm, name) has been selected and recognized during sleep in humans.[23,135–137] Sleeping humans can be aroused according to the relevance of sensory stimuli. Thus, the intensity of arousal and motor activation can differ in response to stimulus modalities. It remains unknown whether unusual or novel oral sensations with oral devices can have a modifying effect on SB genesis or activity through sensory recognition during sleep (see Fig 5-7). It is also unknown whether patients' habituation to intraoral sensation is associated with short-term effects on sleep bruxism.

Can the increase in SB observed in some patients following the insertion of splints be associated with changes in breathing? When patients with mild to moderate OSAS slept with an occlusal splint, the number of apnea/hypopnea events was increased in 50% of patients and snoring became worse.[138] The interincisal distance during sleep is approximately 0–5 mm, which is equivalent to the thickness of an occlusal splint (usually 3–5 mm at the incisor). The insertion of an oral splint might work as a "wedge" that pushes the mandible backward in a way that exaggerates airway narrowing or collapse. In addition, upper airway patency is influenced not only by jaw position but also by sleeping posture. Interestingly, most SB episodes occur in a supine position, which is a risk for airway collapse and apnea.[66–68,78] Importantly, changes in the jaw position relative to cranial and pharyngeal structures can vary greatly between patients under occlusal splint therapy during sleep, e.g., body and neck positions. It is also noted that respiratory disturbances such as apnea and hypopnea can be found in patients with SB and temporomandibular disorders.[109,139] Clinically, it is relevant for clinicians to ask about a history of OSAS and snoring, or to examine upper pharyngeal structures (uvula, tonsil, tongue) when prescribing an occlusal splint.[140,141] After prescription sleep quality and snoring should be reviewed during follow-up interviews to assess whether respiratory disturbance is exaggerated or induced (e.g., sleep disturbance, daytime sleepiness, morning oral dryness). Finally, remember that disturbed sleep is known to be associated with increased pain sensation, fatigue, and mood changes.[142,143]

### *Comment*

Oral splints are frequently used in the management of sleep bruxism. Since the effects of oral splints on SB are variable and unpredictable, oral splints are used for managing orodental consequences rather than to suppress SB activity. In SB management, however, modulations of jaw movement and motor activity by the oral splint during sleep remain poorly understood. In addition, oral splints may have an effect on other oral functions during sleep, such as respiration. Accordingly, the indication for an oral splint should be evaluated on an individual basis in order to avoid unnecessary aggravation of orodental problems, bruxism, and sleep/respiratory disturbance.

## Conclusion

Current knowledge of trigeminal physiology and the results of physiologic studies on bruxism indicate that tooth contacts are a consequence of jaw-closing muscle activation either during wakefulness or during sleep. Teeth in the maxilla and mandible are separated with a space in the resting or quiet condition. Activation of the central nervous system leading to jaw-closing muscle contraction is necessary to initiate bruxism. Thus, peripheral sensory influences are not the only primary factors in initiating bruxism episodes. Current physiologic information is not enough to understand the physiologic mechanisms that link peripheral factors, bruxism activity, and its consequences. Nonetheless, the clinician's main role is to manage and prevent the associated orodental consequences in peripheral structures (teeth, muscle, joint, implant, and prostheses). Clearly, further studies are needed to clarify the role of peripheral sensory factors in bruxism and to define their clinical and biological significance. It is of importance that practitioners clarify the clinical significance of peripheral or occlusal factors in bruxism bearing in mind integrated concepts of physiology and morphology.

### *Acknowledgment*

The author is supported by the Japanese Society for the Promotion of Science.

## References


1. American Academy of Orofacial Pain. Orofacial Pain: Guidelines for Assessment, Diagnosis, and Management. Chicago: Quintessence, 1996.
2. Lobbezoo F, Naeije M. Bruxism is mainly regulated centrally, not peripherally. J Oral Rehabil 2001;28:1085–1091.
3. Lobbezoo F, Rompré PH, Soucy J-P et al. Lack of association between occlusal–cephalometric measures, side imbalance in striatal D2 receptor binding, and sleep-related oromotor activities. J Orofac Pain 2001;15:64–71.
4. Clark GT, Tsukiyama Y, Baba K, Watanabe T. Sixty-eight years of experimental occlusal interference studies: what have we learned? J Prosthet Dent 1999;82:704–713.
5. De Boever JA, Carlsson GE, Klineberg IJ. Need for occlusal therapy and prosthodontic treatment in the management of temporomandibular disorders. I: Occlusal interferences and occlusal adjustment. J Oral Rehabil 2000;27:367–379.
6. Clark GT, Adler C. A critical evaluation of occlusal therapy: occlusal adjustment procedures. J Am Dent Assoc 1985;110:743–750.
7. Okeson JP. Management of Temporomandibular Disorders and Occlusion. St Louis: Mosby, 2003.
8. Ash MM. Paradigmatic shifts in occlusion and temporomandibular disorders. J Oral Rehabil 2001;28:1–13.
9. Luther F. TMD and occlusion part II. Damned if we don't? Functional occlusal problems: TMD epidemiology in a wider context. Br Dent J 2007;202(3):1–6.

10. Lavigne GJ, Khoury S, Abe S, Yamaguchi T, Raphael K. Bruxism physiology and pathopysiology: an overview for clinicians. J Oral Rehabil 2008;35:476–494.
11. Kato T, Thie NM, Huynh N, Miyawaki S, Lavigne GJ. Topical review: sleep bruxism and the role of peripheral sensory influences. J Orofac Pain 2003;17:191–213.
12. Lavigne GJ, Manzini C, Kato T. Sleep bruxism. In: Kryger MH, Roth T, Dement WC (eds). Principles and Practice of Sleep Medicine, ed 4. Philadelphia: WB Saunders, 2005:946–959.
13. American Academy of Sleep Medicine. International Classification of Sleep Disorders. 2nd ed: Diagnostic and Coding Manual. Rochester: Allen Press, 2005.
14. Rugh JD, Harlan J. In: Jankovic J, Tolosa E (eds). Advances in Neurology. New York: Raven Press, 1988: 329–341.
15. Kato T, Blanchet PJ, Montplaisir JY, Lavigne GJ. Sleep bruxism and other disorders with orofacial activity during sleep. In: Chokroverty S, Hening WA, Walters AS (eds). Sleep and Movement Disorders. Philadelphia: Butterworth–Heinemann, 2003:273–285.
16. Kato T, Dal-Fabbro C, Lavigne GJ. Current knowledge on awake and sleep bruxism: overview. Alpha Omegan 2003;96:24–32.
17. Carskadon MA, Dement WC. Normal human sleep: an overview. In: Kryger MH, Roth T, Dement WC (eds). Principles and Practice of Sleep Medicine. Philadelphia: WB Saunders, 2005:13–23.
18. Lavigne GJ, Rompré PH, Montplaisir J. Sleep bruxism: validity of clinical research diagnostic criteria in a controlled polysomnographic study. J Dent Res 1996;75: 546–552.
19. Lavigne GJ, Rompré PH, Poirier G et al. Rhythmic masticatory muscle activity during sleep in humans. J Dent Res 2001;80:443–448.
20. Carskadon MA, Rechtschaffen A. Monitoring and staging human sleep. In: Kryger MHRT, Dement WC (eds). Principles and Practice of Sleep Medicine. Philadelphia: WB Saunders, 2005:1359–1377.
21. Terzano MG, Parrino L, Mennuni G. Phasic Events and Microstructure of Sleep. Lecce, Italy: AIMS, 1997.
22. Terzano GM, Parrino L, Rosa A, Palomba V, Smerieri A. CAP and arousals in the structural development of sleep: an integrative perspective. Sleep Med 2002;3:221–229.
23. Velluti RA. Interactions between sleep and sensory physiology. J Sleep Res 1997;6:61–77.
24. Halasz P, Terzano M, Parrino L, Bodizs R. The nature of arousal in sleep. J Sleep Res 2004;13:1–23.
25. Trulsson M, Johansson RS. Orofacial mechanoreceptors in humans: encoding characteristics and responses during natural orofacial behaviors. Behav Brain Res 2002;135:27–33.
26. Turker KS, Johnsen SE, Sowman PF, Trulsson MA. Study on synaptic coupling between single orofacial mechanoreceptors and human masseter muscle. Exp Brain Res 2006;170:488–500.
27. Trulsson M. Force encoding by human periodontal mechanoreceptors during mastication. Arch Oral Biol 2007;52:357–360.
28. Orchardson R, MacFarlane SH. The effect of local periodontal anaesthesia on the maximum biting force achieved by human subjects. Arch Oral Biol 1980;25: 799–804.
29. van Steenberghe D, de Vries JH. The influence of local anaesthesia and occlusal surface area on the forces developed during repetitive maximal clenching efforts. J Periodontal Res 1978;13:270–274.
30. Turker KS. Reflex control of human jaw muscles. Crit Rev Oral Biol Med 2002;13:85–104.
31. Lund JP. Mastication and its control by the brainstem. Crit Rev Oral Biol Med 1991;2:33–64.
32. Mäntyvaara J, Sjöholm T, Pertovaara A. Perioral and dental perception of mechanical stimulus among subjects with and without awareness of bruxism. Acta Odontol Scand 2000;58:125–128.
33. Ono Y, Suganuma T, Shinya A, Furaya B, Baba K. Effects of sleep bruxism on periodontal sensation and tooth displacement in the molar region. Cranio 2008;26:282–286.
34. Hidaka O, Morimoto T, Kato T et al. Behavior of jaw muscle spindle afferents during cortically induced rhythmic jaw movements in the anesthetized rabbit. J Neurophysiol 1999;82:2633–2640.
35. Goodwin GM, Luschei ES. Discharge of spindle afferents from jaw-closing muscles during chewing in alert monkeys. J Neurophysiol 1975;38:560–571.
36. Svensson P, Arendt-Nielsen L, Houe L. Muscle pain modulates mastication: an experimental study in humans. J Orofac Pain 1998;12:7–16.
37. Arima T, Arendt-Nielsen L, Svensson P. Effect of jaw muscle pain and soreness evoked by capsaicin before sleep on orofacial motor activity during sleep. J Orofac Pain 2001;15:245–256.
38. Lavigne GJ, Rompré PH, Montplaisir J, Lobbezoo F. Motor activity in sleep bruxism with concomitant jaw muscle pain. Eur J Oral Sci 1997;105:92–95.
39. Camparis CM, Formigoni G, Teixeira MJ et al. Sleep bruxism and temporomandibular disorder: clinical and polysomnographic evaluation. Arch Oral Biol 2006;51: 721–728.
40. Rompre PH, Daigle-Landry D, Guitard F, Montplaisir JY, Lavigne GJ. Identification of a sleep bruxism subgroup with a higher risk of pain. J Dent Res 2007;86: 837–842.
41. Nicholson RA, Lakatos CA, Gramling SE. EMG reactivity and oral habits among facial pain patients in a scheduled-waiting competitive task. Appl Psychophysiol Biofeedback 1999;24:235–247.
42. Kubota K, Tanaka R, Tsuzuki N. Muscle spindle activity and natural sleep in the cat. Jpn J Physiol 1967;17: 613–626.
43. Kubota K, Tanaka R. Fusimotor unit activities and natural sleep in the cat. Jpn J Physiol 1968;18:43–58.

44. Klineberg I. Influences of temporomandibular articular mechanoreceptors in functional jaw movements. J Oral Rehabil. 1980;7:307–317.
45. Abe K, Takata M, Kawamura Y. A study on inhibition of masseteric motor fibre discharges by mechanical stimulation of the temporomandibular joint in the cat. Arch Oral Biol 1973;18:301–304.
46. Chase MH. The digastric reflex in the kitten and adult cat: paradoxical amplitude fluctuations during sleep and wakefulness. Arch Ital Biol 1970;108:403–422.
47. Inoue M, Yamamura K, Nakajima T, Yamada Y. Changes in reflex responses of the masseter and digastric muscles during sleep in freely behaving rabbits. Neurosci Res 1999;34:37–44.
48. van der Bilt A, Ottenhoff FA, van der Glas HW, Bosman F, Abbink JH. Modulation of the mandibular stretch reflex sensitivity during various phases of rhythmic open-close movements in humans. J Dent Res 1997;76:839–847.
49. Lobbezoo F, van der Glas HW, Buchner R, van der Bilt A, Bosman F. Jaw-jerk reflex activity in relation to various clenching tasks in man. Exp Brain Res 1993;93: 139–147.
50. Macaluso GM, Pavesi G, De Laat A. Heteronymous H-reflex in temporal muscle motor units. J Dent Res 1998;77:1960–1964.
51. Chase MH, McGinty DJ. Modulation of spontaneous and reflex activity of the jaw musculature by orbital cortical stimulation in the freely-moving cat. Brain Res 1970;19:117–126.
52. Woda A, Pionchon P, Palla S. Regulation of mandibular postures: mechanisms and clinical implications. Crit Rev Oral Biol Med 2001;12:166–178.
53. Graf H. Bruxism. Dent Clin North Am 1969;13:659–665.
54. Peyron MA, Blanc O, Lund JP, Woda A. Influence of age on adaptability of human mastication. J Neurophysiol 2004;92:773–779.
55. Kato T, Akiyama S, Kato Y, Yamashita S, Masuda Y, Morimoto T. The occurrence of spontaneous functional and nonfunctional orofacial activities in subjects without pain under laboratory conditions: a descriptive study. J Orofac Pain. 2006;20:317–324.
56. Michelotti A, Farella M, Gallo LM et al. Effect of occlusal interference on habitual activity of human masseter. J Dent Res 2005;84:644–648.
57. Tsai CM, Chou SL, Gale EN, McCall WD. Human masticatory muscle activity and jaw position under experimental stress. J Oral Rehabil 2002;29:44–51.
58. Yamashita S, Ai M, Mizutani H. Tooth contact patterns in patients with temporomandibular dysfunction. J Oral Rehabil 1991;18:431–437.
59. Rao SM, Glaros AG. Electromyographic correlates of experimentally induced stress in diurnal bruxists and normals. J Dent Res 1979;58:1872–1878.
60. Piquero K, Sakurai K. A clinical diagnosis of diurnal (non-sleep) bruxism in denture wearers. J Oral Rehabil 2000;27:473–482.
61. Glaros AG, Williams K, Lausten L. The role of parafunctions, emotions and stress in predicting facial pain. J Am Dent Assoc 2005;136:451–458.
62. Katase-Akiyama S, Kato T, Yamashita S, Masuda Y, Motimoto T. Specific increase in non-functional masseter bursts in subjects aware of tooth-clenching during wakefulness. J Oral Rehabil 2008;36:91–101.
63. Chase MH, Morales FR. Control of motoneurons during sleep. In: Kryger MH, Roth T, Dement WC (eds). Principles and Practice of Sleep Medicine, ed 4. Philadelphia: Elsevier Saunders, 2005:154–168.
64. Lavigne GJ, Kato T, Kolta A, Sessle BJ. Neurobiological mechanisms involved in sleep bruxism. Crit Rev Oral Biol Med 2003;14:30–46.
65. Okura K, Kato T, Montplaisir JY, Sessle BJ, Lavigne GJ. Quantitative analysis of surface EMG activity of cranial and leg muscles across sleep stages in human. Clin Neurophysiol 2006;117:269–278.
66. Miyamoto K, Özbeck MM, Lowe AA et al. Mandibular posture during sleep in healthy adults. Arch Oral Biol 1998;43:269–275.
67. Schwab RJ, Kuna ST, Remmers JE. Anatomy and physiology of upper airway obstruction. In: Kryger MH, Roth T, Dement WC (eds). Principles and Practice of Sleep Medicine, ed 4. Philadelphia: Elsevier Saunders, 2005: 983–1000.
68. Powell RM, Zander HA. The frequency and distribution of tooth contact during sleep. J Dent Res 1965;44:713–717.
69. Powell RN. Tooth contact during sleep: association with other events. J Dent Res 1965;44:959–967.
70. Baba K, Clank GT, Watanabe T, Chyma T. Bruxism force detention by a piezo electric fil-based recording device in sleeping humans. J Orofac Pain 2003;17:58–64.
71. Trenouth MJ. Computer analysis of nocturnal tooth-contact patterns in relation to bruxism and mandibular joint dysfunction in man. Arch Oral Biol 1978;23:821–824.
72. Huynh N, Kato T, Rompre PH et al. Sleep bruxism is associated to micro-arousals and an increase in cardiac sympathetic activity. J Sleep Res 2006;15:339–346.
73. Macaluso GM, Guerra P, Di Giovanni G et al. Sleep bruxism is a disorder related to periodic arousals during sleep. J Dent Res 1998;77:565–573.
74. von Gonten AS, Palik JF, Oberlander BA, Rugh JD. Nocturnal electromyographic evaluation of masseter muscle activity in the complete denture patient . J Prosthet Dent 1986;56:624–629.
75. Okeson JP, Phillips BA, Berry DTR et al. Nocturnal bruxing events in healthy geriatric subjects. J Oral Rehabil 1990;17:411–418.
76. Trenouth M. The relationship between bruxism and temporomandibular joint dysfunction as shown by computer analysis of nocturnal tooth contact patterns. J Oral Rehabil 1979;6:81–87.
77. Reding GR, Zepelin H, Robinson JE, Zimmerman SO. Nocturnal teeth-grinding: all-night psychophysiologic studies. J Dent Res 1968;47:786–797.

78. Miyawaki S, Lavigne GJ, Mayer P et al. Association between sleep bruxism, swallowing related laryngeal movement and sleep position. Sleep 2003;26:461–465.
79. Kydd WL, Daly C. Duration of nocturnal tooth contacts during bruxing. J Prosthet Dent 1985;53:717–721.
80. Sjöholm T, Lehtinen I, Helenius H. Masseter muscle activity in diagnosed sleep bruxists compared with non-symptomatic controls. J Sleep Res 1995;4:48–55.
81. Ikeda T, Nishigawa K, Kondo K, Takeuchi H, Clark GT. Criteria for the detection of sleep-associated bruxism in humans. J Orofac Pain 1996;10:270–282.
82. Bader GG, Kampe T, Tagdae T, Karisson S, Blomqvist M. Descriptive physiological data on a sleep bruxism population. Sleep 1997;20:982–990.
83. Satoh T, Harada Y. Electrophysiological study on tooth-grinding during sleep. Electroencephalogr Clin Neurophysiol 1973;35:267–275.
84. Tani K, Yoshii N, Yoshino I, Kobayashi E. Electroencephalographic study of parasomnia: sleep-talking, enuresis and bruxism. Physiol & Behav 1966;1:241–243.
85. Kato T, Rompré PH, Montplaisir JY, Sessle BJ, Lavigne GJ. Sleep bruxism: a oromotor activity secondary to microarousal. J Dent Res 2001a;80:1940–1944.
86. Cassisi JE, McGlynn FD, Belles DR. EMG-activated feedback alarms for the treatment of nocturnal bruxism: current status and future directions. Biofeedback Self-Regul 1987;12:13–20.
87. Kardachi BJ, Bailey JO, Ash MM. A comparison of biofeedback and occlusal adjustment on bruxism. J Periodontol 1978;49:367–372.
88. Rugh JD, Johnson RW. Temporal analysis of nocturnal bruxism during EMG feedback. J Periodontol 1981;52: 263–265.
89. Piccione A, Coates TJ, George JM, Rosenthal D, Karzmark P. Nocturnal biofeedback for nocturnal bruxism. Biofeedback Self Regul 1982;7:405–419.
90. Pierce CJ, Gale EN. A comparison of different treatments for nocturnal bruxism. J Dent Res 1988;67:597–601.
91. Nishigawa K, Kondo K, Takeuchi H, Clark GT. Contingent electrical lip stimulation for sleep bruxism: a pilot study. J Prosthet Dent 2003;89:412–417.
92. Jadidi F, Castrillon E, Svensson P. Effect of conditioning electrical stimuli on temporalis electromyographic activity during sleep. J Oral Rehabil 2008;35:171–183.
93. Watanabe T, Baba K, Yamagata K, Ohyama T, Clark GT. A vibratory stimulation-based inhibition system for nocturnal bruxism: a clinical report. J Prosthet Dent 2001;85:233–235.
94. Nissani M. Can taste aversion prevent bruxism? Appl Psychophysiol Biofeedback 2000;25:43–54.
95. Kato T, Montplaisir JY, Guitard F et al. Evidence that experimentally induced sleep bruxism is a consequence of transient arousal. J Dent Res 2003;82:284–288.
96. Arima T, Svensson P, Rasmussen C et al. The relationship between selective sleep deprivation, nocturnal jaw-muscle activity and pain in healthy men. J Oral Rehabil 2001;28:140–148.
97. Kato T, Thie N, Montplaisir J, Lavigne GJ. Bruxism and orofacial movements during sleep. In: Attanasio R, Bailey DR (eds). Dent Clin North Am. Philadelphia: WB Saunders, 2001:657–684.
98. Thie N, Kato T, Bader G, Montplaisir JY, Lavigne GJ. The significance of saliva during sleep and the relevance of oromotor movements. Sleep Med Rev 2002;6: 213–227.
99. Orr WC. Gastrointestinal functioning during sleep: a new horizon in sleep medicine. Sleep Med Rev 2001;5: 91–101.
100. Freidin N, Fisher MJ, Taylor W et al. Sleep and nocturnal acid reflux in normal subjects and patients with reflux oesophagitis. Gut 1991;32:1275–1279.
101. Bremner RM, Hoeft SF, Costantini M et al. Pharyngeal swallowing: the major factor in clearance of esophageal reflux episodes. Ann Surg 1993;218:364–369; discussion 369–370.
102. Marzio L, Grossi L, Falcucci M et al. Increase of swallows before onset of phase III of migrating motor complex in normal human subjects. Dig Dis Sci 1996;41:522–527.
103. Castiglione F, Emde C, Armstrong D et al. Nocturnal oesophageal motor activity is dependent on sleep stage . Gut 1993;34:1659.
104. Miyawaki S, Tanimoto Y, Araki Y et al. Association between nocturnal bruxism and gastroesophageal reflux. Sleep 2003;26:888–892.
105. Herrera M, Valencia I, Grant M et al. Bruxism in children: effect on sleep architecture and daytime cognitive performance and behavior. Sleep 2006;29:1143–1148.
106. Schwab RJ. Genetic determinants of upper airway structures that predispose to obstructive sleep apnea. Respir Physiol Neurobiol 2005;147:289–298.
107. Ferguson KA, Lowe AA. Oral appliances for sleep-disordered breathing. In: Kryger MH, Roth T, Dement WC (eds). Principles and Practice of Sleep Medicine, ed. 4, Philadelphia: WB Saunders, 2005:1098–1108.
108. Villaneuva AT, Buchanan PR, Yee BJ, Grunstein RR. Ethnicity and obstructive sleep apnea. Sleep Med Rev. 2005;9:419–436.
109. Kato T. Sleep bruxism and its relation to obstructive sleep apnea-hypopnea syndrome. Sleep Biol Rhythms 2004; 2:1–15.
110. Okeson JP, Phillips BA, Berry DTR, Cook YR, Cabelka JF. Nocturnal bruxing events in subjects with sleep-disordered breathing and control subjects. J Craniomandib Disord 1991;5:258–264.
111. Sjöholm TT, Lowe AA, Miyamoto K, Fleetham JA, Ryan CF. Sleep bruxism in patients with sleep-disordered breathing. Arch Oral Biol 2000;45:889–896.
112. Ohayon MM, Li KK, Guilleminault C. Risk factors for sleep bruxism in the general population. Chest 2001;119: 53–61.
113. Dao TTT, Lavigne GJ. Oral splints: the crutches for temporomandibular disorders and bruxism? Crit Rev Oral Biol Med 1998;9:345–361.

114. Rugh JD, Solberg WK. Electromyographic studies of bruxist behavior before and during treatment. J Calif Dent Assoc 1975;3:56–59.
115. Rugh JD, Graham GS, Smith JC, Ohrbach RK. Effects of canine versus molar occlusal splint guidance on nocturnal bruxism and craniomandibular symptomatology. J Craniomandib Disord 1989;3:203–210.
116. Solberg WK, Clark GT, Rugh JD. Nocturnal electromyographic evaluation of bruxism patients undergoing short term splint therapy. J Oral Rehabil 1975;2: 215–223.
117. Clark GT, Beemsterboer PL, Solberg WK, Rugh JD. Nocturnal electromyographic evaluation of myofascial pain dysfunction in patients undergoing occlusal splint therapy. J Am Dent Assoc 1979;99:607–611.
118. Okkerse W, Brebels A, De Deyn PP et al. Influence of a bite-plane according to Jeanmonod, on bruxism activity during sleep. J Oral Rehabil 2002;29:980–985.
119. Dube C, Rompre PH, Manzini C et al. Quantitative polygraphic controlled study on efficacy and safety of oral splint devices in tooth-grinding subjects. J Dent Res 2004;83:398–403.
120. van der Zaag J, Lobbezoo F, Wicks DJ et al. Controlled assessment of the efficacy of occlusal stabilization splints on sleep bruxism. J Orofac Pain 2005;19:151–158.
121. Harada T, Ichiki R, Tsukiyama Y, Koyano K. The effect of oral splint devices on sleep bruxism: a 6-week observation with an ambulatory electromyographic recording device. J Oral Rehabil 2006;33:482–488.
122. Baad-Hansen L, Jadidi F, Castrillon E, Thomsen PB, Svensson P. Effect of a nociceptive trigeminal inhibitory splint on electromyographic activity in jaw closing muscles during sleep. J Oral Rehabil 2007;34:105–111.
123. Hasegawa K, Okamoto M, Nishigawa G, Oki K, Minagi S. The design of non-occlusal intraoral appliances on hard palate and their effect on masseter muscle activity during sleep. Cranio 2007;25:8–15.
124. Landry ML, Rompre PH, Manzini C et al. Reduction of sleep bruxism using a mandibular advancement device: an experimental controlled study. Int J Prosthodont 2006; 19:549–556.
125. Bailey JO, Rugh JD. Effect of occlusal adjustement on bruxism as monitored by nocturnal EMG recordings. J Dent Res 1980;59:317.
126. Rugh JD, Barghi N, Drago CJ. Experimental occlusal discrepancies and nocturnal bruxism. J Prosthet Dent 1984;51:548–553.
127. Ash MM. Occlusion: reflections on science and clinical reality. J Prosthet Dent 2003;90:373–384.
128. Lobbezoo F, van der Zaag J, van Selms MK, Hamburger HL, Neaije M. Principles for the management of bruxism. J Oral Rehabil 2008;35:509–523.
129. Amemori Y, Yamashita S, Ai M et al. Influence of nocturnal bruxism on the stomatognathic system. I: A new device for measuring mandibular movements during sleep. J Oral Rehabil 2001;28:943–949.
130. Yugami K, Yamashita S, Ai M, Takahashi J. Mandibular positions and jaw-closing muscle activity during sleep. J Oral Rehabil 2000;27:697–702.
131. Minagi S, Akamatsu Y, Matsunaga T, Sato T. Relationship between mandibular position and the coordination of masseter muscle activity during sleep in humans. J Oral Rehabil 1998;25:902–907.
132. Nishigawa K, Bando E, Nakano M. Quantitative study of bite force during sleep associated bruxism. J Oral Rehabil 2001;28:485–491.
133. Bakke M. Mandibular elevator muscles: physiology, action, and effect of dental occlusion. Scand J Dent Res 1993;101:314–331.
134. Nagels G, Okkerse W, Braem M et al. Decreased amount of slow wave sleep in nocturnal bruxism is not improved by dental splint therapy. Acta Neurol Belg 2001;101: 152–159.
135. Perrin F, Garcia-Larrea L, Mauguiere F, Bastuji H. A differential brain response to the subject's own name persists during sleep. Clin Neurophysiol 1999;110:2153–2164.
136. Lavigne G, Brousseau M, Kato T et al. Experimental pain perception remains equally active over all sleep stages. Pain 2004;110:646–655.
137. Kato T, Montplaisir JY, Lavigne GJ. Experimentally induced arousals during sleep: a cross-modality matching paradigm. J Sleep Res 2004;13:229–238.
138. Gagnon Y, Mayer P, Morisson F, Rompre PH, Lavigne GJ. Aggravation of respiratory disturbances by the use of an occlusal splint in apneic patients: a pilot study. Int J Prosthodont 2004;17:447–453.
139. Smith MT, Wickwire EM, Grace EG et al. Sleep disorders and their association with laboratory pain sensitivity in temporomandibular joint disorder. Sleep 2009;32: 779–790.
140. Bailey DR. Oral evaluation and upper airway anatomy associated with snoring and obstructive sleep apnea. Dent Clin North Am 2001;45:715–732.
141. Lavigne GJ, Goulet JP, Zuconni M, Morrison F, Lobbezoo F. Sleep disorders and the dental patient: an overview. Oral Surg Oral Med Oral Pathol Oral Radiol Endod 1999;88:257–272.
142. Haack M, Mullington JM. Sustained sleep restriction reduces emotional and physical well-being. Pain 2005; 119:56–64.
143. Moldofsky H. Sleep and pain. Sleep Med Rev 2001;5: 385–396.

Chapter 6

# Emotional Factors in the Etiology of Bruxism

*Daniele Manfredini*

## Introduction

Masticatory muscle activities can be divided into functional and parafunctional types. The former are mastication, phonation, deglutition, and all those complex activities grouped under the term "cognitive–behavioral" functions. Parafunctions include bruxism, teeth grinding and clenching, and habits such as biting of nails, objects, and lips, chewing gum, etc.

Bruxism is a stereotyped oral motor disorder characterized by awake and/or sleep-related grinding and/or clenching of the teeth.[1] Bruxism, and parafunctional activities in general, occur in the presence of weakened protective reflexes, and are characterized by enormous occlusal contact forces mainly in a horizontal direction, by a relative occlusal instability, and by isometric muscular contractions. These forces place a great strain on the stomatognathic structures, so pathologic effects of bruxism on these structures are possible and easily comprehensible.

The effect of bruxism with regard to tooth wear, and the relationship between bruxism and temporomandibular disorders (TMD), have been extensively discussed in the literature. Bruxism is considered the most detrimental among all the parafunctional activities of the stomatognathic system, and is a major risk factor for TMD. Nevertheless, there are still many unsolved issues concerning the etiology of bruxism itself.

The etiology of bruxism is certainly a complex and debated issue (see Chapter 4). Most authors suggest a central etiology, but the theory according to which occlusal interferences represent a neuromuscular stimulus capable of triggering such activities has not been abandoned. The study of bruxism is complicated by some diagnostic and taxonomic aspects that have prevented us from achieving an acceptable standardization of diagnosis until recently.

A major concern for researchers approaching this phenomenon is the definition of bruxism itself, which is a term grouping different entities.[2]

For example, sleep and awake bruxism seem to suggest a different pathogenesis, but they are difficult to distinguish clinically.[3] Similarly, a clearer distinction between detected bruxism and perceived bruxism should be made.[4] Unfortunately, bruxism as a pathophysiologic entity can be detected only by means of polysomnographic recordings, the application of which is limited by high cost and the shortage of adequately equipped sleep laboratories.[5]

For these reasons, a set of clinical criteria was developed to screen patients for sleep studies.[6] Although a clinical approach to bruxism diagnosis still remains incomplete, not allowing a distinction between the different types, the criteria present the easiest and most adopted method to gather data in large-sample preliminary studies.

In particular, one of the factors for which pilot data are required is description of temperamental traits that characterize bruxers. According to some authors,[2,7] psychiatric factors could be involved in the etiopathogenesis of bruxism, and parafunctional activities in general. This seems to be supported by reviews suggesting a shift from peripheral (i.e., occlusal) to central (i.e., stress, emotion, personality) regulation theories.[5,8,9]

Many etiological theories have been proposed over the years, but a multifactorial model seems to be the most plausible,[3,10,11] according to which psychosocial and pathophysiological factors interact with morphological–peripheral factors. In this chapter, the role of psychosocial and emotional factors will be discussed.

## Literature Search

A systematic search of the National Library of Medicine's database was performed in April 2007, to identify all peer-reviewed papers in the English literature dealing with the possible relationship between bruxism and psychosocial factors. The search strategy included combinations of the term "bruxism" (which yielded 1947 citations if used alone) with search words "stress", "anxiety", "depression", "psychological factors", and "psychosocial factors". Clinical studies assessing the psychosocial traits of bruxers (by using questionnaires, interviews, and instrumental and laboratory exams) and reviews discussing the contribution of those factors to the etiology of bruxism were included in this review.

Titles and abstracts obtained from the above search were screened according to the inclusion criteria for possible inclusion in the review, and all studies that appeared to meet the above criteria were then retrieved as complete articles. Abstracts providing unclear data were also retrieved as full text articles in order to avoid excluding papers of possible relevance.

The search strategy provided a total of 255 abstracts, including 42 reviews, for the combined search terms "bruxism + stress". Screening of the abstracts showed that 45 papers (9 reviews) were relevant and satisfied the inclusion criteria.

The search terms "bruxism + anxiety" yielded 68 citations, partly overlapping with those identified with "bruxism + stress", and allowed us to retrieve six other relevant citations, of which none was a review. Six further relevant citations (no reviews) were obtained by the terms "bruxism + depression", which yielded a total of 46 citations.

The combined terms "bruxism + psychosocial factors" (22 citations) and "bruxism + psychological factors" (19 citations) were subgroups of the others, and no other relevant citations were retrieved by using these combined search terms.

The search was also extended to related articles in the Medline Plus database, but no other papers satisfying the inclusion criteria were identified. Thus, a total of 57 relevant papers (9 reviews) were obtained as full reports and are discussed in the review.

In this chapter, discussion will start with an appraisal of the available findings about the association between bruxism and stress, which for many years was supposed to be the main etiological theory to explain bruxing behavior. Psychosocial profiles of bruxers, which derive mainly from questionnaire studies adopting several different psychometric tools, are described, followed by presentation of some shortcomings of the current literature and considerations for future research.

## Bruxism and Stress

It is a common opinion that bruxism in general is somehow related to stress. This belief is typical of patients who usually report an increase in their night-time teeth grinding during stressful life periods, and of clinicians who often attribute a patient's bruxing behavior to an increase in stress.

This theory is based on some early case series by Rugh and co-workers, who reported a relationship between stressful daily events and an increase in nocturnal masseter muscle activity.[12–15] In particular, a case report of a young woman whose nocturnal electromyographic (EMG) activity was recorded over a 140-day period and put into the context of her daily pain and stress levels strengthened the conviction that a stress–bruxism association existed.[16] This single case report showed that nocturnal EMG activity increased immediately after stressful events (school exams, meeting with parents, fights with partner, etc.) and that pain levels increased shortly after. At present, the reports by Rugh and co-workers are the only papers in which nocturnal EMG activity is linked to stress. Indeed, as described later in this chapter, successive case studies[17] and experimental work[18,19] have failed to demonstrate such an association.

### *Clinical Data*

Apart from the early reports by Rugh, the bruxism–stress association has been reported by some investigations adopting a clinical and/or self-reported diagnosis of bruxism. Ahlberg and co-workers[20] investigated the association between perceived bruxism and stress experience in the work environment. In a sample of 1,784 employees of a broadcasting company, the authors investigated the frequency of bruxism with a self-assessed questionnire, reporting that frequent bruxers claimed more stress. Subsequent papers by the same group posted similar findings,[21,22] so that the authors claimed that bruxism may reveal an ongoing stress in normal work life.

Another large-population study in which self-assessment was taken as the criterion to diagnose bruxism reported that a "highly stressful life" may be a significant risk factor.[23] These findings supported those of a questionnaire investigation on 511 undergraduate students, who reported more stress in association with bruxism,[24] but they were not in line with those from a similarly designed large-sample study reporting no association between awareness of bruxism and age, gender, marital status, occupation, and stress in general.[25]

With regard to the clinical diagnosis of bruxism, a set of screening-oriented clinical diagnostic criteria was proposed in 1996 by Lavigne and co-workers[6] The criteria were that the patient exhibited, at least five nights a week, grinding bruxism sounds during sleep during the last 6 months, as reported by his/her bed partner, and at least one of the following adjunctive criteria: observation of tooth wear or shiny spots on restorations; report of morning masticatory muscle fatigue or pain; or masseteric hypertrophy on digital palpation. Unfortunately, no paper has addressed the specific issue of the bruxism–stress relationship by adoption of clinical criteria. However, an increase in stress sensitivity with respect to non-bruxers was shown in a group of clinically diagnosed bruxers who fulfilled a battery of tests investigating the whole anxiety spectrum.[26,27]

An animal model study has suggested that emotional stress induces bruxism-like activity in the masseter muscle of rats, which was reduced with anti-anxiety drugs.[28]

Nonetheless, the studies described above do not allow us to draw certain conclusions owing to a number of shortcomings that affect their design and limit the generalization of their findings. The most striking limitation is the subjectivity of the self-report diagnosis of bruxism. Several researchers have shown that patients' self-report of bruxism is not reliable at a diagnostic level, since it may be influenced by both clinician and patient conviction of having a bruxing behavior.[4,29] Furthermore, cross-study comparisons are hardly applicable, since homogeneity of diagnostic criteria for both bruxism and stress levels exist only within work by the same group. Thus, the combination of two parameters whose standardization is difficult at the diagnostic level has prevented us from achieving satisfactory findings with clinical research alone.

### EMG Data

At present, polysomnographic recordings in adequately equipped sleep laboratories represent the standard of reference for the diagnosis of bruxism,[3,5,6] but the approach has found less application than expected because of obvious logistic and economic problems. Portable EMG devices, which record the activity of masticatory muscles during sleep in the habitual environment, reduce costs and limit patients' discomfort, representing an acceptable instrument in the research setting.[19,30]

Unfortunately, only few electromyographic longitudinal investigations have been performed to study the bruxism–stress association.[17-19] Taken together, these studies accounted for a total of 113 patients, with a mean of 15.8 recordings per patient. In general, the available data do not support findings from the early report by Rugh and Harlan,[15] since no relationship was described between EMG-detected sleep bruxism and either experienced stress (the day before the recording night) or anticipatory stress (the day following the recording night).

Pierce and co-workers,[18] in a study on 100 sleep bruxers over a 15-night recording period, found a lack of association between bruxism and stress in 92% of the study population. Watanabe and co-workers[19] found no association of bruxism with any of the daytime self-monitored states (among which were stress levels and sleep quality) of the subjects in a 3-week study of 12 sleep bruxers. These (negative) findings were supported by the single case study by Van Selms and co-workers,[17] which is noteworthy in its attempt to describe fluctuations in daytime and night-time EMG masseter activity over a long time period.

Thus, it seems that available data from EMG-based research do not support the hypothesis of a strict bruxism–stress relationship. This conclusion must be viewed with caution since, as in the case of clinical studies, generalization of results is not possible owing to the paucity of studies, and patients and research groups involved. A more extensive use of portable devices to achieve home EMG recordings is needed, and standardization of bruxism diagnosis and a comparison of results between different investigations should be easier to achieve.

### Stress Diagnosis

The problem of standardization also affects the diagnosis of "stress". Several different criteria have been adopted in the literature, ranging from dichotomic ("stressed" or "not stressed") to ordinal (i.e., nominative rating scales) or numeral (i.e., visual analog scale (VAS) rating) variables. So, interstudy dishomonogeneity should be reduced in future research, possibly with the adoption of a VAS scale, at least until some other assessment instrument has been validated and demonstrated to be superior in both the clinical and research settings.

### Comment

Despite the literature shortcomings, it appears that the clinical and research approaches to the bruxism–stress relationship give opposite indications, with the former suggesting that such a relationship may exist while the latter is unable to demonstrate it in the evidence-based field. At least two biologically plausible reasons can be suggested to explain this controversy.

- The relationship seems to be much more complex than previously imagined, involving many complex psychosocial aspects and disorders, such as anxiety, depression, and personality traits.
- A clearer distinction between sleep and awake bruxism and between grinding and clenching types of bruxism has to be made at the diagnostic level in the attempt to identify the actual pathogenetic pathways underlining these conditions.

These are not mutually exclusive. They will be discussed in the next sections of this chapter.

## Psychosocial Aspects of Bruxism

Despite some controversial aspects, work on the bruxism–stress relationship has seen consistent suggestions that peripheral sensory influences play a minor role in the pathogenesis of bruxism,[9,31] while factors related to the central nervous system (CNS) seem to have much more importance.[3,5] Among these, an interesting issue is that of psychosocial aspects of bruxism and psychiatric disorders associated with it. As with the bruxism–stress studies, the majority of the literature is based on self-reported or clinical diagnosis of bruxism.

The work by Pierce and co-workers[18] was the only EMG study in this field, and found no association between sleep bruxism and personality variables, such as anxiety, depression, and irritability. In contrast, a controlled polysomnographical study of vigilance and reaction time found an increased level of anxiety in sleep bruxers.[32]

Clinically oriented studies have shown that some symptoms related to anxiety disorders have a significantly higher prevalence in bruxers than in non-bruxers,[27,33–35] and that a number of both depressive and manic symptoms of the mood spectrum seem to be present in bruxers.[26,36]

Bruxism has also been associated with emotional tension,[37] psychosomatic disorders,[38] hostility,[39] aggressiveness,[40] apprehension and a tendency to worrying,[41] and psychiatric disorders such as schizophrenia.[42]

In general, results from these studies are supportive of an association of bruxism with a number of psychosocial disorders, and are in contrast with the early results from Harness and Peltier,[43] who found that bruxism was not associated with psychological disturbance as measured by the Minnesota Multiphasic Personality Inventory (MMPI). This investigation was performed on a sample of chronic facial pain patients, thus precluding a comparison with findings from other studies and preventing one from making any conclusion about an actual relationship between bruxism and psychological factors. Indeed, it is well recognized that facial pain is associated with a number of psychiatric and psychosocial disorders.[44–48] Such an association relates mainly to anxiety disorders in the acute stage of pain and depressive disorders in the chronic phase,[49] and does not depend on pain location.[50] Nonetheless, facial pain may be associated with bruxism as well.[51,52]

Thus, the study of bruxism in this context is complicated by the relationships that both bruxism and psychosocial variables have with facial pain. An example supporting this position comes from the study by Camparis and Siqueira,[53] who reported significant differences in the psychosocial profile of bruxers with and without chronic facial pain.

In view of these considerations, a brief discussion of the bruxism–pain relationship may be useful to provide a more comprehensive approach to the study of the role of emotional factors in the etiology of bruxism.

## The Relationship between Bruxism and Pain

It is a common belief among general practitioners that bruxism is a cause of TMD pain, arising from the clinical observation that pain in the muscles of mastication is a frequent accompanying symptom. Nevertheless, pain is not present in *every* bruxer, so the existence of bruxism-related pain is a controversial issue.

Data from the literature come mostly from studies assessing the prevalence of muscular and temporomandibular joint pain in populations of subjects who reported to be bruxers and from investigation of bruxism prevalence in samples of patients with or without facial pain. Even though some support for the association between teeth clenching and facial pain has been provided,[53,54–56] some studies reported no association between bruxism and muscle sensitivity and an association between clenching and joint sounds only.[57,58] Thus, the argument for a cause-and-effect relationship between bruxism and TMD pain is still debated.[51]

At present, there is only one study comparing the prevalence of bruxism in a population of patients with different TMD, as diagnosed with the Research Diagnostic Criteria for TMD, and a control sample of healthy subjects.[52] The clinical diagnosis of bruxism was adopted to perform a large-scale investigation, and an association between bruxism and TMD, and myofascial pain in particular, was reported.

The hypothesis of a clinical association of bruxism with muscle disorders is in agreement with the experimental work of Glaros and co-workers,[59] who demonstrated that sustained low-level parafunctional activities can result in post-training pain in some individuals, and with that of Svensson and Arendt-Nielsen,[60] who reported temporary increases in pain following submaximal clenching. Furthermore, according to Glaros and co-workers,[61] such a low-level activity can also produce arthralgia. Bruxism has often been blamed as the source of traumatic joint load that leads to degenerative joint disease[62] and progressive softening and loss of cartilage.[63,64]

In general, the above findings suggest that an association may exist between bruxism and TMD as a whole, and myofascial pain in particular, but evidence proving the other criteria for a causal relationship is still lacking. An evaluation of the possible cause-and-effect implications of bruxism and TMD pain has to take into account several factors:

- The association must be strong and consistent.
- A dose–response effect should be evident (i.e., the risk of developing TMD increases with the severity of bruxism).
- Possible explanatory pathophysiologic pathways should be identified.
- A temporal relationship should exist between the supposed causal factor and the pathology (i.e., bruxism should be present *before* the onset of TMD symptoms).

Therefore, as with bruxism and stress, it seems that a contrast exists between widely diffused opinions and scientific data.

A dose–response causal relationship between bruxism and TMD pain has been suggested by Molina and co-workers,[55] who reported that severe bruxers had a higher prevalence of specific muscle and joint disorders when compared with mild and moderate bruxers and with a group of non-bruxing TMD patients.

Several hypotheses have been postulated to describe the possible pathophysiologic pathways through which bruxism could induce TMDs, suggesting that parafunctional activities might cause ischemic lesions or traumatic damage in the muscles of mastication and that myofascial pain occurs in bruxers with a low resistance to fatigue.[65]

Nonetheless, the temporal criteria for a causal relationship is hard to demonstrate owing to the daily fluctuations of bruxism events[2,8,66,67] and of TMD symptoms,[68–70] and poor correspondence with the epidemiologic characteristics of the disorders.[51]

Lavigne and co-workers[71] found that bruxers with concomitant jaw muscle pain have fewer episodes per hour of sleep than bruxers without myofascial pain. This suggests that bruxism is not the primary cause of jaw muscle pain, and points to the need to investigate whether the reduced number of bruxism episodes is pain related or whether it is due to an influence of pain on sleep. In line with such findings, a recent investigation found no significant relationship between self-reported bruxism and TMD pain.[72]

Taken together, the findings are a picture of the complexity of the problem, and strengthen the need to achieve a better distinction between the many forms of bruxism, which are probably related at different levels with both psychosocial factors and painful symptomatology.

## Sleep versus Awake Bruxism, and Grinding versus Clenching

Bruxism while awake is commonly characterized by clenching, while sleep bruxism has a combination of clenching and grinding.[2,5] Despite being often grouped together and generically referred to as "bruxism", these disorders may have different etiologies and be influenced by different local and systemic factors. Also, there is some consensus that there is greater association of clenching-type activity during the day with jaw pain compared with sleep grinding.[73–75] Thus it appears logical that efforts should be made to discriminate between sleep and awake bruxism at the etiologic, diagnostic, and therapeutic levels.

The study of relationships between bruxism and stress, psychosocial disorders, and pain is open to severe bias owing to the interrelationships at both single-variable and multi-variable levels. Hence there may be some benefit from an approach that takes into account differences between wake and sleep bruxism, and between grinding and clenching. Indeed, it is likely that divergence of opinions and the contrasting results reported so far might be explained by the heterogeneity of bruxer populations. It might be the reason why the early findings of Rugh and co-workers[12–16] have not been confirmed by successive EMG studies on sleep bruxers.[17–19]

The case reports of Rugh and co-workers described bruxers who were recruited on the basis of the presence of painful symptoms, while subsequent EMG studies included sleep bruxers independent of their complaint of pain in the facial area. The selection of a group of pain-referring bruxers is a possible source of bias affecting the early reports on the bruxism–stress association, since they included a third variable (pain) without assessing its influence on the two variables under study (bruxism and stress). This consideration seems to be strengthened by successive work from the same group,[76] which reported a lack of habituation to experimentally induced stress in subjects with TMD. Such findings, which provided support for the hypothesis that TMD patients and healthy subjects respond differently to stress in terms of habituation to stressful stimuli, have been strengthened by other reports,[77–79] indicating that the stress–bruxism relationship described in the early EMG studies was likely to depend on the inclusion of TMD patients only.

Moreover, patient selection bias may be at the root of differences between findings of studies adopting self-diagnosis of bruxism and those performing EMG recordings in sleep laboratories. Self-referral of bruxism is mainly based on patients' perception of pain in the muscles of mastication in the morning, which is related to daily clenching[80] and not to sleep bruxism.[19]

These observations suggest that the association between bruxism and a number of psychosocial disorders described in many studies may depend on patient selection criteria, which are suited more to detecting daily clenchers rather than sleep bruxers. On the other hand, polysomnographic diagnosis of bruxism actually detects sleep grinders, since increases in muscle potential, to be clearly identified as bruxism, have to be correlated to the loud "grinding sound".[2] Therefore, reported data may actually reflect an association of stress and psychosocial disorders with clenching and not with bruxism as a whole.

This hypothesis was suggested by Olkinuora,[38] who claimed that daytime clenching is a response to stress and that daytime clenchers' scores on psychological tests would be higher in emotional disturbance than subjects who brux and grind their teeth nocturnally. To support this hypothesis, EMG-based work by Rao and Glaros[81] suggested that emotional and situational factors may be important in the etiology of awake bruxism.

Taken together, these observations point toward the suggestion that awake bruxism (clenching) and sleep bruxism (grinding) have to be considered two different disorders.

Sleep bruxism has been repeatedly demonstrated to be part of a complex arousal response of the CNS,[1,8,82–84] occurring during changes in sleep depth, and accompanied by gross body movements, the appearance of K-complexes in the electroencephalogram (EEG), increased heart rate, respiratory changes, peripheral vasoconstriction, and increased muscle activities.[85] Unfortunately, at present there are no definitive findings about the possible influence of emotional factors on such CNS activation, and scarce literature exists about their influence on other parasomnia. Therefore, future studies on sleep bruxism and stress (and/or psychosocial disorders) might benefit from investigation of the other parasomnia, since many considerations expressed for sleep bruxism in this chapter – the poor correspondence between self-reported symptoms and objective findings, the poor correspondence between findings of experimental and clinical studies, and diagnostic difficulties – can be extended to other parasomnias, such as the restless leg syndrome.[86]

In contrast, bruxism during wakefulness (clenching) is likely to be a result of emotional tension or psychosocial disorders that force the subject to respond with a prolonged contraction of masticatory muscles. According to this viewpoint, recent findings of a possible association with the complex spectrum of mood disorders[26,36] are worthy of further investigation. An association between awake bruxism and depression was quite unpredictable, and it was detected almost casually with the administration of a complete battery of tests for the evaluation of two psychopathological spectra, which aimed primarily at evaluating the bruxism–anxiety association.[26] The hypothesis that awake clenching is strictly related to depression, or even being an expression of a depressed mood, is fascinating and found some support in the psychiatric literature – suggesting that bipolar patients are characterized by disturbances in the central neurotransmitter system which may also be involved in the etiology of bruxism.[87,88]

Future work should try to describe common neurological deficits or pathogenetic pathways between manic and depressive disorders and bruxism, if they exist. In this sense, there is a need to clarify the role of some neurotransmitters, and dopamine in particular, which might be key factors in the pathogenesis of both bipolar disorders and bruxism.

Similarly, the actual link between anxiety and stress and awake bruxism has to be better defined. Indeed, awake bruxism may be the result of a transitory anxious reaction to stressful daily events (state anxiety), or a phenomenon related to a more complex psychopathological disorder (trait anxiety). Data based on the use of questionnaires have linked bruxism to both types of anxiety,[26,34,35,81] even though most data come from studies adopting psychiatric instruments that are mainly suitable to detect trait anxiety.

These considerations seem to suggest the existence of an awake bruxism personological profile, strictly related to the sphere of mood and anxiety disorders, even though it has not yet been defined.

Obviously, these aspects are hard to investigate for many reasons. Indeed, the difficulty of diagnosing awake bruxism,[4] in combination with difficulties in standardizing psychosocial diagnoses outside the psychiatric setting,[89,90] and the complexity of the relationships that both variables have with pain,[51,91] makes comparison of results from different studies difficult and represents an obstacle to the design of unbiased investigations.

Nevertheless, although definitive proof is still lacking, there are several indications that the importance of emotional and psychosocial factors is different in awake and sleep bruxism, suggesting that efforts have to be made toward a better definition of these disorders in both etiologic and diagnostic terms.

## Conclusion

The role of emotional factors in the etiology of bruxism is probably one of the most debated issues concerning this disorder. Despite the first studies dating back more than 30 years, definite conclusions cannot be drawn. Factors such as the concurrent presence of pain, which may be strongly linked to psychopathology, act as confounding variables. The selection of heterogeneously diagnosed samples of bruxers is a principal reason for the different findings that have been reported in the literature. Nonetheless, some indications can be suggested to inspire future research.

Despite most data on the etiology and characteristics of bruxism coming from sleep lab studies, there is a paucity of literature on the role of stress and psychosocial disorders in polysomnographically monitored bruxers. These few studies failed to demonstrate an association with any of the investigated psychosocial factors, so dismantling the early hypothesis of a strict bruxism–stress relation.

In contrast, the majority of data concerning an association between psychosocial disorders and bruxism come from studies utilizing a clinical and/or self-report diagnosis of bruxism. In general, these studies showed some sort of association of bruxism with anxiety, stress sensitivity, depression, and other psychological characteristics, apparently in contrast with sleep lab investigations. A plausible explanation is that the latter type of study is more suitable to detect awake bruxism (clenching), while the classical polysomnographic studies focused only on sleep bruxism (grinding). Thus, awake clenching is associated with emotional factors and a number of psychopathological symptoms, while there are no elements to relate sleep bruxism with psychosocial disorders.

Future investigations should be directed toward the achievement of a better distinction between the two forms of bruxism in order to facilitate the design of research studies.

## References

1. De Laat A, Macaluso GM. Sleep bruxism is a motor disorder. Mov Disord 2002;17(2):S67–69.
2. Lobbezoo F, Naeije M. Bruxism is mainly regulated centrally, not peripherally. J Oral Rehabil 2001;28:1085–1091.
3. Bader G, Lavigne GJ. Sleep bruxism: overview of an oromandibular sleep movement disorder. Sleep Med Rev 2000;4:27–43.
4. Marbach JJ, Raphael KG, Janal MN, Hirschkorn-Roth R. Reliability of clinician judgement of bruxism. J Oral Rehabil 2003;30:113–118.
5. Lavigne GJ, Kato T, Kolta A, Sessle BJ. Neurobiological mechanisms involved in sleep bruxism. Crit Rev Oral Biol Med 2003;14:30–46.
6. Lavigne GJ, Romprè PH, Montplaisir JY. Sleep bruxism: validity of clinical research diagnostic criteria in a controlled polysomnographic study. J Dent Res 1996;75: 546–552.
7. Manfredini D, Landi N, Romagnoli M, Cantini E, Bosco M. Etiopathogenesis of parafunctional activities of the stomatognathic system. Minerva Stomatol 2003;52:339–349.
8. Kato T, Thie NM, Montplaisir JY, Lavigne GJ. Bruxism and orofacial movements during sleep. Dent Clin North Am 2001;45:657–684.
9. Kato T, Thie N, Huynh N, Miyawaki S, Lavigne GJ. Topical review: sleep bruxism and the role of peripheral sensory influences. J Orofac Pain 2003;17:191–213.
10. Attanasio R. An overview of bruxism and its management. Dent Clin North Am 1997;41:229–241.
11. Lavigne GJ, Manzini C. Bruxism. In: Kryger MH, Roth T, Dement WC (eds). Principles and Practice of Sleep Medicine. Philadelphia: WB Saunders, 2000:773–785.
12. Rugh JD, Solberg WK. Electromyographic studies of bruxist behaviour before and during treatment. J Calif Dent Assoc 1975;3:56–59.
13. Clark GT, Rugh JD, Handelman SL. Nocturnal masseter muscle activity and urinary catecholamine levels in bruxers. J Dent Res 1980;59:1571–1576.

14. Rugh JD. Psychological stress in orofacial neuromuscular problems. Int Dent J 1981;31:202–205.
15. Rugh JD, Harlan J. Nocturnal bruxism and temporomandibular disorders. Adv Neurol 1988;49:329–341.
16. Rugh JD, Lemke RL (eds). Behavioral Health: a Handbook of Health Enhancement and Disease Prevention. New York: John Wiley, 1984.
17. Van Selms MKA, Lobbezoo F, Wicks DJ, Hamburger HL, Naeije M. Craniomandibular pain, oral parafunctions, and psychological stress in a longitudinal case study. J Oral Rehabil 2004;31:738–745.
18. Pierce CJ, Chrisman K, Bennett ME, Close JM. Stress, anticipatory stress, and psychologic measures related to sleep bruxism. J Orofac Pain 1995;9:51–56.
19. Watanabe T, Ichikawa K, Clark GT. Bruxism levels and daily behaviors: 3 weeks of measurement and correlation. J Orofac Pain 2003;17:65–73.
20. Ahlberg J, Rantala M, Savolainen A et al. Reported bruxism and stress experience. Community Dent Oral Epidemiol 2002;30:405–408.
21. Ahlberg K, Ahlberg J, Kononen M et al. Reported bruxism and stress experience in media personnel with or without irregular shift work. Acta Odontol Scand 2003;61:315–318.
22. Ahlberg J, Savolainen A, Rantala M, Lindholm H, Kononen M. Reported bruxism and biopsychosocial symptoms: a longitudinal study. Community Dent Oral Epidemiol 2004;32:307–311.
23. Ohayon MM, Li KK, Guilleminault C. Risk factors for sleep bruxism in the general population. Chest 2001;119: 53–61.
24. Hicks RA, Conti P. Nocturnal bruxism and self-reports of stress-related symptoms. Percept Mot Skills 1991;72:1182.
25. Melis M, Abou-Atme YS. Prevalence of bruxism awareness in a Sardinian population. Cranio 2003;21:144–151.
26. Manfredini D, Landi N, Romagnoli M, Bosco M. Psychic and occlusal factors in bruxers. Aust Dent J 2004;49:84–89.
27. Manfredini D, Landi N, Fantoni F, Segù M, Bosco M. Anxiety symptoms in clinically diagnosed bruxers. J Oral Rehabil 2005;32:584–588.
28. Rosales VP, Ikeda K, Hizaki K et al. Emotional stress and brux-like activity of the masseter muscle in rats. Eur J Orthod 2002;24:107–117.
29. Chung SC, Kim YK, Kim HS. Prevalence and patterns of nocturnal bruxofacets on stabilization splints in temporomandibular disorder patients. Cranio 2000;18:92–97.
30. Gallo LM, Lavigne GJ, Romprè P, Palla S. Reliability of scoring EMG orofacial events: polysomnography compared with ambulatori recordings. J Sleep Res 1997;6:259.
31. Manfredini D, Landi N, Tognini F, Montagnani G, Bosco M. Occlusal features are not a reliable predictor for bruxism. Minerva Stomatol 2004;53:231–239.
32. Major M, Rompré PH, Guitard F et al. A controlled daytime challenge of motor performance and vigilance in sleep bruxers. J Dent Res 1999;78:54–62.
33. Heller RF, Forgione AG. An evaluation of bruxism control: massed negative practice and automated relaxation training. J Dent Res 1976;54:1120–1123.
34. Da Silva AM, Oakley DA, Hemmings KW, Newman HN, Watkins S. Psychosocial factors and tooth wear with a significant component of attrition. Eur J Prosthodont Restor Dent 1997;5:51–55.
35. Kampe T, Edman G, Bader G, Tagdae T, Karlsson S. Personality traits in a group of subjects with long-standing bruxing behaviour. J Oral Rehabil 1997;24:588–593.
36. Manfredini D, Ciapparelli A, Dell'Osso L, Bosco M. Mood disorders in subjects with bruxing behavior. J Dent 2005;33:485–490.
37. Ramfjord SP. Bruxism, a clinical and electromyographic study. J Am Dent Assoc 1961;62:21–44.
38. Olkinuora M. Psychosocial aspects in a series of bruxists compared with a group of non-bruxists. Proc Finn Dent Soc 1972;68:200–208.
39. Molina OF, dos Santos J. Hostility in TMD/bruxism patients and controls: a clinical comparison study and preliminary results. Cranio 2002;20:282–288.
40. Takemura T, Takahashi T, Fukuda M et al. A psychological study on patients with masticatory muscle disorder and sleep bruxism. Cranio 2006;24:191–196.
41. Fischer WF, O'Toole ET. Personality characteristics of chronic bruxers. Behav Med 1993;19:82–86.
42. Winocur E, Hermesh H, Littner D et al. Signs of bruxism and temporomandibular disorders among psychiatric patients. Oral Surg Oral Med Oral Pathol Oral Radiol Endod 2007;103:60–63.
43. Harness DM, Peltier B. Comparison of MMPI scores with self-report of sleep disturbance and bruxism in the facial pain population. Cranio 1992;10:70–74.
44. Madland G, Feinman C, Newman S. Factors associated with anxiety and depression in facial arthromyalgia. Pain 2000;84:225–232.
45. Mongini F, Ciccone J, Ibertis F, Negro C. Personality characteristics and accompanying symptoms in temporomanibular joint dysfunctions, headache and facial pain. J Orofac Pain 2000;14(1):52–58.
46. Dworkin SF, Sherman J, Mancl L. Reliability, validity, and clinical utility of the Research Diagnostic Criteria for Temporomandibular Disorders Axis II Scales: Depression, Non-Specific Physical Symptoms, and Graded Chronic Pain. J Orofac Pain 2002;16(3):207–220.
47. Yap AUJ, Tan KBC, Chua EK, Tan HH. Depression and somatization in patients with temporomandibular disorders. J Prosthet Dent 2002;88:479–484.
48. Yap AUJ, Dworkin SF, Chua EK et al. Prevalence of temporomandibular disorders subtypes, psychologic distress and pshychisocial dysfunction in asian patients. J Orofac Pain 2003;17(1):21–28.
49. Gatchel RJ, Garofalo JP, Ellis E, Holt H. Major psychological disorders in acute and chronic TMD: an initial examination. J Am Dent Assoc 1996;127:1365–1374.

50. Manfredini D, Bandettini di Poggio A, Romagnoli M et al. Mood spectrum in patients with different painful temporomandibular disorders. Cranio 2004;22(3):234–240.
51. Lobbezoo F, Lavigne GJ. Do bruxism and temporomandibular disorders have a cause-and-effect relationship? J Orofac Pain 1997;11:15–23.
52. Manfredini D, Cantini E, Romagnoli M, Bosco M. Prevalence of bruxism in patients with different research diagnostic criteria for temporomandibular disorders (RDC/TMD) diagnoses. Cranio 2003;21:279–285.
53. Camparis CM, Siqueira JT. Sleep bruxism: clinical aspects and characteristics in patients with and without chronic orofacial pain. Oral Surg Oral Med Oral Pathol Oral Radiol Endod 2006;101:188–193.
54. Moss RA, Lombardo TW, Villarosa GA et al. Oral habits and TMJ dysfunction in facial pain and non-pain subjects. J Oral Rehabil 1995;22:79–81.
55. Molina OF, Dos Santos J, Nelson SJ, Nowlin T. A clinical study of specific signs and symptoms of CMD in bruxers classified by the degree of severity. Cranio 1999;17: 268–279.
56. Ciancaglini R, Gherlone E, Radaelli G. The relationship of bruxism with craniofacial pain and symptoms from the masticatory system in the adult population. J Oral Rehabil 2001;28:842–848.
57. Gavish A, Halachmi M, Winocur E, Gazit E. Oral habits and their association with signs and symptoms of temporomandibular disorders in adolescent girls. J Oral Rehabil 2000;27:22–32.
58. Winocur E, Gavish A, Finkelshtein T, Halachmi M, Gazit E. Oral habits among adolescent girls and their association with symptoms of temporomandibular disorders. J Oral Rehabil 2001;28:624–629.
59. Glaros AG, Forbes M, Shanker J, Glass EG. Effect of parafunctional clenching on temporomandibular disorder pain and propioceptive awareness. Cranio 2000;18:198–204.
60. Svensson P, Arendt-Nielsen L. Effects of five days of repeated submaximal clenching on masticatory muscle pain and tenderness:an experimental study. J Orofac Pain 1996;10:330–338.
61. Glaros AG, Tabacchi K, Glass EG. Effect of parafunctional clenching on temporomandibular disorder pain. J Orofac Pain 1998;12:145–152.
62. Haskin CL, Milam SB, Cameron IL. Pathogenesis of degenerative joint disease in the human temporomandibular joint. Crit Rev Oral Biol Med 1995;6:248–277.
63. Quinn JH. Pathogenesis of temporomandibular joint chondromalacia and arthralgia. Oral Maxillofac Surg Clin North Am 1989;1:47–57.
64. Herb K, Cho S, Stiles MA. Temporomandibular joint pain and dysfunction. Curr Pain Headache Rep 2006;10: 408–414.
65. Lund JP. Pain and the control of muscles. Adv Pain Res Ther 1995;21:103–115.
66. Lavigne GJ, Goulet JP, Zucconi M, Morisson F, Lobbezoo F. Sleep disorders and the dental patient. An overview. Oral Surg Oral Med Oral Pathol Oral Radiol Endod 1999;88:257–272.
67. Lavigne GJ, Guitard F, Romprè PH, Montplaisir JY. Variability in sleep bruxism activity over time. J Sleep Res 2001;10:237–244.
68. Svensson P, Graven-Nielsen T. Craniofacial muscle pain: review of mechanisms and clinical manifestations. J Orofac Pain 2001;15:117–145.
69. Magnusson T, Egermark I, Carlsson GE. Treatment received, treatment demand, and treatment need for temporomandibular disorders in 35-year-old subjects. Cranio 2002;20:11–17.
70. Lobbezoo F, van Selms MKA, Naeije M. Masticatory muscle pain and disordered jaw motor behaviour: literature review. Arch Oral Biol 2006;51:713–720.
71. Lavigne GJ, Romprè PH, Montplaisir JY, Lobbezoo F. Motor activity in sleep bruxism with concomitant jaw muscle pain: a retrospective pilot study. Eur J Oral Sci 1997;105:92–95.
72. Van der Meulen MJ, Lobbezoo F, Aartman IHA, Naeije M. Self-reported oral parafunctions and pain intensity in temporomandibular disorder patients. J Orofac Pain 2006;20:31–35.
73. Pergamalian A, Rudy TE, Zaki HS, Greco CM. The association between wear facets, bruxism, and severity of facial pain in patients with temporomandibular disorders. J Prosthet Dent 2003;90(2):194–200.
74. Glaros AG, Burton E. Parafunctional clenching, pain and effort in temporomandibular disorders. J Behav Med 2004;27:91–100.
75. Glaros AG, Williams K, Lausten L. The role of parafunctions, emotions and stress in predicting facial pain. J Am Dent Assoc 2005;136:451–458.
76. Katz JO, Rugh JD, Hatch JP et al. Effect of experimental stress on masseter and temporalis muscle activity in human subjects with temporomandibular disorders. Arch Oral Biol 1989;34:393–398.
77. Maixner W, Sigurdsson A, Booker D, Fillingim R. Sensitivity of patients with painful temporomandibular disorders to experimentally evoked pain. Pain 1995;63:341–351.
78. Jones DA, Rollmann GB, Brooke RI. The cortisol response to psychological stress in temporomandibular dysfunction. Pain 1997;72:171–182.
79. Ohrbach R. Psychophisiological assessment of stress in chronic pain: comparison of stressful stimuli and of response systems. J Dent Res 1998;77:1840–1850.
80. Dao TTT, Lund JP, Lavigne GJ. Comparison of pain and quality of life in bruxers and patients with myofascial pain of the masticatory muscles. J Orofac Pain 1994;8:350–356.
81. Rao SM, Glaros AG. Electromyographic correlates of experimentally induced stress in diurnal bruxists and normals. J Dent Res 1979;58:1872–1878.

82. Macaluso GM, Guerra P, Di Giovanni G et al. Sleep bruxism is a disorder related to periodic arousal during sleep. J Dent Res 1998;77:565–573.
83. Kato T, Montplaisir JY, Guitard F et al. Evidence that experimentally induced sleep bruxism is a consequence of transient arousal. J Dent Res 2003;82:284–288.
84. Huynh N, Kato T, Romprè PH et al. Sleep bruxism is associated to micro-arousals and an increase in cardiac sympathetic activity. J Sleep Res 2006;15:339–346.
85. Thorpy MJ. Glossary of terms used in sleep disorders medicine. In: Thorpy MJ (ed). Handbook of Sleep Disorders. New York: Marcel Dekker, 1990:779–795.
86. Hornyak M, Riemann D, Voderholzer U. Do periodic leg movements influence patients' perception of sleep quality? Sleep Med 2004;5:596–600.
87. Lobbezoo F, Soucy JP, Hartman NG, Montplaisir JY, Lavigne GJ. Effects of the dopamine D2 receptor agonist bromocriptine on sleep bruxism: report of two single-patient clinical trials. J Dent Res 1997;76:1611–1615.
88. Craddock N, Davè S, Greening J. Association studies of bipolar disorder. Bipolar Disord 2001;3:284–298.
89. Cassano GB, Michelini S, Shear K et al. The Panic–Agoraphobic Spectrum: a descriptive approach to the assessment and treatment of subtle symptoms. Am J Psychiatry 1997;154:27–38.
90. Dell'Osso L, Pini S, Tundo A et al. Clinical characteristics of mania, mixed mania, and bipolar depression with psychotic features. Compr Psychiatry 2000;41:242–247.
91. Rollman GB, Gillepsie JM. The role of psychosocial factors in temporomandibular disorders. Curr Rev Pain 2000;4:71–81.

Chapter 7

# Movement Disorders in the Dental Office

*Frank Lobbezoo, Hans L. Hamburger, and Machiel Naeije*

## Introduction

Patients who suffer from movement disorders – or dyskinesias – involuntarily move either too much (hyperkinesia) or too little (hypokinesia). The term "dyskinesia" originates from the Greek language and literally means "difficulty in moving". Dyskinesias are characterized by an impairment of the power of voluntary movement, resulting in fragmentary or incomplete movements. Most dyskinesias are attributable to a dysfunction of the basal ganglia and related structures, and of the cerebellum. Dopamine-mediated neural circuits (e.g., the extrapyramidal motor system) are frequently involved in the physiopathology of movement disorders. Patients with dyskinesias often suffer from cognitive, motivational, and emotional impairments as well. For reviews, see Kurlan,[2] Müller and co-workers,[3] and Wolters and Van Laar.[4]

There is a need for clear definitions and unambiguous classification systems of the various dyskinesias. From a phenomenologic point of view, dyskinesias can be divided[3] into three main types:

- *akinesia*, an absence or poverty of movements
- *ataxia*, a failure of muscular coordination, resulting in an irregularity of muscular action
- *hyperkinesia*, an abnormally increased motor function.

Hyperkinesias can be subdivided into several subtypes: *tremor* (a trembling or quivering); *dystonia* (a disordered tonicity of muscle); and *jerk* (a sudden reflex or movement). Jerks can be subdivided again into four more types: *tic* (a compulsive, repetitive, stereotyped movement, often resembling a purposeful movement); *chorea* ("dance" in Greek: a ceaseless occurrence of a wide variety of rapid, highly complex, jerky movements that seem well-coordinated but are in fact performed involuntarily); *myoclonus* (a fast, shock-like contraction of a part of a muscle, an entire muscle, or a group of muscles); and *ballism* (a violent, flinging movement).

All of these (sub)types of dyskinesias can, alone or in various combinations, be part of several neurologic disorders, such as Parkinson's disease

This chapter is based on: Lobbezoo and Naeije.[1]

(among others characterized by hypokinesia, tremor, and muscular rigidity).

Further, it is important to note that dyskinesias can differ regarding their *age of onset* (childhood, adolescence, adult), their *etiology* (primary/idiopathic or secondary/iatrogenic), and their *distribution*. The distribution can be focal (one body part involved), segmental (two neighboring body parts involved), multifocal (two or more non-neighboring body parts involved), "hemi" (only one side of the body involved), or generalized (the entire body involved).

Clearly, dyskinesias constitute a complex group of conditions that require the attention of highly skilled medical specialists, including neurologists and psychiatrists, for their diagnosis and treatment.[4] Despite that, dental clinicians are confronted with such disorders as well.

- First, dyskinesias can, at least in part, be located in the orofacial area (for an extensive review, see Jankovic and Tolosa[5]). Reportedly, such orofacial movement disorders may even have "dental" causes and consequences. They can also complicate the "regular" dental management of the patients involved.
- Second, dyskinesias that do not involve the oral or orofacial area can still be a complicating factor in the management of dental problems (e.g., owing to difficulties in stabilizing the head). Unfortunately, literature regarding the dental implications of (oral/orofacial) movement disorders is still scarce, as are curriculum guidelines for dental schools on this subject.

The purpose of the next section, therefore, is to provide a review of the available literature that deals with movement disorders in the dental office.

## Literature Search

As a first step, a Medline search was performed in April 2006, using the National Library of Medicine's Medical Subject Headings (MeSH) database and PubMed. As MeSH terms, "movement disorders" and "dentistry" were used. Both terms were exploded as to include the terms found below these terms in the MeSH tree. Consequently, the term "movement disorders" includes conditions such as Gilles de la Tourette syndrome, Huntington's disease, and Parkinson's disease, while the term "dentistry" represents the entire dental discipline. When Medline was searched with these terms and when the English language was used as a search limit, 112 papers were found, the oldest of them being published in 1963. Fourteen out of these 112 papers were reviews, while the remainder mainly concerned case reports or case series.

As a second step, the selected papers were read as to establish the papers' applicability to this review. Thirty-one papers were thus omitted from the review. The omitted papers dealt, for example, with temporomandibular disorders,[6,7] with the dental treatment of elderly patients in general,[8,9] with the clinical competence of clinicians who are professionally impaired as a result of an accident,[10] with dental fear in a special needs clinic population,[11] or with gait disturbances following iliac crest graft harvesting for intraoral augmentation.[12] The remaining 81 papers yielded an interesting view on the dental implications of movement disorders, which is outlined below.

## Dyskinesias

The selected papers deal with a wide variety of movement disorders, including the following conditions (in alphabetical order): Gilles de la Tourette syndrome, Hallervorden–Spatz disease, Huntington's disease, idiopathic torsion dystonia, oral dyskinesias, palsy, Parkinson's disease, Rett syndrome, and Wilson's disease. Below, these conditions will all be described briefly, along with their dental implications.

### *Gilles de la Tourette Syndrome*

Multiple uncoordinated movements, especially tics of the face, and voice utterances are the main characteristics of Gilles de la Tourette syndrome, a disorder that begins in childhood or adolescence. The typical vocal tics can vary from words to entire phrases, and when coprolalia (involuntary swearing) is present they may sometimes have an embarrassing nature. A characterisic oral feature of Gilles de la Tourette syndrome is self-mutilation, such as intense tongue, lip, and cheek biting.[13,14] In addition, the medications prescribed for the syndrome (e.g., haloperidol, pimozide, clonidine) may have oral side-effects, such as hyposalivation with its adverse consequences for the periodontal and dental tissues.[12]

To illustrate the important contribution of the dentist in the management of the orofacial aspects of Gilles de la Tourette syndrome, a few case reports are summarized. To control his severe tongue biting, a 13-year-old boy was treated with 5–15 mg haloperidol, which was only partly effective. At the age of 16, he was finally managed satisfactorily by wearing dental splints in both the mandible and the maxilla.[15] In a case of upper lip collapse due to severe biting, an acrylic splint was successfully placed in a 13-year-old boy.[16] In another extreme case of self-mutilation, a 4-year-old girl who exhibited self-extraction of teeth and generalized oral and facial pain due to overload, a splint was successfully provided as well.[17] However, a splint failed in another case of Gilles de la Tourette syndrome: a 12-year-old boy lost three of his maxillary incisors despite wearing such a device.[18]

In the dental management of Gilles de la Tourette syndrome, the dentist must be aware of the psychological status, medication regimen, and motor deficits that may influence the dental status and oral hygiene procedures. To that end, the patient's neurologist or psychiatrist should be consulted. In addition, it should be noted that the patient's condition may worsen owing to the stress of the dental visit. Thus, stress should be minimized by creating a safe environment and dividing the dental procedures into small segments. In line with these recommendations, major focus should be put on preventive measures, so that extensive dental treatments can be avoided.[13] If extensive treatments are necessary after all, intravenous sedation with midazolam can be used; in a case of a 13-year-old boy, 6 mg of midazolam successfully inhibited all tics for a total duration of about 30 minutes. In the same patient, a long treatment of about 2.5 hours was successfully completed under general anesthesia.[19]

### *Hallervorden–Spatz Disease*

Characteristic of Hallervorden–Spatz disease is a high deposit of iron in the brain. This rare neurodegenerative disorder has an autosomal-recessive mode of inheritance. The clinical course is variable and includes progressive dystonia, rigidity, chorea, and mental deterioration. As with Gilles de la Tourette syndrome, orodental self-mutilations have been reported. In the case of a 7-year-old boy, these were successfully managed by placement of upper and lower soft polyvinyl bite-guards.[20]

### *Huntington's Disease*

Huntington's disease is a progressive, autosomal-dominant disorder that is mainly characterized by choreatic movements and dementia. It usually has its onset in the fourth or fifth decade of life, but younger individuals (even children under 10 years of age) may be affected.[21] In the orofacial area, grimacing and speech difficulties can occur.[22] In the terminal phases of the disease, dysphagia frequently occurs. Aspiration of food can then lead to death.[23]

Dental treatment of patients with Huntington's disease is hindered by mouth and jaw movements.[24,25] Nevertheless, timing and patience may allow a procedure without sedation, even when the procedure concerns a morphologically difficult endodontic treatment.[26] However, sedation cannot always be avoided, especially when extensive procedures are necessary. In the literature, several cases are described in which suggestions are given for safe anesthetic procedures in the usually frail, elderly, uncooperative, and malnourished Huntington's disease patient.[27–31] As an illustration, an implant–overdenture procedure was successfully carried out under general anesthesia in a 51-year-old male patient, yielding a clear improvement in the patient's chewing function.[32]

### *Idiopathic Torsion Dystonia*

Idiopathic torsion dystonia is an autosomal-dominant disorder with a focal, segmental, or generalized distribution and is characterized by slow, involuntary turning and torsion movements of the neck, trunk, and/or limbs. Also, spasms of the facial, lingual, and masticatory muscles may be present. In that case, major orodental problems may be encountered, such as difficulties in chewing and in wearing full dentures. Edentulous torsion dystonia patients may then benefit from implant-supported overdentures.[33]

Spasmodic torticollis, a non-orofacial, focal torsion dystonia of the neck, may render dental treatment difficult. Adequate sedation can then be achieved with incrementally and intravenously administered midazolam, with a total of 30 mg,[34] an approach similar to the one described by van der Bijl and Roelofse[35] for enabling the dental management of a patient with a generalized spastic nerve/muscle disorder. Spasmodic torticollis itself is frequently managed with injections of botulinum toxin in the neck musculature. As rare oral side-effects of this treatment, salivary stasis and dry mouth have been reported, which are possibly the consequence of paralyzing the smooth muscles of the salivary ducts.[36] Clinicians should be aware of this possibility.

### *Oral Dyskinesias*

Unlike most of the other movement disorders in this review – which are mainly generalized conditions that may also affect the orofacial region or that may influence dental status or management without involving the muscles of the face and masticatory system – some focal dyskinesias exclusively affect the orofacial area. A detailed, clinical overview of this group of conditions can be found in Thomas,[37] and Blanchet and co-workers[38] Below, a brief review of the various oral dyskinesias is given, using the papers of the present Medline search and following the framework suggested by Blanchet and co-workers. According to them, oral dyskinesias can be divided into orofacial dyskinesias and oromandibular dystonias. In turn, both types of oral dyskinesias can be subdivided into three subtypes – idiopathic, tardive, and "dental" disorders – the last two subtypes having an iatrogenic nature.

Orofacial dyskinesias consist of involuntary, mainly choreatic movements of the face, lip, tongue, and jaw. The idiopathic subtype of the disorder may be due to, for example, an underlying psychiatric disease or overdoses of dopamine medications.[38–40] Further, the chronic use of neuroleptica (antipsychotic drugs) may cause tardive diskinesia.[38,40–42] In addition, certain dental conditions, especially edentulousness, and dental procedures like an inadequate prosthesis have been suggested – mainly on the basis of case studies – as possible causes for orofacial dyskinesias.[38–40,43,44] However, as for the "dental" oromandibular dystonias (see below), valid conclusions regarding the existence of a "dental" subtype of orofacial dyskinesias cannot be drawn owing to the poor level of evidence.

Oromandibular dystonias are characterized by excessive, involuntary, and sustained muscle contractions of the lips, tongue, and jaw. Sporadically, idiopathic oromandibular dystonia occurs as an isolated disorder in adults. As a possible underlying cause for this disorder, a defective physiologic inhibitory control of the basal ganglia over the thalamus and brain stem has been suggested.[38] The tardive subtype of oromandibular dystonias is due to a chronic exposure to antipsychotic drugs,[38] while "dental" oromandibular dystonia is thought to be due to dental interventions or orodental traumas.[38] However, it should be stressed that evidence for the existence of this subtype is based mainly on case reports[45] or case series,[46] which makes it difficult to draw valid conclusions or to give recommendation for the prevention of this disorder.

In line with the purported dental causes of orofacial dyskinesias, several papers report improvement of the movement disorder after proper dental rehabilitation. Sutcher and co-workers[47] and Sutcher and Kutz[48] report the successful management of (partially) edentulous patients with orofacial dyskinesia, in whom the existing dentures were replaced with carefully constructed new dentures. As an important step in the treatment, a splint was worn that could be adjusted in the vertical dimension and occlusion until maximum symptom reduction of the movement disorder was achieved. A similar case was described by Mack.[49] Watanabe and co-workers[50] electromyographically monitored the success of their dental treatment of two oral dyskinesia patients. Following meticulous denture work and extraction of "lost" teeth, a remarkable decrease in discharges of the masticatory muscles was detected. In a subsequent series of 22 patients with oral dyskinesia, dental treatment yielded improvement or even disappearance of symptoms in about 75% of the cases.[50] Although the prosthetic approach of oral dyskinesia thus seems promising, Blanchet and co-workers[38] argue that conclusions are hard to draw from these mainly anecdotal papers. Nevertheless, this issue certainly warrants further attention.

The condition where oromandibular dystonia is combined with blepharospasm (i.e., a tonic spasm of the orbicularis oculi muscle, producing a more or less complete closure of the eyelids) is known as Meige syndrome or Brueghel syndrome.[51] This segmental dyskinesia is an adult-onset disorder. Its slow and intense dystonic movements can be triggered by normal activities such as emoting, reading, watching television, fatigue, or speech. In line with the above-described prosthetic alleviation of oromandibular dystonias, a 67-year-old female patient with Brueghel syndrome, who was rehabilitated with oral implants and a mandibular overdenture, showed a remarkable improvement of her masticatory and speech abilities that were sustained during a 5-year follow-up. Even though her blepharospasm worsened, implant-overdenture treatment of edentulous patients with Meige syndrome seems promising with regard to restoration of oral functions.[51]

### *Palsy*

Palsy, or paralysis, may affect the orofacial muscles. Several types of facial palsy can be distinguished, including cerebral palsy, bulbar palsy, and Bell's palsy. Non-progressive brain damage (i.e., an intracranial lesion) may lead to cerebral palsy, usually before the age of 3 years. The condition is characterized by involuntary movements, resulting, *inter alia*, from tremor and chorea. Cerebral palsy patients are difficult to treat for their dental problems, despite case reports on, for example, the successful treatment with implant-supported overdentures of such a patient.[52] Most importantly, the patient's head must be stabilized during treatment.[53] This can be achieved by special head stabilizers[54] or by nitrous oxide inhalation, which reduces the central motor neuron pool excitability to an extent that controllable and comfortable dental management is possible.[55]

Bulbar palsy is mostly seen in patients over 50 years. The condition is due to motor changes in the medulla oblongata and, since it affects respiration, it is fatal. In the orofacial region, the muscles of the lips, tongue, and face are frequently involved, including the masticatory muscles. Consequently, bulbar palsy patients have difficulty in chewing, swallowing, and phonating. One of the first symptoms of this condition may be changes in the retention of dentures. Therefore, by considering all possible causes for ill-fitting dentures, the dental clinician plays an important role in recognizing bulbar palsy.[56]

Bell's palsy is the most common facial palsy and can be present in patients from all age groups. It is a unilateral, facial paralysis with a sudden onset that is caused by a lesion or an inflammation of the facial nerve. Commonly, the herpes simplex virus is involved.[57] Bell's palsy patients mainly suffer from accumulation of food debris in the vestibule and of dental plaque on the affected side. Further, saliva tends to leak from the affected side, which may in turn cause angular stomatitis. A strict oral hygiene protocol should therefore be followed.[14]

### *Parkinson's Disease*

More than 40% of the papers that were selected with the present Medline search deal with Parkinson's disease. Among these papers, some thorough reviews can be found.[14,58–62] From these reviews, it can be learnt that Parkinson's disease is an irreversible, extrapyramidal disorder that usually occurs in the middle and late years of life. The disorder is characterized by hypokinesia, tremor, muscular rigidity, and a shuffling gait. The etiology of the disease is not completely understood. The presence of mercury-containing amalgam fillings, as a suggested dental cause, could not be associated with an increased risk of Parkinson's disease.[63]

In the present concise review, emphasis will be put on the orodental aspects of Parkinson's disease. In the orofacial region, Parkinsonian tremor may affect the tongue and/or the lips, which in turn affects oral functions such as mastication, swallowing, and speech,[64] but not oral perception.[65,66] Interestingly, speech was shown to improve greatly after bilateral chronic stimulation of the subthalamic nucleus.[67] As possible side-effects of the dopamine medications that are frequently prescribed to manage the disease, movements of tongue ("fly-catching") and lips ("pursing") may also be dyskinetic. The face of Parkinson's disease patients is typically expressionless – "mask-like".[14,58–62]

The most commonly encountered oral manifestations of Parkinson's disease are difficulty performing oral hygiene measures, xerostomia, burning mouth/mucositis, difficulty swallowing, drooling of saliva, and less caries (with more teeth) than age-matched controls,[68–76] Most of these oral manifestations are due to changes in salivary flow in relation to the medications of these patients, rather than to the Parkinson's disease itself.[62] The observation of less caries and more teeth was made by Persson and co-workers,[69] who compared 30 patients with a population sample of almost 600 individuals. Although this paper is frequently cited, including in some of the above-mentioned reviews, and although the result was repeated in other studies,[75] some authors question the validity of the observation. Indeed, it seems in contrast with the also frequently encountered, medicine-related xerostomia and the often poor oral hygiene.[61]

Dental treatment of patients with Parkinson's disease requires some special precautions.[62] First, clinicians must be aware of the progressive and multidimensional nature of the disorder; preventive measures and early interventions are desirable so as to prevent extensive procedures during the later phases of the disorder. Walshe,[25] Jolly and co-workers,[58] Collins,[77] Kieser and co-workers,[59] and Alexander and Gage[60] give clear sets of practical advice (e.g., scheduling issues, chair positioning) for practitioners who treat patients with Parkinson's disease. Preventive measures and treatment plans should be compatible with the patient's physical, cognitive, and behavioral abilities. Clear communication with the patient, caregivers, and other healthcare providers is thereby pivotal, as are considerable patience and understanding.[14,78] The dental management of Parkinson's disease patients can, however, be successful only when a multidisciplinary approach is followed, including a dietician and a speech therapist.[61] Optimization of patients' quality of life as well as that of caregivers is one of the most important treatment goals. This sometimes necessitates extra effort on the part of the dental clinician in terms of planning the required procedures so as to meet the needs of the patient and his/her caregiver.[79]

The dental treatment of Parkinson's disease patients is further illustrated by a number of case reports. In one of these, periodontal surgery in a woman with Parkinson's disease was possible only using intravenous sedation with diazepam (Valium) supplemented with $NO/O_2$ inhalation and regular dental anesthesia.[80] In another case, propofol and midazolam were used to obtain sufficient relaxation for a successful dental treatment.[34] As an alternative to sedation, the required level of muscle relaxation for the fabrication of full dentures was achieved by electrical muscle stimulation in yet another case report of a patient with Parkinson's disease.[81] To manage the swallowing difficulties associated with Parkinson's disease, special intraoral training appliances have been designed.[82] Of further interest for the clinician, bite plates of various materials and designs are recommended by several authors to prevent soft tissue biting between meals, to reduce masticatory muscle pain, and to protect the teeth from chattering.[83–85] Finally, since Parkinson's disease patients notably suffer from malfunctioning full dentures, the use of implant-supported overdentures yields a remarkable improvement in their chewing abilities, and thus in their quality of life.[86–89] Regional anesthesia in combination with intravenous midazolam is recommended for such surgical procedures in Parkinson's disease patients.[89]

### *Rett Syndrome*

Rett syndrome is a hereditary, progressive, neurodegenerative disorder that exclusively affects women from birth. Its main oral manifestation is bruxism. Owing to the progressive nature of Rett syndrome, the accompanying bruxism should be treated so as to prevent further attrition and discomfort.[90]

### *Wilson's Disease*

A disordered copper metabolism may lead to the autosomal-recessive disorder Wilson's disease. This is characterized by degeneration of certain parts of the brain, especially the basal ganglia, and may express itself, *inter alia*, by tremor, drooling, and an indistinct speech. When dental restorations are indicated in Wilson's disease patients, copper-containing amalgam alloys should be avoided. Masticatory function and speech benefit most from fixed reconstructions; full dentures without implant support should be avoided.[91–93]

## Conclusion

From the above concise review, it can be gathered that movement disorders may have a profound impact on dentistry. Not only do the majority of generalized dyskinesias have focal manifestations in the orofacial region, but there are also several conditions that exclusively affect the orofacial area. Further, a disorder such as spasmodic torticollis renders dental treatments difficult without having a direct effect on the head and face. The oral manifestations of dyskinesias are in part directly related to the disorder, and in part secondary to the medications that are being used to alleviate the disorder. Practitioners should be able to recognize the oral manifestations and, when they are properly trained, to manage them adequately. When the clinician's training (or experience) falls short, he or she should be able to properly refer the patient to a special needs dental clinic. In most instances, a multidisciplinary approach is necessary, including the medical specialists involved.

From the present review, it can be gathered that implant-supported overdentures are commonly suggested for the oral rehabilitation of these patients. Obviously, when considering such reconstructions, not only should the possible difficulties that may be encountered during the treatment phase be given enough thought, but also the patient's ability (or that of its caregiver) to keep an adequate level of oral hygiene.

The MeSH term "movement disorders" encompasses a whole array of conditions. Only about half of these conditions were included in the present review. Apparently, disorders such as essential tremor (a relatively common familial tremor that includes, *inter alia*, the tongue and head) and Shy–Drager syndrome (a progressive neurodegenerative condition of the central and autonomic nervous systems that may include Parkinsonian-like disturbances and that is characterized by atrophy of the preganglionic lateral horn neurons of the thoracic spinal corda) have so far not been studied in relation to dentistry. Interestingly, the movement disorders branch of the MeSH tree does not include (sleep) bruxism, even though this condition is defined as "a stereotyped movement disorder characterized by grinding or clenching of the teeth (during sleep)".[94] With a prevalence of about 10%,[95] bruxism is undoubtedly the commonest of all movement disorders (a relatively common movement disorder such as Parkinson's disease has a prevalence of only about 100–200 per 100,000 inhabitants[96]).

Clearly, bruxism has been studied and reviewed extensively in relation to dentistry (for reviews outside the present volume, see, e.g., Kato and co-workers,[97] Lavigne and co-workers,[98] and Lobbezoo and co-workers[99]), and this condition was not the subject of the present review. Nevertheless, it may be desirable that the National Library of Medicine (of which the MeSH database is a service) adds "(Sleep) Bruxism" to the movement disorders branch of the MeSH tree, so as to update its controlled vocabulary according to the most recent definition of this condition.

An important issue is related to the level of evidence of the papers that are included in the present review. Most of the included papers are case reports or case series. This is undoubtedly related to the low prevalence of most movement disorders, which makes other study designs with a higher level of evidence difficult to conduct. Although all included papers yield important indications of possible associations and effective treatments, definitive evidence is lacking. A careful interpretation of the findings is therefore warranted. In the field of movement disorders in relation to dentistry, there is a striking lack of methodologically sound studies. In our aging populations, it is a challenge for all of us to improve the quality of this emerging field, for the sake of this sometimes greatly infirm category of patients.

## References

1. Lobbezoo F, Naeije M. Dental implications of some common movement disorders; a concise review. Arch Oral Biol 2007;52:395–398.
2. Kurlan R. Treatment of Movement Disorders. Philadelphia: JB Lippincott, 1995.
3. Müller F, Dichgans J, Jankovic J. Dyskinesias. In: Brandt T, Caplan LR, Dichgans J, Diener HC, Kennard C (eds). Neurological Disorders: Course and Treatment. San Diego, CA: Academic Press, 1996:779–795.
4. Wolters EC, Van Laar T. Bewegingsstoornissen. Amsterdam: VU Uitgeverij, 2003.
5. Jankovic J, Tolosa E. Facial dyskinesias. In: Advances in Neurology, vol 49. New York: Raven Press, 1998.
6. Agerberg G, Carlsson GE. Functional disorders of the masticatory system. II: Symptoms in relation to impaired mobility of the mandible as judged from investigation by questionnaire. Acta Odontol Scand 1973;31:337–347.
7. Solberg WK. Temporomandibular disorders: masticatory myalgia and its management. Br Dent J 1986;160:351–356.
8. Hoad-Reddick G. Organization, appointment planning, and surgery design in the treatment of the older patient. J Prosthet Dent 1995;74:364–366.
9. Chiappelli F, Bauer J, Spackman S et al. Dental needs of the elderly in the 21st century. Gen Dent 2002;50:358–363.
10. Raborn GW, Carter RM. Using simulation to evaluate clinical competence after impairment. J Can Dent Assoc 1999;65:384–386.
11. Martin MD, Kinoshita-Byrne J, Getz T. Dental fear in a special needs clinic population of persons with disabilities. Spec Care Dentist 2002;22:99–102.
12. Joshi A, Kostakis GC. An investigation of post-operative morbidity following iliac crest graft harvesting. Br Dent J 2004;196:167–171.
13. Friedlander AH, Cummings JL. Dental treatment of patients with Gilles de la Tourette's syndrome. Oral Surg Oral Med Oral Pathol 1992;73:299–303.
14. Scully Cbe C, Shotts R. The mouth in neurological disorders. Practitioner 2001;245:539,542–546,548–549.

15. Lowe O. Tourette's syndrome: management of oral complications. ASDC J Dent Child 1986;53:456–460.
16. Shimoyama T, Horie N, Kato T, Nasu D, Kaneko T. Tourette's syndrome with rapid deterioration by self-mutilation of the upper lip. J Clin Pediatr Dent 2003;27: 177–180.
17. Leksell E, Edvardson S. A case of Tourette syndrome presenting with oral self-injurious behaviour. Int J Paediatr Dent 2005;15:370–374.
18. Woody RC, Eisenhauer G. Tooth extraction as a form of self-mutilation in Tourette's disorder. South Med J 1986; 79:1466.
19. Yoshikawa F, Takagi T, Fukayama H, Miwa Z, Umino M. Intravenous sedation and general anesthesia for a patient with Gilles de la Tourette's syndrome undergoing dental treatment. Acta Anaesthesiol Scand 2002;46:1279–1280.
20. Sheehy EC, Longhurst P, Pool D, Dandekar M. Self-inflicted injury in a case of Hallervorden-Spatz disease. Int J Paediatr Dent 1999;9:299–302.
21. da Fonseca MA, Walker PO. Dental management of a child with Huntington's disease: case report. Spec Care Dentist 1993;13:71–73.
22. Starck WJ, Morrissette MP, Chewning LC. Treating a mandibular condylar fracture in a patient with Huntington's disease. J Am Dent Assoc 1992;123:52–58.
23. Moline DO, Iglehart DR. Huntington's chorea: review and case report. Gen Dent 1985;33:131–133.
24. Feeney AW. Dental treatment considerations for patients with Huntington's chorea: a literature review and case report. J Conn State Dent Assoc 1985;59:118–123.
25. Walshe T. Approach to patients with degenerative disorders of the nervous system. Gerodontics 1988;4:156–157.
26. Bradford H, Britto LR, Leal G, Katz J. Endodontic treatment of a patient with Huntington's disease. J Endod 2004;30:366–369.
27. Harmelin W, Cicero J. Systemic problem cases for dentistry under general anesthesia. N Y State Dent J 1967;33: 209–215.
28. Lamont AM. Brief report: anaesthesia and Huntington's chorea. Anaesth Intensive Care 1979;7:189–190.
29. Rodrigo MR. Huntington's chorea: midazolam, a suitable induction agent? Br J Anaesth 1987;59:388–389.
30. Soar J, Matheson KH. A safe anaesthetic in Huntington's disease? Anaesthesia 1993;48:743–744.
31. Cangemi CF, Miller RJ. Huntington's disease: review and anesthetic case management. Anesth Prog 1998;45: 150–153.
32. Jackowski J, Andrich J, Kappeler H et al. Implant-supported denture in a patient with Huntington's disease: interdisciplinary aspects. Spec Care Dentist 2001;21: 15–20.
33. Penarrocha M, Sanchis JM, Rambla J, Sanchez MA. Oral rehabilitation with osseointegrated implants in a patient with oromandibular dystonia with blepharospasm (Brueghel's syndrome): a patient history. Int J Oral Maxillofac Implants 2001;16:115–117.
34. Robb ND, Hargrave SA. Propofol infusion for conscious sedation in dentistry in patients with involuntary movement disorders—a note of caution. Anaesth Intensive Care 1997;25:429–430.
35. van der Bijl P, Roelofse JA. Conscious sedation with midazolam in a dental patient with a spastic nerve/muscle disorder: a case report. Ann Dent 1994;53:37–38.
36. Mann AC. Localised autonomic failure due to botulinum toxin injection. J Neurol Neurosurg Psychiatry 1994;57: 1320.
37. Thomas GA. Abnormal movements of the oral-facial region. Diagnosis, assessment and control. A guide for the dental clinician. Aust Prosthodont J 1988;2:41–45.
38. Blanchet PJ, Rompre PH, Lavigne GJ, Lamarche C. Oral dyskinesia: a clinical overview. Int J Prosthodont 2005;18: 10–19.
39. Koller WC. Idiopathic oral-facial dyskinesia. Adv Neurol 1988;49:177–183.
40. Sutcher H. Prosthetic dentistry in the treatment of movement disorders: dyskinesias and other neurological abnormalities. Med Hypotheses 2001;56:318–320.
41. Kamen S. Tardive dyskinesia. A significant syndrome for geriatric dentistry. Oral Surg Oral Med Oral Pathol 1975; 39:52–57.
42. Mukherjee S, Rosen AM, Cardenas C, Varia V, Olarte S. Tardive dyskinesia in psychiatric outpatients: a study of prevalence and association with demographic, clinical, and drug history variables. Arch Gen Psychiatry 1982;39: 466–469.
43. Sutcher HD, Underwood RB, Beatty RA, Sugar O. Orofacial dyskinesia: a dental dimension. JAMA 1971; 216:1459–1463.
44. Koller WC. Edentulous orodyskinesia. Ann Neurol 1983;13:97–99.
45. Hamzei F, Rijntjes M, Gbadamosi J et al. Life-threatening respiratory failure due to cranial dystonia after dental procedure in a patient with multiple system atrophy. Mov Disord 2003;18:959–961.
46. Ghika J, Regli F, Growdon JH. Sensory symptoms in cranial dystonia: a potential role in the etiology? J Neurol Sci 1993;116:142–147.
47. Sutcher HD, Beatty RA, Underwood RB. Orofacial dyskinesia: effective prosthetic therapy. J Prosthet Dent 1973;30:252–262.
48. Sutcher H, Kutz RA. Facial movement disorders: a progress report. Quintessence Int 1979;10:109–112.
49. Mack PJ. Two-part record blocks: a clinical report. J Dent 1980;8:182–183.
50. Watanabe I, Yamane G, Yamane H, Shimono M. Oral dyskinesia of the aged. II: Electromyographic appearance and dental treatment. Gerodontics 1988;4:310–314.
51. Penarrocha M, Sanchis JM, Rambla J, Guarinos J. Oral rehabilitation using osseointegrated implants in a patient with idiopathic torsion dystonia. Int J Oral Maxillofac Implants 2001;16:433–435.

52. Payne AG, Carr L. Can edentulous patients with orofacial dyskinesia be treated successfully with implants? A case report. J Dent Assoc S Afr 1996;51:67–70.
53. Casamassimo PS. A primer in management of movement in the patient with a handicapping condition. J Mass Dent Soc 1991;40:23–28.
54. Harris FA, Nicholls JI. An automated head stabilizer to facilitate dental care for cerebral palsied patients. J Hosp Dent Pract 1978;12:92–94.
55. Kaufman E, Meyer S, Wolnerman JS, Gilai AN. Transient suppression of involuntary movements in cerebral palsy patients during dental treatment. Anesth Prog 1991;38:200–205.
56. Langer A. Prosthodontic failures in patients with systemic disorders. J Oral Rehabil 1979;6:13–19.
57. Scully C, Felix DH. Oral medicine. Update for the dental practitioner. Disorders of orofacial sensation and movement. Br Dent J 2005;199:703–709.
58. Jolly DE, Paulson RB, Paulson GW, Pike JA. Parkinson's disease: a review and recommendations for dental management. Spec Care Dentist 1989;9:74–78.
59. Kieser J, Jones G, Borlase G, MacFadyen E. Dental treatment of patients with neurodegenerative disease. N Z Dent J 1999;95:130–134.
60. Alexander RE, Gage TW. Parkinson's disease: an update for dentists. Gen Dent 2000;48:572–580.
61. Fiske J, Hyland K. Parkinson's disease and oral care. Dent Update 2000;27:58–65.
62. Dirks SJ, Paunovich ED, Terezhalmy GT, Chiodo LK. The patient with Parkinson's disease. Quintessence Int 2003;34:379–393.
63. Ngim CH, Devathasan G. Epidemiologic study on the association between body burden mercury level and idiopathic Parkinson's disease. Neuroepidemiology 1989;8:128–141.
64. Chavez EM, Ship JA. Sensory and motor deficits in the elderly: impact on oral health. J Public Health Dent 2000;60:297–303.
65. Pow EH, Leung KC, McMillan AS et al. Oral stereognosis in stroke and Parkinson's disease: a comparison of partially dentate and edentulous individuals. Clin Oral Investig 2001;5:112–117.
66. Leung KC, Pow EH, McMillan AS et al. Oral perception and oral motor ability in edentulous patients with stroke and Parkinson's disease. J Oral Rehabil 2002;29:497–503.
67. Gentil M, Garcia-Ruiz P, Pollak P, Benabid AL. Effect of bilateral deep-brain stimulation on oral control of patients with parkinsonism. Eur Neurol 2000;44:147–152.
68. Lantz HJ. Oral complications of parkinsonism. Bull Phila Cty Dent Soc 1977;43:12–19.
69. Persson M, Osterberg T, Granerus AK, Karlsson S. Influence of Parkinson's disease on oral health. Acta Odontol Scand 1992;50:37–42.
70. Kennedy MA, Rosen S, Paulson GW, Jolly DE, Beck FM. Relationship of oral microflora with oral health status in Parkinson's disease. Spec Care Dentist 1994;14:164–168.
71. Clifford T, Finnerty J. The dental awareness and needs of a Parkinson's disease population. Gerodontology 1995;12:99–103.
72. Clifford TJ, Warsi MJ, Burnett CA, Lamey PJ. Burning mouth in Parkinson's disease sufferers. Gerodontology 1998;15:73–78.
73. Anastassiadou V, Katsarou Z, Naka O, Bostanzopoulou M. Evaluating dental status and prosthetic need in relation to medical findings in Greek patients suffering from idiopathic Parkinson's disease. Eur J Prosthodont Restor Dent 2002;10:63–68.
74. ADA Dental Editors Digest. Treating the patient with Parkinson's disease. J Mich Dent Assoc 2003;85:20.
75. Fukayo S, Nonaka K, Shimizu T, Yano E. Oral health of patients with Parkinson's disease: factors related to their better dental status. Tohoku J Exp Med 2003;201:171–179.
76. Nakayama Y, Washio M, Mori M. Oral health conditions in patients with Parkinson's disease. J Epidemiol 2004;14:143–150.
77. Collins R. Special considerations for the dental patient with Parkinson's disease. Tex Dent J 1990;107:31–32.
78. Anonymous. Empathy key to providing care to Parkinson's patient. J Calif Dent Assoc 2003;31:739.
79. Herren C, Abadi B. Urgent denture repair in a medically compromised patient. Gen Dent 2005;53:60–62.
80. Cohen CI. A case report: periodontal surgery in Parkinsonism utilizing intravenous sedation. N Y State Dent J 1978;44:19.
81. Fielding ML. Case report: construction of complete dentures for Parkinson patient. Dent Surv 1977;53:36–37,51.
82. Marron K, Hawker P. Training appliance for swallowing difficulties associated with Parkinson's disease: there can be a catch to it. Med J Aust 1988;148:155–157.
83. Hussein SB. Use of a gum shield for Parkinson's disease patients. Br Dent J 1989;166:320.
84. Durham TM, Hodges ED, Henry MJ, Geasland J, Straub P. Management of orofacial manifestations of Parkinson's disease with splint therapy: a case report. Spec Care Dentist 1993;13:155–158.
85. Minagi S, Matsunaga T, Shibata T, Sato T. An appliance for management of TMJ pain as a complication of Parkinson's disease. Cranio 1998;16:57–59.
86. Applebaum GM, Langsam BW, Huba G. The implant retained UCLA-type clip bar overdenture: a solution to the mandibular edentulous patient affected by Parkinson's disease. Oral Health 1997;87:65–67,69–70,72.
87. Heckmann SM, Heckmann JG, Weber HP. Clinical outcomes of three Parkinson's disease patients treated with mandibular implant overdentures. Clin Oral Implants Res 2000;11:566–571.
88. Chu FC, Deng FL, Siu AS, Chow TW. Implant-tissue supported, magnet-retained mandibular overdenture for an edentulous patient with Parkinson's disease: a clinical report. J Prosthet Dent 2004;91:219–222.

89. Kubo K, Kimura K. Implant surgery for a patient with Parkinson's disease controlled by intravenous midazolam: a case report. Int J Oral Maxillofac Implants 2004;19: 288–290.
90. Magalhaes MH, Kawamura JY, Araujo LC. General and oral characteristics in Rett syndrome. Spec Care Dentist 2002;22:147–150.
91. Mestrom TJ, Spanauf AJ. The dental management of a partially edentulous patient suffering from hepatolenticular degeneration (Wilson's disease). Aust Dent J 1981;26: 153–155.
92. McGuiness JW, McInnes-Ledoux PM, Ferraro EF, Carr JC. Daily release of copper from dental alloy restorations in a patient with Wilson's disease. Oral Surg Oral Med Oral Pathol 1987;63:511–514.
93. Greene MW, King RC, Alley RS. Management of an oroantral fistula in a patient with Wilson's disease: case report and review of the literature. Oral Surg Oral Med Oral Pathol 1988;66:293–296.
94. American Academy of Sleep Medicine. International Classification of Sleep Disorders: Diagnostic and Coding Manual. Chicago, IL: American Academy of Sleep Medicine, 2001.
95. Lavigne GJ, Montplaisir JY. Restless legs syndrome and sleep bruxism: prevalence and association among Canadians. Sleep 1994;17:739–743.
96. Rajput AH, Offort K, Beard CM, Kurland LT. Epidemiological survey of dementia in Parkinsonism and control population. In: Advances in Neurology, vol 40. New York: Raven Press, 1984.
97. Kato T, Thie NM, Huynh N, Miyawaki S, Lavigne GJ. Topical review. Sleep bruxism and the role of peripheral sensory influences. J Orofac Pain 2003;17:191–213.
98. Lavigne GJ, Kato T, Kolta A, Sessle BJ. Neurobiological mechanisms involved in sleep bruxism. Crit Rev Oral Biol Med 2003;14:30–46.
99. Lobbezoo F, van der Zaag J, Naeije M. Bruxism: its multiple causes and its effects on dental implants. An updated review. J Oral Rehabil 2006;33:293–300.

Chapter 8

# Bruxism in Children

*Claudia Restrepo*

## Introduction

Bruxism in children is very common, but the available literature on its diagnosis and treatment is not yet extensive enough for evidence-based clinical practice. Scientific reports about bruxism in children can be found from 1966,[1] dealing with its etiology, diagnosis, and therapies. However, there are many barriers to performing studies in children that would meet the methodologic requirements needed to increase the knowledge in this field. There have been, and still are, difficulties obtaining the written informed consent that allows investigators to probe diagnostic and therapeutic options. The limitations are mainly due to legislation in the countries that have the necessary technology: the laws to protect children do not allow the necessary permissions to develop studies indispensable for increasing the evidence to treat bruxism in children.

## Etiology of Bruxism in Children

Sleep bruxism (SB) is an orofacial movement described as a parafunction in dentistry and as a parasomnia in sleep medicine.[2] It can occur during wakefulness or sleeping and can be voluntary or unconscious. The etiology of sleep bruxism has been defined as multifactorial.[3] It is regulated centrally, but influenced peripherally.[4] This fact means that oral habits,[5] temporomandibular disorders (TMD),[6] malocclusions,[7] hypopnea,[8] high anxiety levels,[9] personality,[10] and stress,[11] *inter alia*,[12] could influence the occurrence of bruxism peripherally. They act as a motor stimulus to the central nervous system, which reacts with an alteration in the neurotransmission of dopamine,[13,14] and the outcome is clenching or grinding of the teeth.

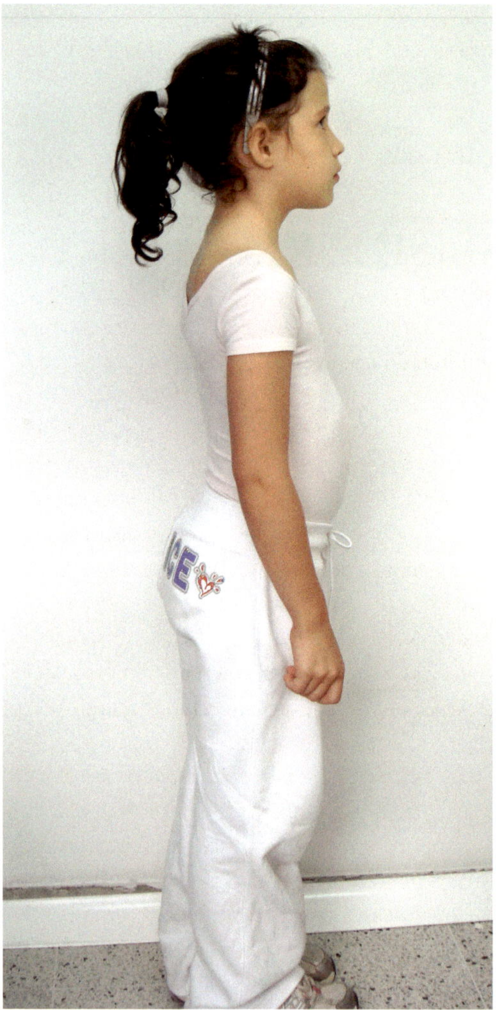

**Fig 8-1** Head and body posture of a bruxist child. Note the kyphosis of the neck and an anterior head posture.

*The physiology in children is different.* Dopamine levels in the brain increase progressively after birth to very high levels in adolescence, when they start to decrease steadily until the age of 30.[15] This makes studies of the etiology of bruxism in children incomparable with the studies in adults. Studies in children are required because the available literature has lacked sufficient scientific rigor thus far.

Children tend to have greater intensity, frequency, and duration of parafunctional habits, such as finger sucking, pacifier sucking, onicophagia, etc. Their presence could be predictive of the same habits during adulthood, although their prevalence and incidence decrease with age.[16] These early parafunctions could lead one to think that children have more risk factors to acquire bruxism than adults.

Neuropsychological disorders are frequently associated with obstructive ventilatory disorders (OVD). Its most severe form, obstructive sleep apnea syndrome (OSAS) is a disorder characterized by repeated episodes of upper airway obstruction associated with hemoglobin desaturation.[17] Its relationships to attention-deficit hyperactivity disorder (ADHD)[18] and to bruxism[19,20] have been probed, but there is not enough evidence to support a relationship between respiration and bruxism.

Oral airway resistance increases with modest degrees of head and neck flexion in healthy adult humans,[21] while in healthy infants, hyperflexion of the head has been shown to affect airflow, airway patency, and pulmonary mechanisms.[22,23] Additionally, sleep bruxism has been correlated with hypopnea[8] and increasing airway patency.[24] More anterior and downward head postures and kyphotic neck have been found in bruxist children, with hyperflexion of the head posture (Fig 8-1).[25] This posture could affect the airflow in the bruxist children and could be part of the etiology of their parafunction. Moreover, this head posture is similar to that described for subjects with hypertrophy of the masticatory muscles[26] and high anxiety levels,[27] both of them characteristics of bruxism.

There is no evidence to prove that bruxism is caused by any kind of parasite. This fact may demystify the paradigm that the grinding of the teeth is due to ameba or any kind of bacteria. Case reports[28] have included bruxism as a *symptom* in children infected with *Cyclospora*, whose microbiological examination showed sporulated oocysts.

## Epidemiology of Bruxism in Children

The prevalence of sleep bruxism is difficult to estimate, since quite often the subjects are unaware of having the disorder[29] and there are many associated factors that can confuse the diagnosis. It is more frequent in the younger generation, with a decline with age.[29] The symptoms recognized in children can persist into adulthood.[16] The literature does not include reliable epidemiological studies specifically focused on the prevalence or incidence of bruxism in children. However, various authors have evaluated the prevalence with questionnaires, and they seem to agree that it ranges from 7% to 88%.[3,30] There is no reported gender difference. Some authors have observed that boys and girls are equally likely to have bruxism; only one study posited that bruxism is more prevalent among boys.[31–33] Children who brux begin at about 4–8 years of age.[3] The incidence of bruxism is higher between 10 and 14 years of age, decreasing afterwards.

Both the questionnaire method and clinical examination of bruxist children could lead to errors in the diagnosis of bruxism. Children who are collaborative could describe symptoms that do not exist, while apprehensive children could report not having symptoms that are really present. Furthermore, the parents do not always know that their children are bruxing, as they are not sleeping close to them and are not with them all day long to detect daytime bruxism.

Some studies during the 1970s asked the scientific community to pay attention to those errors that were affecting the evidence regarding bruxism.[34] They also pointed out that dental wear could give information about bruxism *that already occurred*, but not the current disorder or ongoing damage. Studies of dental wear produced by bruxism in children had not taken into account other factors that can affect wear of the dentition, such as dietary habit and the consistency of the food that is eaten (discussed later in this chapter). Also, endogenous erosion from gastroesophageal reflux, and psychiatric disorders such as bulimia and anorexia, had not been taken into account.

## Factors Associated with Bruxism

### *Anxiety*

An anxiety state is a prominent factor in the development of bruxing behavior in children.[26] However, to study anxiety in children is difficult: most children do not even know what it is to be "anxious".

Several instruments have been used to study anxiety. Although there are scales to measure anxiety in children, and are self-applied,[35] it is important to quantify the child's anxiety also through their parents or carers. Certain questions to the parents and even to the teachers can define the anxiety status of the child better than the child's own opinion of their anxious state. Unfortunately, these types of methods are seldom found in the studies of bruxism in children.[36]

Anxiety is not always positively related to stress.[37] Bruxing adults have been reported to be stressful and to present with headaches, clenching, and/or pain in the neck, back, throat, or shoulders.[38] Signs of bruxism such as headache have been previously related to high anxiety levels.[35] A recent study concluded that children with bruxism are more anxiety prone.[10]

### *Personality*

Activation of dopamine D4 receptors appears to inhibit the functioning of the prefrontal cortex, a brain region implicated in cognitive ability.[39] The 7-repeat allele of the dopamine D4 receptor gene produces less efficient receptors, relative to other alleles, and this may alter the effects of dopamine on cognitive function. Children with persistent antisocial and aggressive personality traits are diagnosed as having disruptive behavior disorder. Van Goozen and co-workers reviewed evidence that antisocial children, and especially those who persisted with this behavior as they grew older, had a range of neurobiologic characteristics such as bruxism.[40] They argued that serotonergic functioning and stress-regulating mechanisms are important in explaining individual differences in antisocial behavior.

Studies of personality traits in bruxist children have been limited. The first report of an attempt to study the relationship between personality and bruxism was the survey by Kuch and co-workers.[41] They did not find any association. However, the study did not include a control group, and the instrument used to evaluate personality was an interview and not a validated assesment. Later, Kampe and co-workers did find a positive relationship between bruxism and personality traits in adults,[38] increasing the controversy. Recently, Restrepo and co-workers, using a more controlled methodology, studied 16 personality traits and found the bruxist children to be more tense than non-bruxist children.[10]

### Hyperactivity and Attention Deficit

Attention-deficit hyperactivity disorder (ADHD) – or "hyperkinetic disorder" as it is officially known in the UK, though ADHD is more commonly used – is generally considered to be a developmental disorder, largely neurologic in nature, affecting about 5% of the world's population.

Dopaminergic neurotransmission[39] is implicated in externalizing behavioral problems, such as aggression and hyperactivity, previously correlated with anxiety and bruxism.[42] The prevalence of bruxism has been evaluated in ADHD children taking medications, ADHD children not taking medications, and controls.[43] The findings show that the children being pharmacologically treated for ADHD show a higher occurrence of bruxism compared to subjects affected by ADHD but not taking medicines, and children without ADHD. It appears that one side-effect of the central nervous system (CNS) stimulants could be bruxism.

### Temporomandibular Disorders

To test temporomandibular disorders (TMD) in children is not easy. The Research Diagnostic Criteria (RDC/TMD) have been developed for scientific evaluation of TMD and are available to researchers and clinicians. The RDC/TMD were developed by a team of international clinical research experts who gathered together to develop, to the largest extent possible, an operationalized system for diagnosing and classifying RDC/TMD, based on the best available scientific data, within the context of a biopsychosocial model. Reliability values ranged from good to excellent for the RDC/TMD clinical exam in children and adolescents. It has been used in children from 10 years old, but its reliability to detect TMD in children under that age has not been reported. Other examinations, such as the one proposed by Bernal and Tsamtsouris,[44] are available, but validity and reliability have not been published.

Temporomandibular joint (TMJ) dysfunction has been generally presumed to be a condition affecting only adults, but there is now enough evidence for its existence in children as well. Study of TMJ dysfunction in children could be important in determining whether early problems predispose patients to craniofacial growth abnormalities, TMJ-related pain, or mandibular dysfunction in adulthood. Surveys have shown that TMJ dysfunction may produce no symptoms in young children. Symptomatic cases may be misdiagnosed as headache or otalgia by the pediatrician or otolaryngologist. The evidence indicates that TMD increase between the primary and the mixed dentition stages,[45] and reach in adolescence a prevalence level close to that found in adults.

The relationship between bruxism with TMD in children is strongly supported,[46] and the existence of an association between TMD and anxiety, depression, and stress (symptoms of bruxism) had been studied earlier,[47] but without demonstrating causality.

Temporomandibular disorders in children and adolescents are often defined on the basis of signs and symptoms, of which the most common are TMJ sounds, impaired movement of the mandible, limitation in mouth opening, preauricular pain, facial pain, headache, and jaw tenderness on movement.[48] Severe pain and dysfunction is a rare combination. One of the possible causal factors suggested for TMD in children is a functional mandibular overload variable, mainly caused by bruxism.

### *Parafunctional Habits*

There is controversy about whether parafunctional habits can be considered to be daytime bruxism. There have not been enough investigations in the field to conclude that any habit – such as sucking, or nail or cheek biting – has the same etiology or pathophysiology in order to be considered bruxism. A sucking habit, for example, develops from an unresolved suction reflex. Its effect on the craniofacial complex could act as a motor stimulus to the CNS, which reacts with an alteration in the neurotransmission of dopamine – and the effect is the clenching or grinding of the teeth.

## Diagnosis of Bruxism in Children

A search of the literature revealed that most of the methods used to diagnose bruxism are indirect: dental wear, anxiety, temporomandibular disorders, etc. The point is that those measurements are not always related to bruxism, so the diagnosis can be mistaken and false positives or false negatives are present.

Different methods and instruments are available to measure the factors indirectly associated with bruxism in children: digital analysis to distinguish pathologic from physiologic wear, psychometric instruments to measure anxiety and stress, methods to detect TMD, electromyography, etc. Polysomnography is a reliable tool, but only useful during the active phase of bruxism; so with a bruxing patient who goes to the polysomnographic exam the day he or she is not in an active phase, the diagnosis is going to be wrong.

Thus far, the most reliable method to diagnose nocturnal bruxism in children is from parents' or carers' reports of the occurrence of bruxism. The problem with this method is that most of the children do not sleep with their parents or close to them, so the parents are not always aware. The other question is: what about daytime bruxism? The studies report daytime bruxism to be a voluntary action, but small children are not aware of what they are doing with their mouth.

More studies are necessary to develop reliable instruments to diagnose bruxism in children. The diagnosis should be multifactorial: questionnaire; oral history-taking (including parents' or carers' reports of grinding sounds); extraoral and intraoral inspection for clinical signs of bruxism; and, in some cases, an electromyographic (EMG) recording of the activity of the masticatory muscles, or even a polysomnographic recording of the sleeping patient. Any single one of these diagnostic tools should not be used in isolation.

## Effect of Bruxism on the Dentition of Children

The effect of bruxism on primary and permanent dentitions is not without controversy. Vanderas and Manetas suggested some years ago[49] that the constant trauma caused by occlusal forces during bruxism made the primary teeth resorb prematurely, accelerating exfoliation of the deciduous teeth. However, there is still no evidence to confirm this hypothesis.

The dentition of children today is generally less worn than in the 1950s, as modern food tends to be softer and processed.[50] The dietary consistency affects craniofacial growth. When food is not hard enough, the teeth do not wear naturally, resulting in insufficient growth of the alveolar base in children. Without adequate stimulation, the arch size is not sufficient for tooth eruption.[51] When brux-

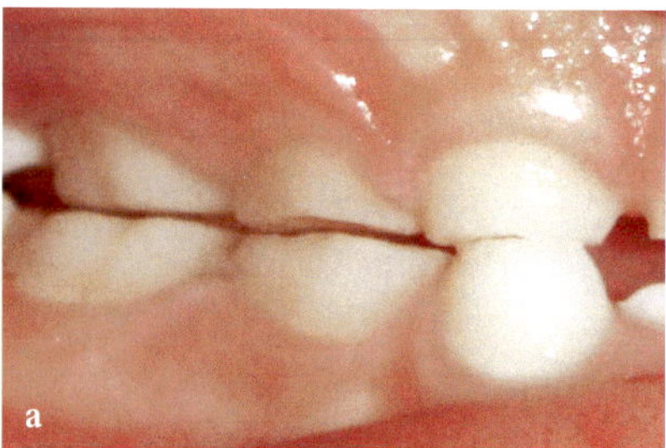


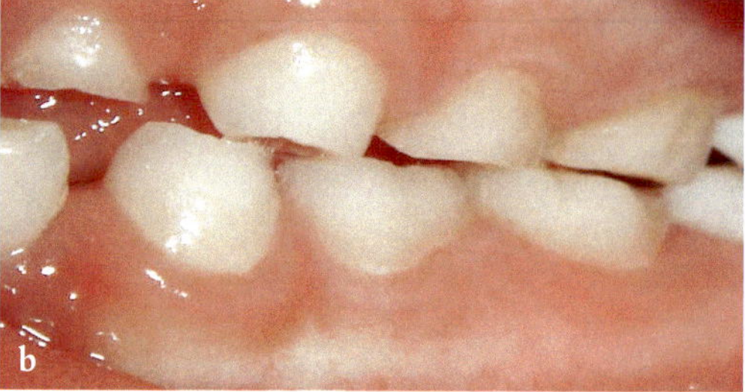


Fig 8-2 **(a and b)** Dental wear, showing flat contacts between the maxillary and mandibular dental arches generated by bruxism.

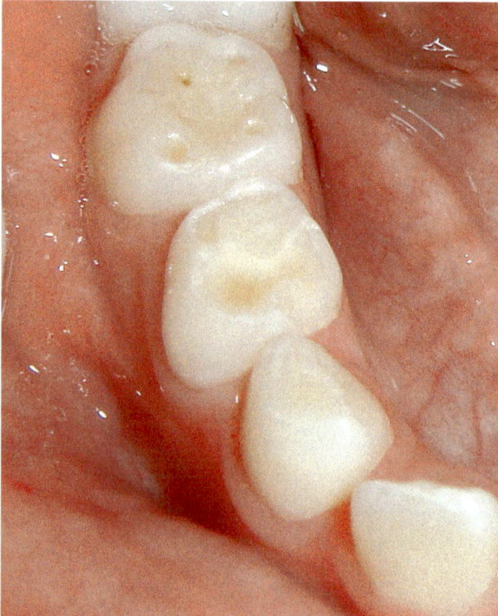

Fig 8-3 Dental erosion in canine and first deciduous molar.

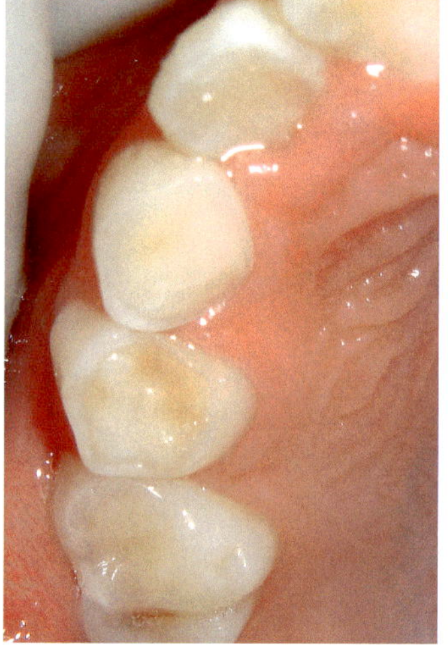

Fig 8-4 Attrition in incisors caused by bruxism, with erosion in canines and deciduous molars.

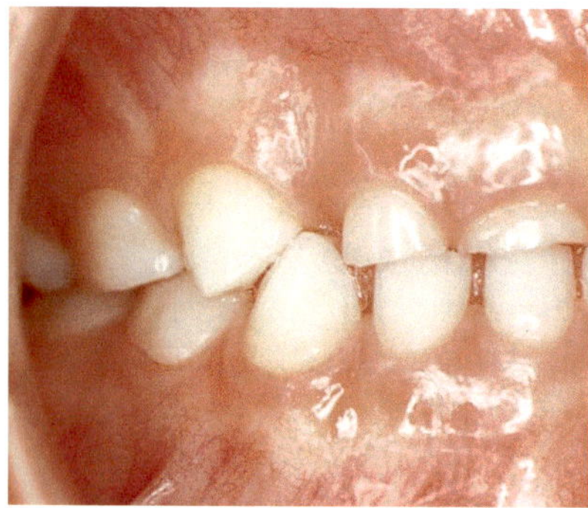

Fig 8-5 Loss of vertical dimension due to dental wear caused by bruxism.

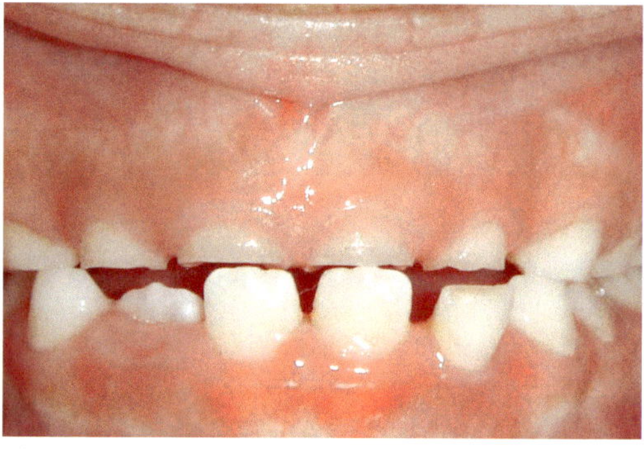

Fig 8-6 Open bite due to dental wear caused by bruxism.

ism occurs, the dental wear is higher, so the contact areas between maxillary and mandibular teeth are bigger and flatter than comes about with natural chewing (Fig 8-2). Those contacts allow horizontal movements of the mandible against the maxilla, and the stimulus to the alveolar bone is higher.[44]

A recent pilot study[52] concluded that the dental wear generated by bruxism allows the masticatory system to exert eccentric and lateral movements that allow the alveolar bone to be stimulated and to grow more. The result is slightly wider dental arches that could lead the bruxist child to have more space in the dental arches to align the teeth. However, further long-term studies are necessary to confirm this possibility.

The attritional effects of bruxism on teeth depends on several factors: type and severity of the parafunction; localization of the teeth and position of the teeth within the arch; intermaxillary relations; number of teeth; cusp heights; mobility; and interdental contacts.[53] Dental wear can be caused, too, by digestive problems and physiologic masticatory functions. Wear of natural teeth depends on variables such as structure and hardness of the enamel, forces applied to the contact surfaces, saliva, and duration of the contacts. Physiologic abrasion occurs during normal function such as mastication and affects the canine ridges, supporting cusps, the molar fossae, and pits. It is difficult to determine whether the dental wear that is found in children is caused by bruxism or by other factors such as diet or endogenous factors. Some evidence is now pointing to the rise in "soft" drink consumption as the most significant factor in the development of tooth wear, causing dental erosion in young people (Fig 8-3). Dental professionals are currently not well prepared to differentiate erosion from attrition. Bruxism may be wrongly stigmatized as the major producer of dental wear (Figs 8-4 to 8-6). Chapter 9 has more information on dental wear.

Modern studies have, if anything, increased the controversy. A survey that included 356 children (aged 6 years) was performed in order to evaluate the prevalence and etiological factors involved with wear of deciduous teeth.[54] The study found no significant correlations between gastroesophageal reflux, tooth-brushing habit, or consumption of citrus-fruit or "soft" drinks and the presence of tooth wear, for all groups of teeth. The wear showed correlation with the presence of bruxism for canines, and with the habit of holding drinks in the mouth before swallowing for incisors. It was concluded that the wear of incisors could be considered physiologic for this age.

## Effect of Bruxism on Craniofacial Morphology

A study was done to investigate the differences between the craniofacial morphologies of bruxers and non-bruxers.[25] The study did not include children, but the bruxing subjects demonstrated dolichocephalic head form and euryprosopic facial type. The study did not find clinically significant differences with the facial morphology of non-bruxers.

There are suggestions that, due to increased occlusal forces, masticatory muscles could become hypertrophied, so the facial morphology could change. This is not supported by the evidence currently available.

## Bruxism in Children with Special Characteristics

Bruxism has been commonly described in children with special characteristics, such as Down syndrome[55] or cerebral palsy.[56] Children with mosaic trisomy were found in one investigation to present the highest bruxism prevalence. Among its symptoms, this type of disorder presents alterations in muscle tone, which sometimes is lower and sometimes higher than in unaffected children. These changes are correlated with other types of variation in brain function that are not necessarily associated with the neurotransmission of dopamine.

The main problem in diagnosing bruxism in this group of children is that the dental wear and parents' description ofbruxism in their children is still the principal tool used to detect the parafunction; and this information is not enough for this group of patients.

## Management of Bruxism in Children

Although there have been investigations of several treatments for bruxism in children,[57,58] there is still a lack of evidence to support therapeutic options that really deal with the etiology of bruxism in this age group. The available evidence is focused on various occlusal, behavioral, and pharmacologic management approaches for bruxism.

Treatment for bruxism is indicated when the disorder causes any one of the following possible consequences: attrition; hypertrophied masticatory muscles; fractures/failures of restorations; premature exfoliation of deciduous teeth; headache; or pain in the masticatory system (TMD).

Small-scale studies have attempted to demonstrate that rigid occlusal splints are effective in the treatment of bruxism in children with primary teeth.[57] Their findings are mainly based on the fact that untreated bruxing children displayed increased wear facets compared with the experimental group. The conclusion that splints are efficient against bruxism is, however, premature, because the bruxism behavior itself was not assessed, only one of its possible consequences. One randomized clinical trial[59] studied children using occlusal splints for two years and compared them to a control group of bruxist children not using the splints. The objective was to determine whether the splints restrict the growth of the maxillary alveolar base, and whether they were useful for the treatment of symptoms of bruxism in children. The findings point to the conclusion that the use of occlusal splints does not restrict the growth of the maxillary alveolar process but is also *not* useful to reduce the symptoms of bruxism.

There is evidence for the positive effect of a combined technique of induced muscular relaxation and competence reaction in 3–6-year-old children who suffer from bruxism.[36] However, bruxism was determined by indirect means, which hampers an unequivocal interpretation of the outcome. Other studies suggested, as an appropriate therapy for diurnal bruxism, self-monitoring – or "habit awareness".[60] These therapies are not reported in children.

Adenotonsillectomy has been considered to reduce bruxism in children with sleep-disordered breathing,[58] but the evidence is still slim. Pharmacologic therapies for bruxism in children, such as with botulinum toxin or dopamine depressors, cannot be found in the literature.

Several local therapies should be considered. Avoiding chewing gum is necessary as the movement of the masticatory muscles could generate a reflex that can be reproduced at night. Sleeping without a pillow generates a better posture and keeps the correct dimensions of the upper airway.[61] Finally, the application of wet heat can help the muscles to relax before going to sleep.

Sleep bruxism is tightly related to sleep habits. Children who watch television or listen to the radio when falling asleep are more prone to bruxism and consequently present more headaches.[62] Evidence suggests that children should take small naps at least once a day, that adults should read aloud to children before putting them to sleep (instead of watching TV with them), and that children should sleep alone.

## References

1. Rosenbaum CH, McDonald RE, Levitt EE. Occlusion of cerebral-palsied children. J Dent Res 1966;45: 1696–1700.
2. Kato T, Thie NM, Huynh N, Miyawaki S, Lavigne GJ. Topical review. Sleep bruxism and the role of peripheral sensory influences. J Orofac Pain 2003;17:191–213.
3. Negoro T, Briggs J, Plesh O, Nielsen I, McNeill C, Miller AJ. Bruxing patterns in children compared to intercuspal clenching and chewing as assessed with dental

models, electromyography and incisor jaw tracing: preliminary study. ASDC J Dent Child 1998;65:449–458.
4. Lobbezzo F, Naeije M. Bruxism is mainly regulated centrally, not peripherally. J Oral Rehabil 2001;28:1085–1091.
5. Castelo PM, Gaviao MB, Pereira LJ, Bonjardim LR. Relationship between oral parasomniaal/nutritive sucking habits and temporomandibular joint dysfunction in primary dentition. Int J Paediatr Dent 2005;15:29–36.
6. Molina OF, dos Santos J, Mazzetto M, Nelson S, Nowlin T, Mainieri ET. Oral jaw behaviors in TMD and bruxism: a comparison study by severity of bruxism. Cranio 2001;19:114–122
7. Sari S, Sonmez H. The relationship between occlusal factors and bruxism in permanent and mixed dentition in Turkish children. J Clin Pediatr Dent 2001;25:191–194.
8. Oksenberg A, Arons E. Sleep bruxism related to obstructive sleep apnea: the effect of continuous positive airway pressure. Sleep Med 2002;3:513–515.
9. Manfredini D, Landi N, Fantoni F, Segù M, Bosco M. Anxiety symptoms in clinically diagnosed bruxers. J Oral Rehabil 2005;32:584–588.
10. Restrepo CC, Vásquez LM, Alvarez M, Valencia I. Personality traits and temporomandibular disorders in a group of children with bruxing behavior. J Oral Rehabil 2008;35:585–593.
11. Tsai CM, Chou SL,Gale EN, Mccall JR. Human masticatory muscle activity and jaw position under experimental stress. J Oral Rehabil 2002;29:44–51.
12. Bayardo RE, Mejia JJ, Orozco S, Montoya K. Etiology of oral habits. ASDC J Dent Child 1996;63:350–353.
13. Lobbezoo F, Soucy JP, Montplaisir JY, Lavigne GJ. Striatal d2 receptor binding in sleep Bruxism: a controlled study with iodine-123-iodobenzamide and single-photon-emission computed tomography. J Dent Res 1996;75: 1804–1810.
14. Lobbezoo F, Soucy JP, Hartman NG, Montplaisir JY, Lavigne GJ. Effects of the d2 receptor agonist bromocriptine on sleep bruxism of two single-patient clinical trials. J Dent Res 1997;76:1610–1614.
15. Haycock JW, Becker L, Ang L et al. Marked disparity between age-related changes in dopamine and other presynaptic dopaminergic markers in human striatum. J Neurochem 2003;87:574–585.
16. Carlsson GE, Egermark I, Magnusson T. Predictors of bruxism, other oral parafunctions, and tooth wear over a 20-year follow-up period. J Orofac Pain 2003;17:50–57.
17. Brunetti L, Rana S, Lospalluti ML et al. Prevalence of obstructive sleep apnea in a cohort of 1207 children of southern Italy. Chest 2001;120:1930–1935.
18. Dillon JE, Blunden S, Ruzicka DL et al. DSM-IV diagnoses and obstructive sleep apnea in children before and 1 year after adenotonsillectomy. J Am Acad Child Adolesc Psychiatry 2007;46:1425–1436.
19. Shur-Fen Gau S. Prevalence of sleep problems and their association with inattention/hyperactivity among children aged 6-15 in Taiwan. J Sleep Res 2006;15:403–414.
20. Grechi TH, Trawitzki LV, de Felício CM, Valera FC, Alnselmo-Lima WT. Bruxism in children with nasal obstruction. Int J Pediatr Otorhinolaryngol 2008;72: 391–396.
21. Amis TC, O'Neill N, Wheatley JR. Oral airway flow dynamics in healthy humans. J Physiol 1999;515: 293–298.
22. Reiterer F, Abbasi S, Bhutani VK. Influence of head-neck posture on airflow and pulmonary mechanics in preterm neonates. Pediatr Pulmonol 1994;17:149–154.
23. Carlo WA, Beoglos A, Siner BS, Martin RJ. Neck and body position on pulmonary mechanics in infants. Pediatrics 1989;84:670–674.
24. Lavigne GJ, Kato T, Kolta A, Sessle BJ. Neurobiological mechanisms involved in sleep bruxism. Crit Rev Oral Biol Med 2003;14:30–46.
25. Velez AL, Restrepo CC, Peláez A et al. Head posture and dental wear evaluation of bruxist children with primary teeth. J Oral Rehabil 2007;34:663–670.
26. Young DV, Rinchuse DJ, Pierce CJ, Zullo T. The craniofacial morphology of bruxers versus nonbruxers. Angle Orthod 1999;69:14–18.
27. Monaco A, Ciammella NM, Marci MC, Pirro R, Giannoni M. The anxiety in bruxer child: a case–control study. Minerva Stomatol 2002;51:247–250.
28. Ponce-Macotela M, Cob-Sosa C, Martínez-Gordillo MN. [Cyclospora in two Mexican children]. Rev Invest Clin 1996;48:461–463.
29. Bader G, Lavigne G. Sleep bruxism; an overview of an oromandibular sleep movement disorder (review). Sleep Med Rev 2000;4:27–43.
30. Milosevic A, Young PJ, Lennon MA. The prevalence of tooth wear in 14-year-old school children in Liverpool. Community Dent Health 1994;11(2):83–86.
31. Reding GR, Rubright WC, Zimmerman SO. Incidence of bruxism. J Dent Res 1966;45:1198–1204.
32. Shetty SR, Munshi AK. Oral habits in children: a prevalence study. J Indian Soc Pedod Prev Dent 1998;16: 61–66.
33. Reding GR, Rubright WC, Zimmerman SO. Incidence of bruxism. J Dent Res 1966;45:1198–1204.
34. Lindqvist B. Bruxism in twins. Acta Odontol Scand 1974;32:177–187.
35. Gorayeb MA, Gorayeb R. Association between headache and anxiety disorders indicators in a school sample from Ribeirao Preto, Brazil. Arq Neuropsiquiatr 2002;60: 764–768.
36. Restrepo CC, Alvarez E, Jaramillo C, Velez C, Valencia I. Effects of psychological techniques on bruxism in children with primary teeth. J Oral Rehabil 2001;28:354–360.
37. White KS, Farrell AD. Anxiety and psychosocial stress as predictors of headache and abdominal pain in urban early adolescents. J Pediatr Psychol 2006;31:582–596.
38. Kampe T, Edman G, Bader G, Tagdae T, Karlsson S. Personality traits in a group of subjects with long-standing bruxing behaviour. J Oral Rehabil 1997;24:588–593.

39. DeYoung CG, Peterson JB, Seguin JR et al. The dopamine D4 receptor gene and moderation of the association between externalizing behavior and IQ. Arch Gen Psychiatry 2006;63:1410–1416.
40. Van Goozen SH, Fairchild G, Snoek H, Harold GT. The evidence for a neurobiological model of childhood antisocial behavior. Psychol Bull 2007;133:149–182.
41. Kuch EV, Till MJ, Messer LB. Bruxing and non-bruxing children: a comparison of their personality traits. Pediatr Dent 1979;1:182–187.
42. Vernalis FF. Teeth-grinding: some relationships to anxiety, hostility, and hyperactivity. J Clin Psychol 1955;11: 389–391.
43. Malki GA, Zawawi KH, Melis M, Hughes CV. Prevalence of bruxism in children receiving treatment for attention deficit hyperactivity disorder: a pilot study. J Clin Pediatr Dent 2004;29:63–67.
44. Bernal M, Tsamtsouris A. Signs and symptoms of temporomandibular joint dysfunction in 3 to 5 year old children. J Pedod 1986;10:127–140.
45. Muhtaro ullari M, Demirel F, Saygili G. Temporomandibular disorders in Turkish children with mixed and primary dentition: prevalence of signs and symptoms. Turk J Pediatr 2004;46:159–163.
46. Hirsch C, John MT, Lobbezoo F, Setz JM, Schaller HG. Incisal tooth wear and self-reported TMD pain in children and adolescents. Int J Prosthodont 2004;17:205–210.
47. Manfredini D, Landi N, Bandettini Di Poggio A et al. A critical review on the importance of psychological factors in temporomandibular disorders. Minerva Stomatol 2003;52:321–330.
48. Barbosa TD, Miyakoda LS, Pocztaruk RD, Rocha CP, Gavião MB. Temporomandibular disorders and bruxism in childhood and adolescence: review of the literature. Int J Pediatr Otorhinolaryngol 2008;72:299–314.
49. Vanderas AP, Manetas KJ. Relationship between malocclusion and bruxism in children and adolescents: a review. Pediatr Dent 1995;17:7–12.
50. Marinelli A, Alarashi M, Defraia E, Antonini A, Tollaro I. Tooth wear in the mixed dentition: a comparative study between children born in the 1950s and the 1990s. Angle Orthod 2005;75:340–343.
51. Simoes WA. Selective grinding and Planas' direct tracks as a source of prevention. J Pedod 1981;5:298–314.
52. Restrepo CC, Sforza C, Colombo A, Pelaez-Vargas A, Ferrario V. Palate morphology of bruxist children with mixed dentition: a pilot study. J Oral Rehabil 2008;35: 353–360.
53. Restrepo C, Pelaez A, Alvarez E, Paucar C, Abad P. Digital imaging of patterns of dental wear to diagnose bruxism in children. Int J Paediatr Dent 2006;16:278–285.
54. Rios D, Magalhães AC, Honórico HM, Buzalaf MA, Lauris JR, Machado MA. The prevalence of deciduous tooth wear in six-year-old children and its relationship with potential explanatory factors. Oral Health Prev Dent 2007;5:167–171.
55. López-Pérez R, López-Morales P, Borges-Yáñez SA, Maupomé G, Parés-Vidrio G. Prevalence of bruxism among Mexican children with Down syndrome. Downs Syndr Res Pract 2007;12:454–459.
56. Peres AC, Ribeiro MO, Juliano Y, César MF, Santos RC. Occurrence of bruxism in a sample of Brazilian children with cerebral palsy. Spec Care Dentist 2007;27:73–76.
57. Hachmann A, Martins EA, Araujo FB, Nunes R. Efficacy of the nocturnal bite plate in the control of bruxism for 3 to 5 year old children. J Clin Pediatr Dent 1999;24: 9–15.
58. DiFrancesco RC, Junqueira PA, Trezza PM et al. Improvement of bruxism after T&A surgery. Int J Pediatr Otorhinolaryngol 2004;68:441–445.
59. Medina I, Restrepo C, Patiño I, Gallego G, Pelaez-Vargas A. Effects of the occlusal splints on the growth of the upper arch in children with primary teeth. ASDC J Dent Child (in press).
60. Ommerborn MA, Schneider C, Giraki M et al. Effects of an occlusal splint compared with cognitive-behavioral treatment on sleep bruxism activity. Eur J Oral Sci 2007;115(2):7–14.
61. Quintero Y, Restrepo CC, Tamayo V et al. Effect of awareness through movement on the head posture of bruxist children. J Oral Rehabil 2009;36:18–25.
62. Zarowski M, Mlodzikowska-Albrecht J, Steinborn B. The sleep habits and sleep disorders in children with headache. Adv Med Sci 2007;52:194–196.

# Part 2

# Effects on the Masticatory System

Chapter 9

# Tooth Wear

*Daniel A. Paesani*

## Introduction

"Tooth wear" is a term referring to different processes which, either individually or in association, lead to the irreversible loss of tooth hard tissue.

Tooth wear is a clinical problem that is increasing all the time. Patients seek professional help for tooth pain and sensitivity, masticatory disorders, and esthetic problems. However, in recent decades, the introduction of caries and periodontal-disease preventive programs has resulted in better tooth survival. This, coupled with increased life expectancy, has led to better natural teeth retention. Consequently, older adults will most likely experience more tooth wear.

Today, there is growing consensus that tooth wear is not the result of just one cause. Quite the opposite, several factors interact along the tooth lifespan and are implicated in tooth wear etiology. However, regardless of whether there is an association between the different etiological factors, it is certain that their effect on teeth over time is cumulative and irreversible. No matter which factor we take to be the principal cause, wear starts immediately after tooth eruption.

When wear of permanent teeth starts at a young age, it may affect an individual for the rest of his or her life, as it forces the clinician to resort to difficult and/or expensive restorative treatments to be undertaken. We can be most helpful to our patients by making an early diagnosis and by immediately taking effective preventive measures after identifying the possible etiologic agent(s). This is even more vital when tooth wear is progressing very quickly.

Tooth wear is, perhaps, the feature most universally associated with bruxism. However, clinicians should be aware that wear is not caused exclusively by parafunctional activity, since there are several processes with different etiologies and mechanisms (excluding caries) which lead to irreversible hard-tissue loss. For this reason, Eccles suggested the use of the generic designation "tooth

*Table 9-1*

Several factors that may cause tooth wear.

| Terminology | Cause of loss of tissue |
|---|---|
| Abrasion | Mechanical process involving foreign objects or substances |
| Demastication | Wearing away of dental tissue as a result of the interaction between food and teeth |
| Attrition | Wearing away of tooth hard tissue as a result of tooth-to-tooth contact |
| Abfraction | Wedge-shaped cervical lesion caused by eccentric occlusal forces (in discussion) |
| Erosion | A chemical or electrolytic process |
| Resorption | A physiologic or pathologic biologic degradation process |

surface loss", when a single etiological factor is difficult to identify.[1] Later, Smith and Knight advocated the use of the term "tooth wear" to embrace all the possible causes and their multiple combinations, with or without a definite etiology.[2]

## Etiology of Tooth Wear

Despite the main subject of this book being bruxism, tooth wear is one of the effects of bruxism and many etiological factors can be associated with it. So a description of all the possible causes of the loss of tooth hard tissue will be provided for completeness. The processes that are considered to be responsible for tooth wear are abrasion, demastication, attrition, abfraction, erosion, and resorption (Table 9-1).

- *Abrasion.* This refers to the wearing away of the tooth's outer covering caused by mechanical forces from a foreign object. Energetic tooth-brushing is the most widely cited example of tooth wear by abrasion. Several factors affect tooth-brushing, including bristle stiffness, length and flexibility of toothbrush handle, abrasivity level, amount and pH of the toothpaste used, energy, hand skill, and the frequency and time devoted to brushing.
- *Demastication.* This refers to the physiologic wearing away of teeth during chewing of an alimentary bolus interposed between the dental arches. The tooth wear level is regulated by the abrasive potential of the chewed food. Today, loss of dental tissue resulting from this process is almost insignificant, since the modern diet, unlike that of our prehistoric ancestors, is not tough and is practically non-abrasive.
- *Attrition.* This refers to tooth wear resulting from contact between opposing teeth, without an exogenous process being involved. It occurs in several levels and extents due to tooth-to-tooth contact during clenching and grinding, deglutition, the last phase of chewing, and during speech. This process not only causes the wearing away of occlusal surfaces and incisal edges, but also causes facets to appear on the proximal surfaces of teeth. During mastication and also during parafunctional clenching, axial forces are exerted on teeth. Periodontal ligament resilience allows teeth to move vertically, which results in friction on the proximal surfaces and subsequent wear of such surfaces. The amount of attrition increases in direct proportion to age.
- *Abfraction.* This refers to the wedge-shaped lesions in the cementoenamel junction area, in the tooth neck. Tooth flexure caused by eccentric occlusal forces during horizontal movements of the jaw has been proposed as etiology, though this remains highly controversial.
- *Erosion.* This is an asymptomatic, gradual tooth-surface loss process caused by an electrolytic or chemical mechanism, without bacteria being involved. The acids causing the erosion are not produced by the oral flora. They may come from ingestion, the environment, or endogenous factors.

- *Resorption*. This is the loss of tooth structure due to a biologic degradation process and the assimilation of substances or structures previously produced by the body. As far as tooth structure is concerned, resorption may be said to be a biologic process by which hard tooth structures are removed due to cementoclastic, ameloclastic, or dentinoclastic activity. This process may be physiologic (e.g., deciduous-teeth root resorption when the tooth formula changes) or pathologic (e.g., root resorption caused by tooth trauma, excessive orthodontic forces, cysts, and tumors).

In this volume we discuss attrition, abrasion, and erosion. Not only are they important in the context of bruxism, their effects are generally confused with one another, making diagnosis difficult. The present chapter will focus on attrition.

## Types of Attrition

Attrition refers to tooth wear by antagonist tooth-to-tooth contacts. Pindborg[3] distinguishes between physiologic attrition, which occurs gradually as a result of mastication, and pathologic attrition, which occurs in localized areas and is caused by parafunctional activity. Very often, when examining patients who show tooth wear, clinicians have to try to distinguish between normal physiologic wear and pathologic wear. Wear is considered to be pathologic whenever the degree of decay prevents teeth from accomplishing their specific function or, without getting to that point, when decay progresses so quickly that it overtakes the patient's life-expectancy.[2] Tooth wear that is accompanied by sensitivity or pain should be considered to be pathologic.

## Physiologic Attrition

### *Attrition in Early Man*

In anthropologic surveys of early human populations, evidence was found of advanced cases of dental attrition. The extent of tooth wear was such that at an age as early as 12 years there was already complete loss of occlusal anatomy.[4] Early humans must have used their teeth in an extremely intensive way. Their diet consisted of wild vegetables (which they probably ate raw and without previously washing them) and the meat from animals. They would grab this food with both hands and tear it with their teeth, probably taking big bites.

Early humans' severe tooth wear has been ascribed to the great amount of abrasive particles in their diet. Uncooked food, plus abrasive agents from the environment (sand, earth, etc.), would compromise the integrity of the tooth anatomy in a very short time. Flattened cusps were characteristic of teeth as early as the second decade of life.[5] The primitive diet required a vigorous masticatory activity, which led to the utmost development of masticatory muscles. The high masticatory forces and the periodontal ligament resilience would have caused teeth to move vertically, and this would gradually wear away the proximal surfaces. Anthropologic studies have shown that prehistoric humans' teeth, rather than having points, had real surfaces in the proximal faces. By action of anterior forces, this interproximal wear would lead to a continuous mesial displacement of all the teeth, which would create enough room for the positioning and alignment of all teeth. There is anthropologic evidence that primitive humans did not suffer from malocclusion and did not have retained teeth.[6,7]

Modern humans gradually modified their eating habits, basing the diet on carbohydrates. They wash, process, and cook food and cut it on a plate by using a knife. This has drastically reduced the abrasiveness, the toughness, and the size of the bites taken into the mouth. This results in reduced tooth wear, and an important decrease in muscle and bony skeleton development.[8] Human beings have had to pay a very heavy price for this important change in their diet: caries and periodontal disease appeared, and there was a high number of malocclusions and retained teeth. The two latter problems have been ascribed to the lesser skeletal development of the jawbones due to their not serving a significant function any more – which led them to be out of proportion to the size of the teeth.[9]

In developed countries, as a consequence of water fluoridation and the introduction of preventive education programs, it has been possible to reduce the prevalence, incidence, and severity of caries and periodontal disease, leading to increased human tooth survival. However, as a result of this, more people and teeth are exposed to the risk of suffering from other dental lesions every day. For this reason, a stronger emphasis is currently being placed on the prevention of tooth hard-tissue noncarious lesions.

### *Attrition in Modern Man*

Today, our diet is practically non-abrasive, so physiologic wear of incisal edges and occlusal surfaces is a process that progresses gradually. Extremely worn teeth are now relatively uncommon in humans; a prevalence of only 2% has been reported.[10,11] However, solving cases of severe attrition is challenging for clinicians, since they represent both a clinical and an esthetic problem.

Not much research has been done on the amount of tooth enamel that naturally wears away per year. The scarce availability of literature on the subject reflects the difficulties involved in the measurement methods used in in-vivo studies. Also, since in modern society physiologic tooth wear is minimal, measurement scales are not sensitive enough for such low values. This affects, too, the study results, which have been highly variable. In a 4-year longitudinal study on models, the amount of annual tooth wear was found to be 15 µm for premolars and 29 µm for molars.[12] Another study reported an annual physiological tooth-wear value of 65 µm, this amount being three times as high in bruxers.[13] In another two-year longitudinal study of 18 subjects, tooth wear was assessed; a volume of 0.04 mm$^3$ and a depth of 10 µm were reported as average annual tooth wear.[14] The authors of this study recommend taking into consideration, when studying tooth wear, the variation in values according to the topographical location of each tooth in the dental arch. The authors report that canines show the greatest wear.

Physiologic tooth wear is directly related to food toughness and the presence of abrasive particles in the food. A group of researchers studied tooth wear in a population of contemporary Australian aborigines whose diet was primitive and also abrasive. They found that, by the age of 25, these aborigines showed such a degree of molar cusp flattening that the dentin was on the verge of pulp exposure.[15] Experiments with animals showed that the presence of abrasive particles in the food causes more tooth wear than the toughness of food itself.[16] The high degree of attrition in Bedouins has been ascribed to the presence of grit and sand from the dry desert in their diet, which is based on cereals.[17] Likewise, individuals exposed to high levels of dust in their workplace, like steelworkers and miners, are prone to accelerated tooth wear.[11]

## Tooth Wear Quantification

The availability of a tool that allows one to quantify tooth wear is vital for both research and for everyday clinical work. Throughout the years, a wide range of indices have been developed, all of them aimed at quantifying the amount of dental tissue lost, and also at longitudinally monitoring a potential progression of the condition. Some authors decided to develop their own indices, probably because they considered the existing indices not to be reliable enough; other authors made modifications to existing indices with the

*Table 9-2*

**Tooth wear index (TWI) from Smith and Knight.**[18]
B = buccal; L = lingual; O = occlusal; I = incisal; C = cervical

| Score | Surface | Criteria |
|---|---|---|
| 0 | B/L/O/I | No loss of enamel surface characteristics |
| | C | No change of contour |
| 1 | B/L/O/I | Loss of enamel surface characteristics |
| | C | Minimal loss of contour |
| 2 | B/L/O | Loss of enamel exposing dentin for less than one-third of surface |
| | I | Loss of enamel just exposing dentin |
| | C | Defect less than 1 mm deep |
| 3 | B/L/O | Loss of enamel exposing dentin for more than one-third of surface |
| | I | Loss of enamel and substantial loss of dentin (but not exposing pulp) |
| | C | Defect 1–2 mm deep |
| 4 | B/L/O | Complete enamel loss + pulp exposure + secondary dentin exposure |
| | I | Pulp exposure or exposure of secondary dentin |
| | C | Defect more than 2 mm deep + pulp exposure + secondary dentin exposure |

aim of improving them. The problem is that the great number of indices plus the many terminologies used makes valid comparison of the different publications almost impossible. Besides, the fact that tooth wear is multifactorial makes the situation even more complicated, since some of these indices are devised to measure the loss of tissue caused by a particular etiology.

Indices may be quantitative or qualitative. The former attempt to objectively measure tooth substance loss by measuring surfaces that represent attrition areas, crown height loss, etc. Qualitative indices are more subjective, and are based on very simplified descriptions made from the findings of clinical examination. They use a descriptive scale that classifies wear as mild, moderate, or severe. Of course, the use of a particular index depends on the specific objective, availability, etc. Objective measurement should be made by resorting to models, since measuring inside the mouth is extremely complicated. From the outset this makes it unsuitable for epidemiology data-gathering, its application being restricted to research studies with a more suitable infrastructure.

A good index should be simple to use and easy to understand; the score should faithfully reflect the loss of tooth substance and should be satisfactorily reproducible – of course, after a period of training and calibration. A "classical" index used in many research studies is the Tooth Wear Index (TWI) by Smith and Knight[18] (Table 9-2), devised to be used regardless of the etiology involved. Later, other authors introduced some modifications to this index.

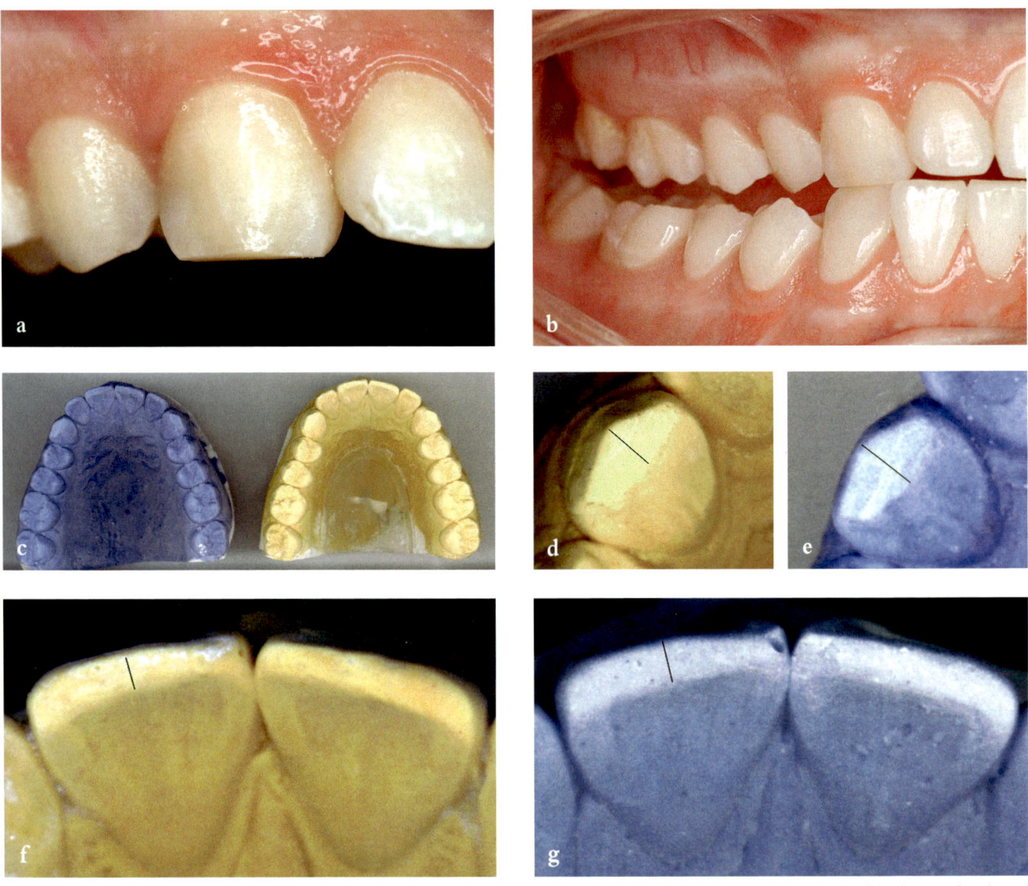

Fig 9-1 **(a)** Maxillary canine showing significant wear caused by bruxism, in a patient who is only 15 years old. **(b)** Occlusal correspondence of the two canines shows wear in both teeth to be reciprocal. **(c)** Scanned models; the yellow model is the initial one, and the blue one was obtained from the same patient 6 months later. Both models are placed with the teeth against the scanner's glass window and scanned at the same time. **(d)** Flattening of the canine cusp tip; the black line shows the width of the wear facet. **(e)** Six months later, wear has increased. **(f)** Initial measurement of right central incisor wear. **(g)** Six months later, incisor wear has increased.

In everyday dental practice, the use of these types of index is very difficult because they demand a great amount of clinical time. When managing patients with tooth wear, general practitioners need to make important decisions, both preventive and therapeutic; but, most importantly, they need a helpful parameter to monitor the potential progression of tooth wear over time. In this respect, comparison between models and pictures of the patient taken at different moments in time is a simple and effective tool to evaluate potential progression of the condition. Pictures are really helpful, since their colors allow dentin to be identified.[19]

It should be remembered that the presence of tooth wear is a historical, cumulative event that does not always imply an active process. For this reason, it is much simpler to identify its etiology in young individuals than in the older age groups. However, identifying tooth wear etiology is difficult also in young patients, since it is generally multifactorial.[20] Though visual inspection alone is

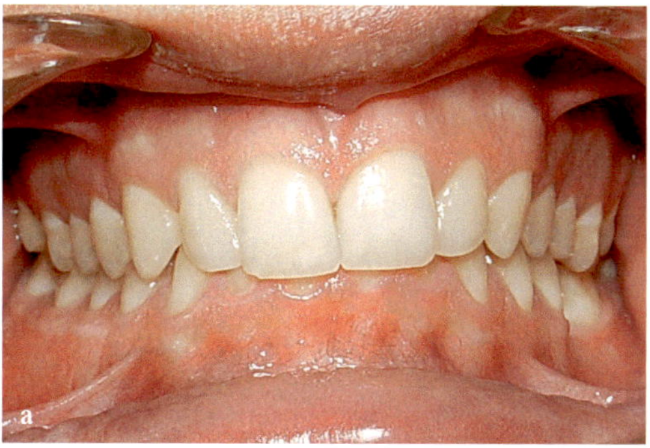

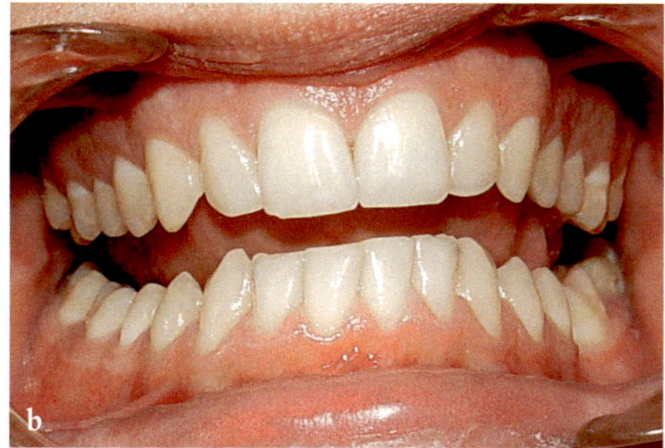

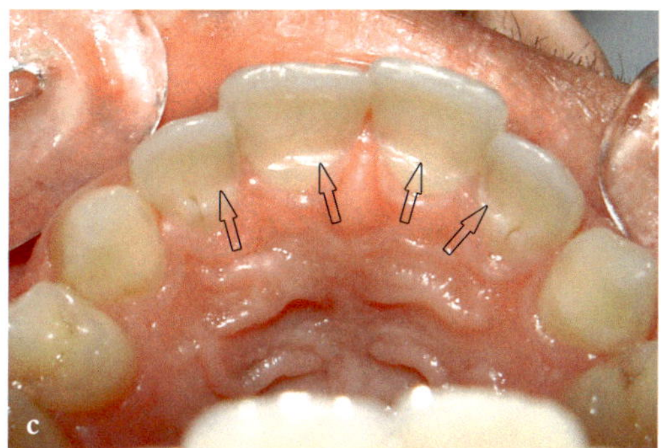

Fig 9-2 **(a)** Non-bruxer with a deep, scissor-like bite. **(b)** Wear is observed in the four incisal edges. **(c)** "Step-like" wear, caused by the recumbent position of the antagonist incisors.

usually sufficient to compare models, these can be scanned at the same scale, which allows images to be zoomed in so as to be more accurately measured. This is a very easy procedure and can be performed in any dental office, since it does not require the use of sophisticated technology (Fig 9-1).

## Factors Involved in Tooth Wear

Tooth wear does not occur in a uniform manner in all patients. Such differences may be ascribed to some intrinsic tooth factors, like enamel thickness and enamel hardness, which depends on its degree of mineralization.[21] It has also been shown that the pH of the oral environment is a factor in the degree of tooth wear. In-vitro attrition in experiments conducted in a hydrochloric acid medium (pH 1.2) was 10 times as great as in experiments conducted in a dry medium.[22] Another reported factor is age, and on this matter there is a high degree of consensus among studies, which demonstrate that tooth wear increases over time.[11,12,20,23–25] A longitudinal study of a group of patients with extensive tooth wear, conducted over a period of 6–10 years, showed that average increase cannot be predicted in proportion to the amount of initial wear.[26]

Some malocclusion variables are also considered to be factors that may contribute to the development of tooth wear by attrition. For example, a deep closed bite can be said to "trap" the jaw, which must make an extensive vertical movement in order to overcome the overbite increase. Clinical trials have shown that deep overbite causes a high degree of incisor wear.[27,28] This is possibly due to the inevitable friction between the anterior teeth, and to the fact that patients with this kind of occlusion have higher incisor bite force.[29] This situation will often be challenging for clinicians, since they are compelled to classify tooth wear as either physiologic

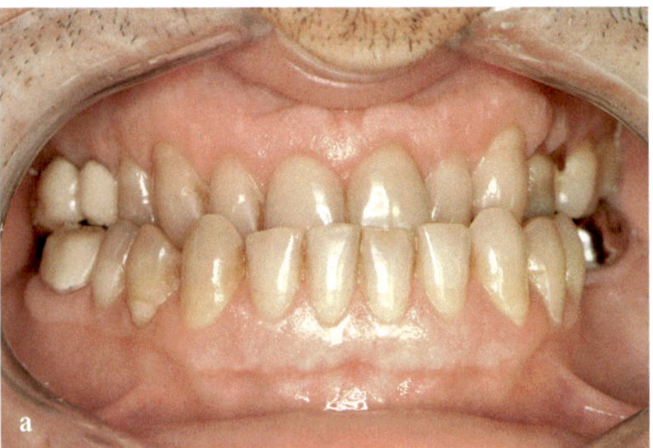


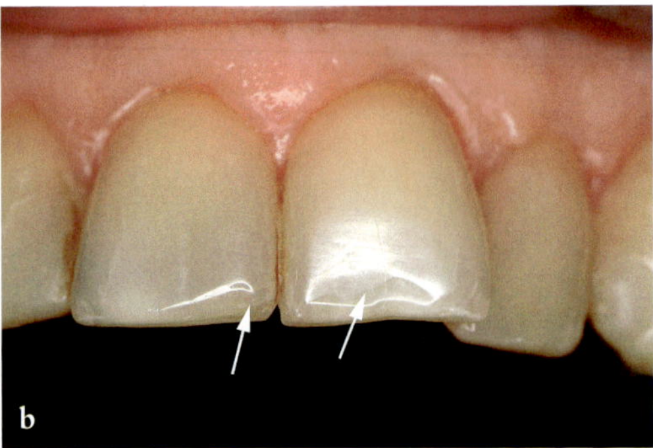


Fig 9-3 **(a)** A 68-year-old non-bruxer with prognathism. **(b)** Physiologic wear of vestibular surfaces (arrows) resulting from the forced occlusion.

or pathological. Figure 9-2 exemplifies and proves what has been said above.

Another malocclusion having special features is prognathism. Mesialization of the jaw causes an inversion of the relation between anterior teeth. Wear occurs on the vestibular face of maxillary incisors and on the lingual face of mandibular incisors. This kind of interdental relationship may contribute to the occurrence of physiologic facets in non-bruxers (Fig 9-3). It has also been suggested that the lack of canine guidance in patients with prognathism predisposes posterior teeth to greater wear.[30,31] Warren and co-workers reported greater incisor wear in patients with Angle class III canine relationship; they also mention that the low prevalence of this malocclusion makes gathering data from a large number of cases impossible, which accounts for the lack of powerful statistics.[32] These authors also reported an association between a posterior crossbite and greater tooth wear.

However, as is always the case with bruxism studies, there are also marked contradictions on this subject. A longitudinal study assessed mixed-dentition wear in 223 teenagers with malocclusion, who then received orthodontic treatment to achieve acceptable occlusion. The same subjects were re-examined 20 years later in order to assess tooth wear. The authors of the study reported a correlation between the deciduous-dentition wear observed in the first exam and the permanent-dentition wear observed in the second exam. However, such correlation was not observed in all the study subjects, but only in the younger ones. Owing to these findings, the authors excluded occlusal factors as the cause of the above-mentioned association, since all the participants had achieved perfect occlusion by means of orthodontic treatment.[33]

Occlusal trauma is another factor that may lead to attrition in the teeth affected. Occlusal load is generally distributed over the maximum dental intercuspation; i.e., over the occlusal table comprising the posterior teeth. However, in patients with unilateral osteoarthritis the occlusal load is usually distributed over the posterior teeth on the affected side. This is due to the lack of articular disc plus the continuous articular remodeling caused by this disease. In the teeth affected by this continuous overload, attrition may occur, without meaning that the patient is a bruxer. Unfortunately, no research has been conducted on this important subject, though it is a common, recurrent fact with this group of patients. Figure 9-4 shows a clinical case as an example of what has been stated above.

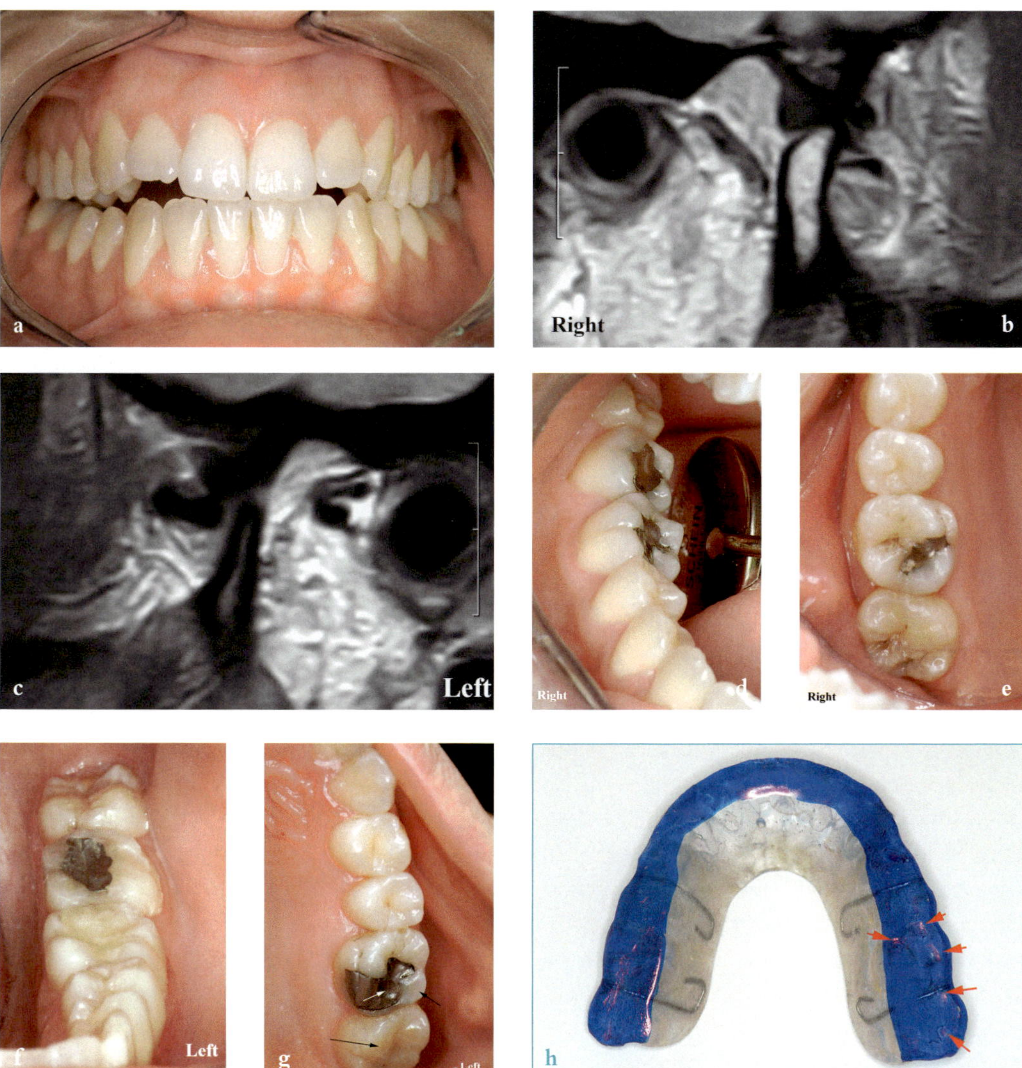


Fig 9-4 **(a)** Non-bruxer (woman) showing occlusal contacts only on the left side. This anomalous interdental relationship is caused by left unilateral osteoarthrosis. **(b)** Magnetic resonance imaging of the normal right temporomandibular joint (TMJ). The disc is normally located between the condyle and the articular eminence during maximum mouth opening; the condyle shows no signs of arthrotic remodeling. **(c)** The left TMJ has limited movement. The disc is displaced in the anterior direction; the condyle shows marked remodeling caused by osteoarthrosis. **(d)** No signs of wear are visible in the teeth of the lower right quadrant. **(e)** The upper right teeth show no signs of attrition either. **(f)** In the mandibular first and second left molars, signs of a significant amount of attrition can be observed. Since it has no antagonist, the third molar is not affected. **(g)** The black arrows indicate attrition in the maxillary cusps; the white arrow indicates wear on the amalgam restoration. **(h)** Splint used by the patient as symptomatic treatment of her condition. Even though occlusal balance was achieved when the splint was made, an overload on the affected side is always observed in control visits.

## Tooth Wear Patterns

A tooth wear pattern is the impression made by the antagonist teeth during the parafunctional movements of the jaw. In people living in a primitive way and in skeletal material obtained in anthropologic surveys, tooth wear was found to occur mainly in the posterior teeth.[34] In contrast, attrition in modern humans occurs mainly and markedly in the anterior tooth area. This has been scientifically demonstrated in children with deciduous teeth,[32,35] in teenagers with mixed dentition or permanent teeth,[36,37] in young adults,[38,39] and in adults of various ages.[11] There is absolutely no doubt, as confirmed by these findings, that tooth grinding in the protrusive and/or lateral direction is the prevailing pattern among bruxers, and its impressions can be observed as sequela mostly in the anterior teeth.

### *Wear During Protrusive Movements*

When there is an anteroposterior or protrusive tooth grinding pattern only, contact between anterior teeth occurs, contact between posterior teeth being considered unusual.[40] The teeth involved in this type of bruxism are the incisors; canine involvement is less than 5%.[30] In patients with Angle class I occlusion, a gap appears between premolars and molars as a result of the Christensen phenomenon, leading, finally, to a loss of tooth structure only in those teeth that interact during this movement. The continuous recurrence of this bruxism pattern will cause incisor crown height to decrease, which, in extremely serious cases, may significantly compromise a person's esthetic appearance. Posterior teeth, which are responsible for vertical dimension (VD), are not in contact during the protrusive movement, and so they will not be affected by wear. Thus, there will be no VD decrease.

When the tooth grinding episode comes to an end, the anterior teeth that were involved in it will show a microscopic loss of enamel and/or dentin. Since the VD has not changed, this slight wear will be offset by a compensatory dentoalveolar eruption mechanism occurring only in the anterior teeth.[41] Something similar occurs in patients with class II, division 2 malocclusions, who suffer from palatal mucosa trauma caused by the continuous dentoalveolar eruption of the incisors.[42] Murphy[7] considers this eruption mechanism to be one of the compensatory mechanisms associated with natural attrition. As a result, wear-affected teeth can maintain a smooth contact with their antagonists in the intercuspal position. Then, this process will repeat itself cyclically as long as this kind of activity continues. As a result of this permanent incisor extrusion, there will be no contact between the posterior teeth during protrusive tooth grinding. Clinically, the uniformity of the gingival festoon line will be disrupted as a result of the continuous dentoalveolar extrusion (Fig 9-5).

In bruxers who wear full prostheses and also show this tooth grinding pattern, this process is obviously different, since eruption is not possible. Thus, during maximum dental intercuspation, the anterior teeth will show a gap which represents the amount of tooth material missing as a result of attrition (Fig 9-6).

All the above explains why there is no VD loss despite the presence of extensive tooth wear. This dental-occlusion dynamic process has been proved by superimposing lateral cephalograms. When compared with subjects not suffering from tooth wear, patients with significant tooth wear (of over a third of crown length) did not show a lower vertical dimension.[43]

### *Wear During Lateral Movements*

Tooth grinding during lateral movements of the jaw mainly involves the canines. Immediately after eruption, during lateral movements of the jaw these will act as a sliding ramp that will prevent posterior teeth from interfering with each other; D'Amico called this mechanism "canine protection".[10] However, canine protection is usually lost

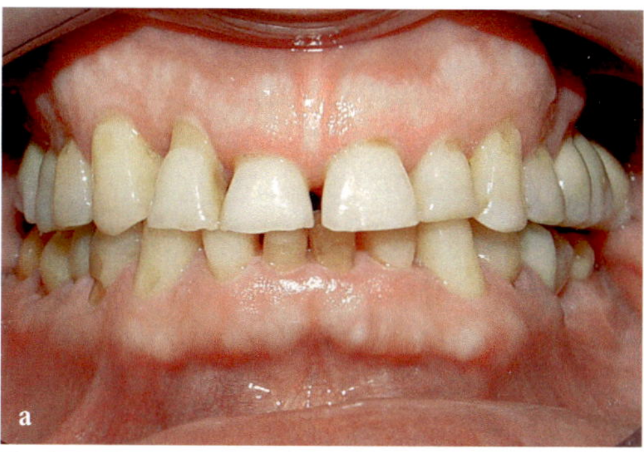

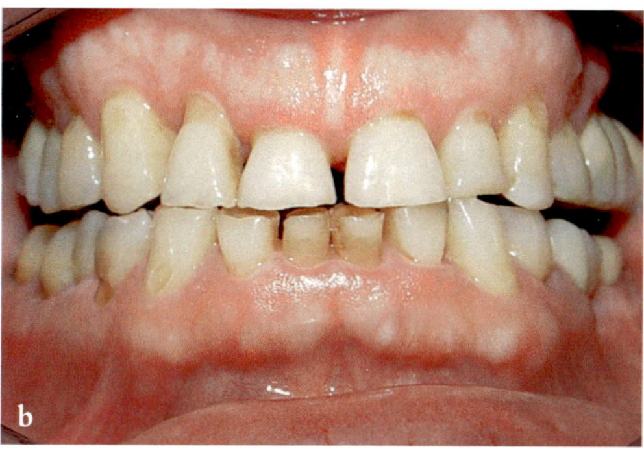

Fig 9-5 **(a)** Patient showing an important loss of hard tissue in his anterior teeth, caused by a combination of bruxism and erosion by gastroesophageal reflux. **(b)** Protrusive bruxism pattern, during which the posterior teeth uncouple. Note the dento-alveolar eruption of the anterior teeth, which shows over the gumline. Marked vestibular exostosis can be seen in both jaw.

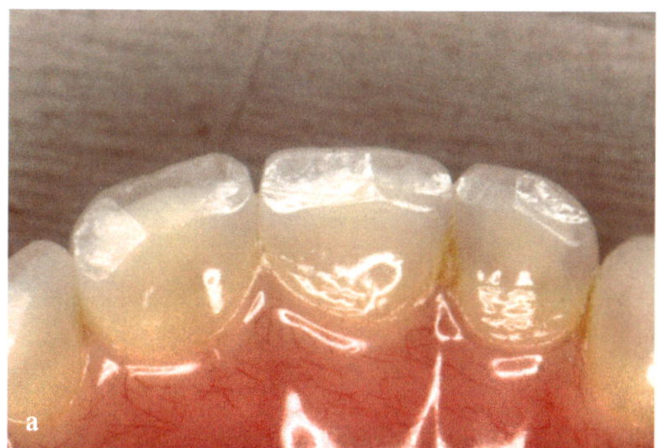

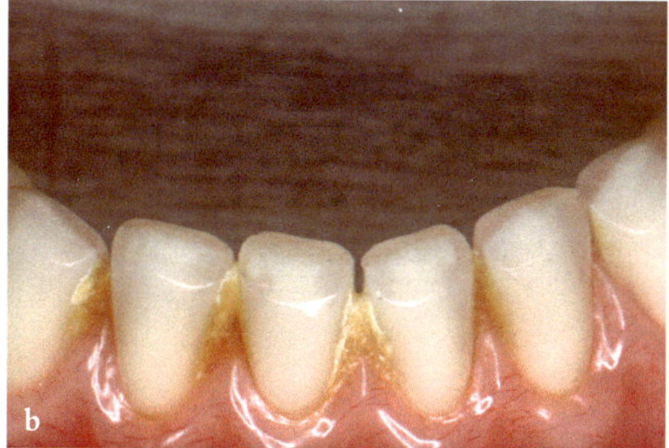

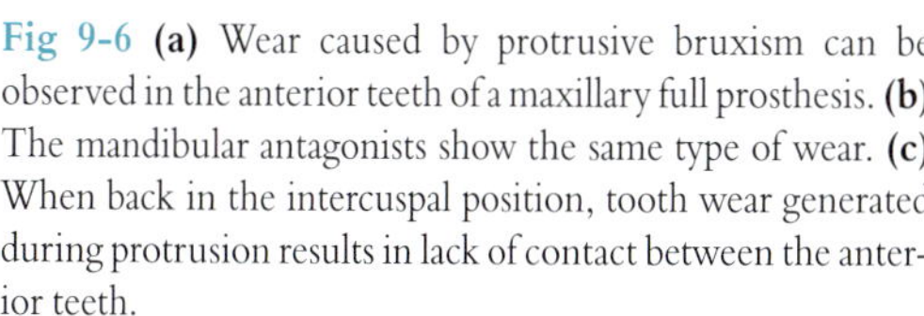

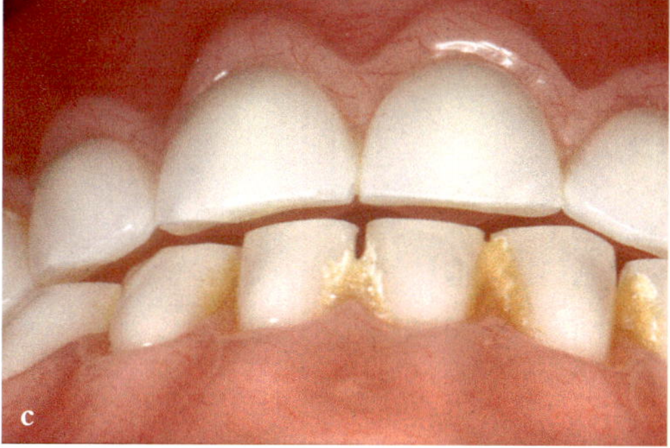

Fig 9-6 **(a)** Wear caused by protrusive bruxism can be observed in the anterior teeth of a maxillary full prosthesis. **(b)** The mandibular antagonists show the same type of wear. **(c)** When back in the intercuspal position, tooth wear generated during protrusion results in lack of contact between the anterior teeth.

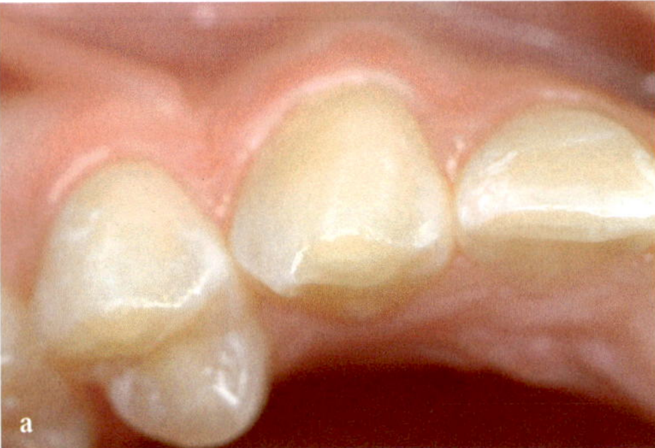

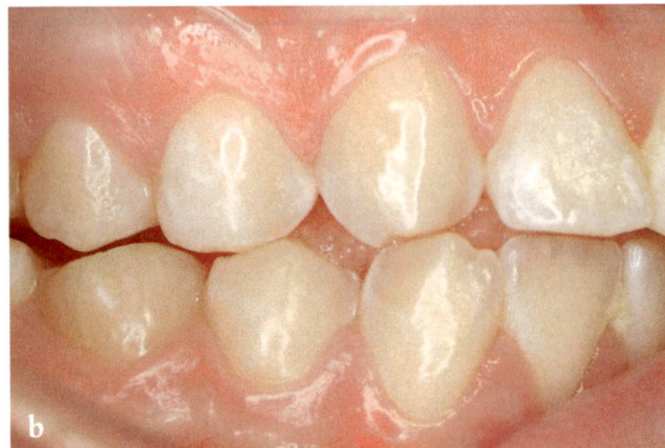

Fig 9-7 **(a)** Attrition can be seen in a canine that erupted only 1 year ago. **(b)** Reproduction of the bruxism pattern causing the wear.

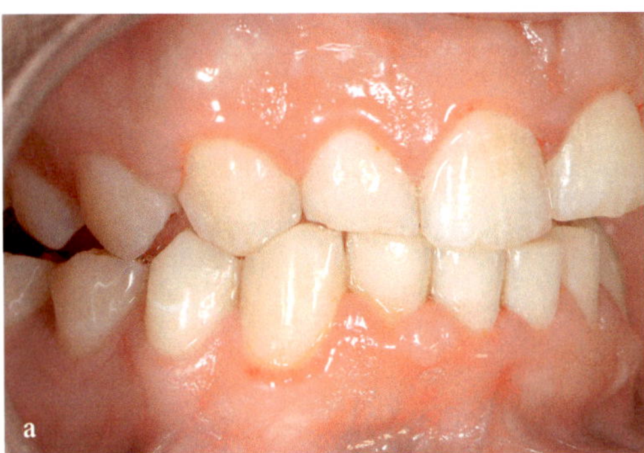

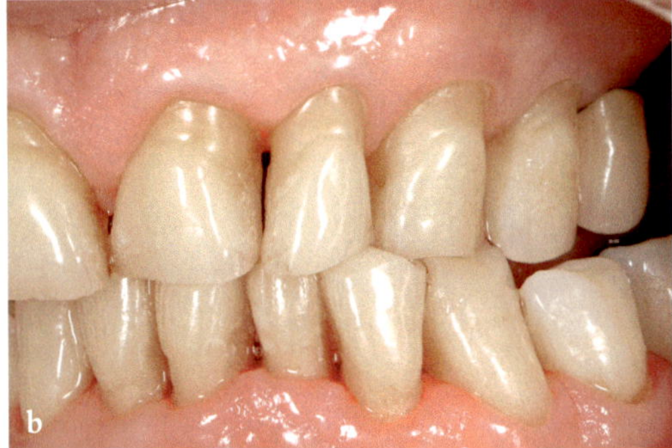

Fig 9-8 **(a and b)** The bruxism pattern was confirmed through the occlusal correspondence of reciprocal wear.

on reaching adult age as a result of canine attrition.[44]

The importance of canine guidance has been proved by a longitudinal study of a population of young dental students. Over the 2-year follow-up, the authors found that only maxillary and mandibular canines were affected by wear, incisors showing the same anatomy they had at the beginning of the study.[45] These findings suggest that incisor wear occurred in the years before canine eruption and that, once they erupted, the canines protected the rest of the teeth.

During bruxing lateral movements, canine wear allows for working-side posterior tooth-to-tooth contact, canine protection becoming a "group function".[46] Scaife[30] points out that tooth wear increases in inverse proportion to the degree of canine protection. Group function during lateral movement is the most common occlusal scheme in adults, as opposed to canine protection, which occurs less commonly.[30,40,44,47,48] Yaffe and Ehrlich[48] consider lateral movement with group function to be a dynamic process, and they describe three stages. The first starts in the maximum intercupation; the second, 1 mm away, laterally; the third, when both canines are in opposition. The occurrence of posterior tooth contact during this movement will vary in location and amount depending on each of these three stages. Contacts tend to decrease from stage 1 to stage 3. The group function allows for the occurrence of posterior tooth-to-tooth contact, generating attrition in the posterior teeth. For this reason, canine attrition is considered to be a factor predisposing to attrition in the posterior sector.[49]

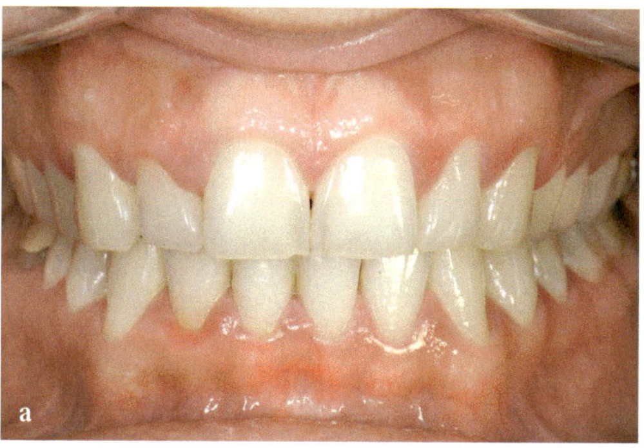


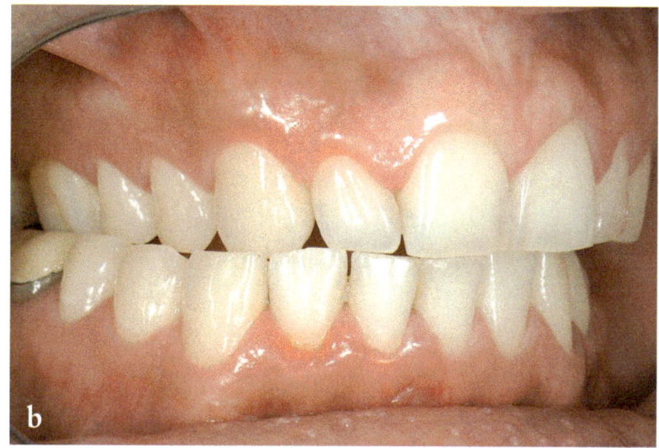


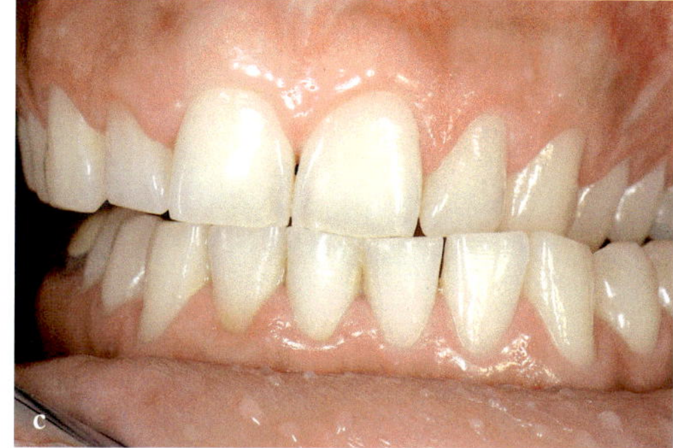


Fig 9-9 **(a–c)** Reproduction of an eccentric bruxism pattern; this patient shows an exaggerated lateral movement in both directions. Note the extreme position of the mandibular canines when the lateral movement is over.

Lateral-grinding bruxism causes wear in those dental structures not involved in the maximum intercuspation scheme. Diagnosing the sequel of this parafunction is relatively easy, since, to a higher or lesser degree, canine cusp tips will be visibly truncated. This grinding pattern, which can often be appreciated early despite the short time elapsed since eruption, can be confirmed through clinical examination of the canine cusp tips (Fig 9-7).

Something similar occurs with incisal edges. The disappearance of incisor mamelons gives dental clinicians a clue to the presence of tooth wear possibly caused by bruxism. If bruxism is suspected, diagnosis should be confirmed by thoroughly examining the relationships between these teeth during eccentric jaw movements. This can be done by examining the models mounted on the articulator, though it is also possible to evaluate these relationships directly in the mouth. If, on comparing antagonist facets of the maxilla and the mandible, wear is found to be reciprocal, such diagnosis will be confirmed (Fig 9-8).

The presence of tooth wear in anterior teeth showing signs of attrition cannot always be confirmed by identifying "normal" horizontal movements. Sometimes, these facets occur during extremely atypical jaw movements, which not even the patient is aware of. We must be on the alert for these situations, especially whenever tooth wear features suggest that bruxism is the main etiological factor involved. Figures 9-9 and 9-10 show patients whose bruxism patterns are demonstrated during extreme lateral movement of the jaw.

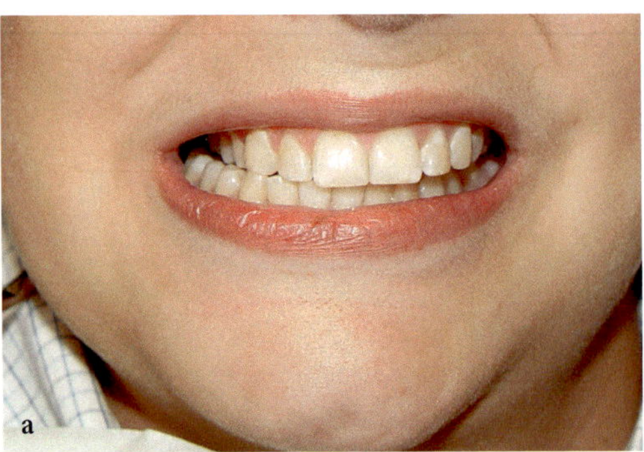

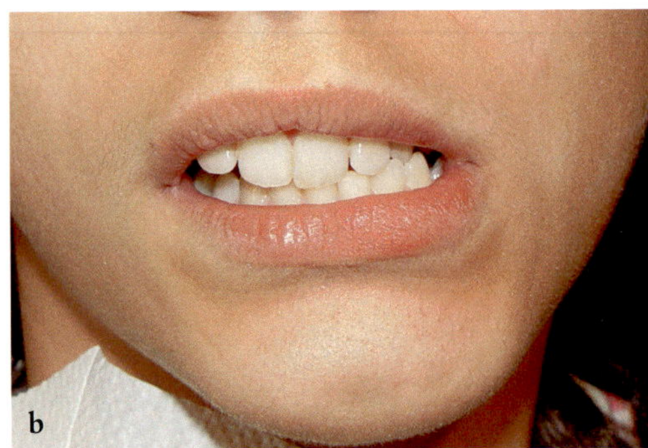

Fig 9-10 **(a and b)** Note the long lateral movement shown by these two teenagers during tooth grinding.

### *Centric Bruxism Pattern*

So far, we have examined attrition caused by eccentric tooth grinding patterns. Centric tooth clenching has been neglected by scientists as an object of study. However, this type of bruxism, which is almost specific to wakefulness, occurs twice as many times as sleep bruxism (tooth grinding), concerning which plenty of research has been conducted. This kind of static or "almost static" bruxism – since some movement occurs, though in the vertical direction – could also leave some sort of a typical scar. No trials have been done to trace the occurrence of dental attrition in patients who show a tooth clenching habit exclusively. However, some clinical observations alert us to the existence of a type of attrition that is different from that described above. Figures 9-11 and 9-12 are two examples of what we consider to be a kind of attrition caused by sustained tooth clenching.

Cavities are commonly seen on some posterior-tooth plastic restorations when centric holding cusps fully articulate over an amalgam or composite. Also, in teeth without restorations, enamel can be affected by this condition – though this cannot be ascribed exclusively to tooth clenching: erosion alone, or erosion in combination with tooth clenching, may be the cause (Fig 9-13).

The mesiopalatal cusps of the maxillary first molar or second molar are generally responsible for the hollowness, restoration fractures and, sometimes, even chipped cusps. Dahl and co-workers[50] assessed tooth clenching force in a study group of patients showing a high degree of attrition (tooth grinders). After comparing the study group with a control group, they found no significant differences between them. The authors concluded that not a big amount of muscle force is needed to cause attrition.[50] Although in an indirect way, this study's findings prove that tooth grinders, who will show a high degree of attrition, belong to a different bruxism subgroup and must be distinguished from exclusive tooth clenchers, who will show a stronger bite force. Muscle power generated during sustained tooth clenching exerts a significant force over the posterior-tooth occlusal table; besides, the more posterior the tooth, the stronger the force exerted.[51]

Maximum bite force is strongly dependent on a patient's facial structure. For example, higher clenching forces have been reported in subjects whose skeletal morphology shows an increased proportion between posterior facial height and anterior facial height (square jaw), when compared to subjects with normal facial proportions.[52,53] This has been challenged by others who, after comparing

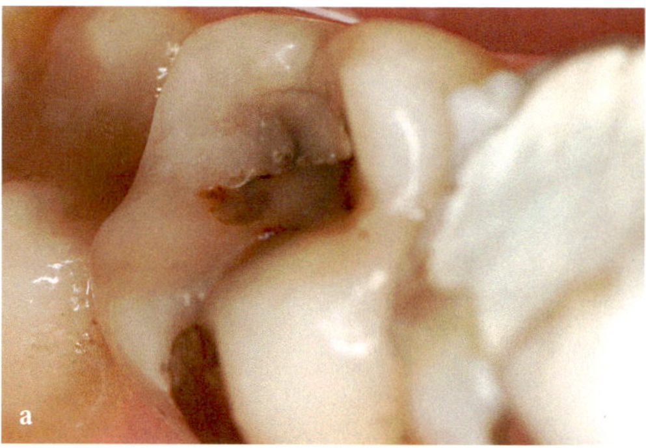

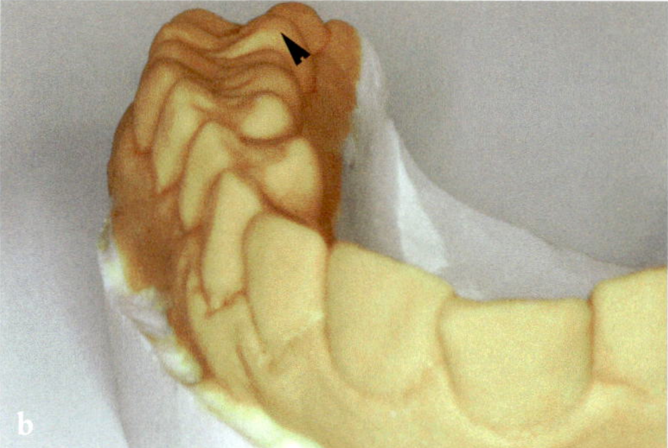

Fig 9-11 **(a)** Deep occlusal wear in a clencher's mandibular second molar which had been restored with composite. **(b)** Extruded antagonist cusp (arrow).

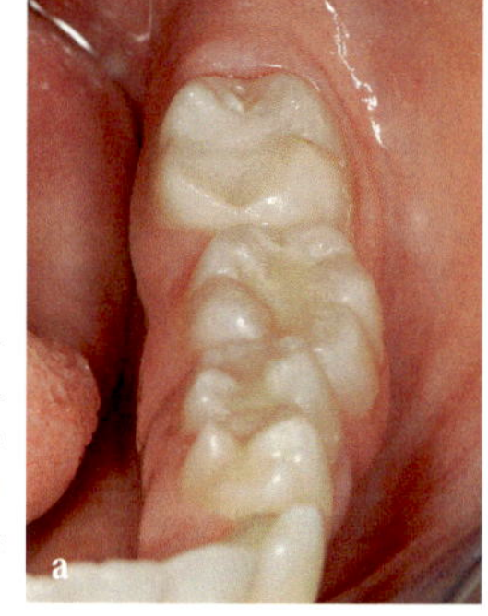

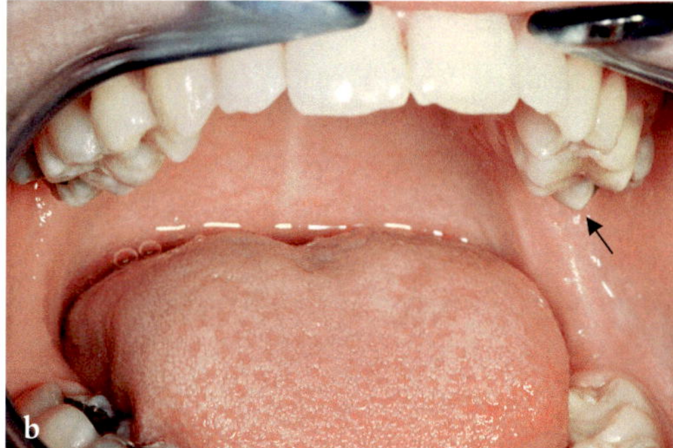

Fig 9-12 **(a)** Wear in a clencher's mandibular second molar which had been restored with composite. **(b)** Note the extrusion of the antagonist (arrow).

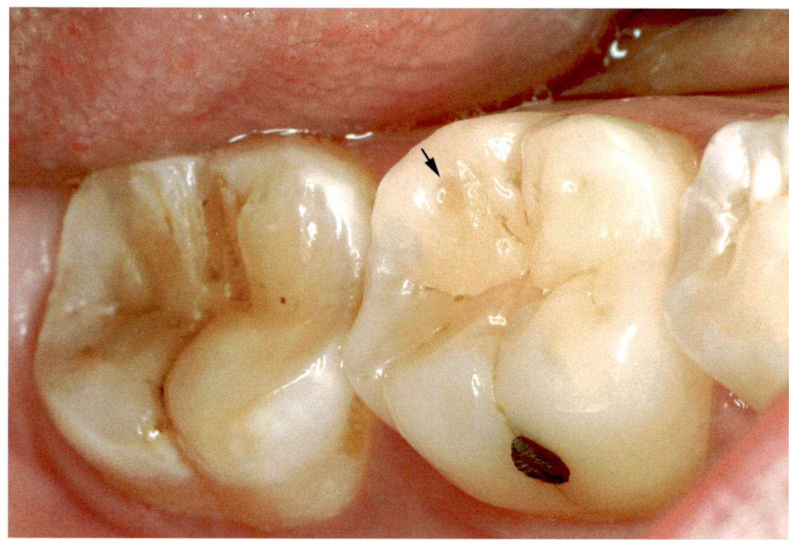

Fig 9-13 Occlusal wear in mandibular molars, caused by intense tooth clenching and increased by erosion. Signs of the action of acid can be observed (arrow).

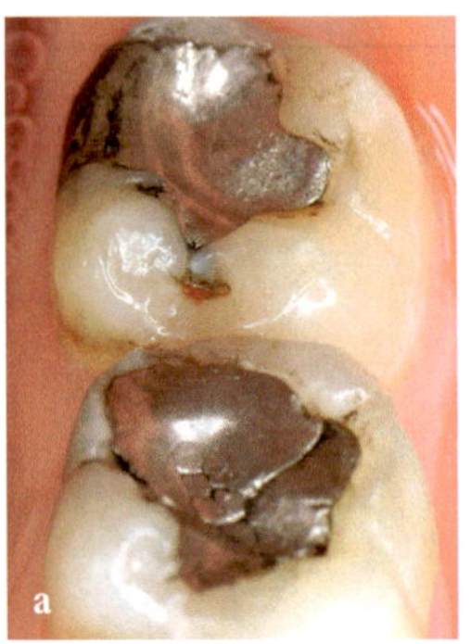

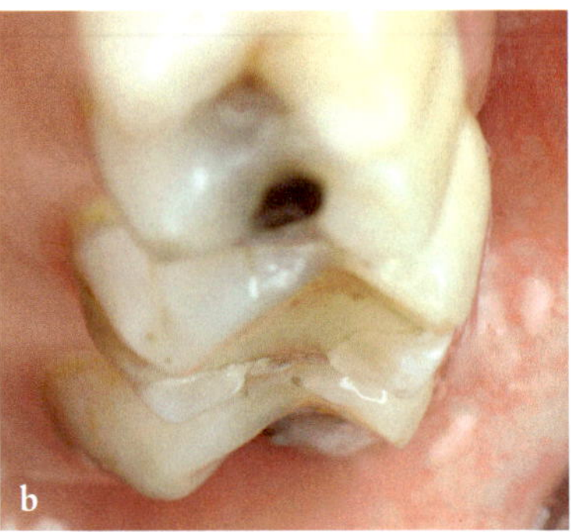

Fig 9-14 **(a)** Marked wear in an amalgam. **(b)** The corresponding extrusion of the antagonist tooth.

bruxers and non-bruxers, claim that both groups have a similar cranial–facial structure.[54] Their study, however, has some methodologic faults: the authors report that 40% of the control population (non-bruxers) presented clinical signs of attrition, from which it may be inferred that the control population, selected through a questionnaire, also included bruxers. The same team of researchers conducted another research study later, and they obtained similar results.[55] However, once again, as with their previous work, we must call into question the fact that subjects with attrition should have been included in the control population, since the inclusion clause stipulated that subjects should show attrition in 90% of their teeth in order to be considered bruxers, or in up to 60% of their teeth to be included in the control population. Such a high percentage value regulating inclusion in the control population will make the control population worthless, since, unquestionably, so much attrition indicates that the control population also included bruxers. Nevertheless, other authors showed, through computed tomography, that brachycephalous patients, who have a short facial height and a small jaw angle, have more developed temporalis and medial pterygoid muscles.[56]

Thus we may conclude that, although there is some disagreement about clenching force, facial biotype, and bruxism, we must be very careful when designing treatment plans for patients with these characteristics. From a preventive point of view, one possibility would be to use rigid restorations instead of plastic ones. The latter have low resistance to attrition, so they are subject to constant wear, which causes the antagonist cusp to slowly and progressively erupt deep into the cavity. On certain occasions, antagonist extrusion is so significant that it interrupts the maxillary of Spee curve considerably, causing a dental occlusion alteration (Fig 9-14).

## Interpretation of Tooth Wear

Tooth wear is unlikely to result from only one factor. Generally, simultaneous erosion, attrition, and abrasion occurs. Of course, some of these factors may be more relevant than others at certain times and according to the specific case. A research study conducted on a population of subjects suffering from excessive tooth wear determined that the main cause was erosion; bruxism was the second most relevant factor.[18] Besides, no abrasion mechanism could be demonstrated as the only cause in the study subjects, and in the few cases involving such a mechanism, this was always in combination with some other factor.

It is vital that dental practitioners be familiar with and able to distinguish between the various processes responsible for tooth wear, since, when

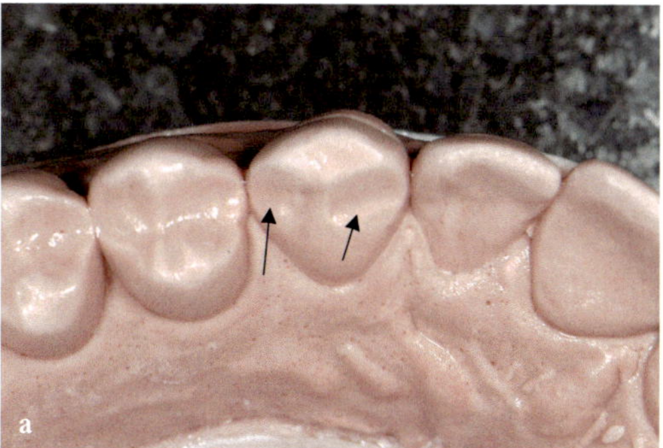

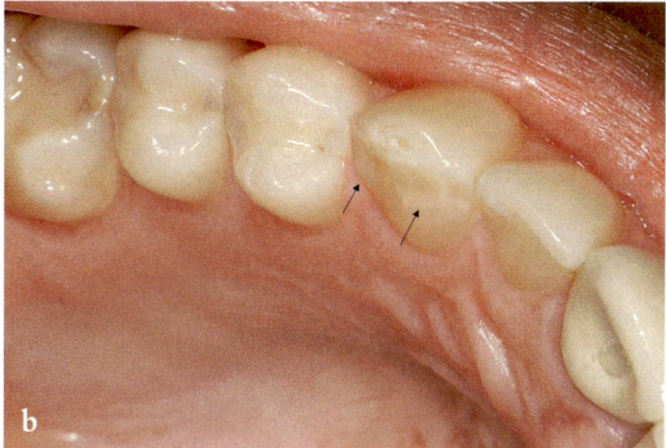

Fig 9-15 **(a)** Step-like attrition in a maxillary canine. The extent of the attrition can be observed perfectly in the model (arrows). **(b)** Clinically, though, it is much less visible.

interacting with bruxism, such processes often cause irreversible lesions in the tooth hard tissue. Being familiar with their origin and mechanism of action helps to manage in a comprehensive way the prevention and early treatment of those factors leading to human tooth decay.

### *Clinical Appearance and Comparison with Erosion*

Identifying the cause of tooth wear is not easy. Often, many etiological agents interact, each of them with their own characteristics. However, some patients' tooth wear pattern may involve only one cause.

Attrition is a mechanism characterized by the "sweep" of hard tissue (enamel and dentin) by antagonist teeth. As a result, reciprocal tooth wear, which is closely related to the potential movements of the jaw, is always to be expected. In order to clinically diagnose attrition, we must examine the specific places where it commonly occurs: anterior-tooth incisal edges, posterior-tooth occlusal surfaces, anterior-tooth palatal surfaces, vestibular surfaces of mandibular anterior teeth, and proximal surfaces (very difficult to observe). Bruxism wear could be compared to the wear generated by a file on a piece of metal or wood.

#### *Incisal edges*

Disappearance of the incisor mamelons is a typical sign of attrition. The edge is turned into a true flattened surface, with a sharp enamel circumferential ridge at the same level as the exposed dentin – it has been considered that enamel, which is harder, supports or protects dentin in this way, which allows for simultaneous wear of both tissues.[57] In contrast, chemical erosion undermines the central area of the incisal edge, creating, in bas-relief between the lingual enamel and the vestibular enamel, a concave slot which corresponds to the eroded dentin. If the patient is requested to make protrusive movements and lack of contact between antagonistic incisors is observed, then this will confirm the impossibility that the crack must have had some mechanical cause.

As is the case with mandibular incisors, maxillary incisor attrition is characterized by flattening of the incisal edges and very sharp enamel ridges. The palatal faces will often show well-circumscribed steps generated by the lower incisal edge.[58] It is difficult to observe such steps in the clinical exam, but they are easily detectable in plaster models (Fig 9-15). Attrition is equally common in maxillary and mandibular anterior teeth. This is not the case with erosion, since mandibular incisors, which are better protected by the action of saliva, are hardly ever affected.[57] The acid affects the maxillary incisal edges, which have a thin, transparent appearance and chipped edges due to the fractures caused by the lack of supporting dentin, which erodes faster (Fig 9-16). Endogenous

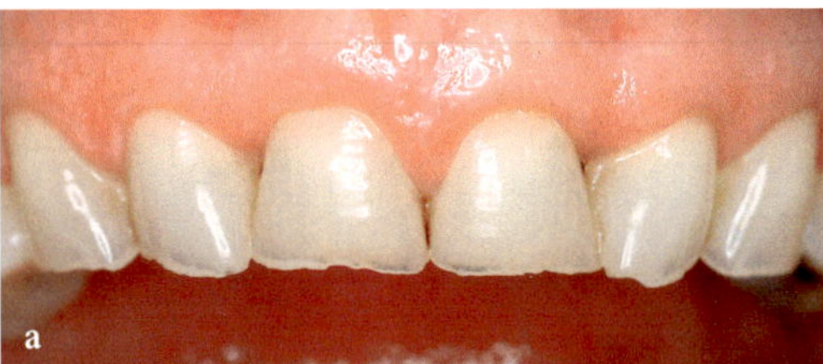

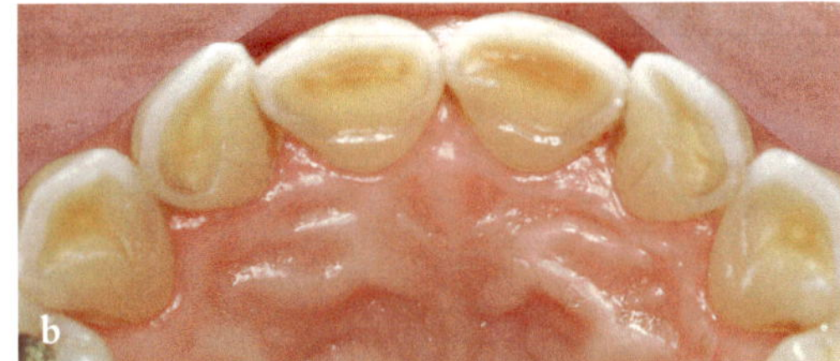

Fig 9-16 **(a)** The lack of supporting dentin accounts for these enamel fractures. **(b)** Palatal view; concave wear reflecting the action of erosion.

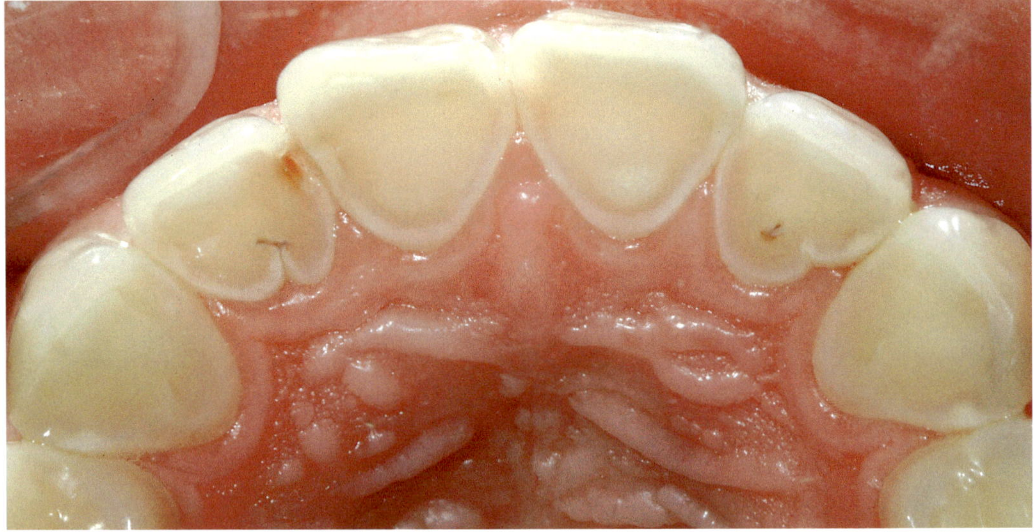

Fig 9-17 Palatal surface erosion in a bulimic patient (woman).

erosion (bulimia, regurgitation, etc.) affects maxillary incisor palatal surfaces in a characteristic way (Fig 9-17). Maxillary incisors have a spoon-like appearance, and a concavity can be seen both longitudinally and transversely. Exposed dentin will typically show a yellowish hue, and it will be surrounded by an enamel circumferential ridge extending up to the gingival crevice.[58]

*Posterior teeth*

Attrition will also cause posterior teeth to flatten proportionately in both the maxillary and mandibular arches. Such flattenings can be easily made to correspond with each other by requesting the patient to perform a lateral movement of the jaw. Typically, molars affected by loss of structure due to erosion will show volcano-shaped lesions or cupped lesions. A yellowish cavity which corresponds to dentin can be seen in the center of the lesion. Erosion will primarily affect mandibular molars, especially the first molar, because it erupts early. Absence of wear on maxillary molars is thought to be related to the protection provided by the saliva from the parotid gland.[59] Note that, for didactic purposes, "pure" lesions corresponding to one or the other of the two mechanisms dealt with are described here; however, in clinical work lesions will not always present in this way.

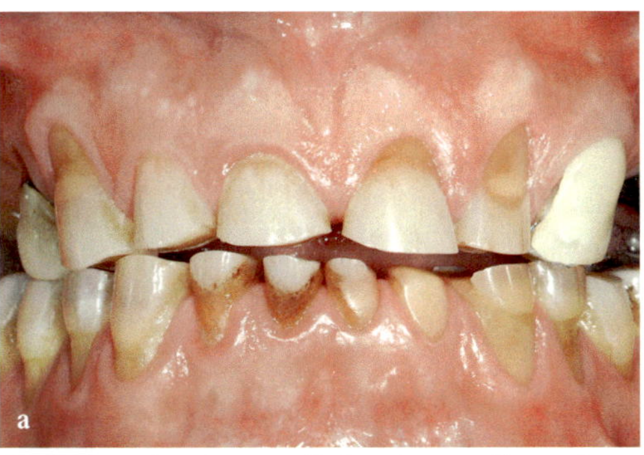

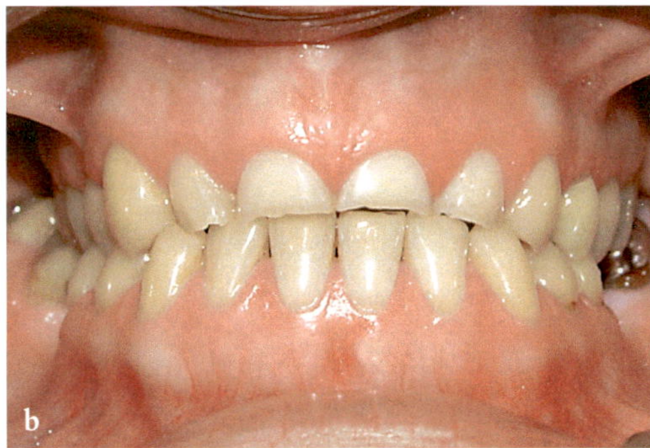

Fig 9-18 **(a)** Attrition caused by bruxism; maxillary and mandibular teeth show a similar amount of wear. **(b)** Erosion caused by bulimia; only maxillary anterior teeth are affected by wear.

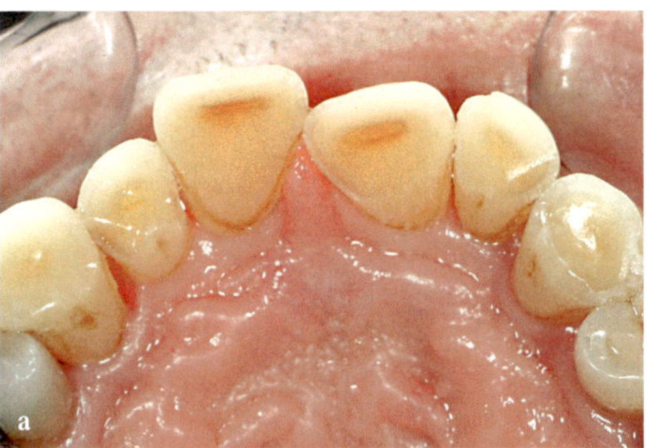

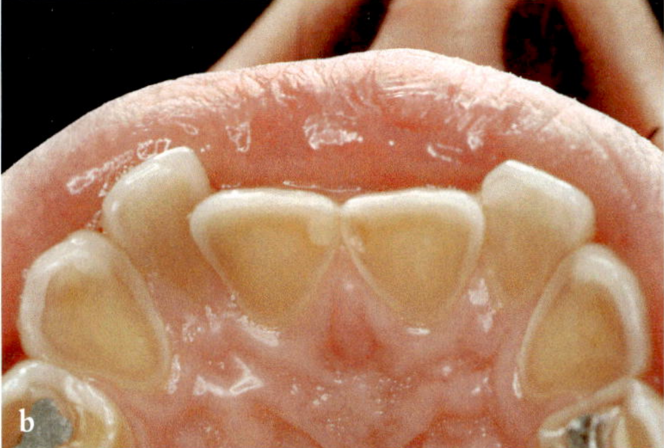

Fig 9-19 **(a)** Attrition in maxillary anterior teeth; a flattened wear pattern can be observed. **(b)** Erosion in maxillary anterior teeth: a concave wear pattern can be observed.

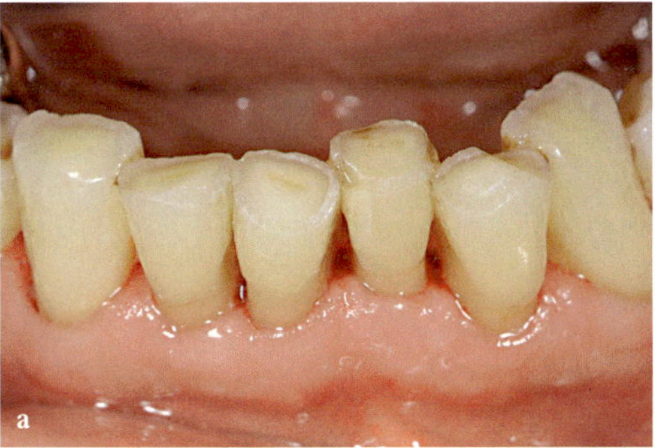

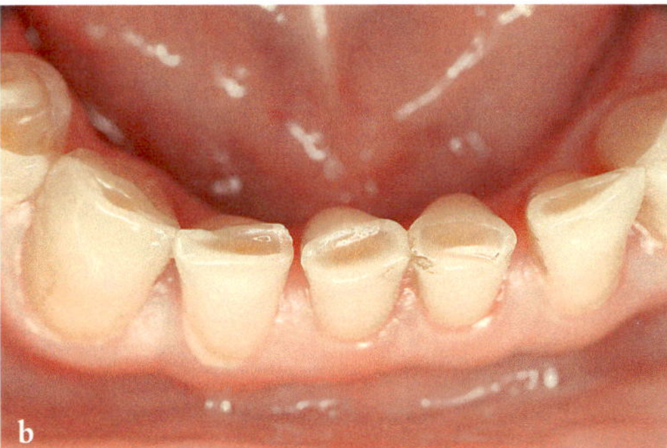

Fig 9-20 **(a)** Attrition in mandibular anterior teeth. **(b)** Erosion in mandibular anterior teeth.

Often, attrition and erosion coexist and interact in the mouth, generating wear patterns that make identification of the source difficult. Figures 9-18 to 9-21 compare attrition and erosion in teeth from different quadrants of the mouth.

In a survey based on models, Woda and co-workers[47] report the existence of functional facets located in the maximum intercupation tooth-contact areas, and of parafunctional facets located some distance away from the maximum intercu-

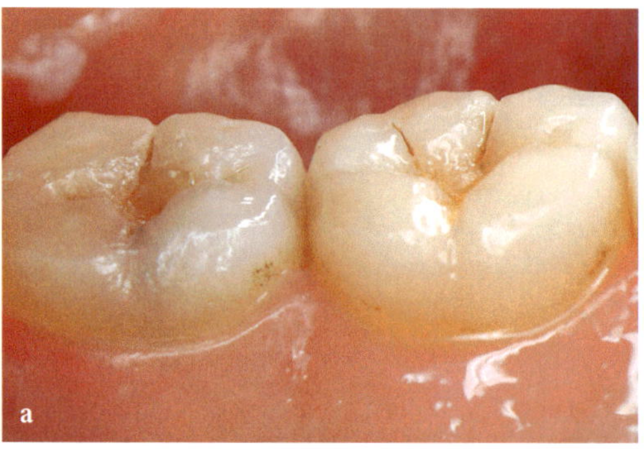


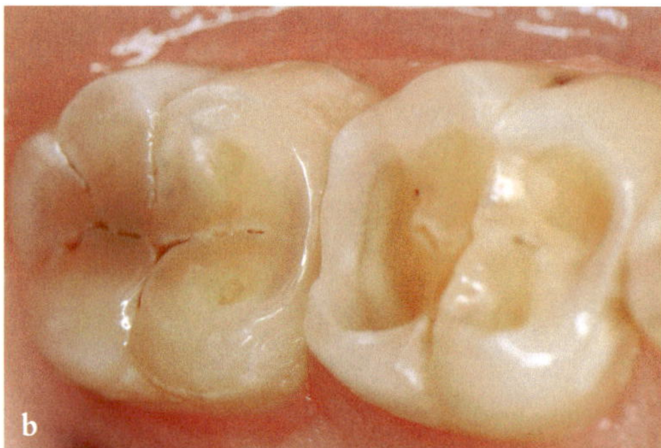


Fig 9-21 **(a)** Attrition in mandibular molars. **(b)** Erosion in mandibular molars.

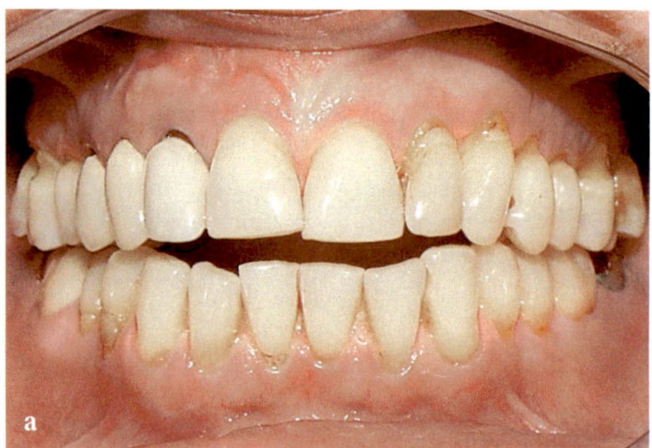


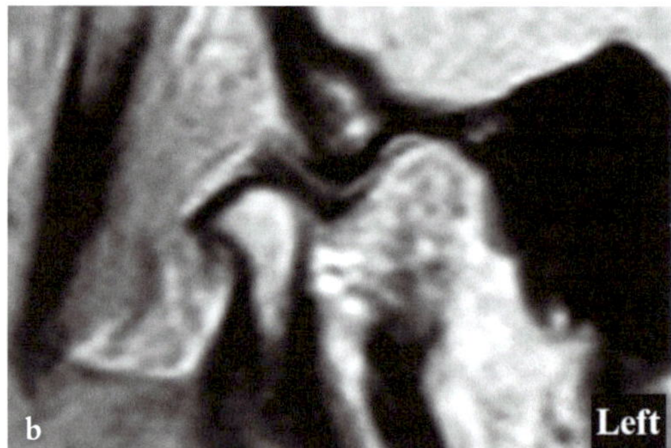


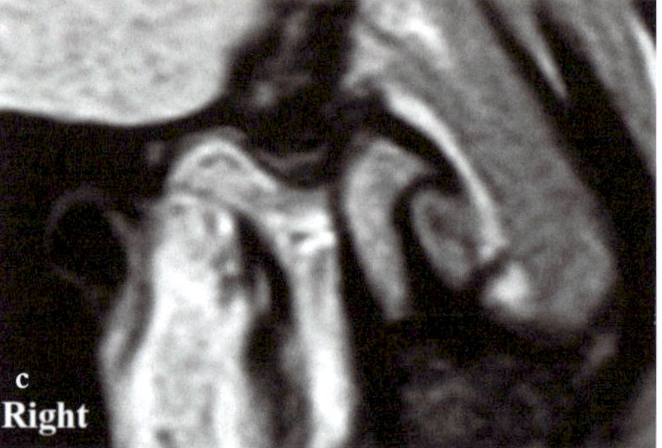


Fig 9-22 **(a)** This bruxer (woman) has osteoarthrosis in both temporomandibular joints and shows progressive open bite. The attrition of the six mandibular anterior teeth cannot be reproduced during any mandibular movement. **(b and c)** Marked osteophytosis can be seen in both condyles, which are affected by osteoarthrosis.

pation. Such parafunctional facets show different characteristics according to their location in anterior or posterior teeth. Anterior teeth will show horizontal facets on the incisal edges and canine cusp tips, away from the maximum intercupation. These facets are likely to be caused by protrusion and lateral movements of the jaw. Vertical facets are located on the palatal faces of maxillary anterior teeth and on the vestibular surfaces of mandibular anterior teeth, in both cases near the intercuspal position. In posterior teeth, facets are distributed in the functional cusps according to working and non-working movements. Since contact distribution in the posterior teeth coincides with the maximum intercupation, the latter is thought to progressively consolidate in accordance with the wear pattern.

Clinical identification of wear by attrition on maxillary incisor and canine palatal surfaces is more difficult. Enamel's white color usually blinds the observer and disguises these scars. Owing to their opacity, plaster models allow for an easier detection.

Sometimes, when evaluating the mandibular dynamics, it may not be possible to verify facet reciprocity between anterior teeth, despite their showing attrition-compatible wear features. One should be on the alert, since such situations may involve a patient who suffers not only from bruxism, but also from some other articular pathology causing an alteration in the maxillary–mandibular relationship. Patients with degenerative arthritis (osteoarthritis) suffer from progressive overbite loss and overjet increase, which results in an open anterior bite[60] (Fig 9-22). In advanced cases, these

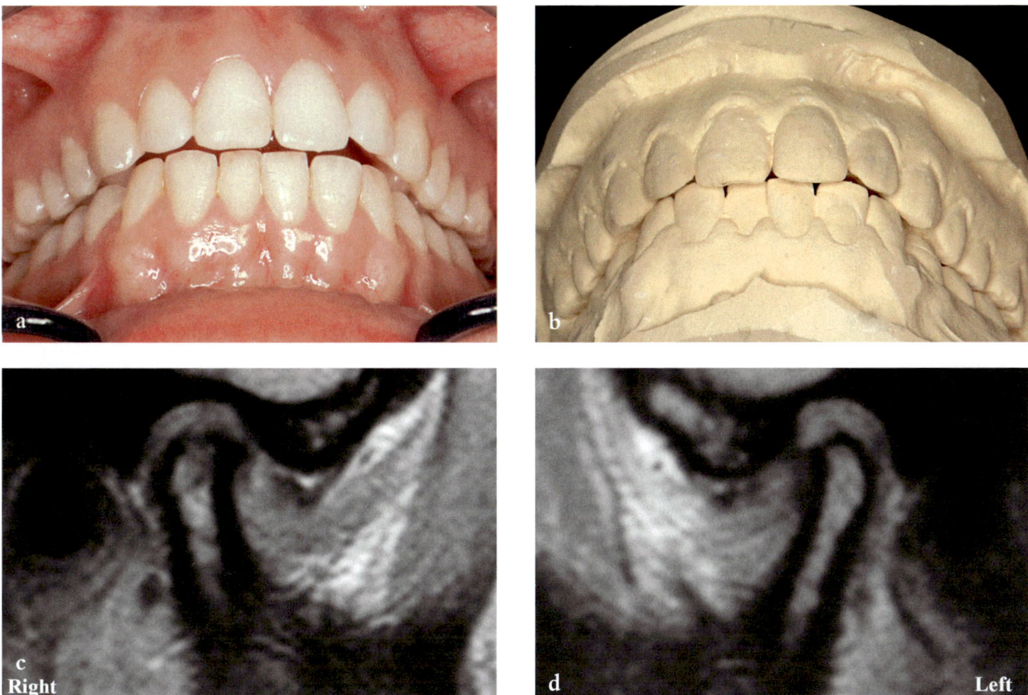


Fig 9-23 **(a)** Osteoarthrosis in a bruxer (woman) who shows symptoms in both temporomandibular joints (TMJs) and a progressive open bite which, according to the patient's account, started 5 months before. **(b)** The models, obtained a year before, confirm the changes that occurred. **(c and d)** MRI of both TMJs shows advanced disc displacements and condyle remodeling (flattening of the left condyle and fresh osteophyte in the right condyle).

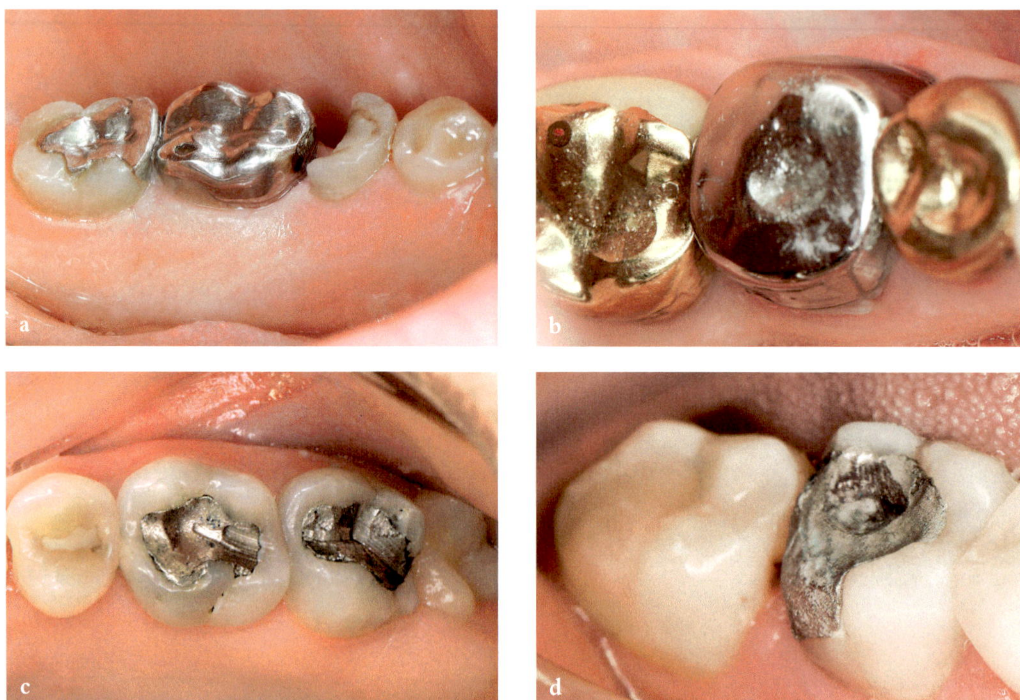

Fig 9-24 **(a–d)** Signs of attrition (bruxism) on metal restorations.

patients may lose the maximum dental intercuspation completely, which makes occlusal correspondence between antagonist teeth very difficult. Sometimes, manually articulating the patient's models not only allows confirmation of the wear pattern but also reveals a change in the three-dimensional position of the jaw (Fig 9-23).

### *Night-guard Examination*

Many people wear night guards, and this number increases every day. Usually, the first contact between a patient and the clinician's office is through a phone call; thus, it is advisable to properly train the staff who answer the phone, so that they ask patients who wear night guards to bring them to the first appointment.

Visual inspection of night guards is really helpful in confirming or excluding the occurrence of sleep bruxism. Some clinicians will label a patient a bruxer simply because the latter's teeth are worn, and they will make a splint for them. Often, although wear may be seen in a patient's natural teeth, when we examine the splint they have been wearing for some time we see no signs of attrition. In this case, another cause for wear may be suspected; it is also possible that the patient used to be a bruxer in the past but no longer has a bruxing habit.

The presence of attrition on the occlusal surface of plastic or rigid restorations and crowns is also evidence of bruxism, and it excludes erosion as the main source of wear (Fig 9-24). The scenario

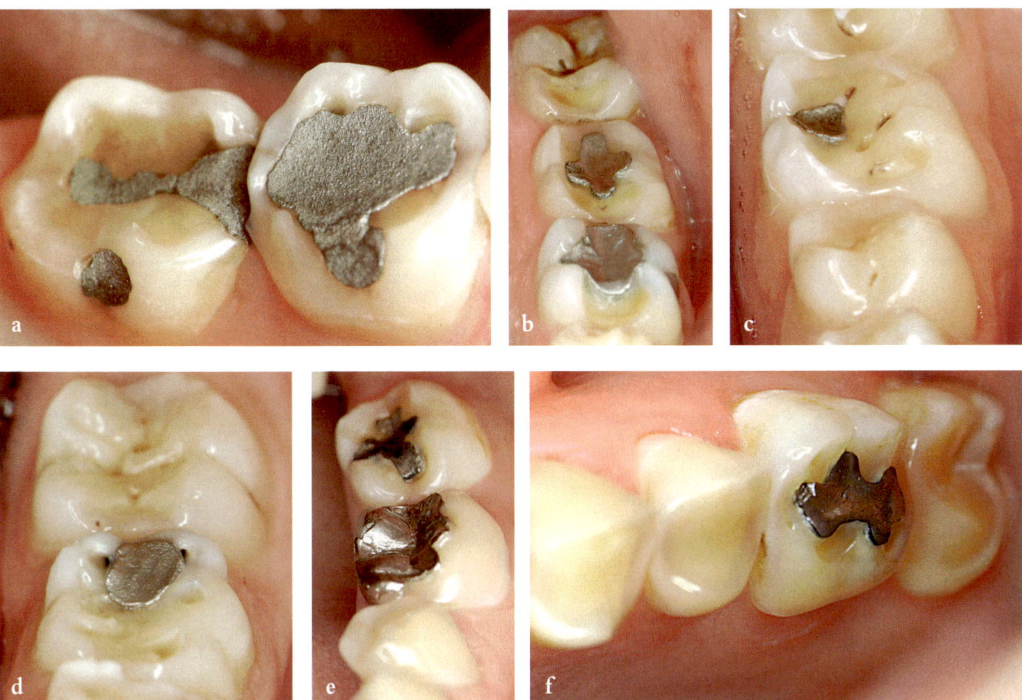


Fig 9-25 **(a–f)** Clinical signs of erosion: metal restorations appear in high relief.

is completely different when we have acid as wear etiology. In these cases, metal restorations that have not been dissolved by the acid appear in high relief (Fig 9-25).

## Conclusion

Perusal of the next chapter, dealing with erosion (another cause of tooth wear, perhaps the most important one), will allow a more complete picture of the subject. Readers will then be empowered not only to identify the true etiological agent involved in tooth wear but also to promptly adopt a preventive strategy to prevent the condition from progressing at a fast pace.

In Table 9-3 we offer a questionnaire model to be handed to patients who suffer from tooth wear. Such questionnaires are very helpful diagnostic tools, since they allow us to collect a significant amount of information which, along with clinical examination, will help us identify the potential cause(s) of dental wear.

*Table 9-3*

**Questionnaire for patients showing tooth wear.**

| BRUXISM | Yes | No | Don't know |
|---|---|---|---|
| Do you grind your teeth when you sleep? | | | |
| Has anybody heard you grind your teeth while you sleep? | | | |
| On waking up, do you usually find that you are clenching your teeth? | | | |
| When you wake up, do you usually have jaw pain or jaw fatigue? | | | |
| When you wake up, do you usually have the feeling that your teeth are loose? | | | |
| When you wake up, do you usually have sore teeth and/or sore gums? | | | |
| When you wake up, do you usually have a temple headache? | | | |
| When you wake up, do you usually have a jaw lock? | | | |
| Have you ever found that you were clenching your teeth in the daytime? | | | |
| Have you ever found that you were grinding your teeth in the daytime? | | | |
| Do you wear some device (night guard) to protect your teeth when you sleep? | | | |
| ABRASION | | | |
| How many times a day do you brush your teeth? | | | |
| How many months does your toothbrush last? | | | |
| Do you use your right hand or your left hand to brush your teeth? | | | |
| When brushing your teeth, do you use a dentifrice (toothpaste) or a tooth gel? | | | |
| Do you use mouthwash? | | | |
| EXOGENOUS EROSION | Yes | No | |
| Environmental factors: | | | |
| Do you usually swim in swimming pools? | | | |
| Do you work in an environment where acid vapors are released into the air? E.g., electroplating, smelting plants, accumulator factories | | | |
| Consumption (indicate whether you eat/drink the following products): | | | |
| Carbonated "soft" drinks (regular or diet) | | | |
| Flavored waters | | | |
| Powder juices prepared with water | | | |
| "Sport" drinks or energy drinks | | | |
| Alcoholic drinks | | | |
| Orange, lemon or grapefruit juice | | | |
| Orange, lemon or grapefruit slices | | | |
| Salads dressed with vinegar or lemon juice | | | |
| A variety of fruits | | | |
| Vitamin C pastilles | | | |

| ENDOGENOUS EROSION | Yes | No | Don't know |
|---|---|---|---|
| Is your pillow wet (drooled on) when you wake up? | | | |
| Do you suffer from gastritis? | | | |
| Do you suffer from hiatus hernia? | | | |
| Do you often feel pain behind your breastbone? | | | |
| Do you usually have an acidity feeling? | | | |
| Do you throw up (vomit) often? | | | |
| Do you belch repeatedly? | | | |
| Do you usually have an acid taste in your mouth? | | | |
| Do you usually suffer from gastroesophageal reflux episodes? | | | |
| Do you usually feel heartburn? | | | |
| Do you usually feel that your mouth is dry, as if you did not have enough saliva? | | | |

## References


1. Eccles JD. Tooth surface loss from abrasion, attrition, and erosion. Dent Update 1982;9:373–381.
2. Smith BG, Knight JK. An index for measuring the wear of tooth. Br Dent J 1984;156:435–438.
3. Pindborg J. Pathology of Dental Hard Tissues. Copenhagen: Munksgaard, 1970.
4. Brace CL. Occlusion to the anthropological eye. In: McNamara JA (ed). The Biology of Occlusal Development. Ann Arbor: Center for Human Growth and Development, 1977:179–209.
5. Beyron HL. Occlusal relations and mastication in Australian aborigines. Acta Odontol Scand 1964; 22:597–678.
6. Begg PR. Stone age man's dentition. Am J Orthod 1954; 40:298–312.
7. Murphy TR. Compensatory mechanism in facial height adjustment to functional tooth attrition. Aust Dent J 1959;4:312–323.
8. Young WG. Anthropology, tooth wear, and occlusion ab origine. J Dent Res 1998;77:1860–1863.
9. Varrela J. Occurrence of malocclusion in attritive environment: a study of a skull sample from southwest Finland. Scand J Dent Res 1990;98:242–247.
10. D'Amico A. Functional occlusion of the natural teeth of man. J Prosthet Dent 1961;11:899–915.
11. Hugoson A, Bergendal T, Ekfeldt A, Helkimo M. Prevalence and severity of incisal and occlusal tooth wear in an adult Swedish population. Acta Odontol Scand 1988; 46:255–265.
12. Lambrechts P, Braem M, Vuylsteke-Wauters M, Vanherle G. Quantitative in-vivo wear of human enamel. J Dent Res 1989;68:1752–1754.
13. Xhonga F. Bruxism and its effect on the teeth. J Oral Rehabil 1977;4:65–76.
14. Pintado MR, Anderson GC, DeLong R, Douglas WH. Variation in tooth wear in young adults over a two-year period. J Prosthet Dent 1997;77:313–320.
15. Molnar S, McKee JK, Molnar IM, Przybeck TR. Tooth wear rates among contemporary Australian aborigines. J Dent Res 1983;62:562–565.
16. Carlsson GE, Hugoson A, Persson G. Dental abrasion and alveolar bone loss in the white rat. Odontol Revy 1967;18:263–268.
17. Russell MD. The distinction between physiological and pathological attrition: a review. J Ir Dent Assoc 1987;33: 23–31.
18. Smith BG, Knight JK. A comparison of patterns of tooth wear with aetiological factors. Br Dent J 1984;157:16–19.
19. Johansson A, Haraldson T, Omar R, Kiliaridis S, Carlsson GE. A system for assessing the severity and progression of occlusal tooth wear. J Oral Rehabil 1993;20:125–131.
20. Nyström M, Könönen M, Alasuusua S, Evälahti M, Vartiovaara J. Development of horizontal tooth wear in maxillary anterior teeth from five to 18 years of age. J Dent Res 1990;69:1765–1770.
21. Lavelle CL. Analysis of attrition in adult human molars. J Dent Res 1970;49:822–828.
22. Kaidonis JA, Richards LC, Towsend GC, Tansley GD. Wear of human enamel: a quantitative in vitro assessment. J Dent Res 1998;77:1983–1990.
23. Silness J, Berge M, Johannessen G. Longitudinal study of incisal tooth wear in children and adolescents. Eur J Oral Sci 1995;103:90–94.
24. Smith BG, Robb ND. The prevalence of tooth wear in 1007 dental patients. J Oral Rehabil 1996;23:232–239.

25. Pergamalian A, Rudy TE, Zaki HS, Greco CM. The association between wear facets, bruxism, and severity of facial pain in patients with temporomandibular disorders. J Prosthet Dent 2003;90:194–200.
26. Carlsson GE, Johansson A, Lundqvist S. Oclusal wear: a follow-up study of 18 subjects with extensively worn dentitions. Acta Odontol Scand 1985;43:83–90.
27. Beyron HL. Occlusal changes in adult dentition. J Am Dent Assoc 1954;48:674–686.
28. Silness J, Johannessen G, Røynstrand T. Longitudinal relationship between incisal occlusion and incisal tooth wear. Acta Odontol Scand 1993;51:15–21.
29. Garner LD, Kotwal NS. Correlation study of incisive biting forces with age, sex, and anterior occlusion. J Dent Res 1973;52:698–702.
30. Scaife RR Jr. Natural occurrence of cuspid guidance. J Prosthet Dent 1969;22:225–229.
31. Seligman DA, Pullinger AG. The prevalence of dental attrition and its association with factors of age, gender, occlusion and TMJ symptomatology. J Dent Res 1988;67: 1323–1333.
32. Warren JJ, Yonezu T, Bishara SE. Tooth wear patterns in the deciduous dentition. Am J Orthod Dentofacial Orthop 2002;122:614–618.
33. Knight DJ, Leroux BG, Zhu C, Almond J, Ramsay DS. A longitudinal study of tooth wear in orthodontically treated patients. Am J Orthod Dentofacial Orthop 1997;112:194–202.
34. Davies TGH, Pedersen PO. The degree of attrition of the deciduous teeth and first permanent molars of primitive and urbanized Greenland natives. Br Dent J 1995;19:35–43.
35. De Vis H, De Boever JA, van Cauwenberghe P. Epidemiologic survey of functional conditions of the masticatory system in Belgian children aged 3–6 years. Community Dent Oral Epidemiol 1984;12:203–207.
36. Egermark-Eriksson I, Carlsson GE, Magnusson T. A long-term epidemiologic study of the relationship between occlusal factors and mandibular dysfunction in children and adolescents. J Dent Res 1987;66:67–71.
37. Hugoson A, Ekfeldt A, Koch G, Hallonsten A. Incisal and occlusal tooth wear in children and adolescents in a Swedish population. Acta Odontol Scand 1996;54:263–270.
38. Kampe T, Hannerz H, Ström P. Facet pattern in intact and restored dentition of young adults: a comparative study. Acta Odontol Scand 1984;42:225–233.
39. Johansson A, Fareed K, Omar R. Analysis of possible factors influencing the occurrence of occlusal wear in a young Saudi population. Acta Odontol Scand 1991;49: 139–145.
40. Ingervall B, Hähner R, Kessi S. Pattern of tooth contacts in eccentric mandibular positions in young adults. J Prosthet Dent 1991;66:169–176.
41. Newman HN. Attrition, eruption, and the periodontium. J Dent Res 1999;78:730–734.
42. Berry DC, Poole DF. Attrition: possible mechanism of compensation. J Oral Rehabil 1976;3:201–206.
43. Crothers A, Sandham A. Vertical height differences in subjects with severe dental wear. Eur J Orthod 1993;15: 519–525.
44. McAdam DB. Tooth loading and cuspal guidance in canine and group function. J Prosthet Dent 1976;35: 283–290.
45. Silness J, Berge M, Johannessen G. A 2-year follow-up study of incisal tooth wear in dental students. Acta Odontol Scand 1995;53:331–333.
46. Beyron HL. Characteristics of functionally optimal occlusion and principles of occlusal rehabilitation. J Am Dent Assoc 1954;48:648–656.
47. Woda A, Gourdon AM, Faraj M. Occlusal contacts and tooth wear. J Prosthet Dent 1987;57:85–93.
48. Yaffe A, Ehrlich J. The functional range of tooth contact in lateral gliding movements. J Prosthet Dent 1987;57: 730–733.
49. Seligman DA, Pullinger AG. The degree to which dental attrition in modern society is a function of age and of canine contact. J Orofac Pain 1995;9:266–275.
50. Dahl BL, Fløystrand F, Karlsen K. Pathologic attrition and maximal bite force. J Oral Rehabil 1985;12:337–342.
51. Tortopidis D, Lyons MF, Baxendale RH, Gilmour WH. The variability of bite force measurement between sessions, in different positions within the dental arch. J Oral Rehabil 1998;25:681–686.
52. Ingervall B, Thilander B. Relation between facial morphology and activity of the masticatory muscles. J Oral Rehabil 1974;1:131–147.
53. Braun S, Bantleon H, Hnat WP et al. A study of bite force. 2: Relationship to various cephalometric measurements. Angle Orthod 1995;65:373–377.
54. Menapace SE, Rinchuse DJ, Zullo T, Pierce CJ, Shnorhokian H. The dentofacial morphology of bruxers versus non-bruxers. Angle Orthod 1994;64:43–52.
55. Young DV, Rinchuse DJ, Pierce CJ, Zullo T. The craniofacial morphology of bruxers versus nonbruxers. Angle Orthod 1999;69:14–18.
56. Weijs WA, Hillen B. Relationships between masticatory muscle cross-section and skull shape. J Dent Res 1984;63: 1154–1157.
57. Teo C, Young WG, Daley TJ, Sauer H. Prior fluoridation in childhood affects dental caries and tooth wear in a South East Queensland population. Aust Dent J 1997;42:92–102.
58. Khan F, Young WG, Daley TJ. Dental erosion and bruxism: a tooth wear analysis from South East Queensland. Aust Dent J 1998;43:117–127.
59. Khan F, Young WG, Law V, Priest J, Daley TJ. Cupped lesions of early onset dental erosion in young southeast Queensland adults. Aust Dent J 2001;46:100–107.
60. Pullinger AG, Seligman DA. Quantification and validation of predictive values of occlusal variables in temporomandibular disorders using a multifactorial analysis. J Prosthet Dent 2000;83:66–75.

Chapter 10

# Dental Erosion

*Daniel A. Paesani*

## Introduction

Dental erosion is the pathologic process whereby dental surface structures are destroyed by the action of acid, without bacteria being involved. Such destruction is gradual, localized, chronic, and irreversible. There is solid scientific proof that erosion, more than attrition and abrasion, is the most important cause of tooth wear.[1–4] Erosion is the result of the action of acids and/or the process of chelation. Erosion can progress slowly and painlessly, but it may also progress at a fast pace, causing the patient to suffer from extreme hypersensitivity. The acids that cause erosion are not produced by the oral flora. Unlike caries, erosion occurs in areas that are free from dental plaque. Based on this definition, Grippo and co-workers suggested that the term "corrosion" be used instead of "erosion", which is the term that has prevailed universally through use and habit.[5]

As a consequence of this process, the tooth surface becomes hypomineralized, and its resistance to wear will decrease significantly. Under these conditions, dentin and enamel will show a lower mechanical resistance to the effects of occlusion and abrasion. Thus, to the wear caused by the erosive process we must add the action of other cofactors (parafunction, mechanical abrasion from tooth-brushing, and demastication) which, acting on the significantly softened tooth structure, will accelerate the general process of wear. Tooth erosion is an irreversible process. In contrast to caries – the early diagnosis of which will allow for enamel remineralization – in the case of erosion no remineralization is possible owing to the lack of a matrix as a consequence of enamel loss.

## Prevalence

Comparing epidemiologic studies is difficult owing to the different analysis parameters, scales, and wear measurement indices used, and to the lack of homogeneity between the study populations. Tooth wear being multifactorial, evaluating erosion's "direct" effects is complicated.

Most studies have been conducted on young individuals, which is only natural because studying children and youths who attend school or college is easier than evaluating groups of adults, who usually do not have enough time to participate in epidemiologic studies.

The results of studies suggest that tooth wear caused by erosion is very common. In fact, it occurs much more commonly than supposed. Järvinen and co-workers[6] reported a prevalence of lesions by erosion of 5% in a population of subjects who regularly visited the dentist's office. Frequency values are said to be on the rise, not only because of the increasing consumption of carbonated "soft" drinks but also because dentists have learned to identify the clinical signs of such lesions. Recent studies conducted in the UK have reported that tooth erosion has a prevalence of 56.3% in 12-year-olds and of 64.1% in 14-year-olds.[7]

Erosion prevalence variations have been related to social status. A study of 4-year-olds conducted in the UK reported an erosion prevalence of 19% in children from households with high socioeconomic status, and only 4% in children from households with low socioeconomic status.[8] In Brazil, the authors of a study of 12-year-old schoolchildren reported an erosion prevalence of 13%, the highest values corresponding to children attending fee-paying schools (21.1%), as opposed to children attending state schools (9.7%).[9] This might be explained by the fact that children with a higher socioeconomic status can buy more "soft" drinks and sweets, which are practically unaffordable for children with a lower socioeconomic status.

Some prevalence variations are due to geographic and cultural differences. A study of 3–5-year-old children in Saudi Arabia reported a deciduous-incisor erosion prevalence of 31%; another survey of a study population with similar characteristics in China reported a prevalence of only 5.7%.[10,11]

Most studies agree that erosion levels are increasing in young individuals, thought to be due to their lifestyle and to changes in nutritional habits.

## Clinical Features and Diagnosis of Erosion

No devices are yet available in clinical practice for the detection of lesions specifically caused by erosion. The clinical features of these lesions are, however, the most important element available to dentists for diagnosis. Although each "insult" affecting the teeth (i.e., attrition, abrasion, and erosion) leaves specific impressions on the teeth, the features of which can be useful for diagnosis, we must recognize that those signs have not been scientifically validated. One of the biggest difficulties is the coexistence of several factors interacting and causing tooth wear. Clinicians will not always be able to isolate only one factor as cause of the wear, which is why the best tools to resort to for accurate determination are clinical experience and personal interviews. Using the questionnaire provided in Chapter 9 from the very beginning is very helpful. This said, it is useful to review some of the typical clinical signs that may lead a practitioner to suspect that tooth wear is being caused by acid.

As a pattern, the clinician should use the anatomic features and the color of normal teeth, and then compare these with the features presented by the patient. Erosion-affected tooth surfaces will show typical features: a smooth, shiny appearance, similar to that of glazed surfaces (they look as if they were "varnished") and rounded margins (Fig 10-1). The palatal surfaces of anterior maxillary teeth show a typical yellowish hue corresponding to the exposed dentin, which is limited by the surrounding enamel's whitish margin (Fig 10-2). Palatal-surface erosion can sometimes be of such magnitude as to mimic a prosthesis carving with a chamfered supragingival shoulder (Fig 10-3). The tongue is likely to play a role in this process: its dorsal surface full of papillae is the ideal topography for retaining the regurgitated acid and for keeping it against the palatal surface of maxillary incisors for a long time.

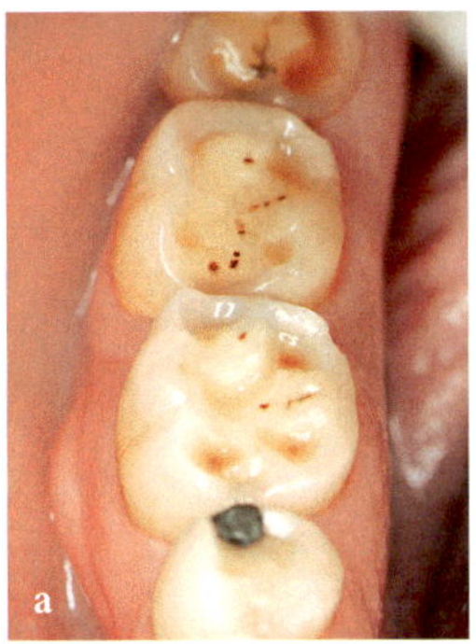

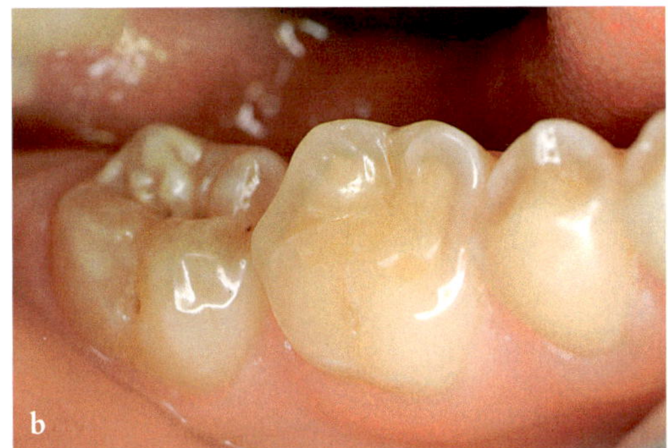

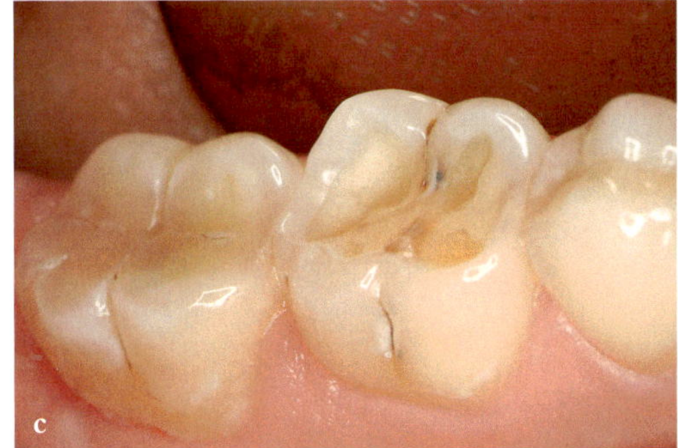

Fig 10-1 **(a–c)** Erosion is characterized by shiny teeth (with a varnished look) and the yellowish hue of exposed dentin; the margins are rounded.

Another specific feature of the erosive process is that the surfaces of restorations, be they plastic or rigid, remain intact and appear in high relief, standing out from the eroded dental surfaces. This happens because acid erodes dental tissues but not the restorations (Fig 10-4). As the process progresses, canine cusp tips round off, ridges flatten, and crevices become less deep, so the typical occlusal topography will slowly disappear (Fig 10-5).

The cupped or volcano-shaped lesions that may be seen in canine, premolar, and molar cusp tips are another sign to help identify erosive lesions. At the bottom of these lesions, the exposed dentin's typical yellowish hue causes it to stand out from the white surrounding enamel (Fig 10-6). Clinical evaluation and analysis of models mounted on the articulator confirm that this kind of wear could not have been caused by grinding of antagonist teeth. The maxillary incisors will appear shortened compared to the mandibular incisors, and incisal edges will appear serrated or chipped (Fig 10-7).

Early-stage erosion diagnosis is very difficult, and determining whether dentin is exposed is even more complicated.[12] Some publications claim that dental erosion is frequently underdiagnosed. Using tooth histology as the "gold standard", a study compared the diagnostic accuracy of pictures and clinical visual inspections.[13] The study focused on the analysis of deciduous-incisor wear by erosion; the incisors were later extracted and studied histologically. Clinical visual inspection and picture analysis showed the same diagnostic accuracy, though when compared with histology both methods underdiagnosed erosion and its magnitude.

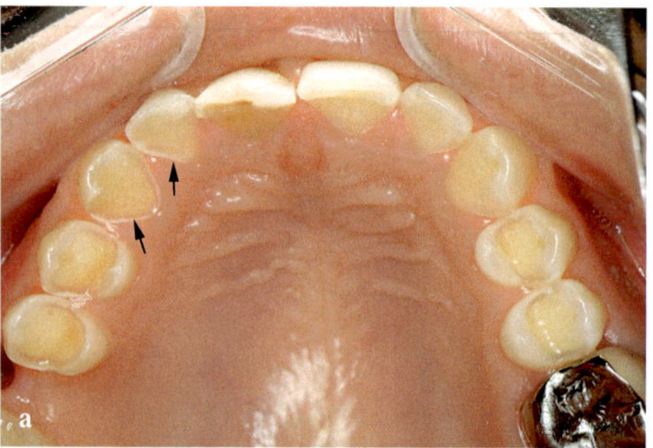

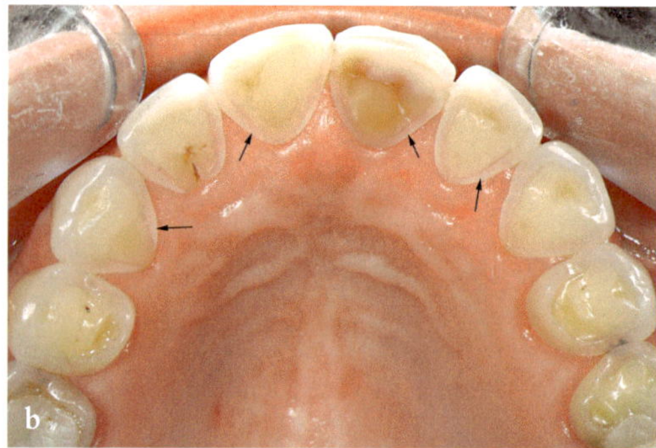

Fig 10-2 **(a and b)** Concave, yellowish palatal surfaces, limited by the enamel's whitish margin (arrows).

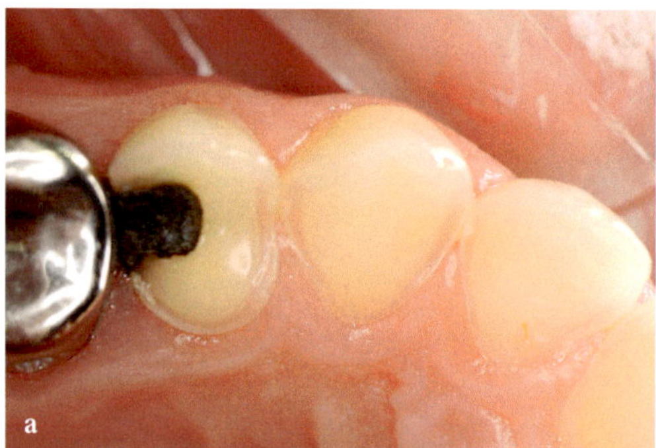

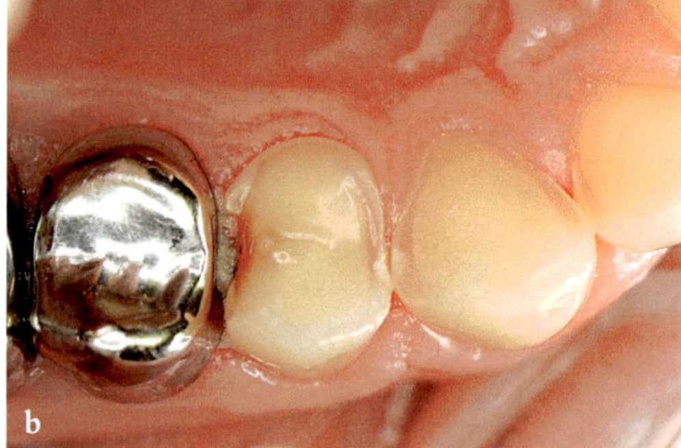

Fig 10-3 **(a and b)** Premolar palatal wear looks like a prosthesis carving with a supragingival chamfered shape.

The presence of stains or pigmentation (caused by tobacco, coffee, tea, etc.) on eroded surfaces suggests old lesions, or that erosion is currently inactive (Fig 10-8).

Today, dental pigmentation surveys are helping to evaluate the results of gastroesophageal reflux treatment. They are a very useful tool for gastroenterologists who treat patients referred by dental practitioners for silent reflux (showing no obvious gastroenterologic signs or symptoms) and who will usually have no parameters for the evaluation of pharmacologic treatment results. Pigmentation analysis is a very effective tool for objectively measuring dental-erosion progression in the short term. Once the pharmacologic treatment is over, the patients are requested to rinse their mouth with tea four times a day for 4 weeks, and then eroded surfaces are clinically evaluated for pigmentation. Figure 10-9 shows erosive lesions on the maxillary incisor palatal surfaces in a teenager. These lesions, along with a drooled-on pillow, were the only signs suggesting potential nighttime gastroesophageal reflux, which was later radiographically confirmed by the gastroenterologist. Following treatment, the presence of pigmentation on the eroded surfaces suggests that treatment was successful.

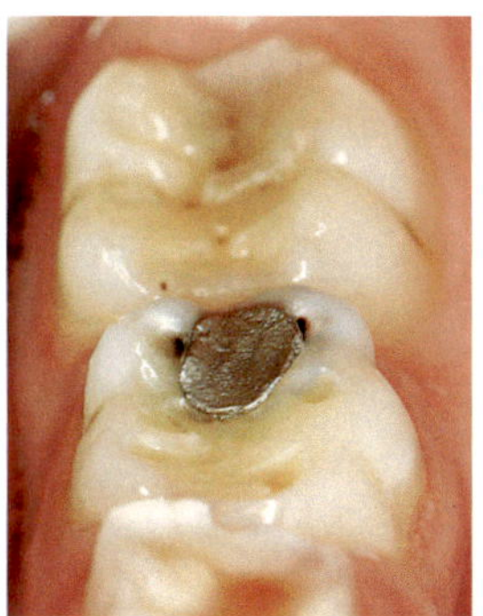

Fig 10-4 Amalgam in high relief.

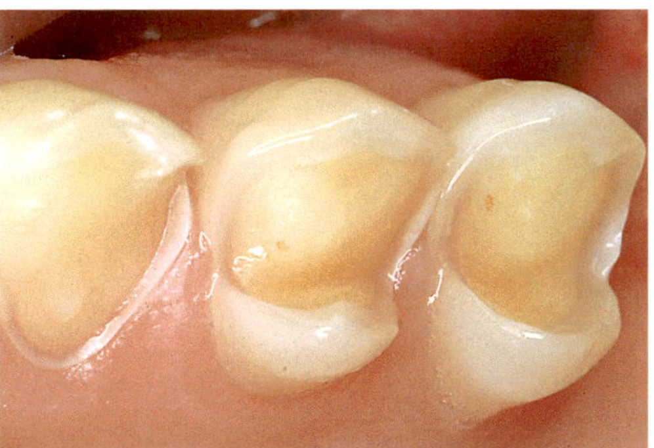

Fig 10-5 Complete loss of the occlusal anatomy.

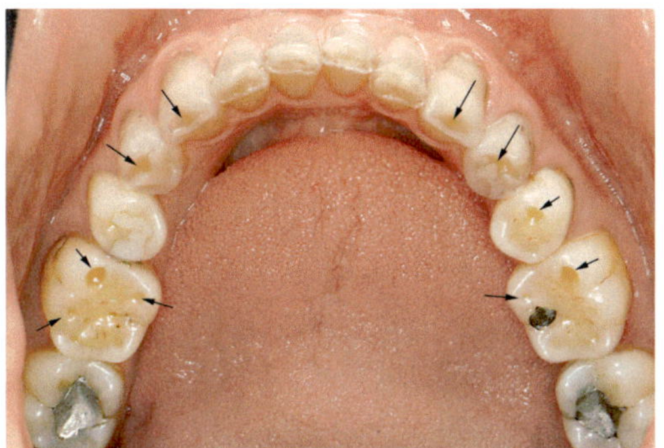

Fig 10-6 Volcano-shaped lesions or cupped lesions, the yellow-colored bottom of which corresponds to dentin (arrows).

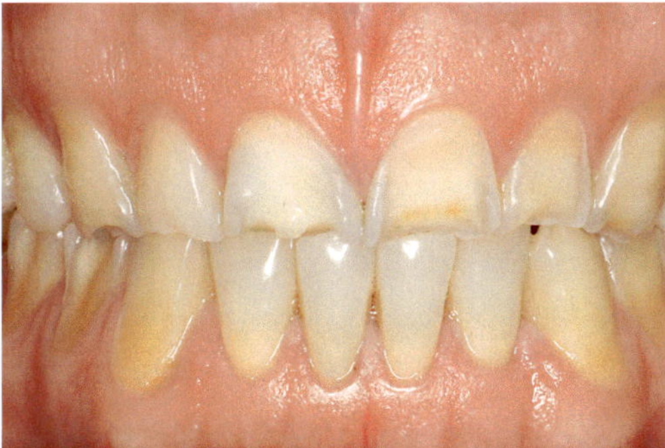

Fig 10-7 Disproportionate wear. Maxillary teeth showing greater wear; the edges have a serrated appearance.

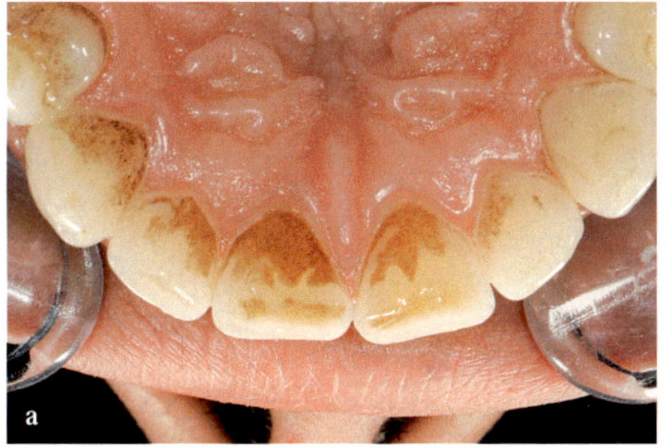

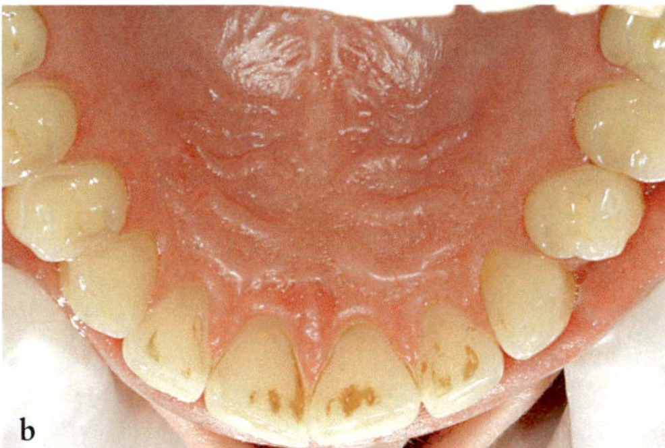

Fig 10-8 **(a and b)** Stains on the eroded teeth indicate that the erosive process is currently inactive.

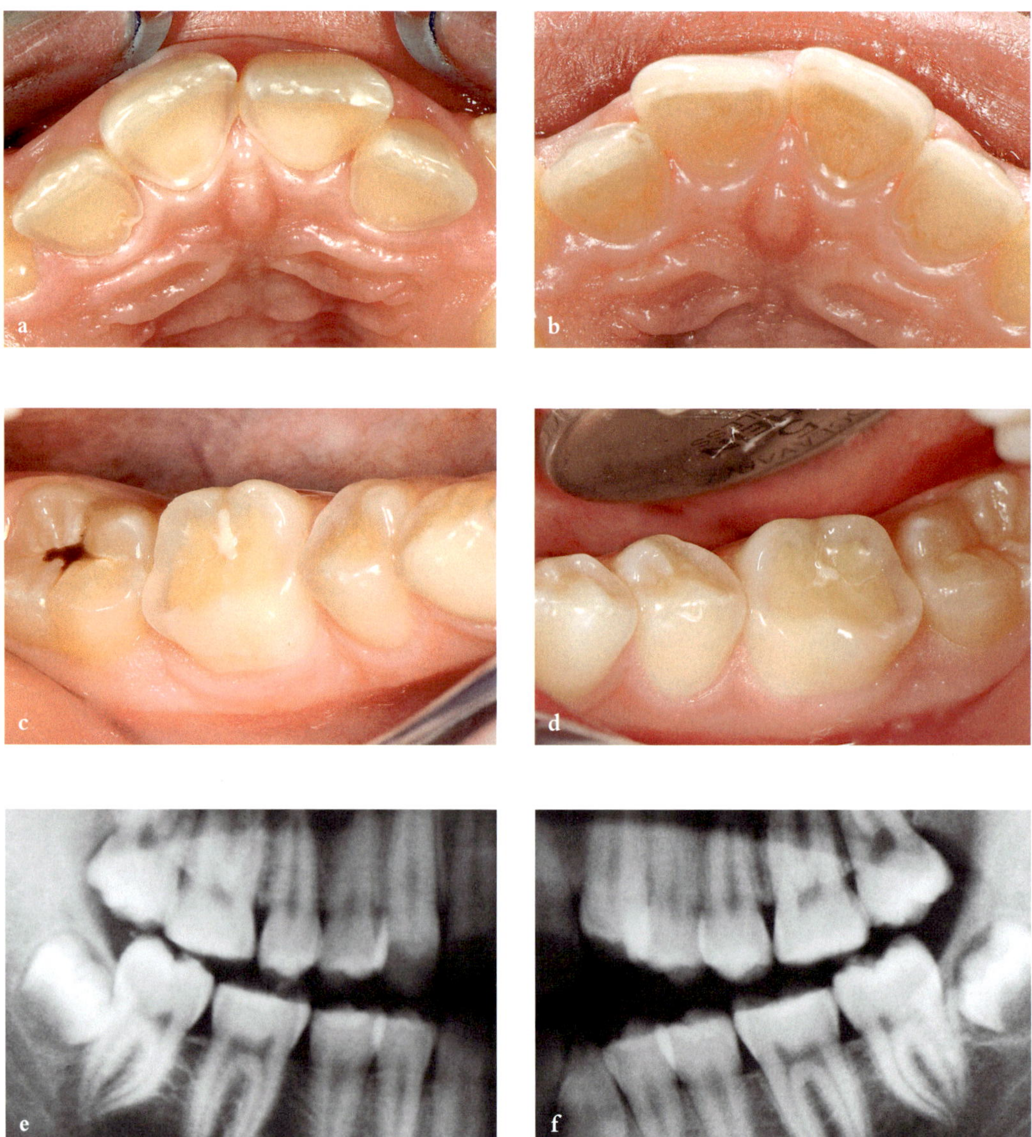

Fig 10-9 **(a)** This 13-year-old shows erosive lesions on the palatal surfaces of incisors. Owing to the absence of symptoms, one gastroenterologist refused to evaluate him. Another gastroenterologist trusted our diagnosis and conducted X-ray studies, which confirmed that the teenager suffered from gastroesophageal reflux. **(b)** This picture taken once the gastroesophageal reflux treatment was over shows how the exposed dentin gets pigmented after reflux regression. **(c and d)** Significant loss of dental hard tissue in first molars. **(e and f)** Radiographs showing anatomic reduction of the four first molars.

## Classification of Erosion according to Its Magnitude

Dental erosion has been assigned three grades of severity, according to the amount of dental-tissue loss:[14]

- Grade 1: Superficial lesion involving enamel only
- Grade 2: Localized lesion affecting less than a third of the tooth, including enamel and dentin
- Grade 3: Generalized lesion affecting more than a third of the tooth, including enamel and dentin.

As mentioned in Chapter 9 on tooth wear, scales and indices are essential tools for scientific research and epidemiologic data gathering, since they allow us to quantify the loss of dental structure. However, they are not relevant for general practitioners. Readers interested in exploring this topic in depth are referred to the literature dealing specifically with dental erosion (e.g., Lussi[15]).

## Classification of Erosion according to Etiology

Dental-surface erosion can be caused by acids from the external environment (exogenous) and/or from the internal environment (endogenous), as well as by acids of unknown origin. Accordingly, we can consider three classes of erosion: exogenous, endogenous, and idiopathic.

### *Exogenous Erosion*

This results from the action of acids coming into the oral cavity from the outside. For an orderly description, we will classify them according to their source: acids from the environment or workplace, acids from food and beverage intake, and acids from pharmaceutical products and oral-hygiene products.

*Workplace acids*

At present, these acids are likely to be the least common cause of exogenous erosion. Breathing in every day, and for many hours, acidic gases and other chemical products released into the workplace air may result in dental erosion. Examples are the chemical industry, an accumulator factory, the electroplating industry, and smelting plant workers. With the improvement of workplace regulations, this cause of dental erosion has decreased significantly. A study reported that factory workers from plants where acids were handled showed less dental erosion when face masks were worn for the protection of the respiratory system.[16]

Professional swimmers going to improperly chlorinated swimming pools every day are at risk, owing to the formation of hydrochloric acid in the water. The literature reports several cases of individuals showing significant generalized erosion in all their teeth. That was the case with a professional team of swimmers who went to the same private-club swimming pool every day: dental erosion was found in 39% of them (23/59). Other club members not using the pool were also examined, and only 3% of them showed erosion (9/295). Twelve percent of club members who frequented the pool but were not professional swimmers showed signs of erosion (46/393). The pH of the pool's water was 2.7, when recommended pH values should range between 7.2 and 8.0. For illustrative purposes, the authors of the study also mention the presence of corrosion in the metallic mixtures under the water and concrete deterioration, resulting from the acidity of the chlorinated gas.[17] Daily contact with the water from these pools for many hours significantly deteriorates people's teeth. For this reason, in the Netherlands, the pH of swimming-pool water is checked daily.[18] In that country only sodium hypochlorite is used for swimming pools, and there is only a 0.14% chance of pool water showing a low pH .[19]

Some publications have reported dental erosion in wine-tasting professionals. Usually, these are employees from state beverage-control commissions (as in Sweden) or those who have full-time jobs in wineries. Their teeth will be in contact with the acid in the wine for many hours a day as they may taste up to 20 different types of wine every day.[20] It has also been reported that wine-tasting professionals resort to hard and frequent tooth-brushing to eliminate the reddish hue left by red-wine tannins, which makes the situation even worse owing to the addition of the abrasive factor. A study of a group of professional enologists conducted in Sweden reported erosion in 74% of cases, the buccal surfaces of the maxillary incisors being most commonly affected.[21]

*Acids from food and beverages*

Undoubtedly, the role that everyday intake plays is very important, since it allows exogenous acids into the body. Dietary acids are considered to be the main etiologic factors governing the development of dental erosion from exogenous sources. Table 10-1 details the pH values of several common foods and beverages.

Manufacturers add certain acids to foods and beverages, examples being malic acid, phosphoric acid, and citric acid. In-vitro and in-situ studies have proved that these acids erode enamel and dentin.[22]

*"Healthy" foods*

A culture of human beauty and image prevails throughout the developed world. This leads many people who want to lose weight to go on diets based on vegetables, fruits, and juices, which are rather acidic. Also, in their quest for a "healthy diet", many become lacto-vegetarian. Lacto-vegetarian diets include large amounts of fruits, juices, and vegetables, and salads usually dressed with vinegar or lemon. Research has been conducted on these diets, owing to their well-known corrosive effects.

For example, in a study of a population of subjects with lacto-vegetarian intake habits, participants were compared by sex and age with a control population of individuals having a normal, varied diet. While control-group subjects did not show dental erosion, erosive lesions had a prevalence of 77% in lacto-vegetarians. In 26.9% of cases, those lesions corresponded to early erosive effects; 19.2% of the lesions corresponded to moderate erosive effects and 30.8% to severe erosive effects. Occlusal faces and incisal edges were the most affected. Such significant levels of erosion resulted from the abundant consumption of salads dressed with vinegar or lemon juice. Lacto-vegetarians will also eat plenty of rough-textured vegetables, fruit juices and honey.[23] Those who consume citrus fruit more than twice a day have also been reported to be at increased risk for erosion – 37 times greater than for those who consume less than that amount.[6] Lussi and co-workers[24] studied a population of Swiss subjects and reported an association between erosion and the consumption of citrus fruit, apples, plums, pears, and their juices. Others also found a link between erosion and an abundant consumption of fruits, juices, and soft drinks.[25] A survey conducted in Cuba found increased dental-erosion frequency in children living near orange-tree plantations: the authors related erosion to abundant consumption of this fruit.[26]

*Wines*

The erosive potential of wine has also been reported. In the School of Dentistry of Adelaide, Australia, the acidity of different types of wine was studied; pHs reported were 3.39 for red wine, 3.15 for white wine, and 3.15 for champagne.[27] Erosion in chronic alcoholics is considered to result possibly from their frequent vomiting rather than from the acidity of alcoholic drinks. However, some suggest that erosion in chronic alcoholics is likely to be caused by the subclinical regurgitations due to the chronic gastritis associated with alcoholism.[28]

*Table 10-1*

**pH values of products commonly consumed.**

| **Product** | | **pH** |
|---|---|---|
| Carbonated soft drinks | Seven Up | 2.3 |
| | Regular Coca-Cola | 2.3 |
| | Diet Coca-Cola | 2.3 |
| | Fanta Orange | 2.5 |
| | Pepsi | 2.3 |
| Waters | Running water | 7.2 |
| | Carbonated mineral water | 5.4 |
| | Non-carbonated mineral water | 7.4 |
| | Dasani Active Lemon | 2.5 |
| Natural fruit juices | Orange juice | 2.8 |
| | Lemon juice | 1.8 |
| | Apple juice | 3.4 |
| "Sport" drinks | Gatorade | 2.9 |
| | Powerade | 3.3 |
| | Fierce | 2.9 |
| | Propel Lemon | 2.8 |
| Energy drinks | Red Bull | 3.4 |
| | Speed | 2.3 |
| Alcoholic drinks | Red wine (Cabernet Sauvignon) | 3.4 |
| | White wine (Chardonnay) | 3.2 |
| | Corona Beer | 4.2 |
| | Cider | 3.1 |
| Infusions | Espresso | 5.5 |
| | Lipton's tea | 6.8 |
| | Iced tea | 3.1 |
| | Cooked Mate tea | 5.5 |
| | Mate tea drunk through tube | 5.5 |
| | Cappuccino | 6.4 |
| Dairy products | Whole milk | 7.0 |
| | Fruity yogurt | 4.1 |
| Fruits | Plum | 3.3 |
| | Peach | 3.5 |
| | Apple | 3.1 |
| | Grapes | 3.8 |
| Other | Tomato ketchup | 3.7 |
| | Mayonnaise | 4.0 |
| | Vinegar | 2.8 |
| | Balsamic aceto | 3.0 |
| | Mustard | 3.6 |
| | Pickles | 2.8 |

*Carbonated "soft" drinks*

Acids enter the oral cavity through carbonated "soft" drinks and fruit juices. "Soft" drink consumption has increased significantly. In the USA, consumption increased 300% in 20 years.[29] This has been shown to be closely related to increased dental erosion.[25] In the US market at the start of this century, 450 brands were sold, and the annual sales volume was over $60 billion.[30] In the USA, annual consumption per capita is estimated to be 200 liters –which surpasses the consumption levels of other drinks such as coffee, beer, milk, and bottled water,[31] the main impact being on children and teenagers. Forty percent of pre-school children drink more than a quarter of a liter per day. The amount is even greater in 12–19-year-olds: females drink more than half a liter and males nearly a liter.[32] In the USA, this is deemed to be a serious problem because these drinks have replaced milk, so that calcium intake has decreased.[33] In American schools, "soft" drinks and fruit juices can be bought from vending machines; pouring rights contracts are signed, by which schools agree to sell products of only one brand exclusively, receiving, in return, an award and incentive payments for greater sales. Pouring rights contracts are a trend in all US school districts; more than $200 million have been paid to schools that entered into such contracts.[34]

The erosive potential of a "soft" drink is thought to depend on several factors, including its low pH, its buffering capacity, and its titratable acidity. While the low pH is responsible for the erosion occurring within the first minutes of drinking, titratable acidity will cause enamel dissolution for a longer time.[35] Fruit juices and fruit-flavoured beverages are based on acidic fruits. Those juices and beverages contain the following acids: citric acid (from oranges), tartaric acid (from grapes), and malic acid (from apples). Vitamin C (ascorbic acid) is usually added, which increases the final acidity.[36] The types of acids (phosphoric and citric) used in classic "cola" drinks as flavor enhancers contribute to the low pH of these drinks,[37] which are also called "carbonated drinks" owing to their content of carbonic acid formed by a carbon dioxide solution. The fact that the pH of these drinks remains low even after letting them settle in a glass (until they lose their effervescence and the carbon dioxide evaporates) proves that their acidity results from the addition of flavoring acids and not from the presence of carbonic acid.

The way beverages are drunk also has an influence on erosion. A greater flow speed will increase surface ion exchange and, consequently, enamel dissolution.[38] The use of a straw may direct the liquid flow to the vestibular surface of the incisors, causing their surfaces to become eroded.[39] Also, keeping the liquid in the mouth for some time before swallowing it will cause surface pH to decrease significantly, which will worsen the erosive process.[40] Swishing "soft" drinks in the mouth before swallowing them will also increase erosion.[38] Temperature is another factor influencing erosion because a rise in temperature will usually accelerate a chemical reaction. This applies to "soft" drinks and fruit juices, whose erosive power increases in direct proportion to the raise in temperature; that is why it is advisable to drink them cold from the fridge or to add ice cubes.[41] When drunk cold, orange juice is less erosive than when drunk at room temperature.[42]

It is generally believed that "Light" or "Diet" versions are not destructive of teeth. However, an in-vitro study showed that they too have an erosive effect, though to a lesser degree than the regular types.[43]

Edwards and co-workers conducted an in-vitro comparative study of the "soft" drinks available in the British market.[44] They measured the initial pH and the amount of sodium hydroxide needed to neutralize the acidity of each of the drinks evaluated. The authors stress that the initial pH value of a drink is not in direct relation with its potential erosive effect. They cite the example of natural fruit juices, whose initial pH, despite not being as low as that of carbonated drinks, requires much more sodium hydroxide to be raised, which evinces the important erosive effect these drinks have on enamel. They also studied the differences between regular "cola" drinks and their corresponding "Light" versions; having found no significant differences between them, the authors concluded that both versions cause dental erosion.

Today, the titratable acidity value (i.e., the total amount of acids present in a solution) is considered to be much more important than the pH value. The acids contained in beverages affect the buffering capacity, and since "soft" drinks are strongly buffered their pH remains low for a long time. This process competes with the buffering capacity of the saliva and alters it; this will cause acidic pH to act on the oral environment for a longer time, boosting erosion.

Dentistry researchers have collaborated with manufacturers by conducting experiments aimed at modifying the chemical composition of these beverages in order to reduce their damaging effects on dentition. Unfortunately, though the goal of reducing erosion was achieved by initial trials, unwanted flavor changes and a lower resistance to bacteriologic decay occurred.[45] Recently, efforts have been made to buffer the erosive effect of "soft" drinks by raising their pH, but they proved unsuccessful.[46] However, the same authors have shown that this can be achieved by modifying the degree of saturation, without the need for pH modification. The addition of calcium and phosphate to orange juice results in saturation with respect to apatite, which prevents erosion.[47] These trials confirm the findings of similar previous research studies.[48] Another group of researchers conducted experiments on the effects of the addition of calcium, phosphate, and fluoride: the erosive effect of orange juice, Sprite and Sprite Light on enamel decreased, but this was not the case with Coca-Cola.[49] Other researchers compared the damaging effect of "soft" drinks, orange juices and "sport" drinks of similar characteristics, with or without calcium, available in the market. Beverages containing calcium caused less adamantine erosion.[50]

Although these experiments showed that enamel dissolution can be reduced by adding minerals to beverages, it is clear that no full preventive effect has been achieved. The fact that many teams of researchers are intensely devoted to studying this topic is a promise of a better future. Nevertheless, it is utopian to think that "soft" drink formula modification can compensate for the replacement of milk consumption.

*Mineral waters*

Studies conducted on the action of mineral water on tooth hard tissues have not found any significant, clinically relevant erosive effects. At first, water carbonation was thought to play a role in the erosive process, but in-vitro comparative studies of carbonated and non-carbonated mineral waters found no differences between them regarding dental-enamel and synthetic-hydroxyapatite dissolution.[51]

Nowadays, there is widespread consumption of flavored mineral waters. People believe these waters to be harmless to teeth, since they contain only a "flavoring" agent. Even worse: since they do not contain sugar, they are thought to be healthier than other beverages. However, it has been shown that fruity flavoring agents strongly affect titratable acidity.[44] The recommendation now is to drink carbonated or non-carbonated mineral waters without flavoring agents. Such waters are innocuous to teeth, which makes them the ideal replacement for acidic "soft drinks", which are the subject of so much controversy.

*"Sport" drinks*

Today, many people engage in a "healthier" lifestyle generally involving the practice of aerobic activities in an intensive and methodical way and a diet rich in fruits and vegetables. Intensive sports practice is generally accompanied by the habit of consuming energy drinks, juices, and carbonated "soft" drinks (all of them having a low pH). Intense physical activity causes the body to lose fluids, which may lead to relative dehydration and reduction in the normal salivary flow. This condition results in a constant need to drink beverages – sugar-sweetened, low-pH beverages – which, in a mouth with diminished salivary flow, boosts the dental erosion mechanism significantly.

The risk of suffering from erosion is four times higher in subjects who consume "sport" or "soft" drinks every day than in subjects who do not consume them.[6] A recent in-vitro investigation compared the erosive power that four beverages have on enamel. Extracted human premolars were submerged in regular Coca-Cola, Diet Coke, Gatorade, and Red Bull. Later, their pH and titratable acidity were measured, and enamel surfaces were observed under optical and electronic microscopes. The four drinks eroded enamel, the erosion caused by Red Bull and Gatorade being significantly greater than the erosion caused by the other two. The authors ascribed the high level of adamantine dissolution caused by Gatorade and Red Bull to the high concentration of refined carbohydrates (sucrose and glucose) contained in these, and to the chelating properties of the sodium citrate contained in Red Bull.[52]

Others relate the erosive effect of "sport" drinks to their citric acid content. In an experiment, citric acid was replaced by malic acid and damage to the enamel diminished.[53] This was confirmed by other researchers, who were able to reduce erosion by adding calcium.[54,55] Recently, an in-vitro study modified the formula of a "sport" drink by adding casein phosphopeptide (amorphous calcium phosphate), which caused its erosive effect to decrease without altering the beverage's flavor.[56]

#### *Herbal tea*

Many people have a habit of drinking plenty of herbal tea. Some of these infusions are made from roses, lemons, peaches, etc. Their pH is generally low, ranging between 2.6 and 3.9, and they are considered to be harmful to individuals with diminished salivary flow.[57] An in-vitro study of fruity teas proved all of them to be erosive agents, since they removed the smear layer.[58] Another team of researchers were able to confirm the acidity of their pH (2.63–4.04) by studying a selection of 44 iced teas. The authors ascribed the low pH of teas to the addition of lemon juice or citric acid.[59] Another study compared the erosive effects of conventional black tea (Typhoo) and herbal tea (Twinings Blackcurrant, Ginseng, and Vanilla). Both of them eroded enamel, herbal tea being five times as erosive as black tea.[60] However, another group of researchers who studied the effect of several fruity teas and iced teas reported opposite results. The authors reported a pH range of 6.2–7.4 (at 45°C) for perfumed teas; iced tea, on the contrary, was found to erode enamel (pH < 4.0). Mouthwash with 5 mL of iced tea caused oral-fluid pH to fall to 4.1–4.9; however, the pH rose to 5.9–7.1 after 2 minutes and to 6.3–7.1 after 5 minutes.[61]

#### *Acids from pharmaceuticals*

Pharmaceutical products with low pH and high titratable acidity may damage teeth. The erosive effect of these drugs may be greater in patients with diminished salivary flow.

#### *Aspirin*

Aspirin is one of the most widely consumed medications in the world, and there are some published reports on its erosive effects. Aspirin is available on the market in the form of powder, pills, and chewable tablets.

Aspirin pills will usually be placed on the tongue and swallowed with the aid of water, but they may also be dissolved in a glass of water and drunk. This method is preferred by people who have a problem swallowing pills. Some will keep the pills between their teeth until they dissolve completely, or they will chew them to accelerate their absorption. The literature warns about the risks of consuming aspirin in these ways, for example, some case reports have described severe erosive lesions occurring on teeth.[62]

Aspirin is available in powder form, and it is advisable to dissolve this in a glass of water and then drink it, or put the powder on the tongue and swallow it with the aid of a glass of water. The literature reports the case of a patient who used to place aspirin powder under the tongue to accelerate absorption; this woman did this up to six times a day for 2–3 years. The authors show how this improper use of acetyl salicylic acid caused such severe dental lesions that all the mandibular teeth required crowns.[63] Another case report is available about a woman who kept aspirin powder behind her teeth; after 6 months her teeth showed severe signs of erosion.[64]

There are also chewable aspirin tablets, and they are available in orange or strawberry flavors, which are the ones the pediatric population prefers. A 1983 study of a group of children suffering from juvenile rheumatoid arthritis reported that erosive dental lesions were observed in those children who chewed aspirin tablets. In contrast, another group of children belonging to the same study population but who swallowed the pills did not show any dental lesions. Interestingly, the authors mention that the children who chewed showed traces of wrapped aspirin in the crevices and cracks of their molars.[65]

An in-vitro pilot study demonstrated the erosive effect of acetyl salicylic acid on enamel and dentin. Then, the authors of the study buffered the acetyl salicylic acid with calcium carbonate, rendering the acid innocuous to tooth structures.[66]

*Vitamin C*

Vitamin C (ascorbic acid) is another pharmaceutical product that may cause erosion. Clinical research studies associated dental erosion prevalence with vitamin C consumption.[67,68] In 1983, Giunta reported the erosive effect of chewable vitamin C tablets on dentition, and provided the example of a patient who chewed such tablets for 3 years.[69] Later, a clinical case was reported of a subject whose chewing vitamin C for a year also resulted in dental lesions. The authors warn physicians and recommend they prescribe tablets that should be swallowed rather than chewed and inform their patients about the risk of chewing tablets.[70] Vitamin C is also available in effervescent tablet form; these tablets must be dissolved in water and are acidic. However, they can be used safely by those people who have normal salivary flow, since contact with the teeth is short.[71] Though not much research has been conducted on chewable vitamin C, it is advisable to avoid chewing these tablets and swallow them instead with a drink.[72]

*Systemic medications*

One publication warns about the use of some chronic-use medications by medically compromised patients.[73] The authors conducted research on the pH and the titratable acidity of eight liquid medicines and two effervescent types which are usually prescribed for long-term use. They reported a low pH and a high titratable acidity in a drinkable solution containing hydralazine hydrochloride which is prescribed to patients suffering from moderate or severe high blood pressure. The other two effervescent medicines evaluated, Phosphate Sandoz and Sandoz K, also proved to be extremely acidic. The authors recommend clinicians to avoid prescribing acidic medicines in the form of effervescent tablets and, whenever possible, to replace them with tablets that should be swallowed.

*Saliva substitutes*

In everyday dental practice it is very common to find patients suffering from xerostomia. The three best known causes of such impairment of the salivary glands are the side-effects of certain medications, the effect of radiotherapy in head and neck cancer patients, and Sjögren's syndrome.

Xerostomia causes speech and mastication problems and it affects the formation of the alimentary bolus and its deglutition. Owing to the dryness in their mouth, patients with xerostomia are constantly drinking in order to lubricate the oral tissues. In the best scenario such patients prefer to drink water, which, though innocuous to the dentition, does not provide protection against acids as does saliva. Other people drink commercial beverages with erosive potential; this compromises hard tissue survival owing to the lack of saliva which can counteract their action.

In fact, people with xerostomia often suffer for a long time without being given minimal preventive advice on how to protect their teeth. The first step is to identify the origin of the mouth dryness. Systemic medications are the most common cause. Such medications include diuretics, antidepressants, antihistamines, antipsychotics, and antihypertensives.[74,75] Once the pharmacologic cause has been identified, the dental practitioner and the patient's own doctor should work together to evaluate the possibility of suspending the medication, reducing its dose, or replacing it by some other medicine.

Special care must be taken whenever saliva substitutes need to be prescribed, since some of these products often have a low pH and have been shown to cause dental demineralization in in-vitro trials.[76] Several saliva substitutes were tested. Glandosane (pH 4.08) and Biotene (pH 4.15) were found to produce significant enamel and dentin loss, which is why the authors recommended their avoidance. The same authors found other products to have important remineralization effects, especially Oralube spray (pH 5.0–7.0) which contains methyl hydroxybenzoate, with the addition of sodium, potassium, magnesium, calcium, chloride, phosphate, and fluoride electrolytes.[77] Oil-based saliva substitutes have recently become available. These modifications introduced by the pharmaceutical industry to saliva substitutes are based on studies that have shown lipids to act as a diffusion barrier inside enamel's organic matrix, thus decelerating the demineralizing process.[78] Experiments have recently been conducted on linseed-based saliva substitutes to which calcium, phosphate, and fluoride were added; a remineralizing effect was demonstrated.[79] Today, neutral-pH saliva substitutes with olive oil at 2% concentration plus fluoride and xylitol (Xerostom) are available in pharmacies. They are available in a full range of products and they have an enamel remineralizing effect.[80]

### *Mouthwashes*

Several studies have evaluated the pH and titratable acidity of mouthwashes and oral deodorants. One of these studies, conducted in vitro, measured the erosive potential of three mouthwashes (Calcusan, Salisan, and Veadent) and a saliva-stimulating tablet (Salivin). As models for comparison, a "sport" drink (Hart-Sport, pH 3.1) known for its erosive effect and a mineral water brand known for its innocuous effect were used. The dissolving potential of Calcusan was four times that of Hart-Sport, and Veadent showed a less strong erosive effect. In contrast, Salisan and Salivin did not cause erosion, and neither did the mineral water brand used as control. The authors ascribed the erosive effect of Calcusan to its content of EDTA (ethylenediaminetetraacetic acid), advertised as an anticalculus agent. They also point out the importance of being aware of the harmful effect that the organic-acid and chelating-acid content of these products has on teeth.[81]

Another research study assessed the pH of several mouthwashes marketed in England. Most of them were found to have acidic pH, in some cases as low as 3.4; only one mouthwash had alkaline pH and another one had an almost neutral pH.[82] An in-situ trial compared the erosive effect of three kinds of acidic mouthwashes: one of them containing acidified sodium chlorite, another containing essential oil components, and a third containing hexetidine. While the three products caused erosion, the first one proved to be the most erosive.[83] Similar results were obtained by other researchers who studied a variety of products marketed in England; their recommendation is that acidic mouthwashes should not be used before tooth-brushing or after an acidic diet intake.[84]

*Dental bleaching agents*

Nowadays there is a widespread desire to have very white teeth, which are associated with health, beauty, and youth. The use of dental bleaching agents is rising as a consequence.

Dental bleaching agents remove organic particle deposits from teeth. They also remove the smear layer, making the teeth more susceptible to erosion. In some cases, an abrasive polishing is performed after the bleaching, and strong chemical products are used that put the integrity of enamel at a higher risk.

The pH of these bleaching agents decreases in inverse proportion to the concentration of hydrogen peroxide they contain. The pH of 26 bleaching agents available on the dental market were researched in a study. The pH ranged between 3.67 (extremely acidic) and 11.13 (extremely alkaline).[85] However, contradictory results were obtained by the different research studies. This may be due to differences between products (acidity and hydrogen-peroxide content differences, perhaps), to the addition of minerals to some products, and to methodologic differences. In-vitro experiments using artificial saliva resulted in enamel microhardness decrease after bleaching with carbamide peroxide at 10% concentration[86] and hydrogen peroxide at 3%.[87] However, others have reported opposite results, and showed that bleaching agents with low concentrations of hydrogen peroxide do not make teeth more susceptible to erosion.[88] An enamel superficial remineralizing effect obtained after bleaching performed with a fluoridated carbamide peroxide gel at 10% has recently been demonstrated.[89] When a similar product without fluoride was used, the remineralization effect was not observed.

It is also necessary to carefully consider the advisability of dental professional cleaning procedures that use abrasive agents for patients showing erosive lesions. Such procedures may represent an additional loss of several microns of enamel per polishing session; thus, tooth susceptibility to erosion will increase as a consequence of the removal of enamel's outer layer, which is rich in fluoride. Since all these procedures are beneficial only from an esthetic point of view, extreme caution must be exercised during their use so as not to increase the tissue loss.

### *Endogenous Erosion*

Endogenous erosion is caused by hydrochloric acid produced by parietal cells of the stomach. The action of gastroesophageal reflux and frequent vomiting causes this acid to reach the oral cavity and erode teeth. Vomiting is the forceful expulsion of the contents of the stomach through the mouth; it is common in many organic pathologies and some psychiatric disorders. Unlike vomiting, regurgitation does not involve diaphragm muscle contraction, and the amount of material expelled is lower.

*Reflux*

In people suffering from gastroesophageal sphincter dysfunction, reflux and regurgitation of acidic content into the mouth frequently occur owing to the increase in stomach pressure or a greater gastric volume. This is even worse in the dorsal recumbent position, since the stomach and the mouth are at the same level, which makes it easier for acid to reach the mouth.

Although there is no fixed critical pH value for teeth, it can be estimated to range between 5.2 and 5.8. Lower pH values trigger an enamel demineralization process[90] and root resorption.[91] Since gastric juice is very acidic (pH 1.0), frequent vomiting and regurgitation produce important lesions in teeth. In the first stage of endogenous erosion, the acids dissolve the palatal surfaces of maxillary anterior teeth. Later, the palatal cusps of premolars and molars become affected; and if the process continues the rest of the teeth will be compromised.

When the acid from the alimentary tract is expelled into the oral cavity, it moves along the dorsal surface of the tongue, which has many papillae and folds, where the hydrochloric acid is retained for some time. Thus, the acid-rich dorsal surface of the tongue, in decubitus position against the palatal surface of the maxillary anterior teeth, is responsible for the erosion of these teeth (Figs 10-10 and 10-11). This phenomenon has been known for 70 years as "perimylolysis",[92] and it has recently been demonstrated in in-vivo studies conducted by a group of British researchers.[93]

Gastroesophageal reflux is a medical condition. Thus, we recommend the reading of Chapter 11, which deals exclusively with this topic and has been written by gastroenterology specialists.

### *Alcohol abuse*

Alcohol abuse is another cause of endogenous erosion. Chronic addiction is a very common condition affecting around 10% of males and 3% of females in the USA.[94] In hard-core chronic alcoholics, erosion is caused not only by the frequent vomiting but also by the chronic gastritis and esophagitis they have, which result in persistent gastroesophageal reflux.[28]

Alcohol abuse is socially frowned upon, which makes it extremely difficult for dental practitioners to discover it in personal interviews because patients will often conceal it. Being able to diagnose alcoholism is very important for dental clinicians, not only because this allows them to relate it to erosion, but also because the treatment plan will need to be based on the assumption that the erosive process will continue.

### *Bulimia and anorexia nervosa*

Expulsion of stomach acids into the oral cavity may be deliberately achieved by subjects suffering from psychiatric disorders such as anorexia nervosa, bulimia, and rumination.

Anorexia is characterized by a strong aversion to food, which results in severe weight loss. This condition springs from a complex interaction of biologic, social, family, and personal factors. Age at presentation is between 12 and 30, and it is ten times as common in women as in men. Anorexics will lose up to 85% of their weight. Anorexia has two clinical variations: self-starvation, and binge-eating followed by purging episodes (laxatives or self-induced vomiting). Patients suffering from anorexia will often deny having a problem. Thus, the diagnostic value of clinical interrogation is scarce. Dental practitioners must identify the condition based on the presence of perimylolysis and emaciation.

It is difficult to distinguish bulimia from anorexia. Like anorexia, bulimia affects mainly women (1:10 ratio), though it presents later than anorexia (at around age 20). Bulimics will engage in binge-eating, followed by induced vomiting. Unlike anorexics, these patients will maintain their normal weight and their physical appearance will not reflect their condition. Figure 10-12 shows the oral status of a bulimic woman who concealed her eating disorder. Finally, the diagnosis for her condition was confirmed by a psychiatric consultation.

### *Rumination*

Rumination is a psychiatric condition that is less common than bulimia and anorexia. It is a special kind of regurgitation in which the content of the stomach is brought up, rechewed, and swallowed again. Unlike bulimia and anorexia, rumination is more common in males (5:1 ratio).[95]

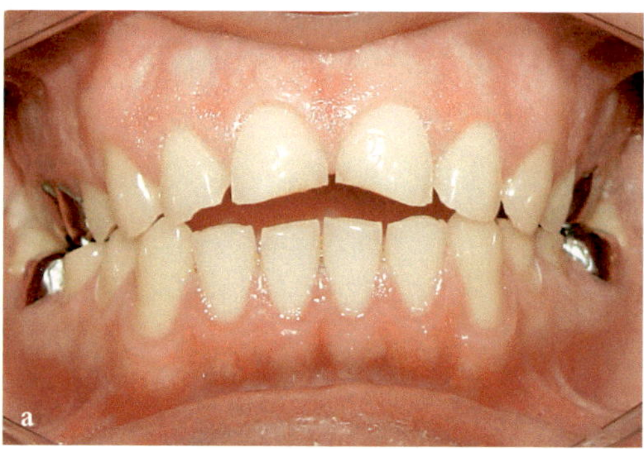

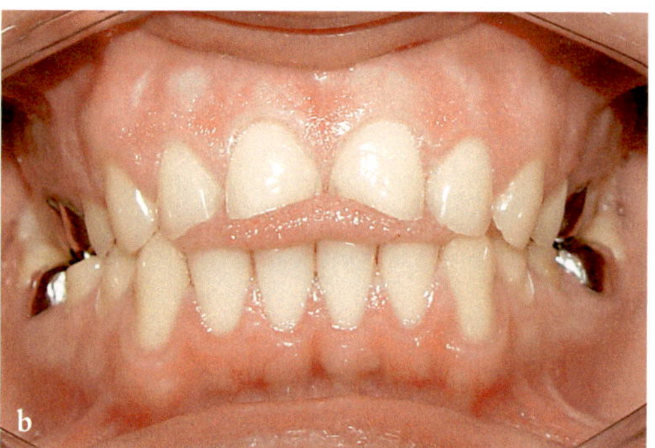

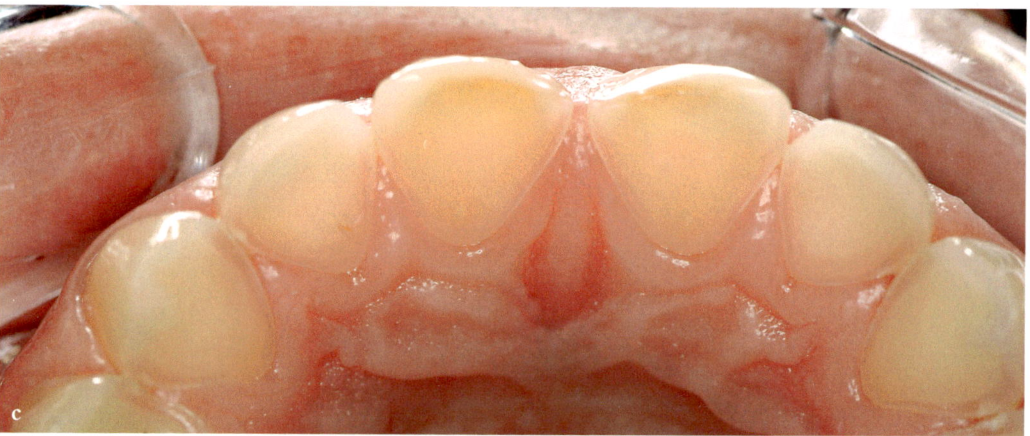

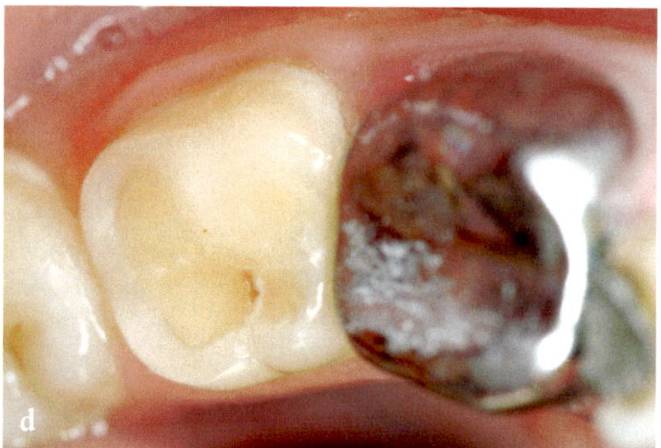

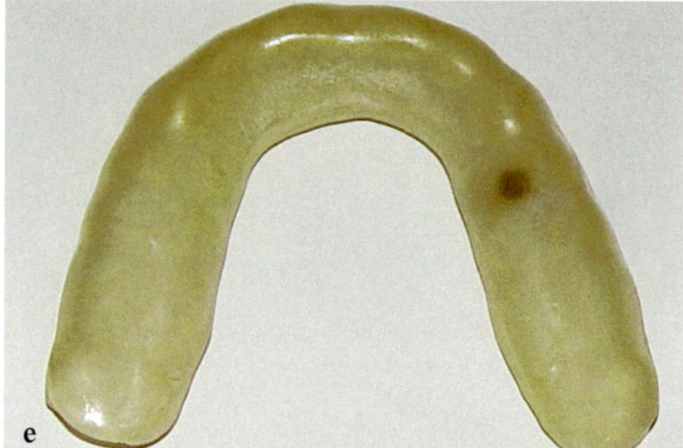

Fig 10-10 **(a–d)** Patient suffering from silent gastroesophageal reflux disease and atypical deglutition. Note the significant wear resulting from the action of the dorsal surface of the tongue against dental hard tissues (perimylolysis). This patient was diagnosed with bruxism by a general dental practitioner. **(e)** The absence of attrition in the patient's nightguard, plus the characteristics of wear, suggests a completely different diagnosis.

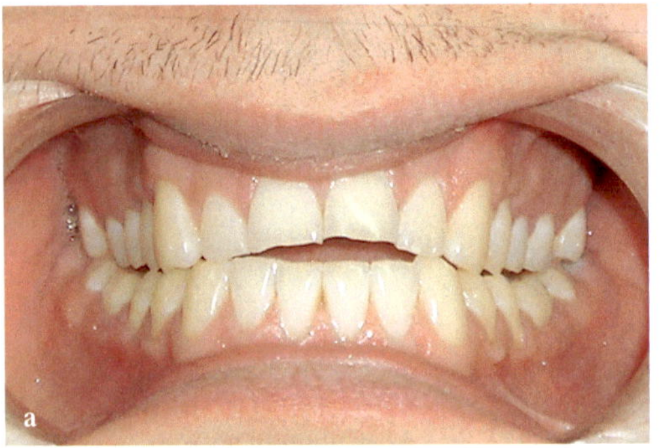

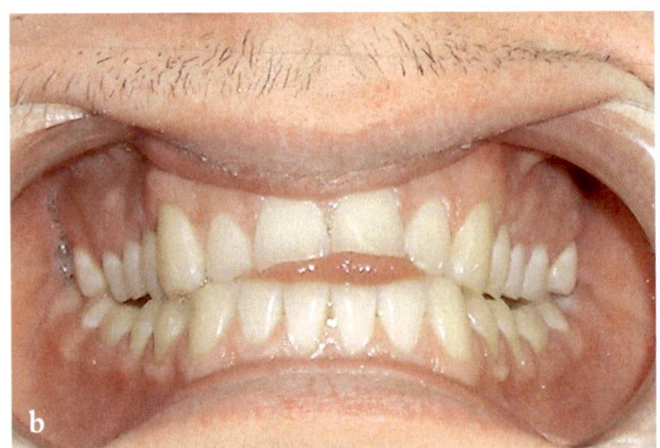

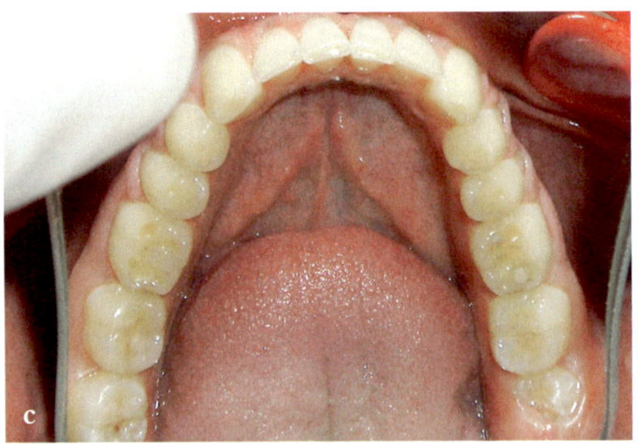

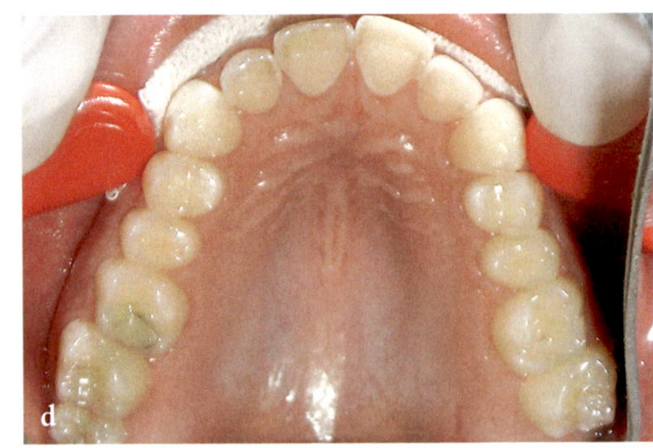

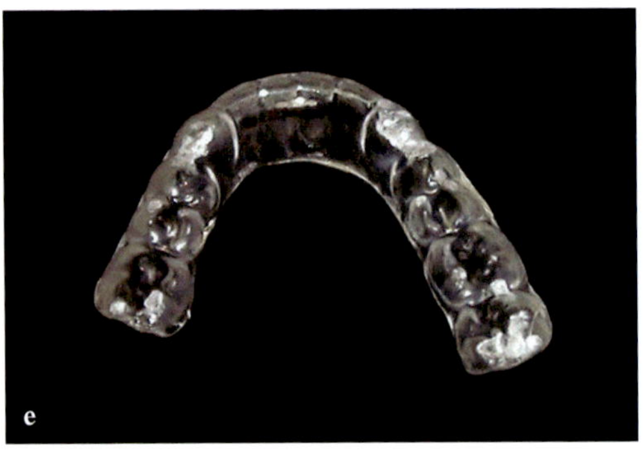

Fig 10-11 **(a–d)** This patient was diagnosed with bruxism. **(e)** Splint wear confirms tooth grinding during sleep. However, as was the case with the patient in Figure 10-10, such were the characteristics of wear as to merit a consultation with a gastroenterologist, who confirmed that the patient was suffering from reflux.

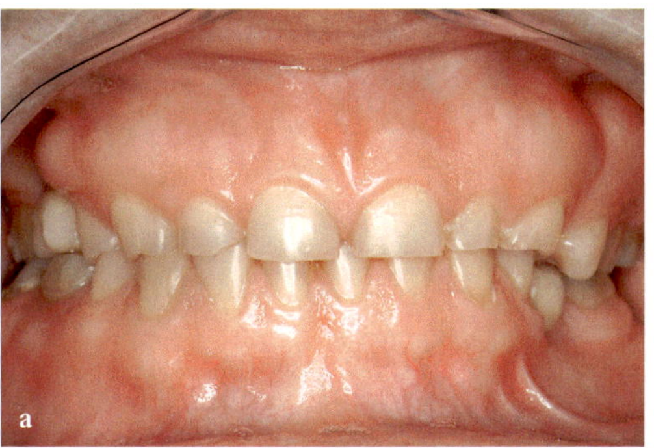


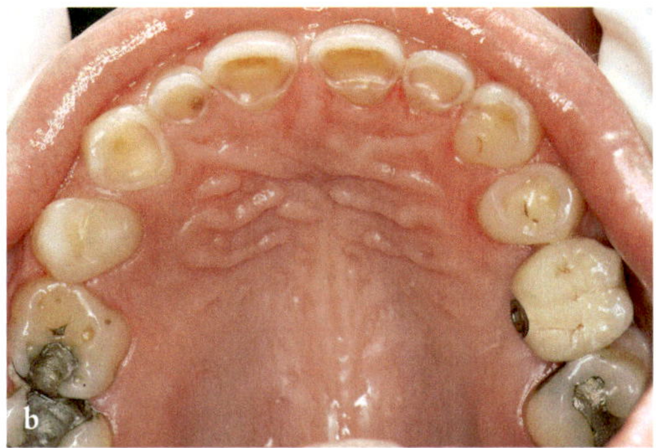


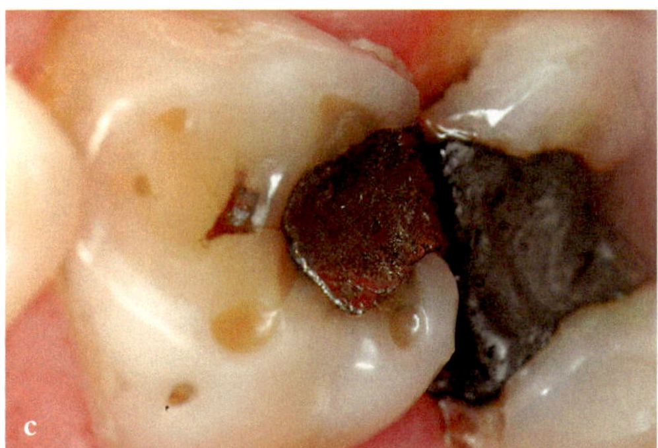


Fig 10-12 **(a–c)** Tooth wear caused by frequent vomiting in a bulimic patient.

### *Idiopathic Erosion*

Many times, in everyday dental practice, patients present with lesions whose features indicate an erosive origin. The curious thing is that history taking will often prove useless in identifying the origin of the acid. No acid content is present in the patient's diet or in his/her workplace environment. Thus, a potential endogenous origin must be considered.

As dental practitioners we need to know how to ask the patient the correct questions in order to identify a possible digestive origin for acid. We ask some very general questions with the aim of finding some clue which justifies referral of the patient to a gastroenterologist. Among other things, in these cases we search for signs: heartburn, epigastric pain, burning, acid taste in the mouth, frequently drooled-on pillow, etc. Usually, despite getting negative answers to all these questions, we will refer the patient to the gastroenterologist anyway, since the kind of tooth wear pattern suggests the involvement of an acid as etiology.

Interestingly, gastroenterologists experience something similar. In the absence of clinical clues (from a gastroenterological point of view) that might make more complex studies worth undertaking, many times they are forced to refer a patient to a dental practitioner. On other occasions, when specialists believe our assumptions to be valid, they will order contrast-enhanced radiographs, endoscopy, or an esophageal pH study, even though the patient's clinical features (from a gastroenterologic point of view) are not such as to justify these studies.

Surprisingly, the results of such studies then reveal the presence of a wide range of alimentary tract pathologies despite their clinical silence. On many occasions, the only clue suggesting such potential alimentary tract anomalies is the presence

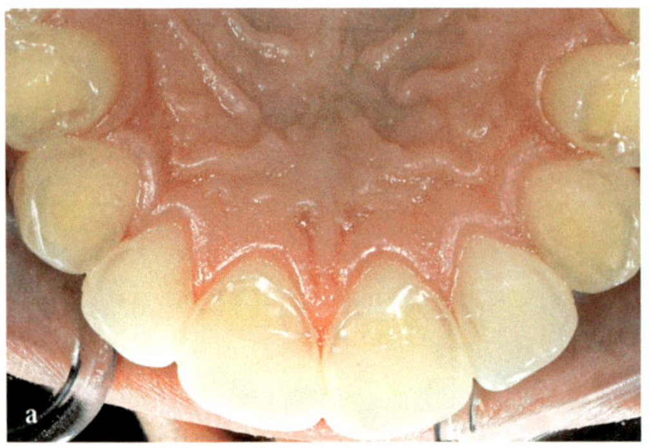

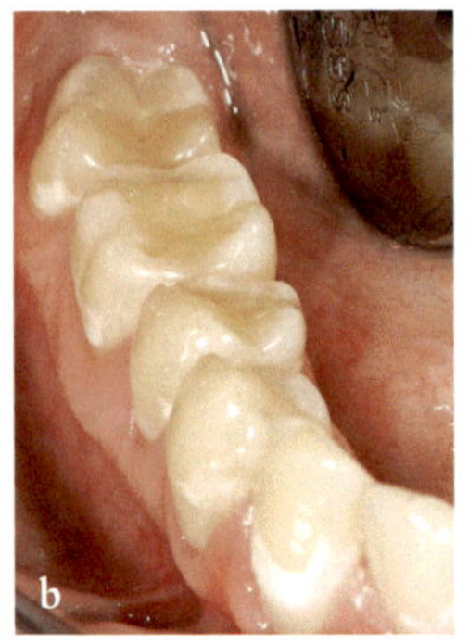

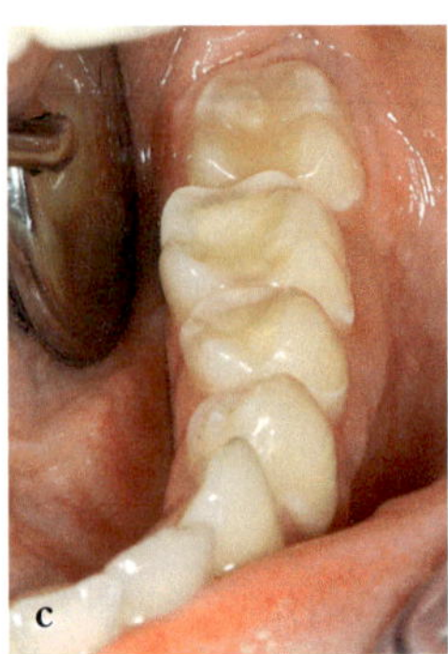

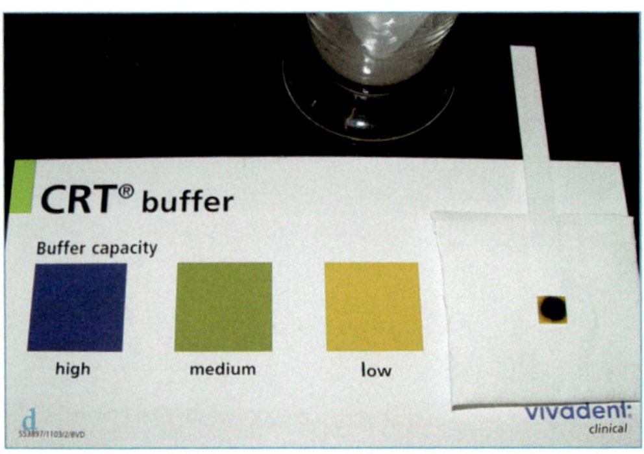


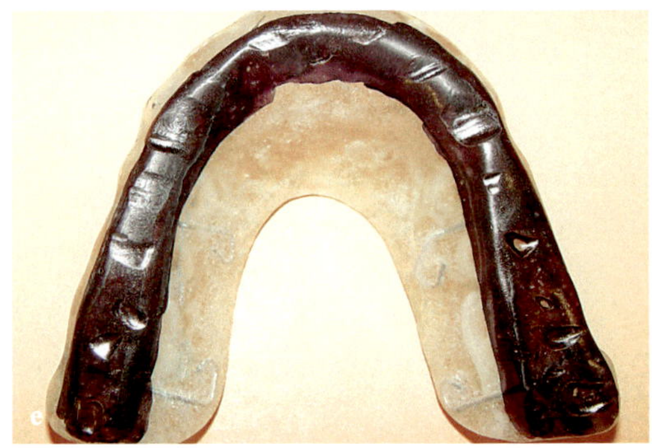

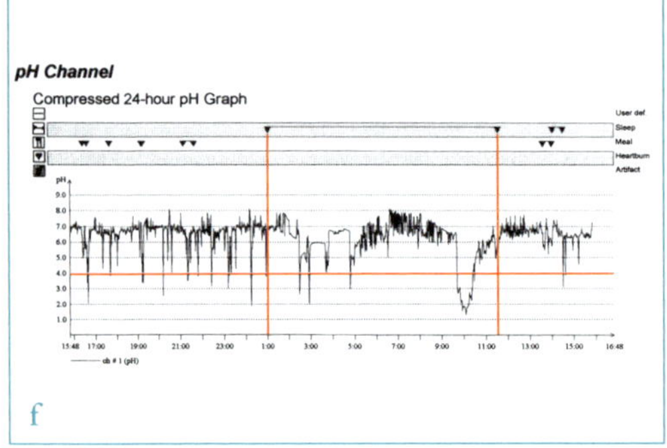


Period Table

| Item | | Total | Upright | Supine | Meal | PostP |
|---|---|---|---|---|---|---|
| Duration of period | (HH:MM) | 24:00 | 13:01 | 10:59 | 01:11 | 08:17 |
| Number of acid refluxes | ( # ) | 32 | 24 | 8 | 8 | 16 |
| Number of long acid refluxes | ( # ) | 2 | 0 | 2 | 0 | 0 |
| Longest acid reflux | (min) | 32 | 1 | 32 | 1 | 0 |
| Total time pH below 4.00 | (min) | 49 | 5 | 44 | 3 | 2 |
| Fraction time pH below 4.00 | ( % ) | 3.4 | 0.7 | 6.6 | 4.2 | 0.4 |
| Symptom Index | ( % ) | n/a | n/a | n/a | n/a | n/a |
| Reflux Index | (refl/hour) | 1.4 | 1.9 | 0.8 | 7.1 | 1.9 |
| EsopHageal Clearance | (min/refl) | 1.5 | 0.2 | 5.1 | 0.4 | 0.1 |

Acid Reflux Detail - HH:MM (length in minutes, minimum value)

| | | | | | |
|---|---|---|---|---|---|
| 16:35 (0.7 3.4) | 16:36 (0.1 4.0) | 16:36 (0.1 3.9) | 16:38 (0.1 2.1) | 17:40 (0.1 3.8) | 19:11 (0.9 3.4) |
| 19:14 (0.2 3.3) | 20:11 (0.2 2.6) | 20:35 (0.1 4.0) | 21:18 (1.0 3.5) | 21:20 (0.1 3.9) | 21:20 (0.1 3.9) |
| 21:47 (0.1 3.8) | 22:23 (0.1 3.6) | 22:25 (0.1 3.2) | 23:09 (0.4 3.1) | 23:10 (0.2 3.8) | 23:11 (0.1 4.0) |
| 23:11 (0.1 3.9) | 23:17 (0.1 3.9) | 00:13 (0.3 1.9) | 00:54 (0.1 3.8) | 02:28 (1.1 2.6) | 02:54 (0.5 2.2) |
| 02:55 (0.3 2.0) | 04:47 (0.1 3.0) | 09:40 (31.7 1.3) | 10:12 (9.8 2.2) | 10:27 (0.2 3.5) | 14:29 (0.1 3.1) |
| 14:30 (0.1 3.7) | 14:36 (0.1 3.9) | | | | |

g

Fig 10-13 **(a–c)** Wear characteristics in this bruxer suggested association with an acid. **(d)** Saliva was evaluated; the results were normal. **(e)** The splint showed signs consistent with sleep bruxism. **(f)** Although the patient had no symptoms of gastroesophageal reflux, the study of esophageal pH confirmed the diagnosis. **(g)** Note that the pH value, as highlighted in the study report, was below 4.0 for 44 minutes (accounting for two reflux episodes) during sleep in the dorsal-recumbent position.

of erosive lesions in teeth. In a study of 40 subjects showing a significant degree of erosion on the palatal surfaces of maxilary incisors, Smith and co-workers were able to provide evidence of this kind of situation.[96] In 36% of cases the patients showed no symptoms, yet they were diagnosed with gastroesophageal reflux by gastroenterologists. Sometimes, we wonder whether the word "idiopathic" is in fact hiding a situation of this kind. The clinical case in Figure 10-13 is an example of this.

## Etiopathogenic Mechanism and Conditioning Factors

The mechanism of erosive lesions occurs at the microscopic level. There is mineral loss, which is very similar to that generated by the acid etching technique used in composite restorations. Regardless of the origin of the acid, this pathology consists of surface demineralization of dental hard tissue, and it may result in complete destruction of teeth.

The factors conditioning the progress of the process are: the pH value of the solution; type of acid; temperature; adhesion to dental structure; amount of titratable acidity (in other words, its buffering capacity); phosphate and calcium concentrations and fluoride content of the aggressive liquid; and the calcium-chelation properties of the drink. Other factors involved are: acid quantity; amount of time the acid remains in the oral cavity; flow speed; surface layer renovation; and personal factors such as the saliva's quality and quantity and the subject's individual characteristics regarding the dental tissues.

### *Acquired Pellicle*

This layer is a biofilm that is free from pathogenic bacteria and covers all the soft and hard tissues of the oral cavity. It originates from the saliva's specific lipids and proteins and it sticks tightly to enamel's outer surface, acting as a barrier which defends teeth from acids.[97] This film plays the role of a selective membrane preventing acids from coming into direct contact with the surface of the tooth. It comprises mucins, proteins and glycoproteins, among which there are several enzymes. One of these enzymes, called "carbonic anhydrase VI", fights erosion by accelerating the neutralization of the hydrogen ions on the surface layers of the teeth. The composition, thickness, and age of the film (maturation time) are factors influencing the degree of protection it may provide against erosion.[98] Amaechi and co-workers showed that the thicker the acquired pellicle, the more it protects teeth from erosion.[99] For this reason, the authors ascribe the high incidence of erosion on the palatal surfaces of maxillary/anterior teeth to the fact that such surfaces are poorly covered with saliva, which is further aggravated by constant sweeping by the dorsal surface of the tongue.

After an acid comes into the oral cavity, in order to get into contact with the mineralized surface of the teeth it must first spread through the acquired pellicle. In early-stage erosion, the acid, after spreading through this pellicle, starts by attacking enamel's surface with its hydrogen ions, which start dissolving the adamantine crystals. At this stage only the surface layer is involved; later, the acid starts seeping in through enamel's cracks and pores, ultimately reaching the prisms and destroying them. This process will cause layer after layer of enamel to deteriorate, from the most superficial to the deepest. The mechanism is not the same for prismatic enamel and non-prismatic enamel. In the case of prismatic enamel, anisotropic dissolution occurs owing to the missing surface, with preferential loss of the interprismatic region or the prism-core region. Non-prismatic enamel is eroded in an irregular fashion; possibly this type of enamel is not so vulnerable to the action of erosion.[100] With regard to dentin, erosion starts in the peritubular region, where it begins by causing dentinal tubules to widen; then, progressive tissue loss occurs, which also affects the intertubular region. When the process progresses at a fast pace, dentin will show signs of hypersensitivity. This is likely to be due to the fact that tertiary dentin formation and dentin tubule obliteration cannot occur at the same pace, which leads to tissue surface loss. Sometimes, the erosive potential exceeds the restoring potential of the pulp/dentin complex, which results in painful complications, pulp inflammation, necrosis and, eventually, periapical processes.[101]

### Critical pH Value for Teeth

A pH value of 5.5 has traditionally been reported to be critical for enamel dissolution; this means that lower values can be expected to trigger a superficial erosive process. However, mineral loss can be triggered by higher pH values.[102] The critical pH for enamel is not a fixed value but a variable one: it is the pH at which a solution is saturated with respect to a particular mineral – in this case, dental hard tissue minerals. The pH of a solution (beverage/food) and its calcium, phosphate, and fluoride content determine the saturation level with respect to the minerals from dental hard tissues. If the pH of the beverage or food solution is higher than the critical value (i.e., if the solution is oversaturated), such solution will tend to precipitate minerals; this is the case with saliva and fluid dental plaque, which are usually oversaturated with respect to teeth and, thus, they will not erode them. In contrast, if the solution's pH is lower than the critical value (i.e., if the solution is not saturated), such solution will trigger a dissolution process (i.e., it will take minerals out from the teeth) which will last until saturation occurs. Once saturated, the aggressive solution will stop demineralizing teeth. Those subjects whose saliva has a low concentration of calcium and phosphate are more vulnerable to the action of acids, since the critical pH for enamel/dentin will be higher. In contrast, saliva that is rich in calcium and phosphate will be able to resist aggressions much better, since the critical pH for teeth will be lower.[103] Despite its acidic pH (4.0), yogurt will not erode dental tissues, because its high content of calcium and phosphate cause it to be supersaturated with respect to teeth.[104] Thus, enamel erosion cannot be induced by any kind of yogurt – fruity yogurts included.

The erosive process will stop and it will not restart until new acids or chelating agents come into the mouth. Also, the amount of drink coming into the mouth with every sip influences erosion, since big volumes can surpass the amount of saliva which is necessary to neutralize the beverage. Besides, some people have a habit of taking a sip of drink and swishing it around the teeth; this has been shown to accelerate erosion.[105] Others have a holding habit, which causes the acid to be in contact with teeth for longer. Dental erosion has been found in children having this habit.[67] Also, the temperature of the drink when coming into the mouth is a factor that affects the erosive process; it has been shown that the higher the temperature of orange juice, "soft" drinks, coffee, and tea, the more the enamel's surface is softened. It is advisable to drink "soft" drinks and juices cold from the fridge; as for cordials (tea and coffee), they should ideally be drunk as cold as possible.[41]

### Action of Acids and Chelating Agents

Dental erosion may be caused by the action of the hydrogen ions liberated by acids; also, by the action of anions which remove calcium – this mechanism is called "chelation". Enamel and dentin consist of minerals, proteins, lipids, and water. The amount of water contained in these tissues is enough for the acid to spread through them and cause erosion; hydrogen ions originate from the dissociation of acid in a watery medium. These hydrogen ions dissolve dental surface minerals. Such is the case of hydrochloric acid, which fully dissociates in water; the resulting hydrogen ion formation rapidly dissolves a tooth's surface. That is the reason why recurrent vomiting in bulimics rapidly erodes the palatal surfaces of anterior teeth. The situation is different with citric acid (orange

*Table 10-2*

**Daily saliva flow – average values (Screbny and Shu[110]).**

| Type of saliva | Function | Hours per day | Flow per minute | Flow per day | Source |
|---|---|---|---|---|---|
| Resting | Protection | Awake: 14<br>Sleep: 8 | Awake: 0.3–0.4 mL<br>Sleep: very scarce | 252–336 mL | ~70% SM + SL<br>~25% parotid gland |
| Stimulated | Mastication | 2 | 1.0–2.0 mL | 120–240 mL | ~50% SM + SL<br>~50% parotid gland |

Total flow is ~372–576 mL/day
SM = submandibular gland; SL = sublingual gland

or lemon juice, etc.), since it has a double-destruction effect on tooth surfaces. In water, this acid dissociates into hydrogen ions – which behave as mentioned – and acidic anions (citrates) – which act as chelating agents, interacting with calcium and removing it from the apatite surface. At a low pH, this acid liberates hydrogen ions, thus causing erosion; in contrast, at a neutral pH its citrates remove calcium from the tooth. At an intermediate pH, as is the case with citrus fruit and its juices, both mechanisms erode teeth at the same time. As we have mentioned, dental erosion does not necessarily require a low pH in order to occur. Another clear example is that of lactic acid, which, at a low pH liberates hydrogen ions very quickly; however, when the pH becomes neutralized, it is its lactate ions which continue removing calcium from dental tissues.[106]

### *Saliva*

Saliva is the most important biologic factor in the fight against erosion. According to Mandel,[107] its main function is to preserve the ecologic balance of the oral cavity. Saliva's functions are many. Mandel lists the following:

- It removes leftover food particles, sugars and acids from the oral cavity.
- Its buffering capacity neutralizes the acids from the intake.
- It reduces the potential of erosive agents.
- It acts as a protective pellicle which prevents the demineralization of enamel's surface layers by acids from the intake.
- Owing to its content of calcium and phosphate, it maintains a state of supersaturation near tooth surfaces.
- It provides the calcium, the phosphate, and the fluorides needed for the early remineralization of enamel.

Saliva contains 99% water plus a variety of electrolytes, including calcium, potassium, magnesium, bicarbonate, and phosphates. It also contains proteins, immunoglobulins, mucins, enzymes, and nitrogenated components such as ammonia and urea. These components have different functions. Bicarbonate, phosphate, and urea are responsible for pH modulation and saliva's buffering capacity. Mucins and proteins have a cleansing function, and, along with other oral microorganisms, they are involved in dental plaque metabolism. Calcium, phosphate, and proteins maintain tooth insolubility and determine demineralization and remineralization. Enzymes, proteins, and immunoglobulins have an antibacterial function.[108,109]

According to Screbny and Shu,[110] total daily saliva secretion ranges between 372 and 576 mL (Table 10-2). Stimulated saliva accounts for 38% of this amount; the rest is unstimulated saliva, which accounts for 62% of the total saliva and averages 252–336 mL. The submandibular and sublingual glands secrete 70% of the unstimulated saliva, while parotid glands secrete 25%. Upon stimulation, these percentages will change, and 50% of the saliva will be secreted by the parotid glands.

Although the minor salivary glands, which are present throughout the mouth, secrete saliva in very small amounts, such saliva has a very important moistening function.[110] In normal conditions, saliva is always present in the mouth. A limited amount (~0.8 mL) of residual saliva remains throughout the oral cavity after each deglutition.[111] Average salivary flow varies significantly from individual to individual. An unstimulated saliva rate of more than 0.1 mL/min is considered to be a normal value.[112] With regard to stimulated saliva, 1 mL/min is considered to be the minimum normal volume.[113] Salivary secretion is regulated by the circadian rhythm: it decreases during sleep and increases during wakefulness.

The pH of normal saliva ranges between 6.7 and 7.4, which means it is almost neutral. These values are dependent on bicarbonate concentration. Bicarbonate is the most important buffer, since it spreads over the plaque and buffers acidity. This mechanism operates in a more efficient way during the secretion of an abundant stimulated salivary flow. When salivary flow is low, the amount of bicarbonate decreases; thus, the pH becomes lower and there is reduced buffering capacity. Phosphate is an important buffer during the secretion of unstimulated saliva.[114]

The saliva of patients suffering from erosion has lower calcium and phosphorus content, when compared to the saliva of control subjects. This has been related to scarce unstimulated saliva flow. Patients whose unstimulated flow is less than 0.1 mL/min have a five times higher risk of erosion than patients with higher rates.[6]

When people having normal saliva secretion levels consume acidic drinks, these are neutralized in the mouth within about 10 minutes, and the tip of the tongue's pH remains low during the first 2 minutes only.[115] In contrast, in those subjects with a low saliva secretion level, pH values may remain low for about 30 minutes.[116]

Figure 10-14 shows a female patient with a history of radiation to the pterygomaxillary fossa as treatment for a tumor. The radiotherapy affected the salivary glands, and within just 11 months she developed erosive lesions.

About 30% of the population show some level of oral dryness. Patient complaints of dryness are not a reliable sign for assessing the functional status of the salivary glands. Some patients will not notice that they have less saliva until their salivary flow has decreased by 50%.[117] Four parameters have been suggested for the clinical identification of salivary gland hypofunction: dry lips; dry buccal mucosa; absence of saliva on palpation; and high index values of caries, missing teeth, and restored teeth.[118] Undoubtedly, drug intake is the commonest cause of reduced salivary flow. Medications that may cause this problem include antidepressants, anticholinergics, anti-Parkinson drugs, antihistamines, antipsychotics, antihypertensives, minor tranquilizers, and diuretics. Of course, we must also mention the specific pathologies of the salivary glands.

People with less saliva will usually drink a great number of acidic drinks to compensate for mouth dryness. This aggravates the erosive effect of such beverages, due to the lack of buffering capacity associated with scarce saliva. Something similar occurs to people who engage in intensive sport activities daily. A significant amount of body fluids are lost during exercise – saliva among them – which results in oral dryness. Some sports people will consume many drinks advertised as "sport" or "energy" drinks. These products are generally acidic and, because of the poor buffering capacity of the pH typical of a dry mouth, they will progressively affect enamel. Even worse is that other people, when feeling their mouth is dry, will suck

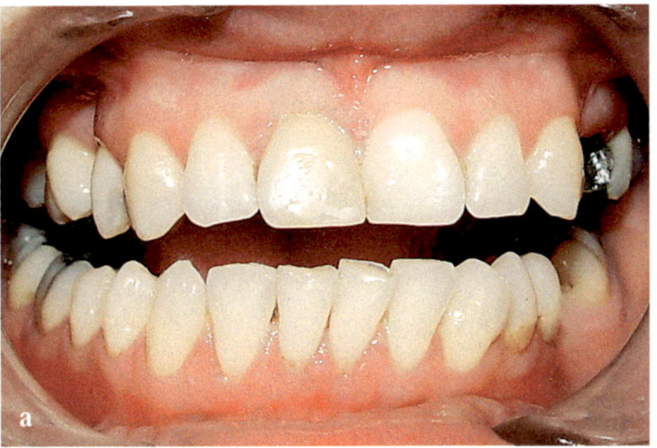

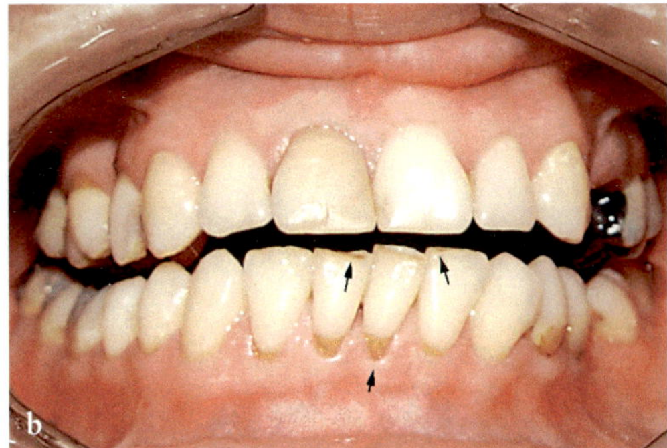

Fig 10-14 **(a and b)** Erosion caused by impairment of the salivary glands after radiotherapy for a tumor.

a lemon to stimulate the secretion of saliva. The stimulatory effect of citric acid on saliva has recently been shown by a research study: a 0.38 mL/min flow of unstimulated saliva increased to 1.87 mL/min after three drops of citric acid at 4% concentration were applied on the tongue's dorsum.[119] As an example of exogenous erosion, Järvinen[6] reports on the case of a subject with reduced stimulated salivary secretion who had the habit of consuming citrus fruit three times per week in order to stimulate salivation.

The clinical case depicted in Figure 10-15 concerns a young rugby player who trained intensively and consumed "energy" drinks to compensate for mouth dryness. In addition he sucked two lemons every day.

In the fight against erosion, there is no doubt that saliva's most important function is that of creating the acquired pellicle. The acquired pellicle protects enamel from the demineralization process caused by acids, though a recent research study has shown that its protective effect on dentin tissue is limited.[120]

In an in-situ study, a piece of enamel was stuck on an acrylic splint covering the palate with the aim of measuring enamel erosion with the microscope after daily intake of 11 glasses of orange juice. For comparison, the same experiment was conducted on another group of subjects who drank water instead of juice. The authors reported a higher level of enamel erosion in those who consumed orange juice than in those who consumed water. Then, the same experiment was conducted *in vitro*. Erosion measurements were 10 times as high as those registered in the mouth, which proves saliva's important remineralizing effect.[121]

In short, saliva can be said to be the most important biologic factor in the fight against erosion. A good salivary flow helps to prevent and reduce dental hard tissue dissolution. In contrast, a poor buffering capacity due to scarce salivary secretion facilitates the erosive process. The measurement of saliva parameters can be easily performed in the dental office by using techniques that are described later in this chapter.

### *Tooth Structure Variations*

Regardless of the type of acid and its titratable acidity, temperature, and exposure time, there are other individual factors that can modify the erosive process and its magnitude. In-vivo clinical trials of human teeth subject to the acidic effect of lemon juice have shown significant variations that may be ascribed to differences in the composition and degree of hardness of teeth, which are dependent on the fluoride content and the degree of mineralization.[122]

Erosion also differs according to whether it develops in deciduous teeth or permanent teeth. Children are more predisposed to dental erosion

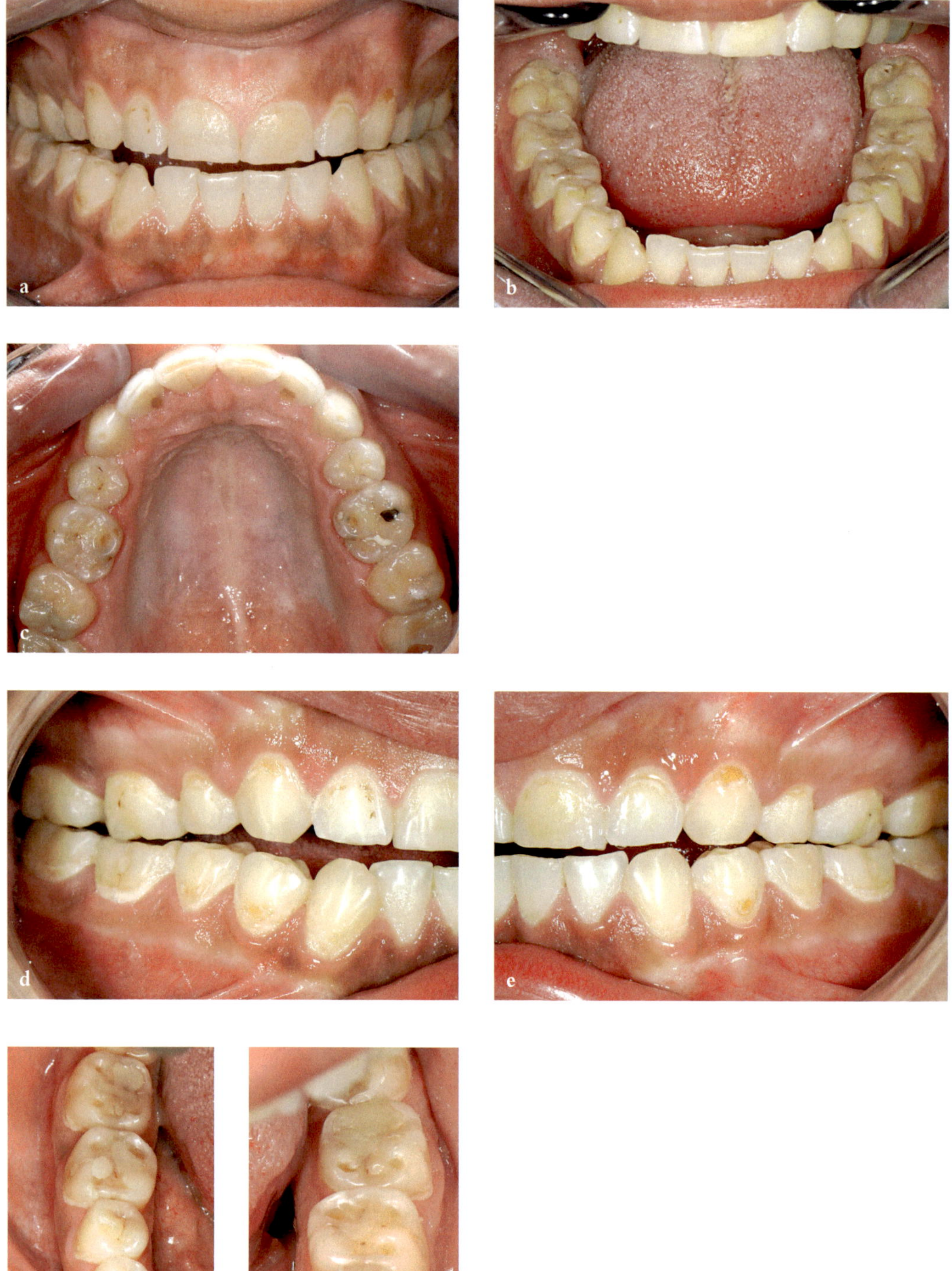


Fig 10-15 **(a–g)** This 22-year-old sportsman shows significant erosive wear which compromised all his teeth.

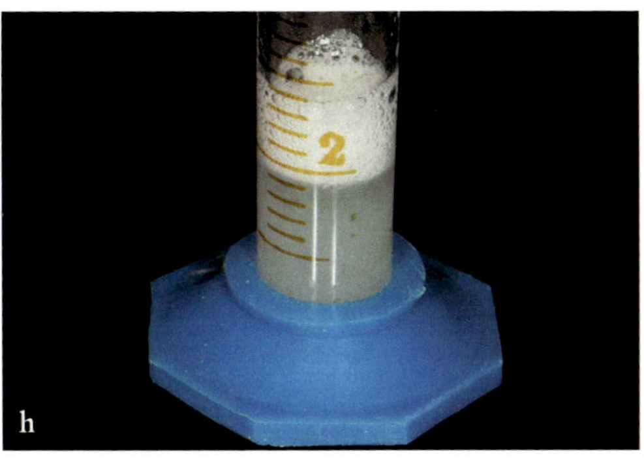

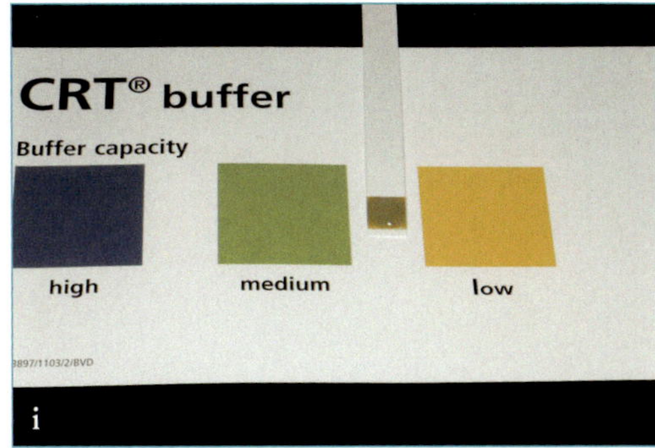


**Fig 10-15 (h and i)** His saliva was scarce; buffering capacity was deficient. During the intensive training sessions, he would drink Gatorade, and he was in the habit of sucking two lemons every day. Note the large amounts of dentin exposed on the vestibular surfaces.

than adults, because their salivary flow is lower.[122] Besides, children's diet is usually richer in acidic drinks.[7,25] With regard to potential deciduous and permanent teeth differences in susceptibility to erosion, research studies have been contradictory in their findings. Some authors report deciduous teeth's enamel to be less hard[123] and erosion to progress 1.5 times as fast in deciduous teeth as in permanent teeth;[42] others have not confirmed such differences.[124,125] Perhaps, the fact that deciduous teeth are smaller than permanent teeth and enamel is less thick in the former, are factors causing erosion that reaches the level of dentin more quickly than in the latter.[126] Finally, it seems, the higher prevalence of tooth wear in children may be ascribed to the combined action of erosion, abrasive wear, and attrition.[127]

### *Erosion and Caries*

Despite their etiopathogenic mechanisms being very similar (apatite-crystal dissolution), rarely do erosion and caries occur simultaneously. Caries occurs in places where dental plaque accumulates; in contrast, erosion occurs in places that are free from dental plaque.[100] In the erosive process, the teeth will literally be bathed in acid, while in the case of caries the acid is produced by the microorganisms inside the plaque. In patients with endogenous erosion and who regurgitate or vomit constantly, teeth are recurrently attacked by the contents of the stomach (pH 1.0); the same happens with exogenous erosion due to the recurrent intake of acidic beverages and food (pH 2.3/4.0). However, rarely do these subjects have caries. In general, caribacteria will not survive in extremely acid environments. A pH value lower than 4.2 has been shown to interrupt the cariogenic metabolism of *Streptococcus mutans*.[128] This explains why erosion and caries will not coexist on the same tooth surface.

A study compared the structure of the exfoliated deciduous teeth of children who drank orange juice for 12–18 months; then such teeth were compared with similar teeth of children who did not recieve any beverage at school. The former children's exfoliated teeth showed signs of erosion, but, curiously, these children showed a lower caries index in their permanent teeth.[129] Such research studies confirm what we usually see in daily dental practice – that patients whose teeth are damaged by erosion hardly ever show caries (Figs 10-16 and 10-17).

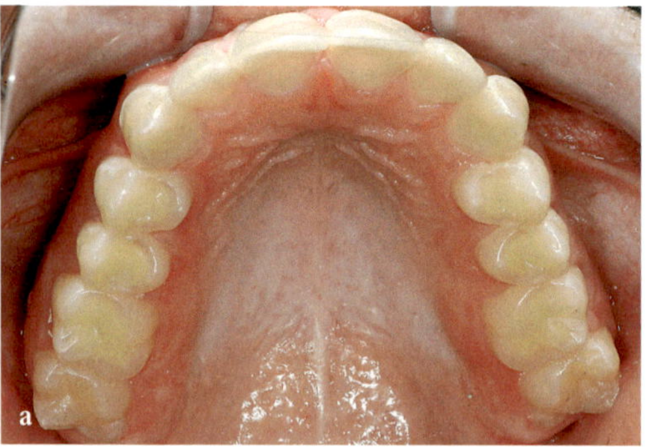

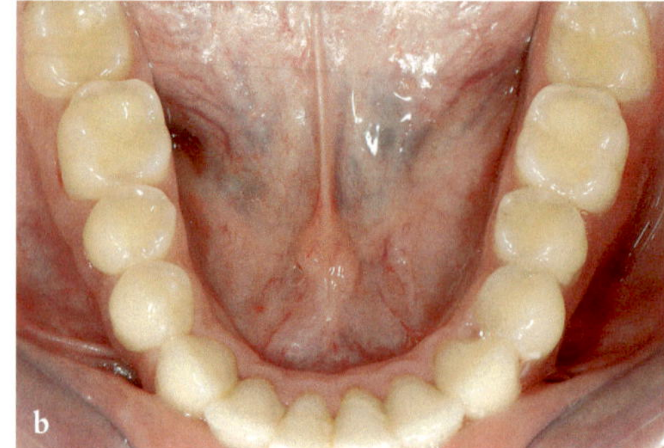

Fig 10-16 **(a and b)** Despite the exposed dentin, no caries will develop.

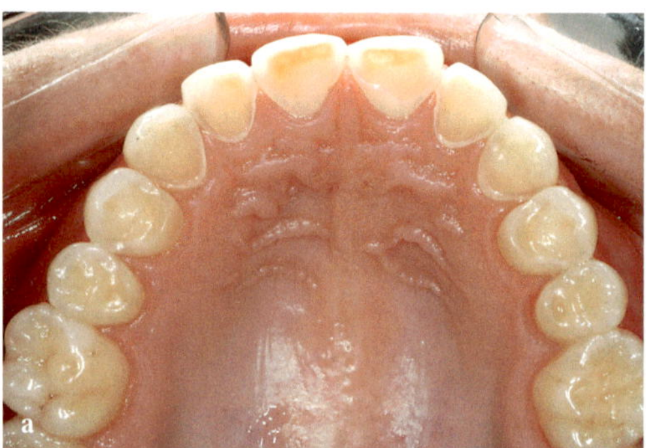

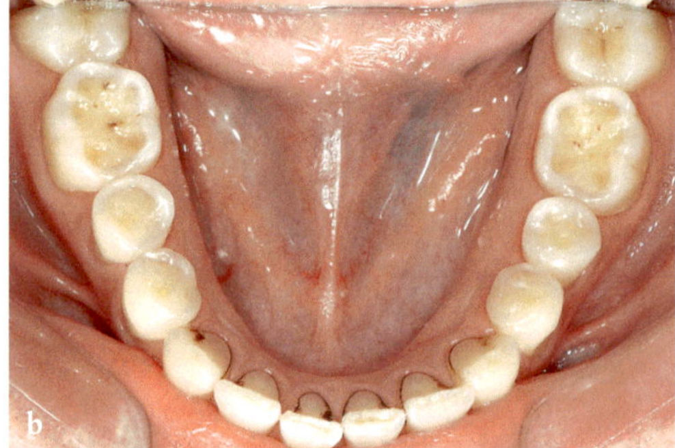

Fig 10-17 **(a and b)** The exposed dentin's yellowish hue and the loss of occlusal ridges and crevices are signs of erosion, which in this case affects many teeth. However, these patients will hardly develop caries.

## Salivary Secretion and Buffering Capacity Quantification

Saliva can easily be studied in any dental office by means of a simple test; this allows the clinician to assess how efficiently it protects against erosion. Performing a saliva test should be included in the diagnosis protocol for patients who show multiple-etiology tooth wear and, especially, for patients showing accelerated wear with clinical evidence of erosion.

The best treatment plan for worn teeth is to control the etiologic agent causing such wear. A simple saliva test, and evaluating intake, hygiene habits, potential alimentary-tract alterations, and parafunctions will provide valuable information that is essential for diagnosis and for devising a dental-wear preventive strategy.

### *Patient Preparation*

One hour prior to the test, patients should abstain from:

- eating and drinking (water excluded)
- chewing gum
- smoking
- brushing the teeth
- using a mouthwash.

### *Objectives and Techniques*

The factors to evaluate are: (1) functioning of minor lip salivary glands; (2) resting saliva amount and quality (viscosity, flow rate, pH); and (3) stimulated saliva amount and quality (flow rate, pH, buffering capacity).

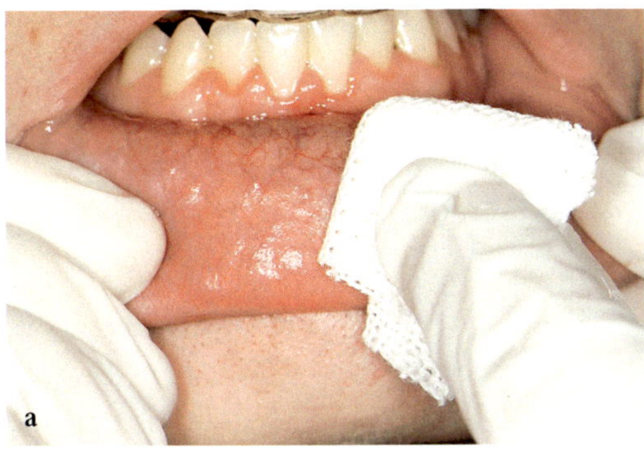

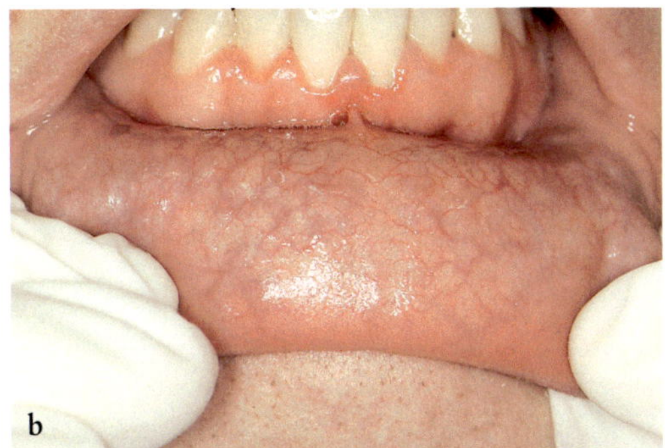

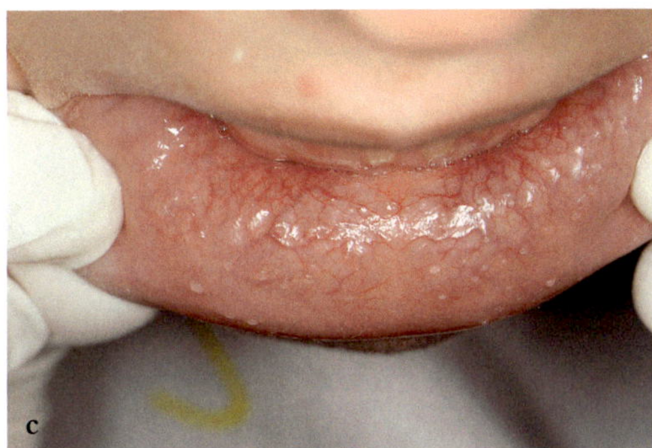

Fig 10-18 Lip gland evaluation. **(a)** The mucosa is dried with gauze. **(b)** The lip is turned outward and kept in that position. **(c)** After 1 minute, small saliva drops can be observed.

*Lip salivary glands*

The functioning of minor lip salivary glands can be assessed by means of a simple test. Despite secreting small volumes of saliva, these small glands are very important for oral cavity lubrication. With good light and the patient comfortably seated on the dental chair, the clinician will proceed to turn the patient's lower lip outward and to gently dry the mucosa. Then, he or she will measure the time elapsed before the small lip glands begin to secrete small saliva drops which will make the mucosa look shiny. The time required for this procedure is 1 minute (Fig 10-18).

*Study of unstimulated saliva*

Unstimulated (resting) saliva has the very important role of preserving the integrity of oral tissues, since it is the saliva covering the teeth for the longest time. Although unstimulated saliva values have been shown to vary widely from individual to individual, they are quite stable. Salivary flow values below the normal range suggest a depression of the basal activity of glands.[110] Flow rate, pH value, and viscosity can be evaluated on a sample of such saliva.

*Unstimulated saliva flow*

Unstimulated saliva is secreted without physiologic stimuli being involved. The patient is asked to accumulate saliva in the mouth for 5 minutes without swallowing it, and to keep the tongue still on the mouth floor. Once the 5 minutes have elapsed, the patient is requested to spit the accumulated saliva into a graduated container. The amount of saliva thus obtained is measured. Unstimulated saliva above 0.1 mL is considered to be normal; this was

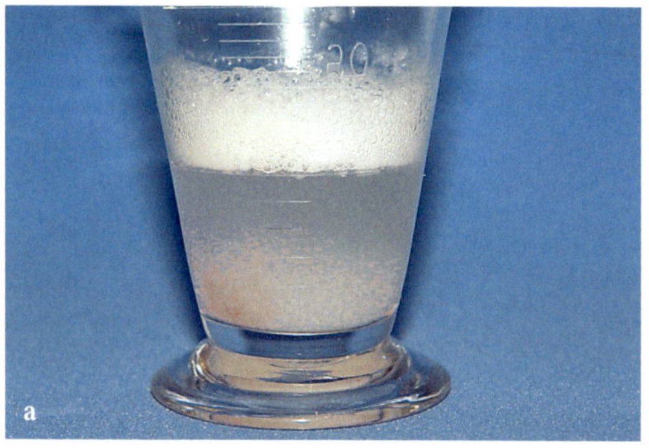
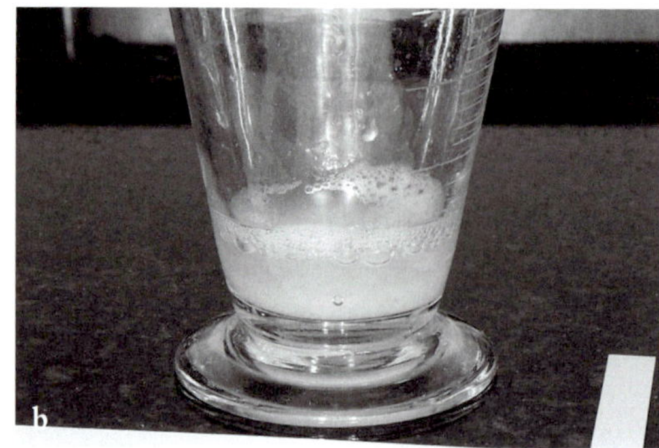
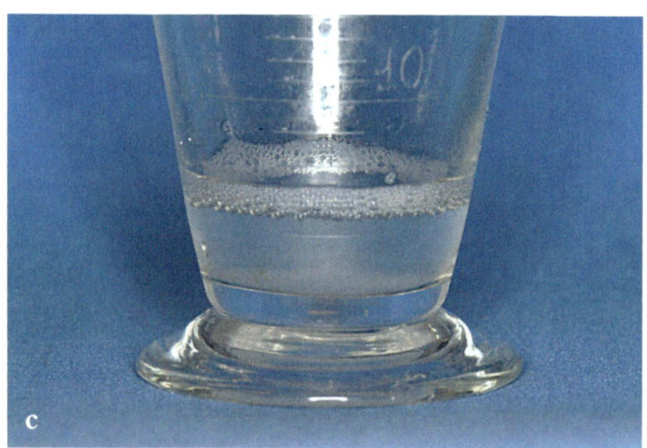
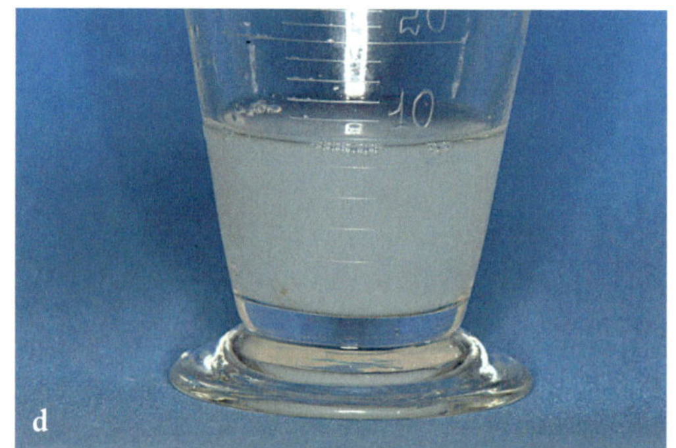
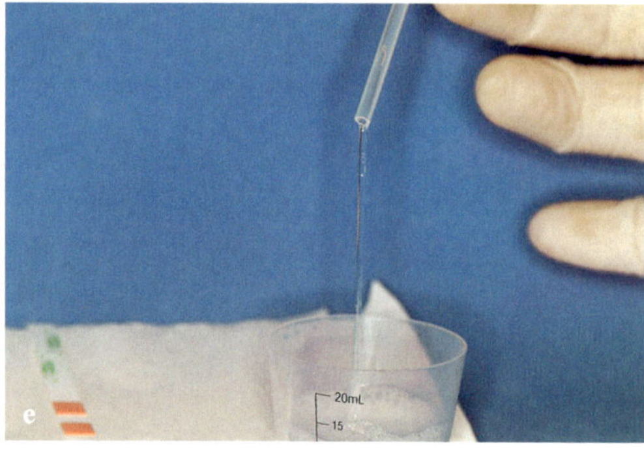

Fig 10-19 **(a–e)** Different types of saliva.

determined according to the results obtained in data-gathering from the general population.[112]

*Unstimulated saliva viscosity*

This test consists of observing the appearance of the saliva contained in a glass receptacle. Clear, watery saliva has normal viscosity. Saliva with sticky residues and bubbles has increased viscosity (Fig 10-19).

*Unstimulated saliva pH*

As will be seen later in this section, pH can be measured by using commercially available colorimetric test kits. Examples of these are CRT buffer Ivoclar (Vivadent, Lichtenstein) and Saliva-Check (GC Corp, Tokyo). Alternatively, an electronic pH meter can be used (Twin pH B-212: Horiba, Tokyo).

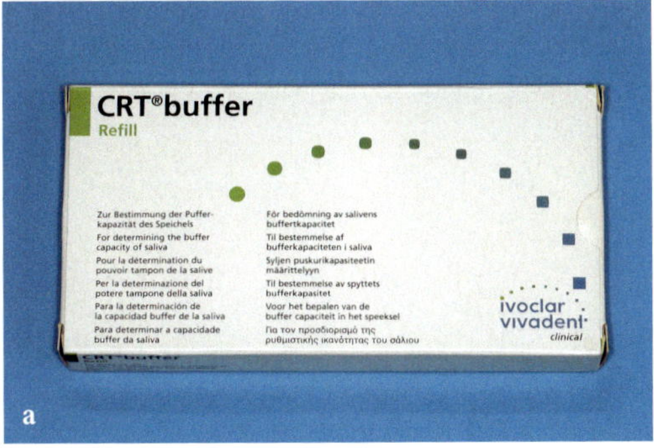


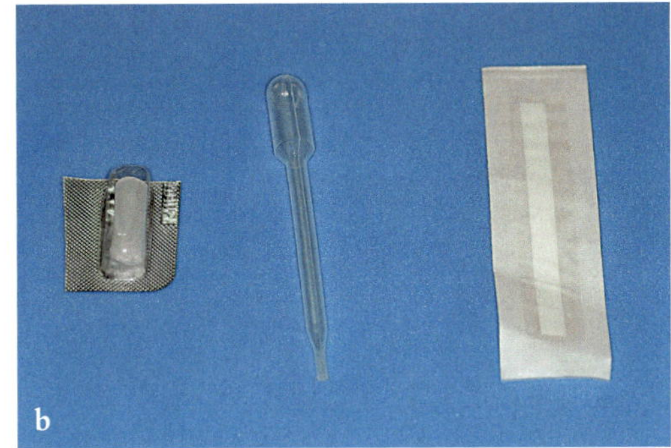

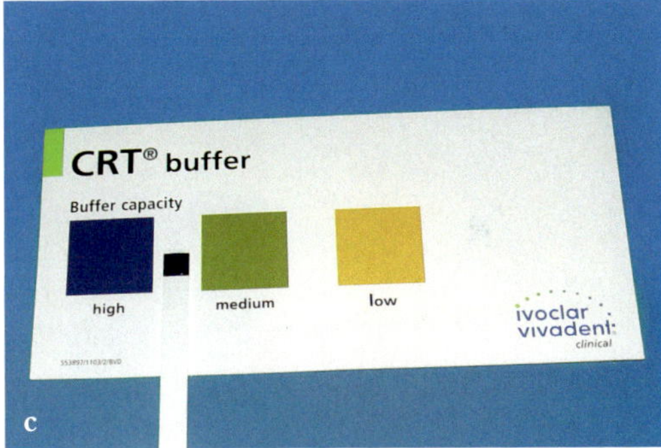


Fig 10-20 **(a–c)** The CRT Buffer system.

*Study of stimulated saliva*

Stimulated saliva plays a specific role during mastication and deglutition. Flow values below the normal range are considered to be indicative of a failure of the gland to respond to exogenous stimuli.[110] Apart from salivary flow measurement, pH and buffering capacity against acids can be evaluated.

*Stimulated saliva flow*

The patient, comfortably seated in an upright, relaxed position, starts stimulating the secretion of saliva by chewing a paraffin pellet for a whole minute so as to soften and homogenize it; the saliva accumulated in the mouth should be discarded. From this moment onwards, the patient will keep on chewing for 5 minutes in order to stimulate saliva secretion (a timer will be of help to control the time). The patient should spit the saliva into a calibrated container every now and then. Once the 5 minutes have elapsed, the total amount of saliva secreted is measured. The resulting value must be divided by 5 to obtain the average amount of saliva secreted per minute. Normal values for adults are above 1 mL/min. Values below 0.7 mL/min are considered to be a risk factor. Values ranging between 1.0 and 0.7 mL/min are considered to be borderline.[113]

*Stimulated saliva pH and buffering capacity*

The next step is the evaluation of pH and buffering capacity. As has already been mentioned, this test can be done by using kits obtained from dental shops or by using a pH meter.

The CRT Buffer system consists of strips of test paper containing a weak acid that must be neutralized by saliva's buffering capacity (Fig 10-20). Using one of the pipettes included in the kit, a

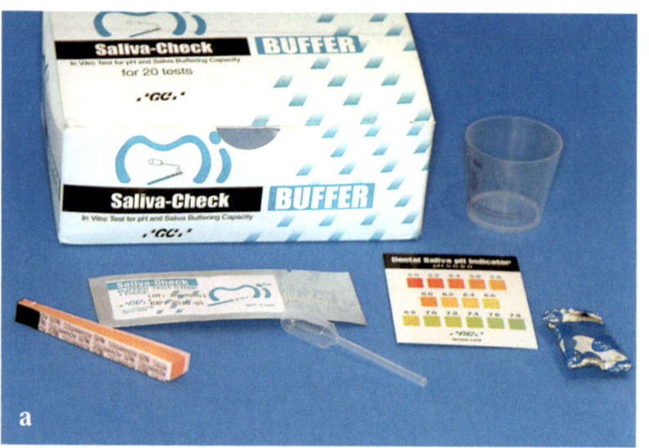


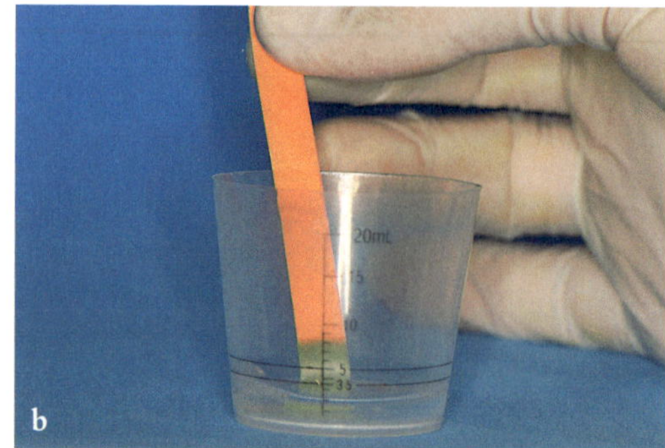


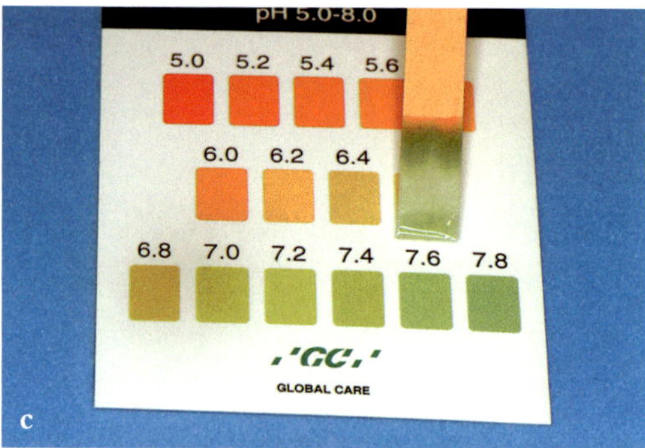


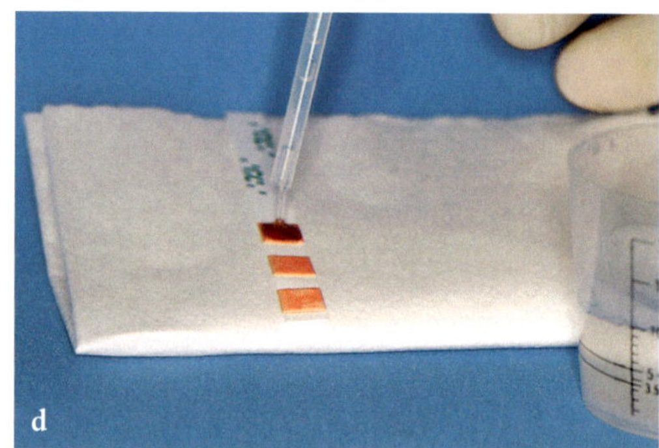


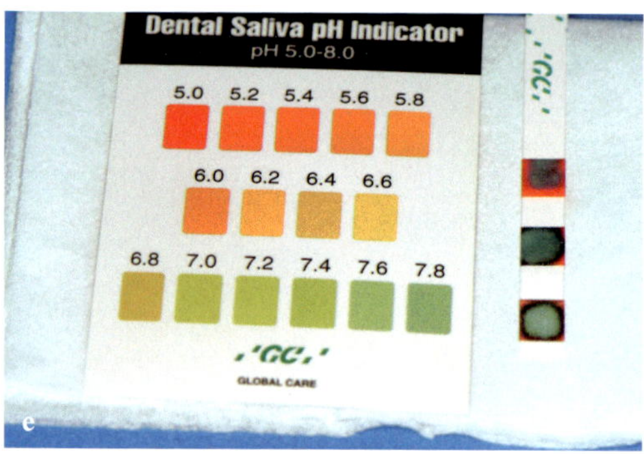


**Fig 10-21** **(a–e)** The Saliva-Check system.

drop of saliva is applied to the test paper, which contains an acid and a pH indicator. Saliva dissolves acid, which causes pH to be low at the beginning of the test; if the saliva has a buffering capacity, the pH will increase and the test paper's color will change. Yellow indicates a pH value of 4.0 or below, which means that saliva has not been able to increase the pH; this represents a risk factor for the patient. Green indicates a low-normal buffering capacity. Blue indicates a good buffering capacity. A research study compared the results obtained with this method with the results obtained with an electronic pH meter; significant correlation between both methods was reported.[130]

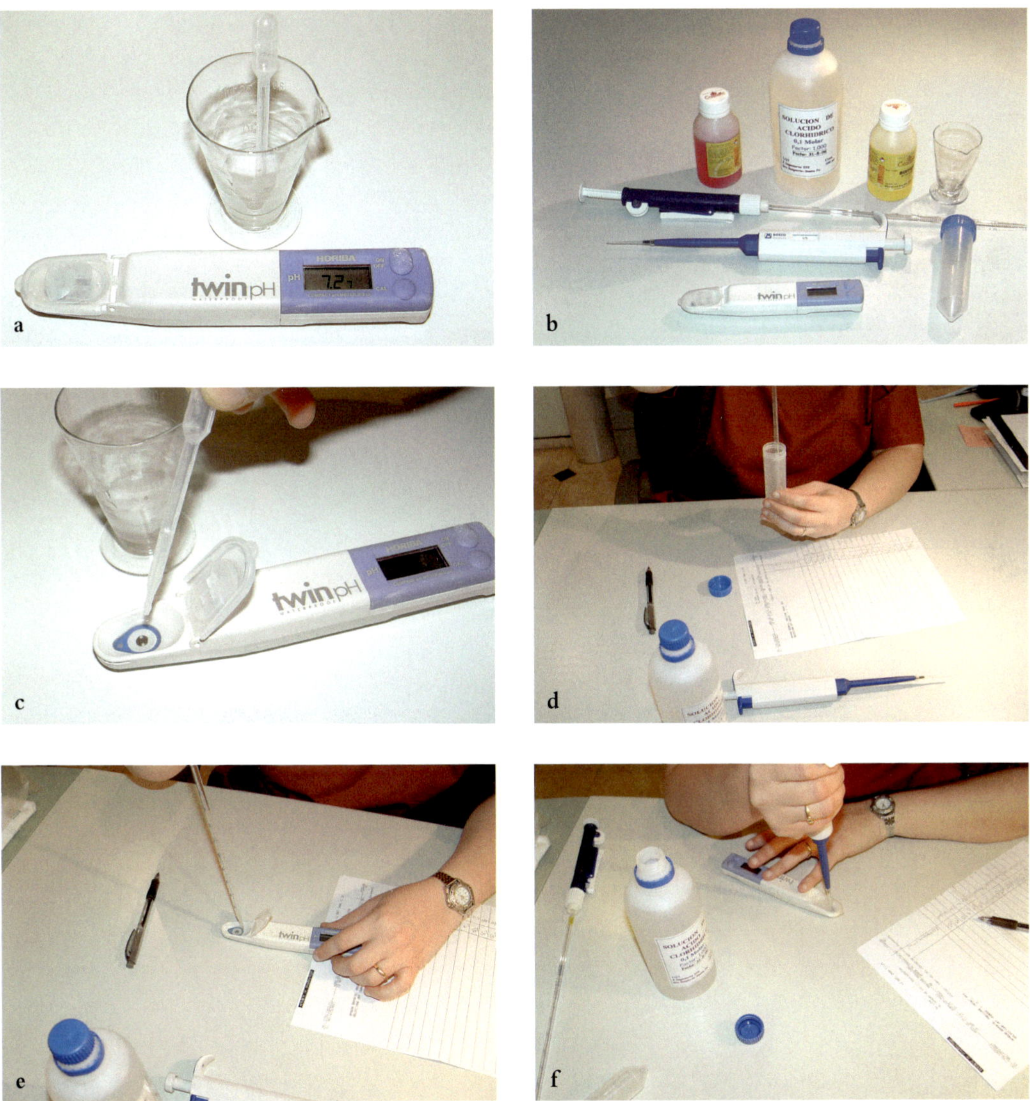


Fig 10-22 **(a–f)** Equipment needed in order to study saliva by using a pH meter. The saliva is placed in a pH meter; then its reaction to each addition of acid is measured.

The Saliva-Check system is another commercially available option (Fig 10-21). This method allows one to measure saliva's buffering capacity and pH by making color comparisons. The kit includes a color-coded sheet which allows one to determine pH values by color comparison and by using a graduated scale increasing by 0.2 units from 5.0 up to 8.0. Also, buffering capacity can be tested with another strip by means of colorimetric comparison. As with CRT Buffer, this method classifies the buffering capacity into "very low", "low", and "high" (or "normal").

Electronic pH meters allow quantification of saliva's pH and buffering capacity (Fig 10-22). To measure pH, a sample of saliva should be placed in the receptacle containing the sensor; then the results will be shown in the liquid crystal display. The buffering capacity is tested by adding a titratable acid to a saliva sample to check whether the saliva reacts and neutralizes the acid. A hydrochloric acid solution at 0.1 mol/L concentration is used as the aggressor agent. Using a graduated pipette, a 0.5 mL sample of the stimulated saliva obtained earlier is placed into the pH meter's receptacle; once the saliva is stable, the initial pH value is obtained. Then a 10 μL drop of acid is added with a micro-graduated pipette; after the stabilization, pH will fall. This procedure should be repeated eight times, and pH values should be recorded each time; such pH values will gradually decrease, since saliva will gradually lose its acid neutralization capacity. It is advisable to store the pH values in a spreadsheet (e.g., Excel) and to print charts representing a specific curve for each saliva.

The pH value registered when the added acid reaches 50 μL is the one that determines the buffering capacity of that saliva (Fig 10-23). A pH below 4.5 indicates poor saliva quality, a value between 4.5 and 5.5 indicates average quality, and a value above 5.5 indicates that the saliva has a good buffering capacity.[131] The same procedure may be used to test unstimulated saliva; however, it has been suggested that stimulated saliva should be used, since it is more consistent with oral health.[131]

Identifying individuals whose saliva's buffering capacity shows alterations and identifying the aggressor acid's source allows the adoption of preventive measures: modification of intake habits and methods of hygiene, salivary secretion stimulation, etc. Finally, we should emphasize that a multidisciplinary strategy involving dental practitioners, saliva specialists, and gastroenterologists working as a team should be used in the management of patients showing accelerated tooth wear.

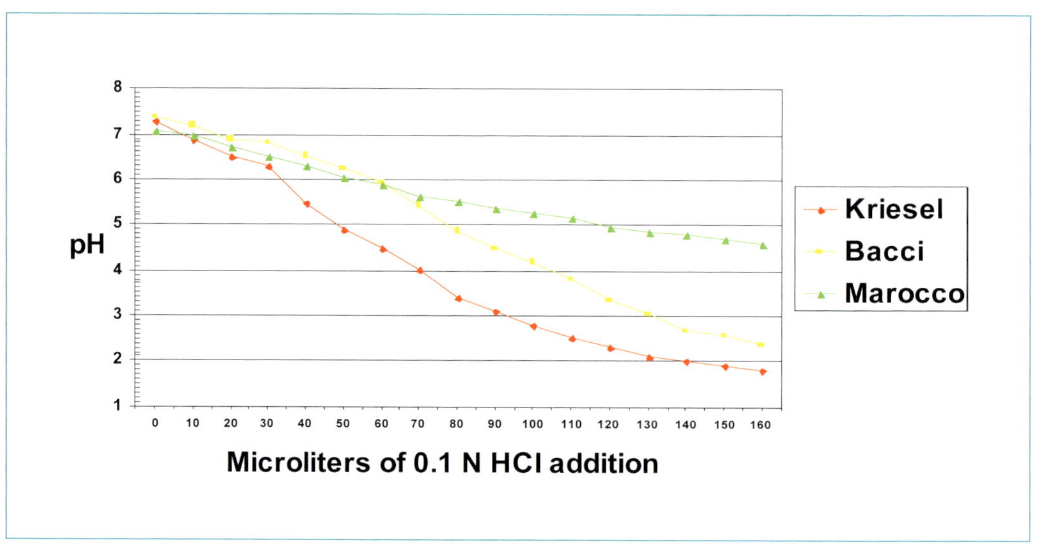


Fig 10-23 Chart showing the saliva reactions of three individuals. The red line represents the patient from Figure 10-10.

## References


1. White DK, Hayes RC, Benjamin RN. Loss of tooth structure associated with chronic regurgitation and vomiting. J Am Dent Assoc 1978;97:833–835.
2. Smith BG, Knight JK. A comparison of patterns of tooth wear with aetiological factors. Br Dent J 1984;157:16–19.
3. JärvinenV, Meurman JH, Hyvarinen H, Rytömaa L, Murtomaa H. Dental erosion and upper gastro intestinal disorders. Oral Surg Oral Med Oral Pathol 1988;65: 298–303.
4. Aine L, Baer N, Maki M. Dental erosion caused by gastroesophageal reflux disease in children. J Dent Child 1993;60:210–214.
5. Grippo JO, Simring M, Schreiner S. Attrition, abrasion, corrosion and abfraction revisited: a new perspective on tooth surface lesions. J Am Dent Assoc 2004;135: 1109–1118.
6. JärvinenV, Rytömaa L, Heinonen O. Risk factors in dental erosion. J Dent Res 1991;70:942–947.
7. Dugmore CR, Rock WP. The progression of tooth erosion in a cohort of adolescents of mixed ethnicity. Int J Paediatr Dent 2003;13:295–303.
8. Millward A, Shaw L, Smith A. Dental erosion in four year-old children from differing socio-economic backgrounds. J Dent Child 1994;61:263–266.
9. Peres KG, Armenio MF, Peres MA, Traebert J, De Lacerda JT. Dental erosion in 12-year-old school children: a cross-sectional study in Southern Brazil. Int J Paediatr Dent 2005;15:249–255.
10. Al-Malik MI, Holt RD, Bedi R. Erosion, caries and rampant caries in preschool children in Jeddah, Saudi Arabia. Community Dent Oral Epidemiol 2002;30:16–23.
11. Luo Y, Zeng XJ, Du MQ, Bedi R. The prevalence of dental erosion in preschool children in China. J Dent 2005;33:115–121.
12. Ganss C, Klimek J, Lussi A. Accuracy and consistency of the visual diagnosis of exposed dentine on worn occlusal/incisal surfaces. Caries Res 2006;40:208–212.
13. Al-Malik MI, Holt RD, Bedi R, Speight PM. Investigation of an index to measure tooth wear in primary teeth. J Dent 2001;29:103–137.
14. Eccles JD. Dental erosion of nonindustrial origin: a clinical survey and classification. J Prosthet Dent 1979;42: 649–653.
15. Lussi A. Dental Erosion: From Diagnosis to Treatment. Basel, Switzerland: Karger, 2006.
16. Kim HD, Douglass CW. Associations between occupational health behaviors and occupational dental erosion. J Public Health Dent 2003;63:244–249.
17. Centerwall BS, Armstrong CW, Funkhouser LS, Elsay RP. Erosion of dental enamel among competitive swimmers at a gas-chlorinated swimming pool. Am J Epidemiol 1986;123:641–647.
18. Scheper WA, van Nieuw Amerongen A, Eijkman MA. Oral condition in swimmers. Ned Tijdschr Tandheelkd 2005;112:147–148.
19. Lokin PA, Huysmans MC. Is Dutch swimming pool water erosive? Ned Tijdschr Tandheelkd 2004;111:14–16.
20. Gray A, Ferguson MM, Wall JG. Wine tasting and dental erosion: case report. Aust Dent J 1998;43:32–34.
21. Wiktorsson AM, Zimmerman M, Angmar-Månsson B. Erosive tooth wear: prevalence and severity in Swedish winetasters. Eur J Oral Sci 1997;105:544–550.
22. Zero DT. Etiology of dental erosion: extrinsic factors. Eur J Oral Sci 1996;104:162–177.
23. Linkosalo E, Markkanen H. Dental erosions in relation to lactovegetarian diet. Scand J Dent Res 1985;93:436–441.
24. Lussi A, Schaffner M, Hortz P, Suter P. Dental erosion in a population of Swiss adults. Community Dent Oral Epidemiol 1991;19:286–290.
25. Millward A, Shaw L, Smith AJ, Rippin JW, Harrington E. The distribution and severity of tooth wear and the relationship between erosion and dietary constituents in a group of children. Int J Paediatr Dent 1994;4:151–157.
26. Krünzel W, Cruz MS, Fischer T. Dental erosion in Cuban children associated with excessive consumption of oranges. Eur J Oral Sci 2000;108:104–109.
27. McIntyre JM. Erosion. Aust Prosthodont J 1992;6:17–25.
28. Robb ND, Smith BGN. Prevalence of pathological tooth wear in patients with chronic alcoholism. Br Dent J 1990;169:367–369.
29. Cavadini C, Siega-Riz AM, Popkin BM. US adolescent food intake trends from 1965 to 1996. Arch Dis Child 2000;83:18–24.
30. Derived from website www.nsda.org/softdrinks/history/ in 2001.
31. Putram JJ, Allshouse JE. Food Consumption, Prices, and Expenditures, 1970–97. Washington, DC: Food and Consumers Economic Division, Economic Research Services, US Department of Agriculture, 1999.
32. Harrack L, Stay J, Story M, Soft drinks consumption among US children and adolescents: nutritional consequences. J Am Diet Assoc 1999;99:436–441.
33. Miller GD, Jarvis JK, McBean LD. The importance of meeting calcium needs with foods. J Am Coll Nutr 2001;20(2 Suppl):168S–185S.
34. American Academy of Pediatrics. Soft Drinks in Schools. Committee on School Health. Pediatrics 2004;113: 152–154.
35. Jensdottir T, Holbrook P, Nauntofte B, Bouchwald C, Bardow A. Immediate erosive potential of cola drinks and orange juices. J Dent Res 2006;85:226–230.
36. Touyz LZ. The acidity (pH) and buffering capacity of Canadian fruit juice and dental implications. J Can Dent Assoc 1994;60:454–458.
37. Sorvari R, Rytomaa I. Drinks and dental health. Proc Finn Dent Soc 1991;87:621–631.

38. Moss SJ. Dental erosion. Int Dent J 1998;48: 529–539.
39. Mackie IC, Blinkhorn AS. Unexplained losses of enamel on upper incisor teeth. Dent Update 1989;16:403–404.
40. Johansson AK, Lingström P, Infeld T, Birkhed D. Influence of drinking method on tooth-surface pH in relation to dental erosion. Eur J Oral Sci 2004;112:484–489.
41. Barbour ME, Finke M, Parker DM et al. The relationship between enamel softening and erosion caused by soft drinks at a range of temperatures. J Dent 2006;34: 207–213.
42. Amaechi BT, Higham SM, Edgar WM. Factors influencing the development of dental erosion in vitro: enamel type, temperature and exposure time. J Oral Rehabil 1999;26:624–630.
43. Steffen JM. The effects of soft drinks on etched and sealed enamel. Angle Orthod 1996;66:449–456.
44. Edwards M, Creanor S, Foye R, Gilmour W. Buffering capacities of soft drinks: the potential influence on dental erosion. J Oral Rehab 1999;26:923–927.
45. Grenby TH. Lessening dental erosive potential by product modification. Eur J Oral Sci 1996;104:221–228.
46. Barbour ME, Parker DM, Allen GC, Jandt KD. Human enamel dissolution in citric acid as a function of pH in the range 2.30 to 6.30: a nanoindentation study. Eur J Oral Sci 2003;111:258–262.
47. Barbour ME, Parker DM, Allen GC, Jandt KD. Human enamel erosion in constant composition citric acid solutions as a function of degree of saturation with respect to hydroxyapatite. J Oral Rehabil 2005;32:16–21.
48. Larsen MJ, Nyvad B. Enamel erosion by some soft drinks and orange juices relative to their pH, buffering effect and contents of calcium phosphate. Caries Res 1999;33:81–87.
49. Attin T, Weiss K, Becker K, Buchalla W, Wiegand A. Impact of modified acid soft drinks on enamel erosion. Oral Dis 2005;11:7–12.
50. Hara AT, Zero DT. Analysis of the erosive potential of calcium-containing acidic beverages. Eur J Oral Sci 2008;116:60–65.
51. Parry J, Shaw L, Arnaud MJ, Smith AJ. Investigation of mineral waters and soft drinks in relation to dental erosion. J Oral Rehabil 2001;28:766–772.
52. Owens BM, Kitchens M. The erosive potential of soft drinks on enamel surface substrate: an in-vitro scanning electron microscopy investigation. J Contemp Dent Pract 2007;7:11–20.
53. Meurman JH, Härkönen M, Näveri H et al. Experimental sports drinks with minimal dental erosion effect. Scand J Dent Res 1990;98:120–128.
54. Hooper S, West NX, Sharif N et al. A comparison of enamel erosion by a new sports drink compared to two proprietary products: a controlled, crossover study in situ. J Dent 2004;32:541–545.
55. Venables MC, Shaw L, Jeukendrup AE et al. Erosive effect of a new sports drink on dental enamel during exercise. Med Sci Sports Exerc 2005;37:39–44.
56. Ramalingam L, Messer LB, Reynolds EC. Adding casein phosphopeptide-amorphous calcium phosphate to sports drinks to eliminate in-vitro erosion. Pediatr Dent 2005; 27:61–67.
57. Angmar-Månsson B, Oliveby A. Herbal tea: an erosion risk? pH, buffer capacity and fluoride concentration of herbal tea. Tandläkartidningen 1980;72:1315–1317.
58. Rees JS, Loyn T, Rowe W, Kunst Q, McAndrew R. The ability of fruit teas to remove the smear layer: an in-vitro study of tubule patency. J Dent 2006;34:67–76.
59. Behrendt A, Oberste V, Wetzel WE. Fluoride concentration and pH of iced tea products. Caries Res 2002;36: 405–410.
60. Brunton PA, Hussain A. The erosive effect of herbal tea on dental enamel. J Dent 2001;29:517–520.
61. van Nieuw Amerongen A, van den Kaijbus PA, Veerman EC. [Influence of teas with fruit aroma and ice teas on pH and buffer capacity of saliva.] Ned Tijdschr Tandheelkd 2004; 111:80–84.
62. Grace EG, Sarlani E, Kaplan S. Tooth erosion caused by chewing aspirin. J Am Dent Assoc 2004;135:911–914.
63. McCracken M, O'Neal SJ. Dental erosion and aspirin headache powders: a clinical report. J Prosthodont 2000; 9:95–98.
64. Bull AW, Corbett JR. Erosion: case report. Aust Dent J 1968;13:164.
65. Sullivan RE, Kramer WS. Iatrogenic erosion of teeth. J Dent Child 1983;50:192–196.
66. Rogalla K, Finger W, Hannig M. Influence of buffered and unbuffered acetylsalicylic acid on dental enamel and dentine in human teeth: an in-vitro pilot study. Methods Find Exp Clin Pharmacol 1992;14:339–346.
67. O'Sullivan EA, Curzon ME. A comparison of acidic dietary factors in children with and without dental erosion. J Dent Child 2000;67:186–192.
68. Al-Malik MI, Holt RD, Bedi R. The relationship between erosion, caries and rampant caries and dietary habits in preschool children in Saudi Arabia. Int J Paediatr Dent 2001;11:430–439.
69. Giunta JL. Dental erosion resulting from chewable vitamin C tablets. J Am Dent Assoc 1983;107:253–256.
70. Passon JC, Jones GK. Atypical dental erosion: a case report. Gerodontics 1986;2:77–79.
71. Meurman JH, Murtomaa H. Effect of effervescent vitamin C preparations on bovine teeth and on some clinical and salivary parameters in man. Scand J Dent Res 1986; 94:491–499.
72. Hays GL, Bullock Q, Lazzari EP, Puente ES. Salivary pH while dissolving vitamin C-containing tablets. Am J Dent 1992;5:269–271.
73. Nunn JH, Ng SK, Sharkey I, Coulthard M. The dental implications of chronic use of acid medicines in medically compromised children. Pharm World Sci 2001;23:118–119.
74. Atkinson JC, Wu AJ. Salivary gland dysfunction: causes, symptoms, treatment. J Am Dent Assoc 1994;125: 409–416.

75. Cassolato SF, Turnbull RS. Xerostomia: clinical aspects and treatment. Gerodontology 2003;20:64–77.
76. Meyer-Lueckel H, Kielbassa AM. Use of saliva substitutes in patients with xerostomia. Schweiz Monatsschr Zahnmed 2002;112:1037–1058.
77. Kielbassa AM, Shohadai SP, Schulte-Mönting J. Effect of saliva substitutes on mineral content of demineralized and sound dental enamel. Support Care Cancer 2001;9:40–47.
78. Featherstone JD, Rosenberg H. Lipid effect on the progress of artificial carious lesions in dental enamel. Caries Res 1984;18:52–55.
79. Meyer-Lueckel H, Tschoppe P, Kielbassa AM. Linseed based saliva substitutes and their effect on mineral dissolution of predemineralized bovine dentin in vitro. J Dent 2006;34:751–756.
80. Wiegand A, Gutsche M, Attin T. Effect of olive oil and olive-oil-containing fluoridated mouthrinse on enamel and dentin erosion in vitro. Acta Odontol Scand 2007;65: 357–361.
81. Rytömaa I, Meurman JF, Franssila S, Torkko H. Oral hygiene products may cause dental erosion. Proc Finn Dent Soc 1989;85:161–166.
82. Bhatti SA, Walsh TF, Douglas CW. Ethanol and pH levels of proprietary mouthrinses. Community Dent Health 1994;11:71–74.
83. Pontefract H, Hughes J, Kemp K, Yates R, Newcombe RG, Addy M. The erosive effect of some mouthrinses on enamel: a study in situ. J Clin Periodontol 2001;28: 319–324.
84. Pretty IA, Edgar WM, Higham SM. The erosive potential of commercially available mouthrinses on enamel as measured by quantitative light-induced fluorescence (QLF). J Dent 2003;31:313–319.
85. Price R, Sedarous M, Hiltz G. The pH of tooth-whitening products. J Can Dent Assoc 2000;66:421–426.
86. Basting RT, Rodriguez AL Jr, Serra MC. The effect of 10% carbamide peroxide, carbopol and/or glycerin on enamel and dentin microhardness. Oper Dent 2005;30: 608–616.
87. Lopez GC, Bonissoni L, Baratieri LN, Vieira LC, Monteiro S. Effect of bleaching agents on the hardness and morphology of enamel. J Esthet Restor Dent 2002;14: 24–30.
88. Pretty IA, Edgar WM, Higham SM. The effect of bleaching on enamel susceptibility to acid erosion and demineralization. Br Dent J 2005;12:285–290.
89. Attin T, Betke H, Schippan F, Wiegand A. Potential of fluoridated carbamide peroxide gels to support post-bleaching enamel re-hardening. J Dent 2007;35:755–759.
90. Driessens FC, Theuns HM, Borggreven JM, van Dijk JW. Solubility behavior of whole human enamel. Caries Res 1986;20:103–110.
91. Weiger R, Kuhn A, Löst C. Effect of various types of sodium perborate on the pH of bleaching agents. J Endod 1993;19:239–241.
92. Holst JJ, Lange F. Perimylolysis. A contribution toward the genesis of tooth wasting from nonmechanical cases. Acta Odontol Scand 1939;1:36–48.
93. Gregg T, Mace S, West NX, Addy M. A study in vitro of the abrasive effect of the tongue on enamel and dentine softened by acid erosion. Caries Res 2004;38:557–560.
94. Christen AG. Dentistry and the alcoholic patient. Dent Clin North Am 1983;27:341–361.
95. Mayes SD, Humphrey FJ, Handford HA, Mitchell JF. Rumination disorder: differential diagnosis. J Am Acad Child Adolesc Psychiatry 1988;27:300–302.
96. Smith BG, Barlett WD, Robb ND. The prevalence, etiology and management of tooth wear in the United Kingdom. J Prosthet Dent 1997;78:367–372.
97. Mandel ID. The role of saliva in maintaining oral homeostasis. J Am Dent Assoc 1989;119:298–304.
98. Hannig C, Hannig M, Attin T. Enzymes in the acquired enamel pellicle. Eur J Oral Sci 2005;113:2–13.
99. Amaechi BT, Higham SM, Edgar WM, Milosevic A. Thickness of acquired salivary pellicle as a determinant of the sites of dental erosion. J Dent Res 1999;78:1821–1828.
100. Meurman JH, ten Cate JM. Pathogenesis and modifying factors of dental erosion. Eur J Oral Sci 1996;104:199–206.
101. Meurman JH, Drysdale T, Frank RM. Experimental erosion of dentin. Scand J Dent Res 1991;99:457–462.
102. Birkhed D. Sugar content, acidity and effect on plaque pH of fruit juices, fruit drinks, carbonated beverages and sports drinks. Caries Res 1984;18:120–127.
103. Dawes C. What is the critical pH and why does a tooth dissolve in acid? J Can Dent Assoc 2003;69:722–724.
104. Kargul B, Caglar E, Lussi A. Erosive and buffering capacities of yoghurt. Quintessence Int 2007;38:381–385.
105. Shellis RP, Finke M, Eisemburger M, Parker DM, Addy M. Relationship between enamel erosion and liquid flow rate. Eur J Oral Sci 2005;113:232–238.
106. Featherstone JDB, Duncan JF, Cutress TW. A mechanism for dental caries based on chemical processes and diffusion phenomena during in-vitro caries simulation on human tooth enamel. Arch Oral Biol 1979;24:101–112.
107. Mandel ID. The functions of saliva. J Dent Res 1987;66: 623–627.
108. Edgar WM. Saliva: its secretion, composition and functions. Br Dent J 1992;172:305–312.
109. Roth G, Calmes R (eds). Salivary glands and saliva. In: Oral Biology. St Louis: CV Mosby, 1981:196–236.
110. Screbny LM, Shu WX. The use of whole saliva in the differential diagnosis of Sjögren's syndrome. Adv Dent Res 1996;10:17–24.
111. Edgar WM. Saliva and dental health. Clinical implications of saliva: report of a consensus meeting. Br Dent J 1990;169:96–98.
112. Humphrey SP, Williamson RT. A review of saliva: normal composition, flow, and function. J Prosthet Dent 2001;85:162–169.

113. Ericsson V, Hardwick L. Individual diagnosis, prognosis and counseling for caries prevention. Caries Res 1978;12 (Suppl 1):94–102.
114. Lagerlof F, Oliveby A. Caries-protective factors in saliva. Adv Dent Res 1994;8:229–238.
115. Meurman J, Rytömaa I, Kari K, Laakso T, Murtomaa H. Salivary pH and glucose after consuming various beverages, including sugar-containing drinks. Caries Res 1987;21:353–359.
116. Tenovuo J, Rekola M. Some effects of sugar-flavored acid beverages on the biochemistry of human whole saliva and dental plaque. Acta Odontol Scand 1977;35:317–330.
117. Dawes C. Physiological factors affecting salivary flow rate, oral sugar clearance, and the sensation of dry mouth in man. J Dent Res 1987;66:648–653.
118. Navazesh M, Christensen C, Brightman V. Clinical criteria for the diagnosis of salivary gland hypofunction. J Dent Res 1992;71:1363–1369.
119. Engelen L, de Wijk RA, Prinz JF, van der Bilt A, Bosman F. The relation between saliva flow after different stimulations and the perception of flavor and texture attributes in custard desserts. Physiol Behav 2003;78:165–169.
120. Hannig C, Becker K, Häusler N et al. Protective effect of the in-situ pellicle on dentin erosion: an ex-vivo pilot study. Arch Oral Biol 2007;52:444–449.
121. West NX, Maxwell A, Hughes JA et al. A method to measure clinical erosion: the effect of orange juice consumption on erosion of enamel. J Dent 1998;26:329–335.
122. Mannerberg F. Effect of lemon juice on different types of tooth surface: a replica study in vivo. Acta Odontol Scand 1962;20:153–164.
123. Crossner CG, Hase JC, Birkhed D. Oral sugar clearance in children compared with adults. Caries Res 1991;25: 201–206.
124. Johansson AK, Sorvari R, Birkhed D, Meurman JH. Dental erosion in deciduous teeth: an in-vivo and in-vitro study. J Dent 2001;29:333–340.
125. Maupome G, Aguilar-Avila M, Medrano-Ugalde H, Borges-Yañez A. In-vitro quantitative microhardness assessment of enamel with early pellicles after exposure to an eroding cola drink. Caries Res 1999;33:140–147.
126. Hunter ML, West NX, Hugues JA, Newcombe RG, Addy M. Erosion of deciduous and permanent dental hard tissue in the oral environment. J Dent 2000;28: 257–263.
127. Lussi A, Kohler N, Zero D, Schaffner M, Megert A. A comparison of the erosive potential of different beverages in primary and permanent teeth using an in-vitro model. Eur J Oral Sci 2000;108:110–114.
128. Michalek SM, McGhee JR. Oral streptococci with emphasis on Streptococcus mutans. In: McGhee JR, Michalek SM, Casell GH (eds). Oral Microbiology. Philadelphia: Harper & Row, 1982:679–690.
129. Stabholz A, Raisten J, Markitziu A et al. Tooth enamel dissolution from erosion or etching and subsequent caries development. J Pedod 1983;7:100–108.
130. Kitasako Y, Moritsuka M, Foxton RM et al. Simplified and quantitative saliva buffer capacity test using a hand-held pH meter. Am J Dent 2005;18:147–150.
131. Moritsuka M, Kitasako Y, Burrow MF, Ikeda M, Tagami J. The pH change after HCl titration into resting and stimulated saliva for buffering capacity test. Aust Dent J 2006;51:170–174.

# Chapter 11

# Gastroesophageal Reflux as a Cause of Dental Erosion

*Sergio Fuster and Carlos Gianoni*

## Introduction

Although the effects of reflux of stomach contents on the esophagus and the upper respiratory tract had been well known by gastroenterologists and general practitioners for many years, little attention was paid to the effects of such contents on the oral cavity, and reflux had never been related to tooth wear from erosion.

In 1935, Winkelstein[1] was the first to suggest that reflux was the cause of esophageal damage. Later in the 1930s, Bargen and Austin[2] and Holst and Lange[3] suggested the possibility that some cases of dental erosion might be caused by gastroesophageal reflux. But it was not until a little more than 10 years ago that the works of Järvinen,[4] Meurman and co-workers,[5] Taylor and co-workers,[6] and Scheutzel[7] confirmed that an association between reflux and tooth wear existed in more than 30% of the cases in their series.

## Anatomophysiology of the Upper Digestive Tract

From the mouth to the anus, the digestive system comprises a tube – the digestive tract – with which several exocrine and endocrine glands, such as the salivary glands, the liver and the pancreas, are associated.

The first part of the digestive tract comprises the mouth and the pharynx. Here, food is broken down by the process of chewing, and is mixed with saliva to form the alimentary bolus; also, the salivary glands produce some enzymes which start the digestive process.

Once the alimentary bolus has been formed, by means of a complex and well-coordinated neck muscle neuromuscular process, deglutition of the bolus occurs, and food is prevented from entering the respiratory tract and sent to the esophagus. The esophagus is a tubular structure approximately 25 cm long, with a cervical portion, a thoracic portion, and an abdominal portion. It forces the alimentary bolus into the stomach by means of

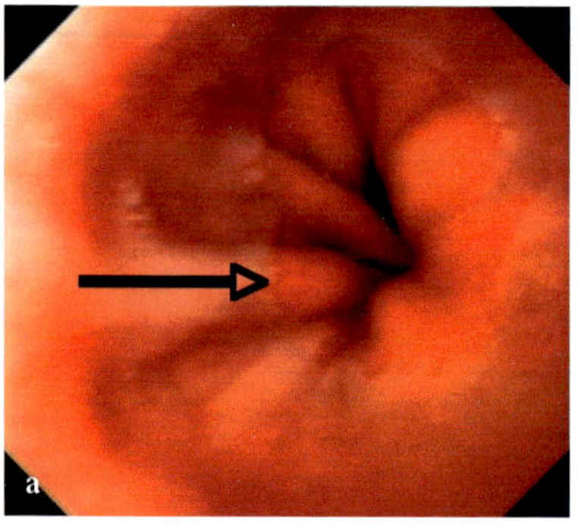


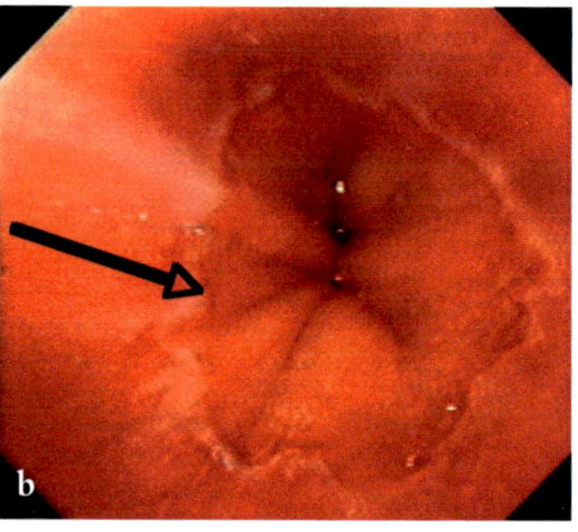


Fig 11-1 **(a and b)** Endoscopic images of a normal esophagus, where the Z line (arrow) corresponding to the transition between the esophageal epithelium and the gastric mucosa can be clearly seen.

coordinated muscle movements called "peristalsis". Reflux of food and gastric juice is prevented by two high-pressure zones in the esophagus – the upper esophageal sphincter (UES) and the lower esophageal sphincter (LES) – and by means of forward peristalsis. The UES is located at the level of the cricopharyngeus muscle, 20 cm away from the maxillary dental arch; the LES is located in the abdominal esophagus area, where the organ runs through the diaphragm and its pillar muscles. When in the resting state, the esophagus behaves as a virtual cavity closed at both ends by a tonic contraction of the UES and the LES. During deglutition, both sphincters relax and a coordinated, sequential activity – primary peristalsis – begins, which carries the degluted content to the stomach. Once the bolus reaches its destination, another tonic contraction of the UES and the LES prevents the content from going back up into the esophagus. If this should happen anyway, or if bits of degluted material remain halfway down the esophagus, waves are generated which propel them to the stomach; this is called "secondary peristalsis".

The esophagus is lined by an exquisitely sensitive epidermoid–epithelium mucosa which is chiefly supplied by the 10th cranial nerve. This epidermoid mucosa changes abruptly to secretory columnar mucosa in the esophageal–gastric junction, the area of the transition known as the "Z line" (Fig 11-1).

The stomach is a dilated portion of the digestive tract, a fully abdominal, elastic organ capable of storing multiple alimentary boluses and of expanding up to the pelvis area if necessary in order to accept significant volumes of food in a short time. Well-differentiated in terms of function, the regions of the stomach are as follows (Fig 11-2).

- The fundus is the upper part of the stomach. It acts as a reservoir for the food it receives through the esophagus and has the capability of adjusting to its content without increasing the tension of the walls.
- The body is the mid-part. Along with the fundus and by means of contractions, it allows for the content to travel to the distal part.
- The antrum, or antrum–pyloric region, shows more muscular activity and is in charge of transforming food into smaller particles, more suitable for being transported into the duodenum by means of more intense contractions.

One valve allows entrance of the bolus into the stomach and another one allows emptying of the stomach. The former, called the "cardiac sphincter", is located in the upper, posterior area of the stomach, where the esophagus ends. The latter valve is the "pyloric sphincter". It is much more pronounced and has greater muscular strength than the cardiac sphincter. The stomach secretes

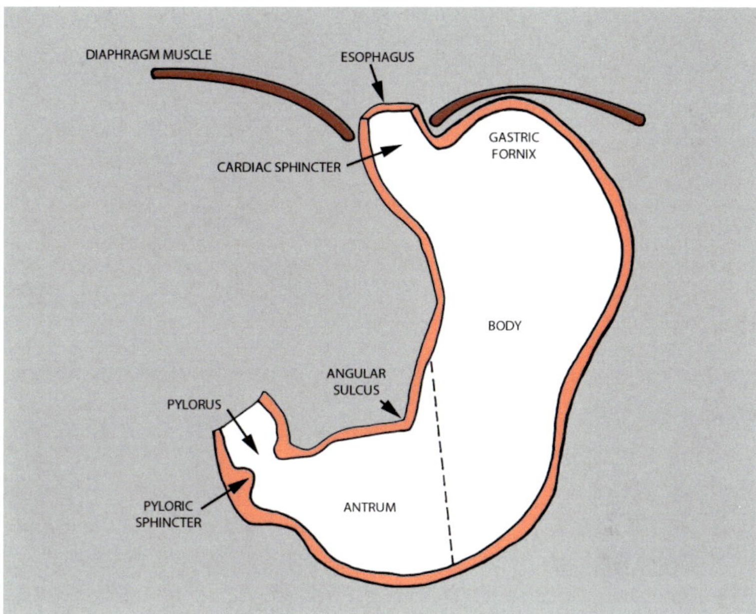


Fig 11-2 Anatomic structure of the stomach.

digestive juices and the only elements it can absorb quickly are monosaccharides and alcohol. The digestive secretions of the stomach mainly contain a great volume of hydrochloric acid and peptic enzymes, which create a highly acidic environment; usually the pH of these secretions ranges from 1 to 2, with small time-dependent variations. The volume of these secretions is highly variable, and even under empty stomach conditions extending for a period of 8 hours, such volume will always range from 20 to 100 mL.

Physiologically, after the last bite of food has been swallowed, the stomach will spend at least an hour mixing and secreting gastric juices without emptying and with the esophageal and pyloric sphincters closed. Only after this secretion and mixing process (which usually lasts more than an hour) does the gastric antrum begin to make movements that cause the bolus to travel to the pylorus and the duodenum – at a rate of approximately 10 mL of bolus material per movement, thus starting the gastric emptying process (Figs 11-3 and 11-4).

Gastric emptying rate in normal subjects is influenced by the physical and chemical features of the food consumed, by environmental and body factors, and by positional, neurogenic, and hormonal factors. For example, cold food has a slower gastric emptying than warm food (e.g., potatoes); liquids have a faster gastric emptying than solid food; carbohydrates have a faster gastric emptying than protein; and complex fats have the slowest gastric emptying. A cold environment and hypothermia delay emptying; the right lateral decubitus position accelerates it. Anticholinergic drugs and plain muscle relaxants cause gastric emptying to slow down. All the conditions that delay gastric emptying can potentially cause reflux. When there is cardiac sphincter incompetence, postprandial mixing movements produce high intragastric pressure, which may surpass UES pressures and cause postprandial reflux even when the person is in the upright position. If the person is also in a dorsal decubitus position, the biggest gastric volume moves to the fornix and it is more likely to reflux back up into the esophagus and the mouth.

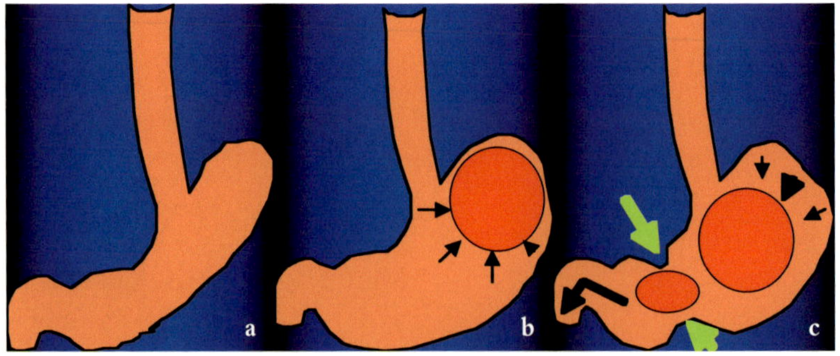


Fig 11–3 Gastric physiology: **(a)** empty; **(b)** food redistribution; **(c)** emptying.

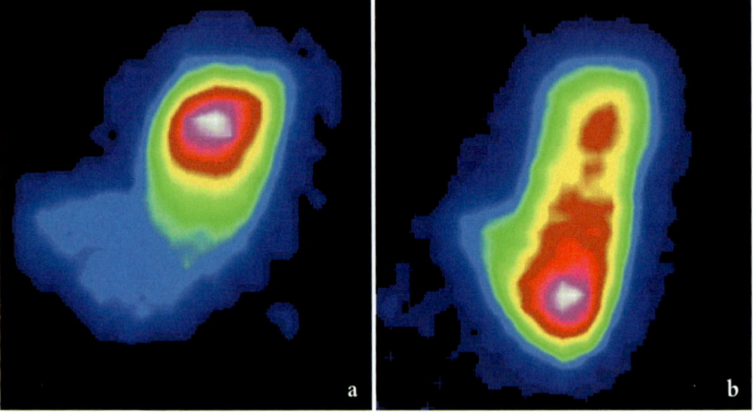


Fig 11–4 Scintigraphic study showing: **(a)** proximal accumulation; **(b)** redistribution and subsequent emptying.

## Definition of Reflux

From a pathophysiologic point of view, gastroesophageal reflux (GER) is defined as the return of the contents of the stomach and/or the duodenum into the esophagus. It is a physiologic phenomenon which, in normal conditions, occurs after eating and is asymptomatic. It occurs several times a day and is related to transient relaxations of the lower esophageal sphincter. When the number and duration of daily reflux episodes increase, symptoms and/or lesions appear in the mucosae which result in gastroesophageal reflux disease (GERD).

Such reflux may consist of food recently consumed, or of gastric content under empty stomach conditions, or both at the same time. Sometimes, subjects are aware of reflux, but most of the time the sensory system will not detect it; this will depend on the physical–chemical properties of the reflux material, the distance traveled by it, and esophagus sensitivity. The shorter the distance traveled by the reflux material, the less chance it has of being detected. When the material reaches the mouth, it is easily detectable by exteroceptive sensors. Sometimes it may reach the upper airway without being detected and cause respiratory disorders such as cough, bronchial spasms, pharyngitis, etc.

Reflux is usually non-permanent and occurs intermittently during the day and at night-time, depending on the pathology causing it and on the patient's habits. It occurs more frequently at night and when the person is in the dorsal decubitus position; also after consumption of plentiful, greasy food and carbonated drinks, and when there is abdominal hyperpressure from abdominal exercises or weight-lifting exercises. Mint and smoking also increase it.

Passive gastroesophageal reflux as an entity – which we are dealing with in this chapter – is completely different from vomit, which involves much more noticeable muscular, digestive tract, and abdominal wall movements.

As agreed in the Genval Workshop Report,[8] the designation "gastroesophageal reflux disease (GERD)" should include all subjects who are at risk of organic complications secondary to gastroesophageal reflux, or whose quality of life is being altered by symptoms ascribable to such a condition that has been confirmed to be benign.

Although the prevalence of reflux in the population depends on the method of study used, from an epidemiologic point of view GERD is deemed to be a very common pathology in the west. So much so that, in 1976, Nebel and co-workers,[9] from the western coast of the USA, found that 14% of their study subjects suffered from "heartburn" once a week. MaCarthy[10] showed that 44% of the people throughout the USA had that same symptom once a month. Locke and co-workers,[11] working in the Mayo-Olmstead Clinic, found that heartburn occurred weekly in 19.8% of the community studied. In a study carried out in Argentina using the same method as the one used in the Mayo Clinic, Chiocca and co-workers[12] found the weekly prevalence of heartburn in 836 study subjects to be 23%. In Finland, Isolauri and Laippala[13] reported that heartburn and acid regurgitation occurred weekly in 15% of their study subjects.

The disease is deemed to be more prevalent in the west[14–17] than in the east; Taiwan and Japan are an exception.[18]

The most common complications of gastroesophageal reflux are hematemesis and peptic stenosis, the incidence of which ranges from 1% to 1.5%. Only 10% of patients suffering from chronic gastroesophageal reflux develop Barrett's esophagus (BE) or intestinal metaplasia, while the incidence of adenocarcinomas in BE is 0.4–0.5% per year.

## Pathophysiology of Reflux

Gastroesophageal reflux disease is a multifactorial entity caused by alterations in the defensive and aggressive mechanisms of the esophagus. The antireflux barrier is composed of the crural diaphragm and the LES. Both of them constitute the sphincter mechanism of the esophageal–gastric junction. If this mechanism fails, reflux occurs. The moving upward of the contents of the stomach depends on the resistance offered by the body of the esophagus and on the clearance mechanisms (saliva and esophageal peristalsis[19]). The resistance offered by the esophageal mucosa and gastric emptying time also play a defensive role. The aggressor agent is determined by the quality of the reflux material – gastric juice and/or duodenal juice (HCl, pepsin, conjugated bile salts);[20,21] when the reflux material comprises both gastric juice and duodenal juice it is more aggressive.

The mechanisms that cause reflux are believed to be:

- hypotensive LES[22]
- increased intra-abdominal pressure
- transient LES relaxations.

Four decades ago, the antireflux barrier was thought to depend on an adequate LES pressure. Subsequent studies have shown the existence of a significant pressure value superimposition, both in control subjects and in patients with GERD, even at different times of the day. However, it has been shown that patients with pathologic reflux usually have a hypotensive sphincter. Pressures below 6 mmHg are currently considered to be associated with pathological reflux.

The increase in intra-abdominal pressure caused by effort, physical activity, and (mainly) obesity will boost the production of reflux. Fur-

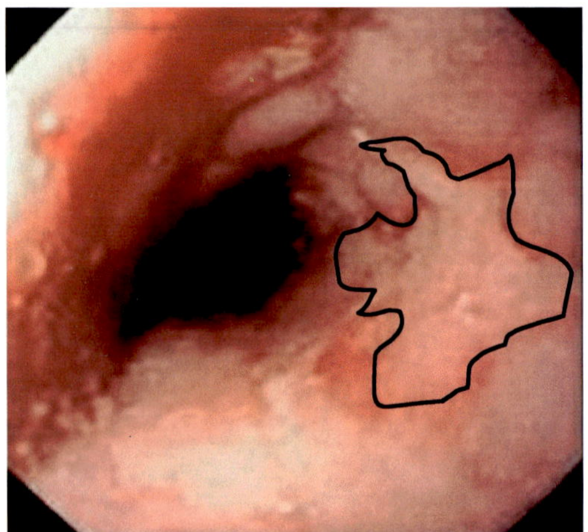

Fig 11–5 Endoscopy image of an esophageal ulcer.

ther aggravation will occur when there is a hypotensive sphincter.

Transient LES relaxations are those sphincter relaxations not provoked by deglutition. They are considered to be the main determining factor of gastroesophageal reflux both in normal subjects and in subjects affected by the disease.[22–25] Transient relaxations occur due to submaximal pharyngeal stimuli (not inducing deglutition) or to gastric fundus distention. Fifty percent of patients suffering from GERD show delayed gastric emptying; this will result in a bigger number of transient relaxations, with the consequent occurrence of reflux during such relaxations.[26]

There is controversy about the relationship between *Helicobacter pylori* and GERD. According to some published works, this bacterium can aggravate GERD; according to others, it can make it less severe. Others consider that *H. pylori* does not have an effect on the degree of severity and the treatment of the disease.[27–29]

Based on the above, the presence of gastroesophageal reflux can be ascribed to diseases inherent to the esophagus and the stomach; that is, hiatal hernia, LES incompetence, connective tissue diseases (especially scleroderma), diabetes, and alcoholism; as well as repeated pregnancy, obesity, ascites, diabetic and alcoholic gastroparesis, and effects secondary to chronic drug intake, without previous symptoms.

## Clinical Manifestations of Reflux

GERD has typical symptoms, atypical or extradigestive symptoms, and alarm symptoms.

*Heartburn* is a retrosternal burning sensation which can reach the throat, caused by the moving upward of the gastric content. Its intensity is variable and it will depend on the sensitivity of each patient. Heartburn and *acid regurgitation* are considered to be cardinal symptoms of GERD; when both are present, specificity is 80%, but sensitivity is low. The degree of severity and the frequency of these symptoms do not allow one to predict the extent of the esophageal mucosa lesion. It is believed that around 30–40% of patients with heartburn have endoscopic esophagitis; the rest do not show epithelial damage – an entity known as "non-erosive gastroesophageal reflux disease".[30,31] Reflux may remain asymptomatic over long periods of life and, despite this fact, cause irreversible lesions in the esophagus of these patients.

The most common digestive pathology is *esophagitis* (erosion, esophageal ulceration, peptic stenosis, and metaplasia),[32,33] which sometimes hinders normal food intake. These diseases may be very symptomatic, but sometimes they may have a torpid progression with absence of significant symptoms (Fig 11-5).

At other times, such chronic reflux causes changes to occur in the lower esophagus which result in the replacement of epidermoid epithelium by gastric or intestinal metaplasia. This is known as Barrett's disease[34] and it is a risk factor for neoplastic degeneration. The lower-esophagus intestinal metaplastic mucosa must progress through three stages of dysplasia – low, moderate, and high – before developing into adenocarcinoma; these changes take a long time to occur.

That is why early detection of this condition entails treatment, in order to prevent the natural progress of the disease.

The so-called "atypical symptoms" and extra-digestive manifestations of reflux – particularly the respiratory ones – are shown in Table 11-1. They are not always accompanied with typical reflux symptoms or erosive esophagitis symptoms; frequently, they are the only manifestation of the disease.[35]

In children, *torticollis, food rejection, recurrent abdominal pain,* and *irritability* should be considered as probable manifestations of gastroesophageal reflux.

*Dysphagia, weight loss,* and *anemia* are considered to be alarm symptoms. In these cases, patients should be thoroughly evaluated in order to exclude esophageal cancer from Barrett's epithelium. When no ulcero-peptic disease is present, *epigastric pain* which is relieved by antacids may be due to reflux.

Gastroesophageal reflux is considered to be the second most common cause of non-cardiogenic chest pain after coronary disease; GER accounts for more than 50% of cases.[36] This etiology is suspected when non-cardiogenic chest pain has little relation with physical effort, occurs when the subject is in the decubitus position (especially at night), is associated with the postprandial period or with deglutition, and/or is relieved by antacids or by adopting an upright position.

Patients with coronary failure may have reflux, which can be worsened by the drugs used in the treatment of such coronary failure – nitrites and calcium-channel blockers. The performance of a therapeutic diagnostic test with a double dose of proton pump inhibitor (PPI) is currently advised.

*Table 11-1*

**Extra-digestive manifestations associated with gastroesophageal reflux disease.**

Epigastric pain
Non-cardiogenic chest pain
Respiratory manifestations:
- chronic cough
- hoarseness and aphonia
- pharyngitis
- laryngitis
- aryngeal spasm
- larynx cancer
- globus hystericus
- sleep apnea
- asthma
- idiopathic pulmonary fibrosis

Dental erosion
Idiopathic chronic hiccups
Sialorrhea
Lingual burning sensation
Halitosis

## *Reflux and Respiratory Symptoms*

In 1892, Sir William Osler[37] was the first to observe that there is risk of asthma when eating late at night. This association has been more recently confirmed by the frequent findings of hiatal hernia or reflux on radiographs. Today, the new diagnostic technologies available provide further confirmation. Although reflux is associated with multiple respiratory pathologies, as shown in Table 11-1, it is most commonly and markedly associated with asthmatic manifestations, bronchial spasms, intermittent irritative cough, and recurrent pharyngitis and laryngitis. Pathologic gastroesophageal reflux may produce respiratory manifestations; the precipitating mechanisms can be the aspiration mechanism,[35,38–41] the reflex mechanism[42,43] (from increased vagal tone, which would produce bronchial hyperreactivity as a consequence of esophageal acidification), or it may be secondary to respiratory disease (Figs 11-6 and 11-7).

These manifestations are very common in both children and adults of both sexes, and they occur at any age, mostly without associated digestive symptoms.[35] This causes the patients to visit many

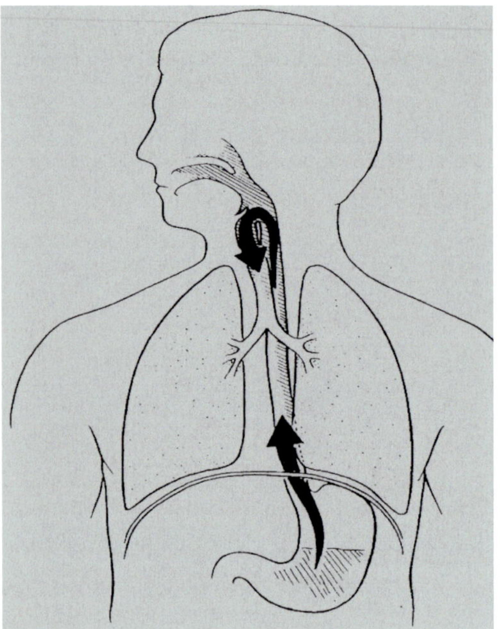

Fig 11–6 Pathophysiologic mechanism of the respiratory symptoms produced by gastroesophageal reflux.

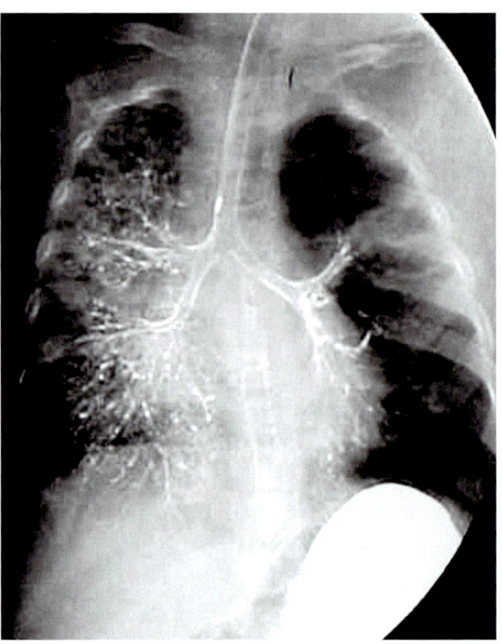

Fig 11–7 Aspiration bronchogram (presence of the contrast material inside the respiratory tract).

respiratory disease specialists, neumologists, ENT specialists, and allergists, and sometimes they will be wrongly diagnosed as allergic. Often these patients will undergo multiple symptomatic respiratory treatments, with different results. Eventually, some informed specialist who is attentive to detail will consider reflux as the probable cause, will evaluate these patients and treat them, team-working with the pneumologist when there are associated diseases. In this way, symptoms will be relieved.

The association of asthma with gastroesophageal reflux must be suspected in cases of adult-onset asthma, night-time bronchial spasms, and no previous history of allergies. Adult asthmatics have been reported to have pathologic gastroesophageal reflux in 20–90% of cases; a lower percentage has reflux esophagitis.[44–47] Fifty percent of asthmatics with gastroesophageal reflux do not show gastroesophageal reflux symptoms. The intensity of the symptoms is not related to the degree of severity of asthma; however, the greater the severity of asthma, the more severe is the reflux. Despite the evident association between these two diseases, the differential diagnosis can often be difficult, because it is not easy to distinguish between reflux-induced asthma and gastroesophageal reflux-exacerbated asthma.

Fifty percent of patients with chronic cough have gastroesophageal reflux in the distal esophagus and, to a lesser extent, in the proximal esophagus.[48,49] Making a diagnosis is not easy, since endoscopy results and prolonged pH-metry results are usually normal in these patients, and minimal acid exposure may precipitate the symptom. Cough crises may be so severe (sometimes associated with vomiting) that, whenever they occur while these patients are in the decubitus position, they will not be able to sleep at night and will opt to sleep in a seated position. Extreme cases have been reported in which cough, vomiting, and retching crises resulted in a detached retina and momentary vision loss.

Through cineradiology, patients with idiopathic pulmonary fibrosis have been shown to suffer from gastroesophageal reflux and hiatal hernia more often than the control group.[50]

Laryngitis is frequently associated with gastroesophageal reflux; 20% of patients have endoscopic esophagitis. The proximal esophagus of patients who have laryngeal symptoms has been exposed to reflux for a longer time and a higher percentage of episodes occur in this region.[51,52] Posterior laryngitis is the characteristic lesion, but also edema, erythema, granulomas, or ulceration may be seen.[53] Proton pump inhibitors (PPIs) relieve symptoms and laryngeal lesions by 50% and 100%, respectively. The association between gastroesophageal reflux and laryngeal cancer has not been conclusively demonstrated.[54,55]

A high percentage of sleep apnea episodes affecting children and adults may be related to reflux; thus, it is advisable that these patients undergo prolonged pH-metry studies. In patients with pathologic reflux, globus hystericus is likely to be related to the laryngeal irritation caused by the reflux material.

All these extra-digestive manifestations of gastroesophageal reflux – provided, of course, that gastroesophageal reflux has been proven to be the cause of the problem – are successfully treated by inhibiting acid secretion. When patients showing such severe symptoms cannot be compensated by medical treatment, antireflux surgery is indicated, which has a high success percentage.

### *Other Clinical Manifestations of Reflux*

Gastric content pH is normally not higher than 2.0, and it usually ranges from 1.0 to 1.5; thus, it is very harmful for the mucosae and also, as shown by Schweizer-Hirt and co-workers,[56] for dental enamel.

Also, in some cases, brought back to the stomach by bile, variable amounts of bile salts (another agent that erodes mucosae and dental enamel) can be present in the gastric content. This is commonly seen in patients who have undergone colecistectomy.

Clinical manifestations of the presence of acid in the oral cavity can vary. Sometimes, only a nonspecific feeling of oral hyperesthesia and burning exists (which is more marked on the tongue), without the presence of a specific anatomopathologic lesion. In most cases, the occurrence of such manifestations is likely to be related to severe gastroesophageal reflux. Dental erosion is considered to be the main manifestation of GERD in the oral cavity; sometimes, it may be the only clinical sign of the disease. Tooth involvement starts with subtle enamel changes, which progress until dentin is affected; this causes significant loss of dental tissue. The association between dental erosion and acid reflux has been observed in both children and adults. Muñoz and co-workers[57] demonstrated the relationship between GERD, the degree of severity of dental erosion, and the presence of a higher number of dental pieces affected.

As shown by prolonged pH-metry studies, patients with dental erosion had greater acid exposure, regardless of the degree of severity of such exposure. As is the case with other extra-digestive manifestations, endoscopic findings did not correlate with this pathology.

The location of erosion from gastroesophageal reflux seems to be different from the location of erosion caused by other etiological factors, especially in the maxilla and mandibular regions. Also, erosion from gastroesophageal reflux has been reported to be more frequently associated with pathologic gum recession. Cebrián Carretero and co-workers[58] suggest that splints be used during sleep for diagnostic and therapeutic purposes. Apart from gastroesophageal reflux, much less common causes of dental erosion from intrinsic acid (in this case, from vomiting) exist.

*Table 11-2*

**Method of study of gastroesophageal reflux disease.**

| Morphologic | Functional |
|---|---|
| Esophageal transit radiography esophagogram<br>Esophagogastroduodenal serial radiography under radioscopy<br>Esophagogastroduodenal endoscopy with biopsy | Esophageal 24-hour pH-metry<br>Esophageal manometry<br>Gamma camera<br>Impedanciometry<br>BilitecTM 2000 |

## Diagnosis of Reflux

Today, gastroenterologists can resort to different procedures for studying these patients and confirming the presence of reflux, evaluating the damage to the mucosa caused by such reflux, staging the disease, and analyzing reflux material pH, the number and duration of reflux episodes per day, and the time of the day at which they occur.

As we have mentioned, typical gastroesophageal reflux symptoms are highly sensitive in diagnosing the disease.[59–61] The methods for studying and confirming the presence of reflux in these patients can be classified into morphologic and functional (Table 11-2).

An esophagram is useful for identifying reflux esophagitis morphological changes and their complications, such as stenosis and ulceration. It also allows one to document hiatal hernia or esophageal shortening.[62]

The oldest and most cost-effective non-invasive method is barium-meal contrast-enhanced dynamic radiography (Fig 11-8). This allows well-trained radiologists to demonstrate the presence of contrast reflux going back from the stomach into the esophagus by performing provoking maneuvers (changes in position, increased abdominal pressure, Trendelenburg position, cold water intake, etc.). Patients with dysphagia should be evaluated first with this method. Moderate or severe esophagitis can be diagnosed through dynamic radiography with a high degree of accuracy.[63]

Although in most cases well-trained radiologists will detect reflux, there are some sporadic reflux cases in which radiologists are not successful in provoking reflux at the time of the study despite performing radiologic maneuvers.

In general, onset of reflux occurs in the first years of life, and the condition remains intermittently throughout life, regardless of its symptoms. As adults (sometimes very young ones) these patients will usually show some alterations in the esophageal mucosa, which range from non-erosive mild inflammation to intestinal metaplasia and dysplasia. Videoendoscopy with biopsy is the method of choice for imaging the aggression of reflux against the esophageal mucosa of patients with chronic reflux and for evaluating the status of the mucosa. However, since the non-erosive form of GERD accounts for 30–40% of cases, a negative endoscopy does not exclude the presence of GERD.[64,65]

Whenever lesions are observed, multiple biopsies at different levels are indicated in order to detect Barrett's epithelium, determine the scheduling of follow-ups, and prevent potential complications, such as esophageal adenocarcinoma. Biopsies are an invasive procedure and they are usually performed under anesthetic sedation; they have a

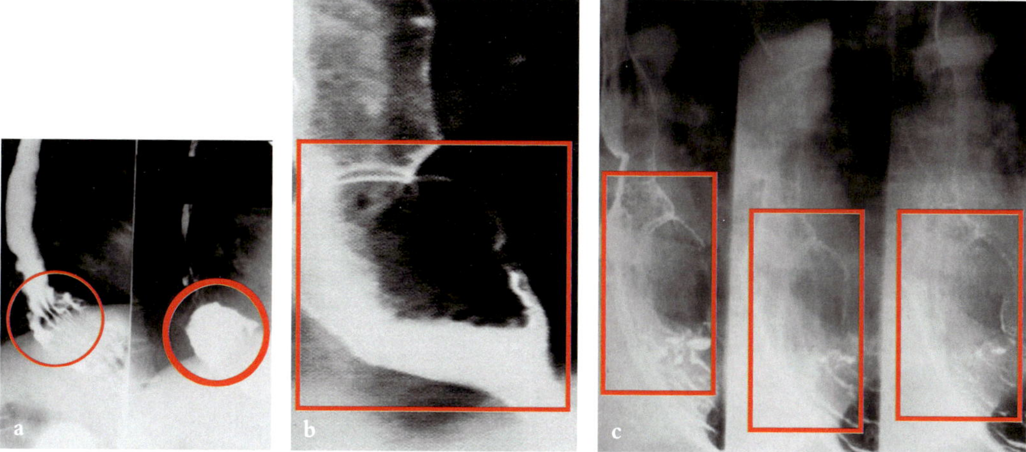


Fig 11–8 **(a–c)** Contrast-enhanced esophagograms showing hiatal hernias from gliding. Hiatal hernias result from the gliding along of the upper proximal portion of the stomach through the diaphragm hiatus towards the thorax.

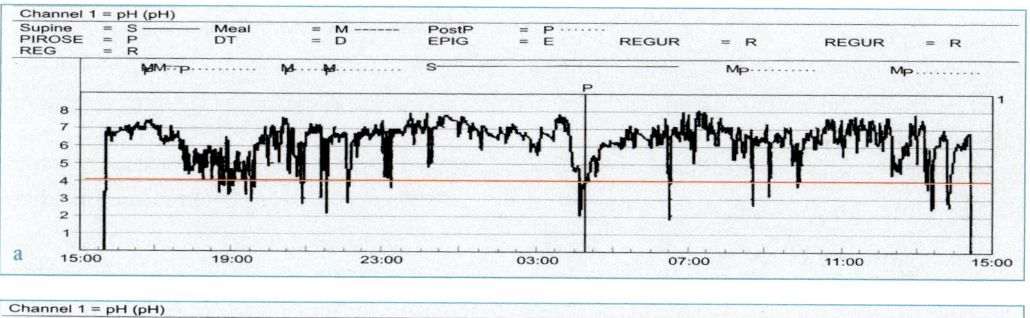


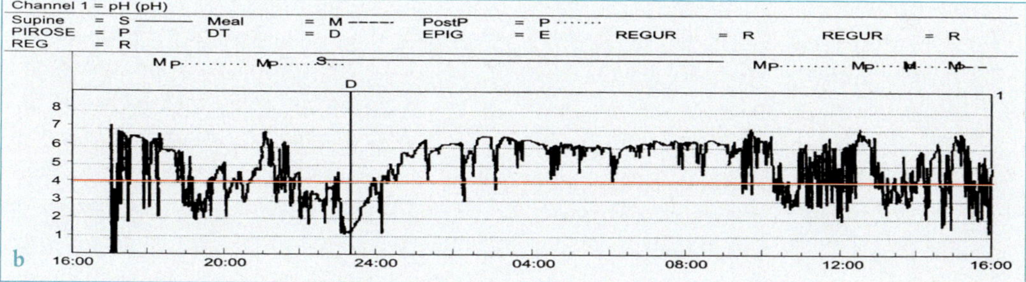


Fig 11–9 **(a)** Normal pH-metry reading. The values are shown above the red line, and correspond to a pH value of 4. **(b)** Pathologic pH-metry reading, with pH values falling below 4 (red line).

short duration and they allow one to record images, take pictures, and compare stages.

Capsule endoscopy is another technique for visualizing the esophageal mucosa. This device is swallowed and it starts transmitting good-resolution radio telemetry pictures to an external receiver.

When no lesions exist in the mucosa, biopsy is not helpful for confirming or excluding pathologic reflux.[66] Then, functional studies are indicated in order to confirm the presence of GERD.

Approximately 50 years ago, gastroduodenal pH measurement studies were carried out for the

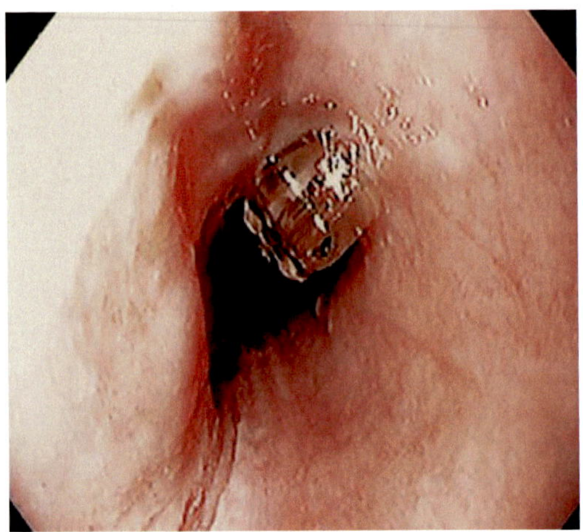

Fig 11–10 Endoscopy image of electrode attached to the esophageal wall.

first time.[67,68] In 1969, Spencer was the first researcher to describe the continuous intraesophageal pH measurement technique of using a glass electrode.[67] Halfway through the 1970s, Johnson and DeMeester described a simplified method for measuring esophageal pH in 24 hours and for quantitative analysis of abnormal exposure to acid.[69] This method consists of measuring the pH of the esophagus at different levels from its lower third to its upper third by means of a catheter with one or several sensors. The catheter reaches the esophagus through the nose and is connected to an ambulatory recording device which allows the patient to move as usual, eat, lie down, work, etc. Acid reflux episodes with a pH lower than 4 can thus be measured and their duration can be quantified (Fig 11-9) They can also be correlated with other symptoms and the time of occurrence can be accurately determined, which allows one to relate them to the activity the patient was engaged in (dorsal recumbent position or dorsal decubitus position, abdominal effort, etc.).

Other devices are available for pH measurement which are even more sophisticated. Recently, the use of the catheter-free pH monitoring system, Bravo (Medtronic: Shoreview, MN), has been approved by the US Food and Drug Administration. This new system measures esophageal pH by means of a capsule which is attached to the esophageal mucosa, 5 cm above the esophageal–gastric junction, through endoscopy. The capsule detects esophageal reflux and data are transmitted via radio-frequency telemetry to an external recording system (Fig 11-10).[70]

This system extends intraesophageal pH data collection to 48 hours, which allows for better identification of patients with abnormal exposure to acid and increases the number of recorded symptoms associated with reflux events.[71]

Even more sophisticated procedures can be indicated for complex cases that are difficult to diagnose or treat; for example, esophageal manometry, impedanciometry, and radioisotopic gamma-camera reflux study.

The first esophageal manometry was done in 1883. From then onwards, this technique has evolved, with the development of probes with three catheters and eight catheters with pneumatic–hydraulic pumps, solid-state catheters with integrated pressure transducers, miniature polygraphs with digitalized manometric traces, and computerized analysis (Fig 11-11). Also 24-hour ambulatory monitoring has been performed.

Despite these technological advances, the clinical usefulness of conventional stationary manometry in GERD is limited. The advantage lies in the detection of ineffective esophageal motility or other motor disorders and LES incompetence.[72,73]

Manometry allows evaluation of the motility of the esophagus during the physiologic act of deglutition. Based on this, manometry has the ability to establish:

- location, resting pressure, and relaxation (presence, absence, or incompleteness) of UES and LES
- presence or absence, amplitude, speed, and duration of peristaltic waves
- anti-peristaltic waves
- other types of contractions – mass, segmentary, or spontaneous.

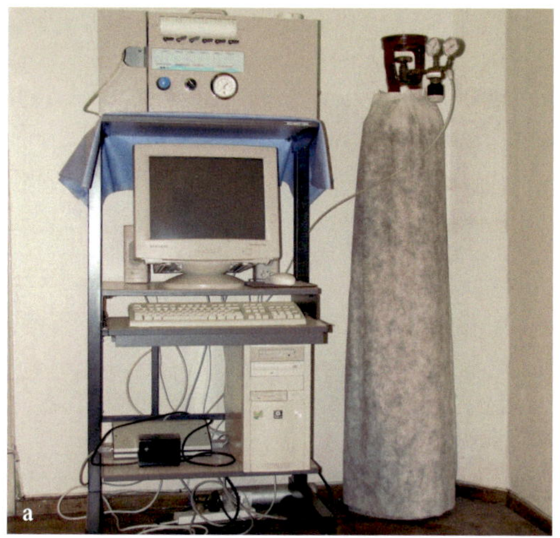

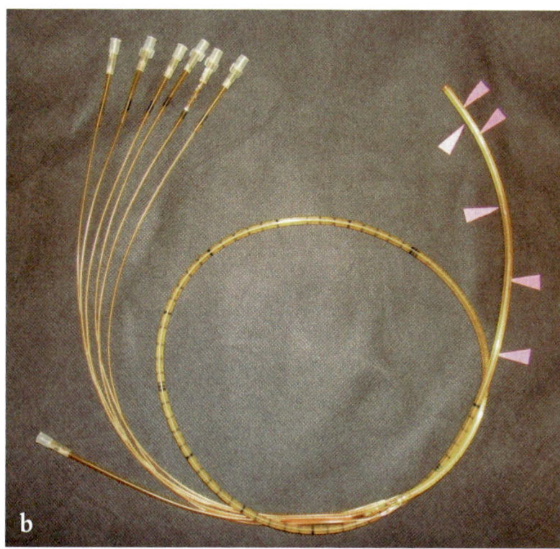

Fig 11-11 **(a)** Manometry equipment and six-channel pneumohydraulic pump. **(b)** Six-channel Arndorfer probe for manometry.

Although this method cannot be used for diagnosing reflux, it is indicated – as stated by the guidelines from the American Gastroenterological Association – for presurgical evaluation of some patients, and for excluding the association of reflux with other primary or secondary esophageal motor disorders (Fig 11-12).[72]

In 1991, Silny[73] described a new technique that is on the increase for GERD diagnosis: intraluminal electrical impedance (Fig 11-13). This technique can be combined with manometry and pH-metry measurements, and it provides data on the presence, physical characteristics, and proximal extension, distribution, and clearance of reflux material in the esophagus, plus information on the motor function of the esophagus.[74–76] The testing requires a short period of time (2–3 hours), and the parameters evaluated are reflux composition (gas, liquid, mixed) and proximal extension of reflux (in cases of liquid reflux). The technique can detect acidic and non-acidic GER. It can be used for diagnosing patients who had refractory symptoms during medical treatment. This method also allows evaluation of symptoms with or without medication. It can also correlate symptoms with acid or non-acid events. It quantifies the reflux pattern

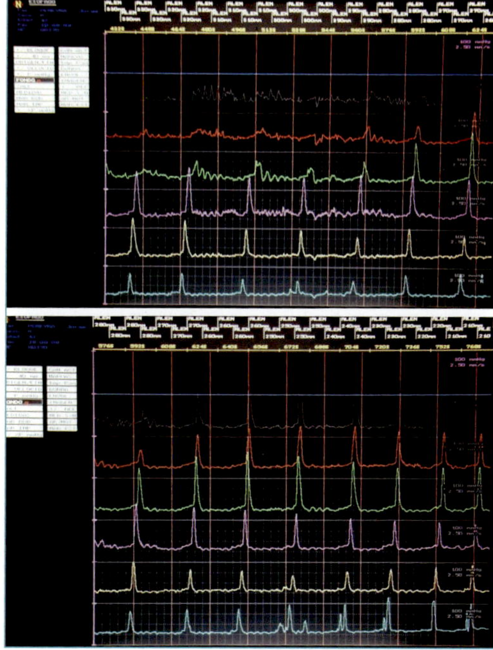

Fig 11-12 Esophageal manometry readings.

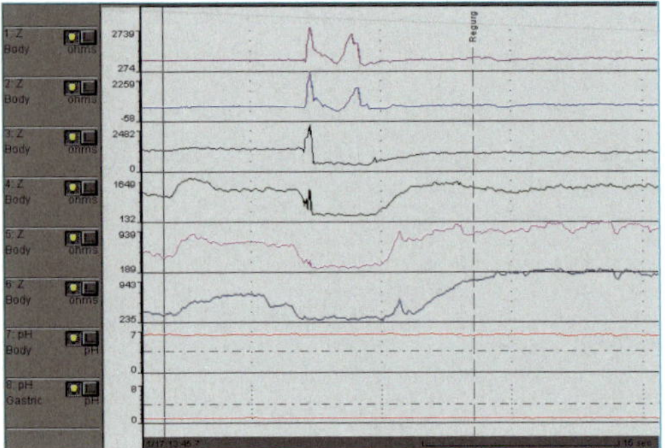

Fig 11-13 Impedanciometry reading.

and correlation of symptoms also in the postprandial period. Finally, it has the ability to diagnose supra-esophageal reflux.

In 1976, Fischer and co-workers[77] were the first to use radioactive material to detect GERD. They used orange juice marked with Tc-99. Once the patient has swallowed the marked liquid, they adopt the dorsal recumbent position in front of a gamma camera which quantifies radioactivity in the regions of interest – esophagus and stomach. The images can be inspected visually, and transit curves and esophageal emptying curves can be obtained.[77,78]

A technique which uses positron-emission tomography with Tc-99 markers has been recently described. This allows detection of erosive esophagitis in patients with suspected GERD. A study compared the endoscopy results and the results of this technique, and the latter was found to have high sensitivity and specificity.[79]

BilitecTM 2000 (Medtronic, USA) is an ambulatory monitoring device which detects duodenogastroesophageal reflux by taking advantage of the optical properties of bilirubin. Its use is limited to research protocols, and its clinical usefulness is still questionable.[80]

## Role of Dental Practitioners in Diagnosing Reflux

Dental practitioners play an important role in the early detection of dental erosive lesions non-ascribable to exogenous causes, since they will counsel the patient on the need for medical evaluation of his or her digestive system, confirmation of the presence or absence of reflux through specific techniques, identification of the possible etiology of reflux, evaluation of the current status of the condition, and choice of a suitable treatment among the many efficient methods currently available. The role of professional clinicians in the health system is of cardinal importance, since they allow for the diagnosis and treatment of a condition which, on many occasions, has erosive tooth wear as its only symptom. And their role would be even more far-reaching if they could issue an early warning to parents of children who show reflux-related changes, since this pathology commonly begins at birth but, unfortunately, it is not detected until complications arise in adolescence and adult years.

## Treatment of Reflux

Treatment goals are:

- symptom relief
- lesion cicatrization
- avoidance of recurrence
- prevention of complications (stenosis, ulcer, Barrett's esophagus, etc.)
- restoration of quality of life.

In order to alleviate or correct reflux, hygiene and dietary measures should first be adopted. Examples are raising the headboard of the bed by 10–15 cm, avoiding consumption of quantities of greasy food, chewing slowly, and avoiding going to bed before more than two hours have elapsed since eating.[81–83] In obese or overweight patients, weight loss will help reduce the intensity and frequency of symptoms.[84–86] It is advisable to avoid chocolate, carbonated drinks, coffee, and acidic foods (tomatoes, citrus fruit). Smokers and alcohol drinkers should quit their habits. Abdominal exercises, reducing girdles, and corsets should be avoided.

The intake of some drugs (e.g., calcium-channel blockers and bronchodilators) should be carefully re-evaluated. These drugs can cause direct irritation of the esophageal mucosa by stimulating gastric secretion, delaying gastric emptying, increasing gastric and intra-abdominal pressure and, consequently, increasing transient relaxations of the LES.

Although no controlled studies are available on the strict adoption of these measures, and bearing in mind that these hygiene and dietary requirements should be complied with throughout the whole life, they could worsen quality of life even more. Nevertheless, doctors should instruct patients to avoid precipitating factors of GER.

Antacids (aluminum hydroxide), alginates[87,88] (they are usually sold with antacids), and sucralfate are less potent drugs with short-lived effects, but their effectiveness in rapidly relieving symptoms has been demonstrated. They are indicated for the treatment of patients with mild sporadic symptoms, and for pregnant women.

Prokinetic agents are used in the management of this disease. These drugs increase LES pressure and improve esophageal clearance, gastric emptying, and antroduodenal coordination. Included among these drugs are metoclopramide,[89] domperidone, cisapride,[90,93] cinitapride, mosapride,[91–93] and etopride, which have different intensities of action.

$H_2$-antagonists (cimetidine, ranitidine, and famotidine) block acid secretion and reduce the frequency and severity of reflux episodes. These are fast-acting drugs, but early tolerance to their effects is developed and the dose to be prescribed is higher than the dose prescribed for peptic ulcer disease. They relieve the symptoms of mild forms of the disease.

Proton pump inhibitors (PPIs) are the "gold standard" medication for the treatment of GERD; they act on the stomach wall cells, thus blocking the production of acid. They have been used for this purpose for more than 20 years. The anti-secretion effect is achieved progressively, and peak level is reached 72–96 hours after the beginning of treatment. These drugs are so effective that, on administration of certain dosages, they can maintain a gastric content pH value of 4 or over, with very scarce side-effects. PPIs include omeprazole, lanzoprazole, rabeprazole, pantoprazole, and esomeprazole.[94–100] They will rapidly relieve symptoms and heal a high proportion of esophageal lesions. PPIs should be used for treating severe esophagitis or recurrent esophagitis, since they have been shown to effectively prevent the recurrence of symptoms and mucosa lesions.[101–106]

Antireflux surgery is indicated for patients who will not respond to medical treatment or for patients with specific indications. Before surgery and the type of technique to be used are decided on, thorough functional evaluation of the esophagus must be carried out through prolonged pH-metry and manometry. In some cases, studies which evaluate gastric secretion and gastric emptying should be considered, since this can also influence the surgical decision-making process and the choice of the surgical technique to be used.[107]

Although several surgical techniques are available which may solve this pathology, they all tend to close the pillar muscles of the diaphragm at the level where the esophagus crosses the esophageal hiatus of the diaphragm, and to generate some valve system within the stomach which can prevent reflux of the gastric content.[107] The logical thing to do would be to adapt the technique to the motor characteristics of the esophagus; this approach was called "tailored antireflux surgery" by DeMeester et al.[108] Conventional surgery has been reported to heal 59–95% of cases,[109] with good long-term results.

Laparoscopy has been used for the treatment of GERD since 1991. The advantage of this technique is that it allows for shorter post-surgical (pain) recovery times and shorter post-surgical hospital stays. Clinical improvement ranges from 78% to 100%.[110–112]

Currently, both techniques have low mortality rates, but morbidity – mainly dysphagia and gas bloat – ranges from 6% to 31%.[113,114]

## Conclusion

From the clinical point of view, the aim of the treatment is to relieve pain or reflux symptoms (acidity, heartburn, recurrent cough, etc.), to repair mucosa lesions caused by reflux before diagnosis was made, and to achieve lesion cicatrization, dilate stenosis, remove severe dysplasias, etc. While patients can subjectively evaluate pain or symptom relief in a few days or weeks, at least 8 weeks are needed in order to achieve true healing of esophageal erosive lesions – the amount of time needed depends on the degree of severity of the lesions and the strength and suitability of the treatment chosen.

Our main concern is for patients who show dental erosion as the only manifestation of reflux confirmed by some reliable method, and who are being treated with antireflux drugs; since these patients do not have other lesions or specific symptoms, it is difficult to establish right dosage and the period of time the drug should be taken. Considering that reflux is a mostly chronic condition, when we detect abrasive dental erosion from reflux we should ask ourselves, "Is it wise to treat these patients with drugs all their life?", and "Would it be reasonable to resort to antireflux surgery when abrasive dental erosion from reflux is the only manifestation?" The challenges which gastroenterologists and dentists currently face are to find a simple way to assess tooth wear as early as possible, to evaluate patients and treat them if they suffer from reflux, to adjust the dosage of the antireflux drugs prescribed by monitoring the pH of saliva at different times of the day, and to have some simple, affordable method at their disposal that allows evaluation of treatment outcomes.

## References


1. Winkelstein A. Peptic esophagitis: a new clinical entity. JAMA 1935;104:206.
2. Bargen JA, Austin LT. Decalcification of teeth as a result of obstipation with long continued vomiting: report of a case. J Am Dent Assoc 1937;24:1271–1273.
3. Holst JJ, Lange F. Perimylolysis: a contribution towards the genesis of tooth wasting from non-mechanical causes. Acta Odontol Scand 1939;1:36–49.
4. Järvinen V, Meurman JH, Hyvàrinen H, Rytòmaa I, Murtòmaa H. Dental erosion and upper gastrointestinal disorders. Oral Surg Oral Med Oral Pathol 1988;65: 298–303.
5. Meurman J, Toskala J, Nuutinen P, Klementi E. Oral and dental manifestations in gastroesophageal reflux disease. Oral Surg Oral Med Oral Pathol 1994;78:583–589.
6. Taylor G, Taylor S, Abrams R, Mueller W. Dental erosion associated with asymptomatic gastroesophageal reflux. J Dent Child 1992;59:182–185.
7. Scheutzel P. Etiology of dental erosion: intrinsic factor. Eur J Oral Sci 1996; 104:178–190.
8. Dent J, Brun J, Fendrick A et al, on behalf of the Genval Workshop Group. An evidence-based appraisal of reflux disease management: the Genval Workshop Report. Gut 1999;44(Suppl 2):S1–15.
9. Nebel OT, Fornes M, Castell DO. Symptomatic gastroesophageal reflux: incidence and precipitating factors. Am J Dig Dis 1976;21:953–956.
10. McCarthy D. Living with chronic heartburn: insights into its debilitating effects. Gastroenterol Clin North Am 2003;32:1–9.
11. Locke GR, Talley NJ, Fett SL et al. Prevalence and clinical spectrum of gastroesophageal reflux: a population-based study in Olmstead County, Minnesota. Gastroenterology 1997;112:1448–1456.
12. Chiocca JC, Olmos J, Salis GB, Soifer LO, Rios H. Prevalence of gastroesophageal reflux in Argentina: epidemiological nationwide study. Gastroenterology 2000; 118(4)(Suppl 2), A2591.
13. Isolauri J, Laippala P. Prevalence and symptoms suggestive of gastroesophageal reflux in an adult population. Ann Med 1995;27:67–70.
14. Chang CS, Poon SK, Lien HC. The incidence of reflux esophagitis among the Chinese. Am J Gastroenterol 1997; 92:666–671.
15. Diab FH, Izraiq MI. Frequency of gastroesophageal reflux disease (GERD): complications in a Middle-Eastern population. ASGE Meeting. G Int End 1998;47(6):A167.
16. Ho KY, Kang JY, Seow A. Prevalence of gastrointestinal symptoms in a multiracial Asian population, with particular reference to reflux-type symptoms. Am J Gastroenterol 1998;93:1882–1886.

17. Kashiwagi Y, Rurukawa N, Koyama T et al. The prevalence of gastroesophageal reflux disease in Japan: prospective evaluation with endoscopy in 5629 subjects. Gastroenterology 1998;114(Suppl):G0688.
18. Yeh C, Hsu CT, Ho HCS. Erosive esophagitis and Barrett´s esophagus in Taiwan: a higher frequency that expected. Dig Dis Sci 1997;42:702–706.
19. Katz P. Esophageal motility abnormalities: a clinician's perspective. AGA Postgraduate Course. Gastroenterology 1999;93–101.
20. Vaezi MF, Richter J. Role of acid and duodenogastric reflux in esophageal mucosal injury: a review of animal and human studies. Gastroenterology 1995;108:1897–1907.
21. Vaezi M F, Richter J. Role of acid and bile reflux in gastroesophageal reflux disease. Gastroenterology 1996;111: 1192–1199.
22. Dent J, Holloway RH, Toouli J, Doods WJ. Mechanisms of lower esophageal sphincter incompetence in patients with symptomatic gastro esophageal reflux. Gut 1998;29: 1020–1028.
23. Mittal RK, McCallum RW. Characteristics and frequency of transient relaxations of the lower esophageal sphincter on patients with reflux esophagitis. Gastroenterology 1988;95:593–599.
24. Sifrim D, Janssens J, Vantrappen G. Transient lower esophageal sphincter relaxations and esophageal body muscular contractile response in normal humans. Gastroenterology 1996;110:659–668.
25. Sifrim D, Vantrappen G, Janssens J. Permissive role of the esophageal body during transient LES relaxation (TSLESRs). Neurogastroenterol Motil 1994;6:171.
26. McCallum RW, Berkowitz DM, Lerner E. Gastric emptying in patients with gastroesophageal reflux. Gastroenterology 1981;80:285–291.
27. Labenz J, Malfertheiner. Helicobacter pylori in gastroesophageal reflux disease: causal agent, independent or prospective factor? Gut 1997;41:277–280.
28. Schenk BE, Kuipers EJ, Klinkenberg-Knol EC et al. H. pylori, GERD and efficacy of omeprazole therapy. Gastroenterology 1997;112:A282.
29. Vicari JJ, Peek RM, Falk GW et al. The seroprevalence of cagA-positive Helicobacter pylori strains in the spectrum of gastroesophageal reflux disease. Gastroenterology 1998;115:50–57.
30. Klauser AG, Schindelbeck NE, Muller Lissner SA. Symptoms in gastro-esophageal reflux disease. Lancet 1990; 335:205–208.
31. Shi G, des Varannes SB, Scarpignato C, Le Rhun M, Galmiche JP. Reflux related symptoms in patients with normal oesophageal exposure to acid. Gut 1995;37: 457–464.
32. Ollyo JB, Lang F, Fontollet CH et al. Savary's new endoscopic grading of reflux-oesophagitis: a simple, reproducible, logical, complete and useful classification. Gastroenterology 1990;9:A00.
33. Lundell LR, Dent J, Bennett JR et al. Endoscopic assessment of esophagitis: clinical and functional correlates and further validation of the Los Angeles classification. Gut 1999;45:172–180.
34. Sampliner RE. Practice guidelines on the diagnosis, surveillance and therapy of Barrett's esophagus. The Practice Parameters Committee of the American College of Gastroenterology. Am J Gastroenterol 1998;93:1028–1932.
35. Barish CF, Wu WC, Castell DO. Respiratory complications of gastroesophageal reflux. Arch Intern Med 1985;145:1882–1888.
36. Cherian P, Smith LF, Bardham KD. Esophageal test in the evaluation of non cardiac chest pain. Dis Esophagus 1995;8:129–133.
37. Osler W. The Principles and Practice of Medicine. New York:, D. Appleton & Co., 1892.
38. Tuchman D N, Boyle JT, Pack AI, Scwartz J et al. Comparison of airway response following tracheal or esophageal acidification in the cat. Gastroenterology 1984;87:872–881.
39. Little FB, Koufman JA, Kout RI. Effect of gastric acid on the phatogenesis of subglottic stenosis. Ann Otol Rhinol Laryngol 1985;94:516–519.
40. Crausaz FM, Favez G. Aspiration of solid food particles into lungs of patients with gastroesophageal reflux and chronic bronchial disease. Chest 1988;93:376–378.
41. Chernow B, Johnson LF, Janowitz WR, Castell DO. Pulmonary aspiration as a consequence of gastroesophageal reflux: a diagnostic approach. Dig Dis Sci 1979;24:839–844.
42. Mansfield LE, Stein MR. Gastroesophageal reflux and asthma: a possible reflex mechanism. Ann Allergy 1978;41:224–226.
43. Mansfield LE, Hameister HH, Spaulding HS, Smith NJ, Glab N. The role of the vagus nerve in airway narrowing caused by intraesophageal hydrochloric acid provocation and esophageal distention. Ann Allergy 1981;47:431–434.
44. Kiljander TO, Salomaa ER, Hietanen EK et al. Gastroesophageal reflux in asthmatics. Chest 1999;116:1257–1264.
45. Klinkenberg-Knol EC. Otolaryngologic manifestation of gastro-esophageal reflux disease. Scand J Gastroenterol 1998;33(Suppl 225):24–28.
46. Sontag SJ, O'Conell S, Khandelwal A. Most asthmatics have gastroesophageal reflux with or without bronchodilator therapy. Gastroenterology 1990;99:613–620.
47. Sontag SJ, Skorodin M, O´Conell S et al. Ambulatory 24- hour esophageal pH monitoring in patients with asthma. Gastroenterology 1984;86:A1261.
48. Irwin RS, French CL, Curley FJ et al. Chronic cough due to gastroesophageal reflux. Chest 1993;104:1511–1517.
49. Waring JP, Lacayo L, Hunter J et al. Chronic cough and hoarseness in patients with severe gastroesophageal reflux disease: diagnosis and response to therapy. Dig Dis Sci 1995;40:1093–1097.

50. Mays E, Dubois J, Hamilton G. Pulmonary fibrosis associated with tracheobronchial aspiration. Chest 1976;69: 512–515.
51. Jacob P, Karilas PJ, Herzon G. Proximal esophageal pHmetry in patients with " reflux laryngitis". Gastroenterology 1991;100:305–310.
52. Shaker R, Milbrath M, Junlong R et al. Esophagopharyngeal distribution of refluxed gastric acid in patients with reflux laryngitis. Gastroenterology 1995;109:1575–1582.
53. Koufman JA. The otolaryngologic manifestations of gastroesophageal reflux disease: a clinical investigation of 225 patients using ambulatory 24-hour pH monitoring and an experimental investigation of the role of acid and pepsin in the development of laryngeal injury. Laryngoscope 1991;101:1–78.
54. Chen MY, Ott DJ, Casolo BJ et al. Correlation of laryngeal and pharyngeal carcinomas and 24-hour pH monitoring of the esophagus and pharynx. Otolaryngol Head Neck Surg 1998;119:460–462.
55. Ward PH, Hanson DG. Reflux as an etiological factor of carcinoma of the laryngopharinx. Laryngoscope 1988;98: 1195–1199.
56. Schweizer-Hirt CM, Schait A, Schmid R et al. Erosion und Abrasion des Schmelzes: Eine experimentelle Studie. Schweiz Mschr Zuhnheilk 1978;88:497–529.
57. Muñoz JV, Herreros B, Sanchiz V et al. Dental and periodontal lesions in patients with gastro-oesophageal reflux disease. Dig Liver Dis 2003;35:461–467.
58. Cebrián Carretero JL, López-Arcas-Calleja JM. Gastroesophageal reflux diagnosed by occlusal splint tintion. Med Oral Patol Oral Cir Bucal 2006;11:E26–28.
59. Locke GR, Talley NJ, Weaver AL, Zinsmeister AR. A new questionnaire for gastroesophageal reflux disease. Mayo Clin Proc 1994;69:539–547.
60. Carlsson R, Dent J, Bolling-Sternevald E, Johnsson F et al. The usefulness of a structured questionnaire in the assessment of symptomatic gastroesophageal reflux disease. Scand J Gastroenterol 1998;33:1023–1029.
61. Shaw M, Talley N, Beefe T et al. Initial validation of a diagnostic questionnaire for gastroesophageal reflux disease. Am J Gastroenterol 2001;96:52–57.
62. Wallace C, Wu MB. Ancillary tests in the diagnosis of gastro esophageal reflux disease. Gastroenterol Clin N Am 1990;19:671–683.
63. Ott DJ, Gelfand DW, Wu WC. Reflux esophagitis: radiographic and endoscopic correlation. Radiology 1979;130: 583–588.
64. Carlsson R, Dent J, Watts R et al. Gastro-esophageal reflux disease in primary care: an international study of different treatment strategies with omeprazole. International GORD Study Group. Eur J Gastroenterol Hepatol 1998;10:119–124.
65. Vieth M, Haringsma J, Delarive J et al. Red streaks in the esophagus in patients with reflux disease: is there a histomorphological correlate? Scand J Gastroenterol 2001;36: 1123–1127.
66. Schindbeck NE, Wiebecke B, Klauser AG et al. Diagnostic value of histology in non-erosive gastro-esophageal reflux disease. Gut 1996;39:151–154.
67. Spencer J. Prolonged pH recording in the study of gastroesophageal reflux. Br J Surg 1969;56:912–914.
68. De Caestecker JS, Heading RC. Esophageal pH monitoring. Gastroenterol Clin N Am 1990;19:645–669.
69. Johnson LF, DeMeester TR. Twenty-four hour pH monitoring of the distal esophagus: a quantitative measure of gastroesophageal reflux. Am J Gastroenterol 1974;62:325–332.
70. Streets CG, DeMeester TR, Peter JH et al. Clinical evaluation of the Bravo probe: a catheter-free ambulatory esophageal pH monitoring system. Gastroenterology 2001;120:A35.
71. Remes-Troche JM, Ibarra J, Carmona R, Valdovinos MA. Performance, tolerability and symptoms related to prolonged pH monitoring using the Bravo system in Mexico. Am J Gastroenterol 2004;99(S15):A42.
72. Kahrilas PJ, Clouse RE, Hogan WJ. American Gastroenterological Association Technical Review on the Clinical Use of Esophageal Manometry. Gastroenterology 1994; 107:1865–1884.
73. Silny J. Intraluminal multiple electric impedance procedure for measurement of gastrointestinal motility. J Gastroenterol Motil 1991;3:151–162.
74. Tutuian R, Vela M, Shay S, Castell D. Multichannel intraluminal impedance in esophageal function testing and gastroesophageal reflux monitoring. J Clin Gastroenterol 2003;37:206–215.
75. Castell DO, Vela MF. Combined multichannel intraluminal impedance and pH-metry: an evolving technique to measure type and proximal extent of gastroesophageal reflux. Am J Med 2001;111(Suppl 8A):157–159S.
76. Sifrim D, Holloway RH, Silny J et al. Composition of the postprandial refluxate in patients with gastroesophageal reflux disease. Am J Gastroenterol 2001;96:647–655.
77. Fischer RS, Malmud LS, Roberts GS et al. Gastroesophageal (GE) scintiscanning to detect and quantify GE reflux. Gastroenterology 1976;70:301–308.
78. Kjellen G, Brudin L, Hakansson HO. Is scintigraphy of value in the diagnosis of gastro esophageal reflux disease? Scand J Gastroenterol 1991;26:425–430.
79. Hsu CH, Shiun SC, Hsu NY et al. Using non-invasive radionuclide imaging to detect esophagitis in patients with gastro esophageal reflux disease. Hepatogastroenterology 2003;50:107–109.
80. Vaezi MF, LaCamera RG, Richter JE. Validation studies of Bilitec 2000: an ambulatory duodenogastroesophageal reflux monitoring system. Am J Physiol 1994;267: G1050–1057.
81. Becker DJ, Sinclair J, Castell DO. A comparison of high and low fat meals on postprandial esophageal acid exposure. Am J Gastroenterol 1989;84:782–786.

82. Johnson LF, DeMeester TR. Evaluation of elevation of the head of the bed, betanechol, and antacidfoam tablets on gastroesophageal reflux. Dig Dis Sci 1981;26:673–680.
83. Stanciu C, Bennett JR. Effects of the posture on gastro-esophageal reflux. Digestion 1977;15:104–109.
84. Lundell L, Ruth M, Sandberg N et al. Does massive obesity promote abnormal gastroesophageal reflux? Dig Dis Sci 1995;40:1632–1635.
85. Wilson LJ, Ma W, Hirschowitz BI. Association of obesity with hiatal hernia and esophagitis. Am J Gastroenterol 1999;94:2840–2844.
86. Fischer BL, Pennathur A, Mutnick JL, Little AG. Obesity correlates with gastroesophageal reflux. Dig Dis Sci 1999;44:2390–2394.
87. Sunderland A, Dettmar PW, Pearson JP. Alginates inhibit pepsin activity in vitro: a justification for their use in gastro-oesophageal reflux disease. Gastroenterology 2000;118:4A347.
88. Mazure PA, Sferco AN, Chiocca JC. Acción de los alginatos sobre el reflujo en las hernias hiatales. Acta Gastroent Latinoam 1974;6:69–72.
89. Lazaroni FA, Chiocca JC, Salis GB et al. Acción del bromuro de metoclopramida y del clorhidrato de metoclopramida sobre el esfínter esofágico inferior y la peristalsis del tercio inferior del esófago. Acta Gastroent Latinoam 1979;9:15–22.
90. Goldin GF, Marcinkiewicz M, Zbroch T et al. Esophagus protective potencial of cisapride: an additional benefit for gastro-esophageal reflux disease. Dig Dis Sci 1997;42: 1362–1369.
91. Ruth M, Hamelin B, Rohss K, Lundell L. The effect of mosapride, a novel prokinetic, on acid reflux variables in patients with gastro-oesophageal reflux disease. Aliment Pharmacol Ther 1998;12:35–40.
92. Suyama T, Tokubayashi F, Omatsu Y et al. Accelerating effect of AS-4370 (mosapride) on gastric emptying time (double sampling test method) and its clinical efficacy on chronic gastritis accompanied by epigastric symptoms. Jap Arch Intern Med 1993;40(7):175–183.
93. Carlsson L, Amos GJ, Andersson B et al. Electrophysiological characterization of the prokinetic agents cisapride and mosapride in vivo and in vitro: implications for proarrhythmic potential? J Pharmacol Exp Ther 1997; 282:220–227.
94. Richter JE, Kahrilas P, Johanson J et al. Efficacy and safety of esomeprazole compared with omeprazole in GERD patients with erosive esophagitis: a randomized controlled trial. Am J Gastroenterol 2001;96:656–665.
95. Rohss, K, Rydholm H et al. Esomeprazole 40<ts>mg provides more effective acid control than lanzoprazole 30<ts>mg. Gastroenterology 2000; 118,4:A344.
96. Sandmark S, Carlsson R, Fausa O et al. Omeprazole or ranitidine in the treatment of reflux esophagitis: results of a double-blind, randomized, Scandinavian multicentre study. Scand J Gastroenterol 1988;23:625–632.
97. Vantrappen G, Rutgeerts L, Schurmans M, Coenegrachts JL. Omeprazole (40<ts>mg) is superior to ranitidine in short-term treatment of ulcerative esophagitis. Dig Dis Sci 1988;33:523–526.
98. Hatlebakk JG, Berstad A, Carling L et al. Lanzoprazole versus omeprazole in short-term treatment of reflux esophagitis: results of a Scandinavian multicentre trial. Scand J Gastroenterol 1993;28:224–228.
99. Corinaldesi R, Valentini M, Belaiche J et al. The European Pantoprazole Study Group. Pantoprazole and omeprazole in the treatment of reflux esophagitis: a European multicentre study. Aliment Pharmacol Ther 1995;9: 667–671.
100. Castell DO, Richter JE, Robinson M et al. Efficacy and safety of lanzoprazole in the treatment of erosive reflux esophagitis. The lanzoprazole group. Am J Gastroenterol 1996;91:1749–1757.
101. Mossner J, Koop H, Porst H et al. One-year prophylactic efficacy and safety of pantoprazole in controlling gastro-esophageal reflux symptoms in patients with healed reflux oesophagitis. Aliment Pharmacol Ther 1998;11: 1087–1092.
102. Gough AL, Long RG, Cooper BT et al. Lansoprazole versus ranitidine in the maintenance of treatment of reflux esophagitis. Aliment Pharmacol Ther 1996;10: 529–539.
103. Vigneri S, Termini R, Leandro G et al. A comparison of five maintenance therapies for reflux esophagitis. N Engl J Med 1995;333:1106–1110.
104. Plein K, Hotz J, Wurzer H et al. Prevention of relapse in gastro-esophageal reflux disease (GERD): a randomized double blind, long term multicentre study using 20 mg or 40 mg pantoprazole. Digestion 1998;59 (Suppl 3):600.
105. Lauritsen K, Jaup B, Carling S et al. Efficacy of pantoprazole compared with omeprazole in prevention of relapse of reflux esophagitis: double-blind, randomized multi-center trial. Gastroenterology 2000;118(4):A333.
106. Thjodleifsson B, Beker JA, Dekkers C et al. Rabeprazole versus omeprazole in preventing relapse of erosive or ulcerative gastroesophageal reflux disease: a double-blind multicenter, European trial. The European Rabeprazole Study Group. Dig Dis Sci 2000;45:845–853.
107. Stein, H J, Feussner H, Siewert JR. Management of gastroesophageal reflux disease 1995. Surgical therapy of gastroesophageal reflux: which patient, which procedure, which approach? Dis Esophagus 1994;7:239–244.
108. DeMeester TR, Bonavina L, Albertucci M. Nissen fundoplication for gastroesophageal reflux disease. Ann Surg 1986;204:9–20.
109. Donahue P, Bombeck CT, Samelson S et al. The floppy Nissen fundoplication: effective long-term control of pathologic reflux. Arch Surg 1985;120:663–668.
110. Waring JP, Hunter JG, Oddsdottir M et al. The preoperative evaluation of patients considered for laparoscopic antireflux surgery. Am J Gastroenterol 1995;90:35–38.

111. Patti MG, Arcerito M, Pellegrini CA et al. Minimally invasive surgery for gastroesophageal reflux disease. Am J Surg 1995;170:614–617.
112. Perdikis G, Hinder RA, Wetscher GJ. Nissen fundoplication for gastroesophageal reflux disease: laparoscopic Nissen fundoplication, technique and results. Dis Esophagus 1996;9:272–277.
113. Ireland AC, Holloway RH, Tooli J et al. Mechanisms underlying the antireflux action of the fundoplication. Gut 1993;34:303–308.
114. Siewert J R, Stein HJ. Nissen fundoplication for gastroesophageal reflux disease: technical details, long-term outcome and causes of failures. Dis Esophagus 1996;9: 278–284.

Chapter 12

# Controversies on the Effects of Bruxism

*Daniel A. Paesani*

## Introduction

Concept controversy is common in all scientific disciplines. Bruxism as a phenomenon is no exception. The aim of this volume is to clarify rather than add to the existing confusion. In this chapter, some of these controversies will be described and the literature will be reviewed. This will allow the reader to become aware of both the evidence and the discrepancies and to draw his or her own conclusions in order to adopt a specific stance toward the clinical situations he or she will have to deal with in everyday dental practice. The chapter will cover the effects of bruxism on dentition, on the soft tissues, and on bone.

## Effects on the Dentition

### *Progressive Dental Crowding*

*(Refer to the case studies in Figures 12-1 to 12-7.)*
Undoubtedly, progressive disruption of dental occlusion is a problem that affects both the health and the esthetic appearance.

Quite frequently, people with a complete, mature dentition present with progressive misalignment of the anterior teeth; in the scientific literature, this is known as "late anterior crowding". Misalignment will usually develop in the mandible; however, though on a smaller scale, it may also develop in the maxillary teeth. This has become a subject of concern to many orthodontists, since crowding also frequently reoccurs following corrective treatments of the primary malocclusion. There is much discussion about the origin of this anomaly. The suggested causes include: force exerted from the posterior segment due to physiologic mesial drift; the anterior component of the force of occlusion on mesially inclined teeth; mesial vectors of muscular contraction; and the presence of a developing third molar.[1] Other potential etiologic factors are: late mandibular growth, skeletal morphology and complex growth patterns, soft tissue maturation, periodontal forces, dental morphology, occlusal factors, and connective tissue changes.[2]

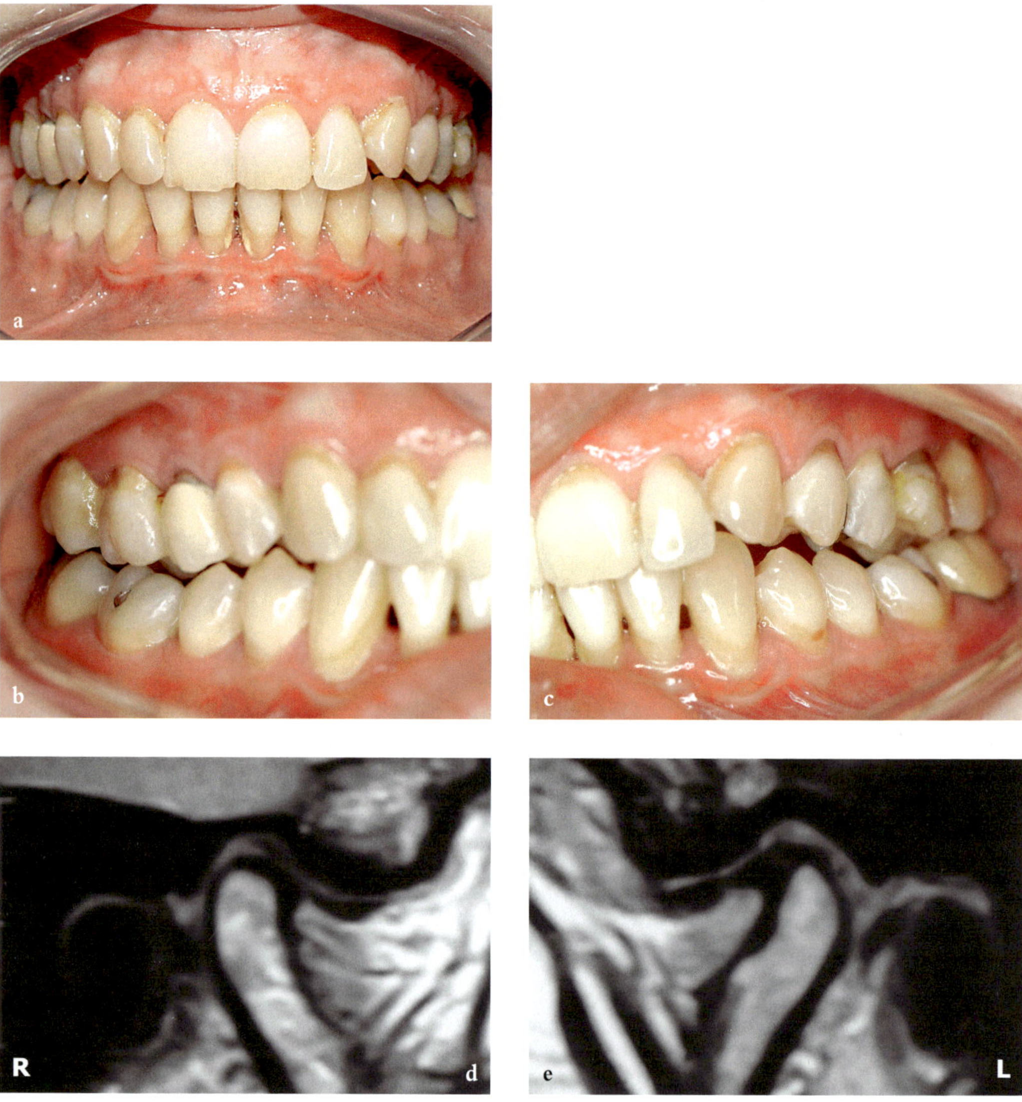


Fig 12-1 **(a–c)** Bruxer (woman) showing progressive vestibularization of the left maxillary lateral incisor. Loss of maximum dental intercuspation secondary to degenerative arthritis can be seen. There is complete lack of contact in the right quadrant, and only the left second molars are occluding. **(d)** Magnetic resonance imaging (MRI) of the right temporomandibular joint (TMJ) anterior disc: there is displacement, and the glenoid fossa has a flattened appearance. **(e)** MRI of the left TMJ: the condyle is small and arthritic, and an osteophyte can be seen on its anterior edge.

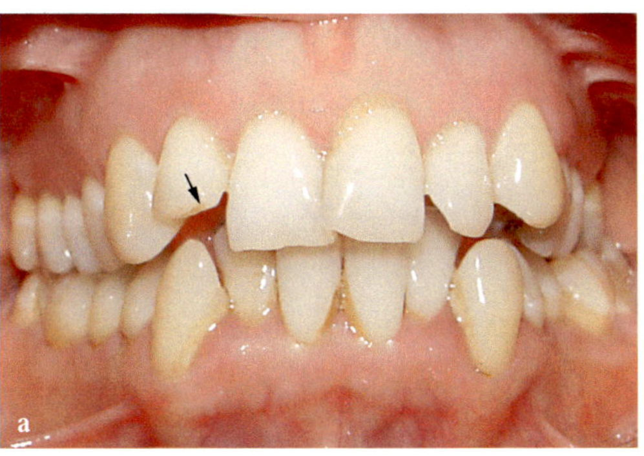


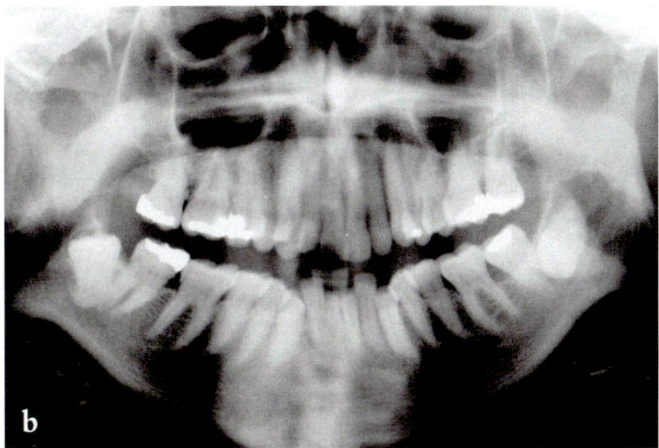


Fig 12-2 **(a)** Progressive maxillary and mandibular incisor crowding. There is no contact between the attrition facet in the maxillary lateral incisor (arrow) and antagonist teeth during mandibular movements. **(b)** Panoramic radiograph showing significant degeneration in both condyles.

Since the factors potentially involved are so many, and most of them are not directly related to the aim of this volume, we will deal only with the potential effect of bruxism on the disruption of dental occlusion.

Periodontists have dealt extensively with this subject, and it seems they do not agree as to whether bruxism should be considered one of the causes of pathologic tooth migration (PTM).[3] This tooth migration has been defined by Carranza[4] as tooth displacement that occurs when the balance among the factors that maintain physiologic tooth position is disturbed by periodontal disease. Its prevalence is high in populations suffering from periodontal disease – it has been reported to be 55.8%.[5] Diagnosing PTM is not difficult, since the patients themselves will usually present to the dental clinician owing to the development of a diastema between their maxillary incisors; usually, such diastemas will progressively increase in size. Periodontal disease, occlusal trauma, pressure exerted by soft tissues (cheeks, tongue, and lips), apical and periodontal inflammation, and a variety of oral habits are mentioned among PTM's etiologic factors.[3] It is only logical to assume that bruxism generates enough orthodontic forces to be able to move certain teeth, and, in fact, some authors have considered this to be possible.[4,6,7] Southard and co-workers[8] consider the increase in interproximal forces as a result of parafunction to be one of the causes of tooth alignment disruption. In protrusive bruxism simulations, mandibular incisor displacements were observed which ranged from 100 to 700 µm, depending on the amount of force exerted during the simulation. These same researchers obtained similar results in lateral bruxism simulations.[9] However, a study of a population of patients suffering from periodontal disease failed to demonstrate PTM association with tooth wear and bruxism identified by means of questionnaries.[5]

### *Anterior Component of Force*

Though first postulated by Edward Angle at the beginning of the 20th century, the anterior component of force (ACF) was objectively demonstrated for the first time by Osborn in 1961, and later confirmed by Picton in 1962.[10,11] However, in 1989, Southard and co-workers claimed that they were the first to have scientifically measured the ACF.[12] These authors suggest that ACF is likely to result from the mesial inclination of posterior teeth that are loaded with occlusal forces; such occlusal forces are then transmitted to the anterior segment through the contact point. Considerable forces were reported by these authors: 5 lbf at the level of

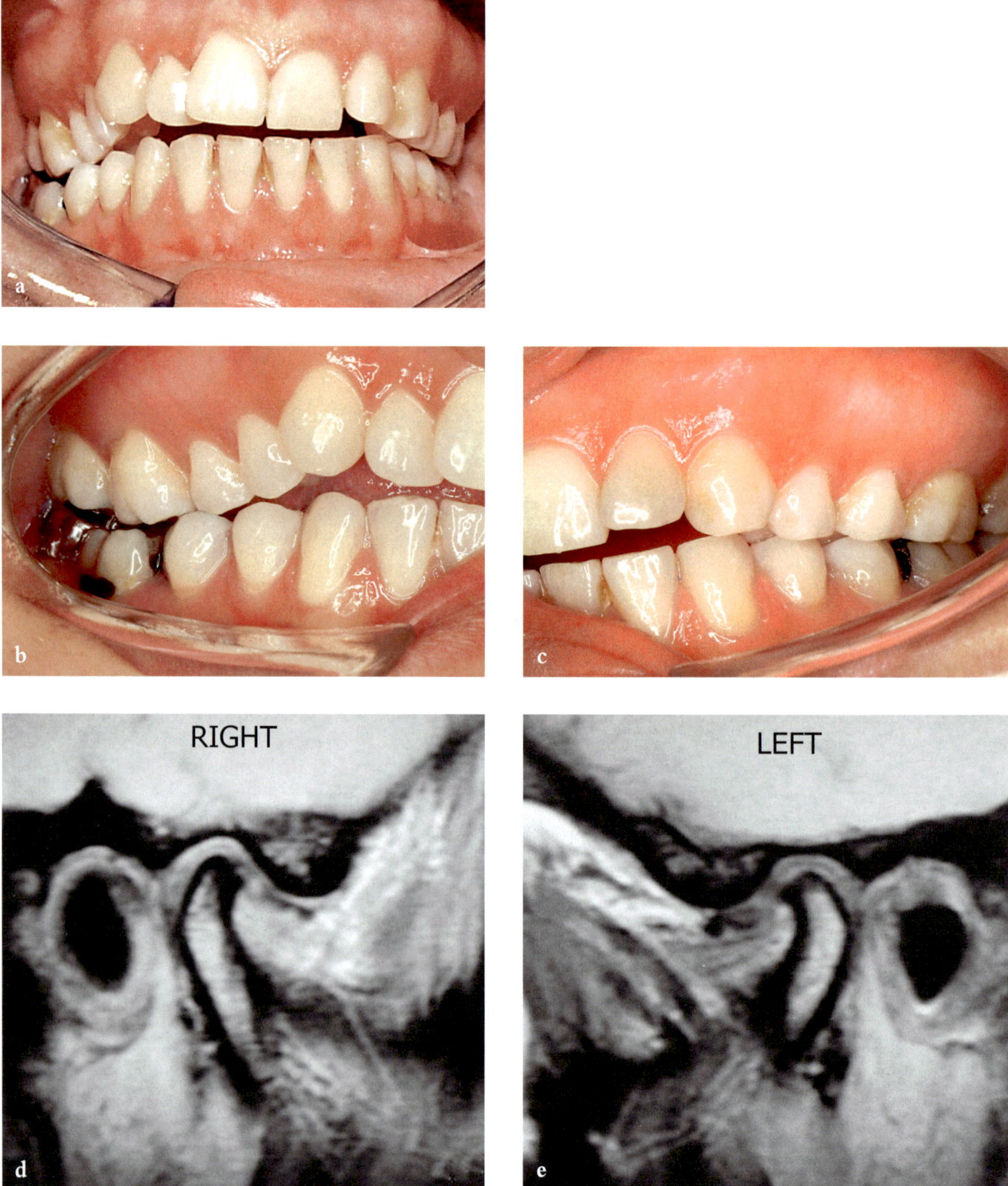


Fig 12-3 **(a)** Intercuspal position alteration and incisor crowding. **(b)** The right hemi-arch lacks occlusal contacts. **(c)** Over-occlusion in left teeth. **(d)** Magnetic resonance imaging (MRI) of the right temporomandibular joint (TMJ): condyle bone marrow sclerosis is observed, and the disc has been displaced forward and the condyle rests on the retro-discal tissues. **(e)** MRI of the left TMJ: significant condyle sclerosis and osteophytosis is seen, and the disc is anteriorly displaced.

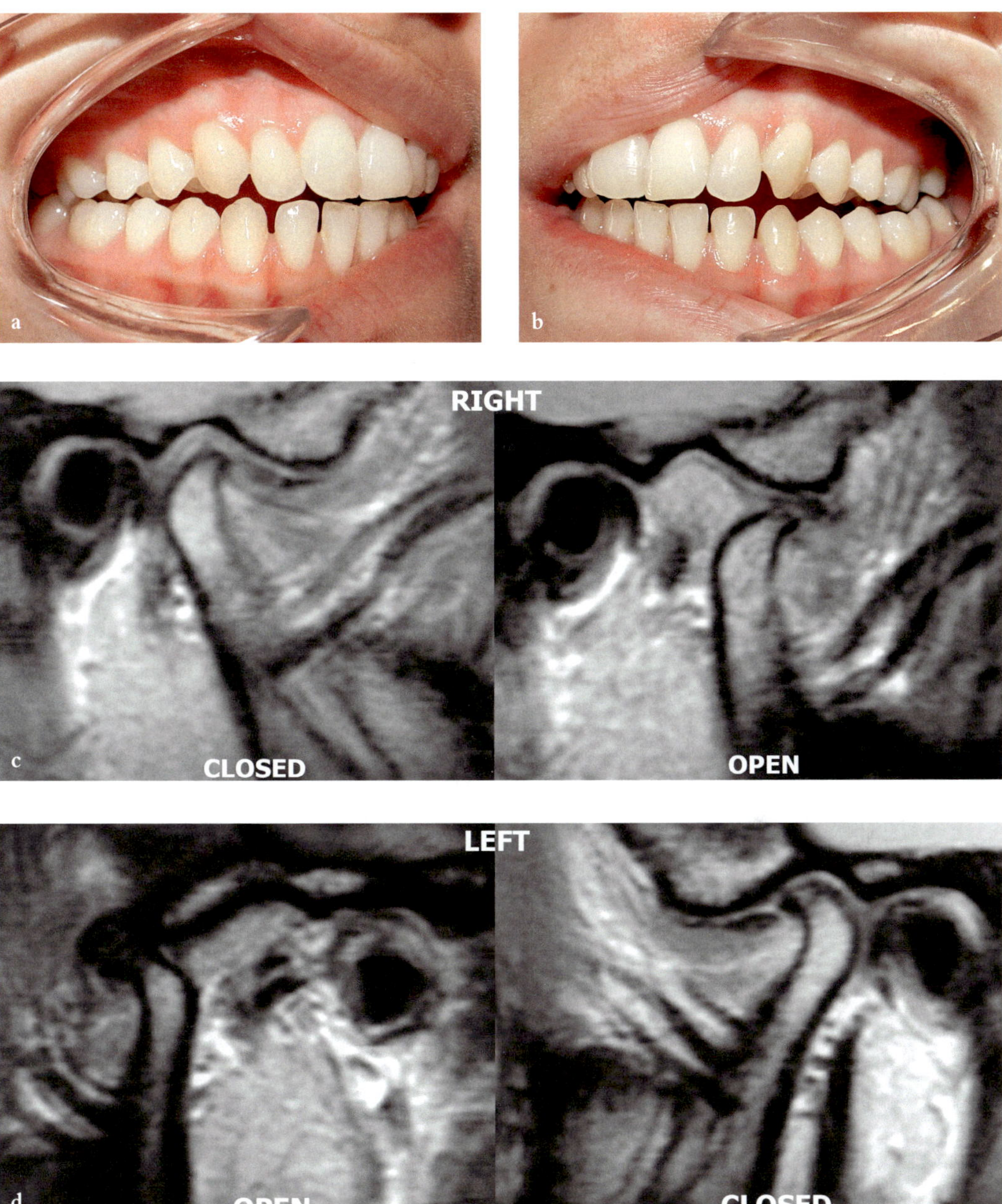


Fig 12-4 **(a)** Intercuspal position alteration. Contact exists only at the level of the second molar; also maxillary incisor crowding is present. **(b)** Occlusal contact only at the level of the second molar. **(c)** Non-reducible disc displacement; an osteophyte is seen in the anterior pole of the condyle. **(d)** Non-reducible disc displacement; an osteophyte is seen in the anterior pole of the condyle.

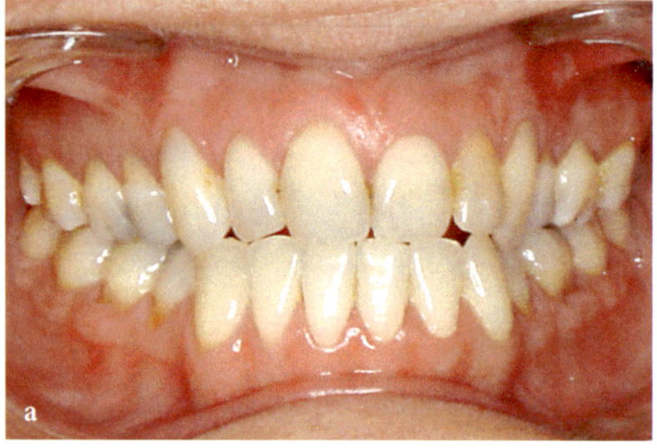

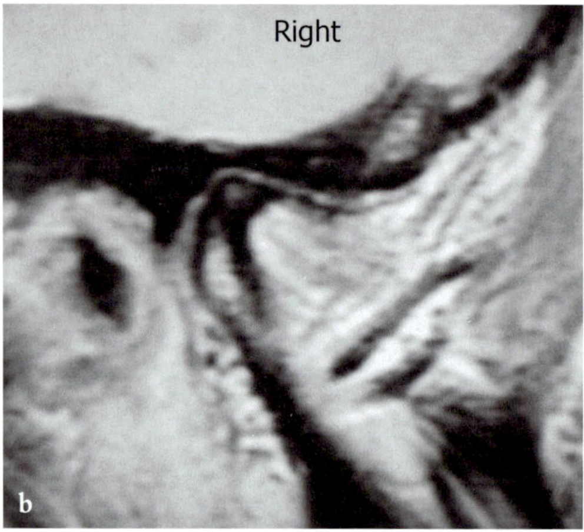


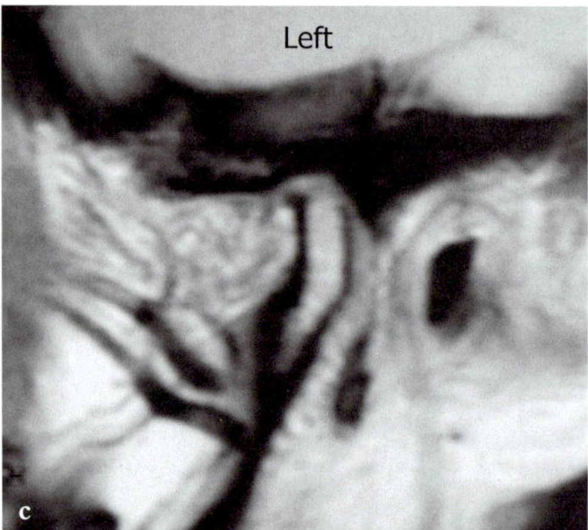


Fig 12-5 **(a)** Progressive displacement of the left maxillary lateral incisor and overbite loss. **(b)** There is significant arthritic remodeling of the condyle, and a displaced, non-reducible disc. Glenoid cavity flattening can be seen. **(c)** Arthritic condyle; displaced, non-reducible disc. The glenoid fossa has a flattened appearance.

the premolars, and 1 lbf at the level of the canines. These values were obtained while having the participants exert a bite force of just 20 lbf over the second molars. The authors also showed that ACF increases in direct proportion to the increase in clenching forces.[13] Others also showed that interdental contact point forces increase in direct proportion to the increase in maximum-intercuspation bite force.[14] It should be noted that the maximum voluntary clenching force values reported in the literature range between 75 and 150 lbf,[15] and that dental clenching forces will usually double during sleep.[16] In a subsequent study, Southard and co-workers related ACF with anterior-segment crowding.[17] This was later confirmed by another team of researchers who conducted a similar study.[18]

In the trial carried out by Southard and his team, increase in interproximal force occurred in teeth on the contralateral side. The authors deem this to be a transmission of forces that crossed the dental midline through the contact points.[12] However, the same result was obtained by another researcher in a trial carried out on subjects with an incomplete dental arch due to missing teeth; this author ascribed the results he obtained to the distortion of both jawbones caused by the clenching forces.[19] The deformation of the jaws during tooth clenching has been demonstrated by means of a computerized three-dimensional model using finite elements.[20] The jawbones may become deformed owing to the muscle forces exerted in function and, especially, in parafunction – it has been shown that the mandibular arch width decreases during unilateral and bilateral tooth clenching.[20,21] Contact point forces vary during mastication and according to the time of day, location in the arch, and type of tooth. This has been ascribed to multifactorial physiologic variations.[22] However, others have denied that distortion of the jaws occurs, or at least they consider such distortion to be clinically irrelevant owing to the low distortion values found.[23]

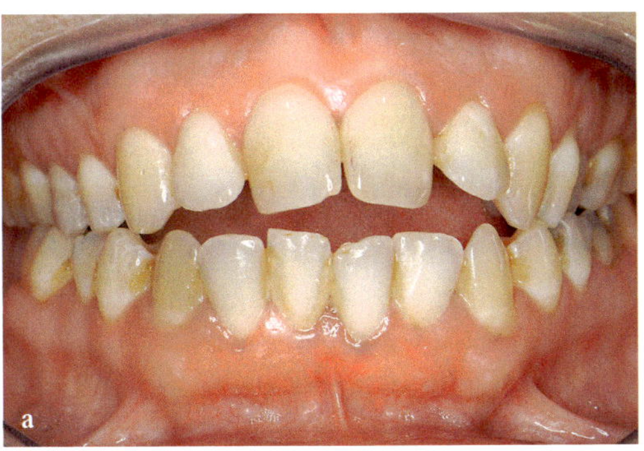
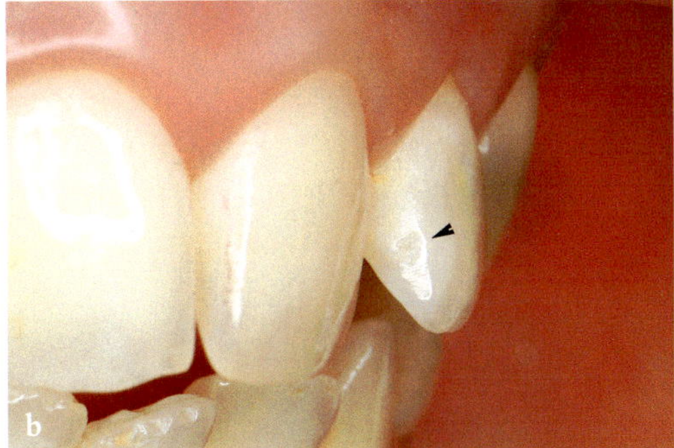

Fig 12-6 **(a)** Patient with osteoarthritis who describes progressive disruption of maxillary and mandibular incisors. **(b)** An interproximal facet (arrow), which is a sign of the movement undergone by the incisor.

Clearly, whatever the originating mechanism may be, when sustained tooth clenching occurs, the force exerted by the teeth increases at the level of the contact point, which generates a force component that will make such teeth drift mesially. Even though some authors have mentioned bruxism as one of the causes of crowding and/or anterior tooth mesial migration, in fact no research studies are available on the bruxism hypothesis. As we have seen in Chapter 1, bruxism of the clenching type during wakefulness occurs twice as often as bruxism of the grinding type during sleep; this means that the number of people who spend many hours a day challenging the stability of teeth in their arches is great. During maximum tooth clenching in the maximum dental intercuspal position, the number of occlusal-contact point surfaces distributed over the teeth in the arches increases relative to the number of occlusal contact-point surfaces existing during the jawbone smooth-contact position. This means that the masticatory system is prepared to handle a proper distribution of these forces by increasing the number of force-dissipation surfaces along the teeth.[24] The studies show that the individual clenching force of each tooth increases as we move posteriorly along the arches.[25] In everyday practice we must deal with patients in whom such a mechanism distributing forces over all the teeth in the arch fails, so that the strong bruxism forces are exerted on a few teeth only (sometimes, on one tooth only). Sometimes the teeth are able to adjust to these atypical situations (intrusion, wear); at other times they just give in (death of pulp tissue, fractures, etc.). It should also be considered possible that these individual occlusal loads will create an important anterior component of force which will boost crowding or a simple dental migration.

The masticatory system is perfectly well prepared to adjust to different physiologic requirements; but, of course, it needs some time for this. Thus, compensatory migration occurs to offset slow contact-point wear, and compensatory extrusion occurs to offset progressive occlusal-surface physiologic wear. If this did not happen, maximum intercuspation would fail to exist and to be maintained throughout life. Some conditions will significantly alter the different components of the masticatory system; this may cause such natural adjustment mechanisms to become overburdened and thus fail to maintain a compensatory status. Subjects with severe malocclusion (i.e., an occlusal abnormality that does not have a dental source but is produced by a severe change in the position of the jaws resulting from degenerative arthritis) are commonly seen in clinics that provide services to patients with temperomandibular disorders (TMD). Such changes in the position of the

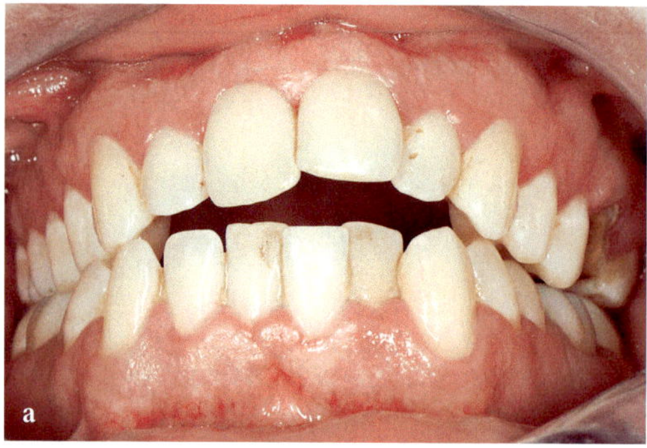


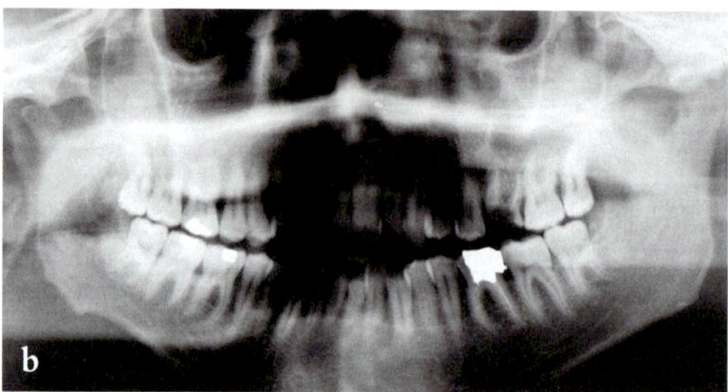


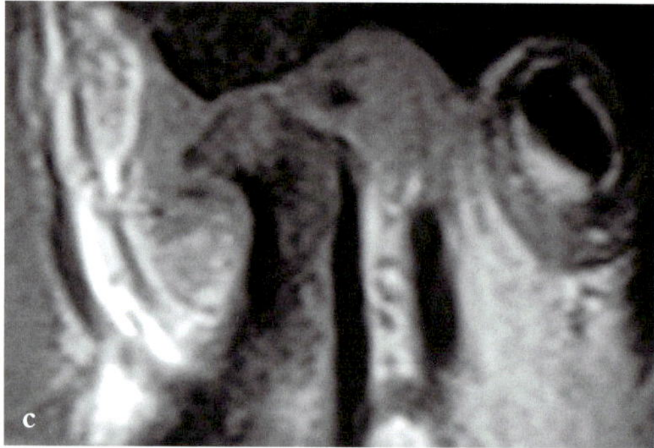


Fig 12-7 **(a)** Significant occlusal alteration and progressive incisor crowding. Occlusal contact occurs only in the right quadrant, possibly related to temporomandibular joint (TMJ) osteoarthritis on that side. **(b)** Panoramic radiograph showing significant size asymmetry between both condyles. **(c)** In this magnetic resonance imaging (MRI) study, the extent of condyle deformation can be appreciated; there is also significant fossa flattening.

jaws occur faster than that of the teeth in their effort to maintain maximum intercuspation. Usually, patients will present with occlusions such that "maximum intercuspation" is present on one tooth only, or on a few, sometimes unilaterally and sometimes bilaterally. If to this we add the fact that many of these patients have the habit of clenching their teeth during wakefulness without noticing it, we will have a perfect replica of the trial carried out by Southard and co-workers.[12]

Although a positive relationship has been reported between the ACF and dental crowding, it is also true that no research studies have been able to demonstrate higher crowding incidence in patients with malocclusion secondary to degenerative arthritis. In this chapter, some case reports are presented to better illustrate the various situations just described. It is to be hoped that, in the future, the scientific method will provide enough evidence to confirm or reject this simple clinical observation (Figs 12-1–12-7).

### *Non-carious Cervical Lesions*

These lesions of the cervical area of the tooth have many names, which are usually in accordance with the different etiologic theories concerning their origin. The names most frequently used in the literature are: non-carious cervical lesion (NCCL), cervical wedge-shaped defect, cervical erosion, cervical abrasion, idiopathic cervical erosion and abfraction. There are three main hypotheses regarding their origin: (1) dental hard tissue abrasion due to tooth brushing; (2) the forces exerted by the dental occlusion; and (3) endogenous or exogenous chemical erosion.

Clinically, there are two types of lesion:

- dish-shaped – flat, shallow, and with ill-defined borders
- wedge-shaped or deep-crevice-shaped – with sharp, well-defined borders.

Shallow lesions are more common than wedge-shaped lesions (Fig 12-8).[26] These two types of shape could correspond to different etiologies or could represent different stages of the same lesion.[27]

Through ultrastructural visualizations, some authors claim that deep-creviced lesions and wedge-shaped lesions are preceded by shallow lesions.[28] Others consider that deep lesions with sharp borders have an occlusal etiology, while shallow-shaped lesions represent abrasion from tooth brushing.[29] Sometimes these lesions are asymptomatic, but on other occasions significant touch tenderness and thermal-change sensitivity occurs. Through electron microscopy, it has been shown that the absence of sensitivity in some of these lesions is associated with their slow progress.[27] In contrast, symptomatic lesions are due to the exposure of dentinal tubules, which remain open.[30]

Reported prevalence values range between 5% and 85%, maxillary premolars being the teeth most commonly affected. The incidence and severity of NCCLs increase with the patient's age.[27,29,31–37]

*Abrasion from tooth brushing*

Going back in time a little bit, NCCLs used to be considered "cervical lesions caused by abrasion"[38] (Fig 12-9). The results of research studies on oral hygiene are extremely contradictory. It has been shown that the tooth-brushing method, the force exerted, and the abrasive power of toothpaste are important factors influencing the development of NCCLs.[31,39,40] While cervical abrasion has been ascribed by some authors to toothbrush bristle hardness,[41] others claim that soft toothbrushes are the ones that boost abrasion, since they carry more toothpaste.[42] Also, toothpaste abrasiveness has been related to wear. According to Litonjua and co-workers,[43] toothpaste plays a major role, while toothbrushes play a secondary role. Radentz and co-workers[44] claim that the tooth-brushing method and frequency are not relevant to the development of NCCLs, but they consider that toothbrush bristle hardness and the three teeth to which the toothbrush is applied first – the ones where the biggest amount of toothpaste is concentrated – play an important role. In contrast, others reject the idea of toothpaste having an abrasive effect, and ascribe such abrasive effect to toothbrushes.[45] The results of studies conducted in the lab and in situ suggest that the amount of wear produced by toothpastes is clinically insignificant.[46,47]

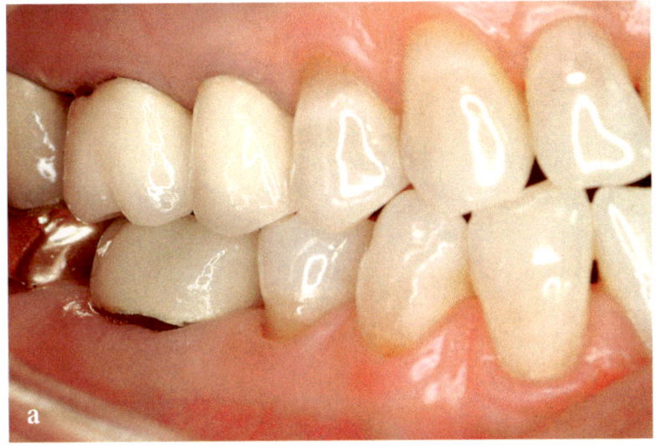

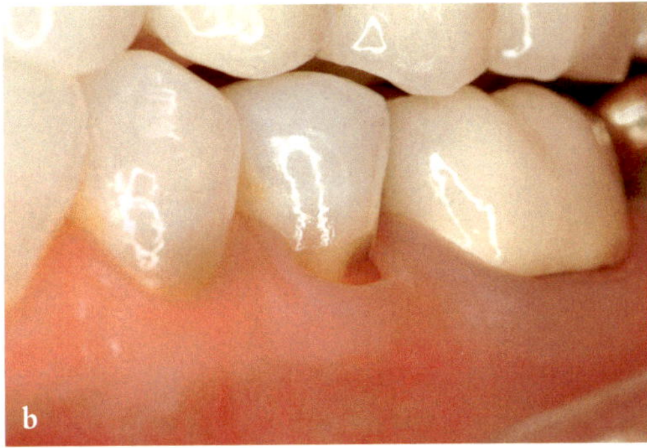

Fig 12-8 **(a)** Dish-shaped, shallow lesion with ill-defined borders. **(b)** Wedge-shaped, deep lesion with well-defined borders.

A higher oral hygiene level has been associated with NCCLs.[31] Individuals who brush their teeth more than twice a day show a greater number of NCCLs.[39] However, another study reports that 40% of teeth with NCCLs belonged to individuals showing a great amount of plaque on the vestibular surfaces of their teeth.[48] Also, Bergström and Eliasson have reported NCCLs in subjects whose oral hygiene was poor.[49]

Since men generally exert more manual force than women, one would expect that NCCLs would be more frequent in men; however, the prevalence is the same for both genders.[31,39,44] If tooth brushing caused NCCLs, it would be reasonable to assume that, 90% of people being right-handed, such lesions would be more preva-

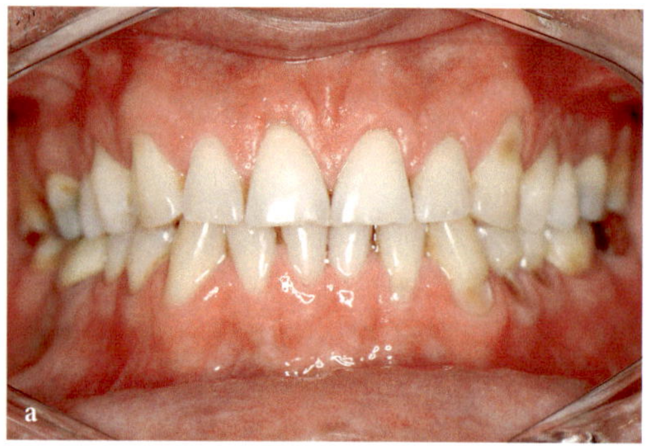


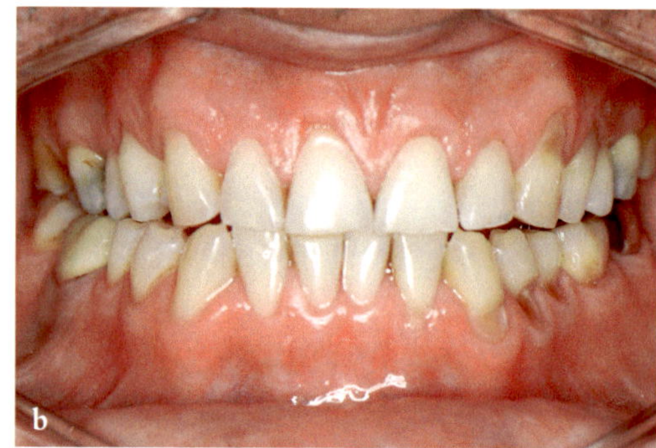


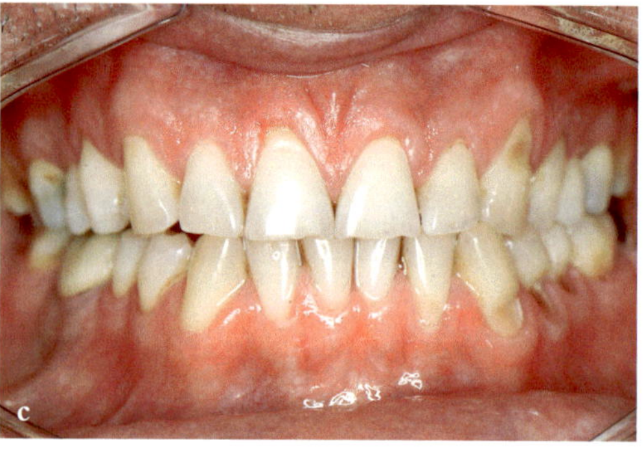


Fig 12-9 **(a)** Bruxer with non-carious cervical lesions (NCCLs). Shallow lesions are more prevalent in the maxilla; in contrast, wedge-shaped lesions prevail in the mandible. This is a right-handed patient with an excessively hard tooth-brushing habit. **(b)** During right lateral movement, group function occurs; however, there are no signs of lesions. **(c)** During left lateral movement, group function occurs and there are NCCLs.

lent on the left side of the mouth. However, NCCLs have not been found to prevail on one side of the mouth.[37] The fact that some teeth showing NCCLs are placed next to other teeth that are completely free of these lesions puts the idea of tooth brushing having a traumatic effect into question, since it is difficult to understand why it will affect certain teeth without affecting those next to them.[27] Though not frequent, the presence of NCCLs on the lingual surfaces of teeth – a place where toothbrushes have very limited access – is another contradiction.[50] Though rare, these lesions are subgingival, and they occur in areas where the toothbrush cannot reach.[51–53] They have even been reported in animals.[54] It is also difficult to account for the fact that only a few NCCL cases are associated with gum abrasion despite gums being tissues that are easily ulcerated by hard tooth brushing. However, others have reported less gum recession in control teeth than in teeth with NCCLs; this has been ascribed to tooth brushing.[33]

In short, in accordance with the literature on oral hygiene, it is highly unlikely that tooth-brushing effects alone can be the main cause of NCCLs.

### *Dental occlusion*

NCCLs have been ascribed to bruxism.[55,56] In 1984, Lee and Eakle distinguished between cervical lesions caused by erosion and cervical lesions of unknown origin (or "idiopathic"). While the former do not have sharp borders, the latter are markedly wedge-shaped. The authors hypothesize that the possible etiologic factor involved in the development of these wedge-shaped lesions – which they call "cervical lesions from occlusal

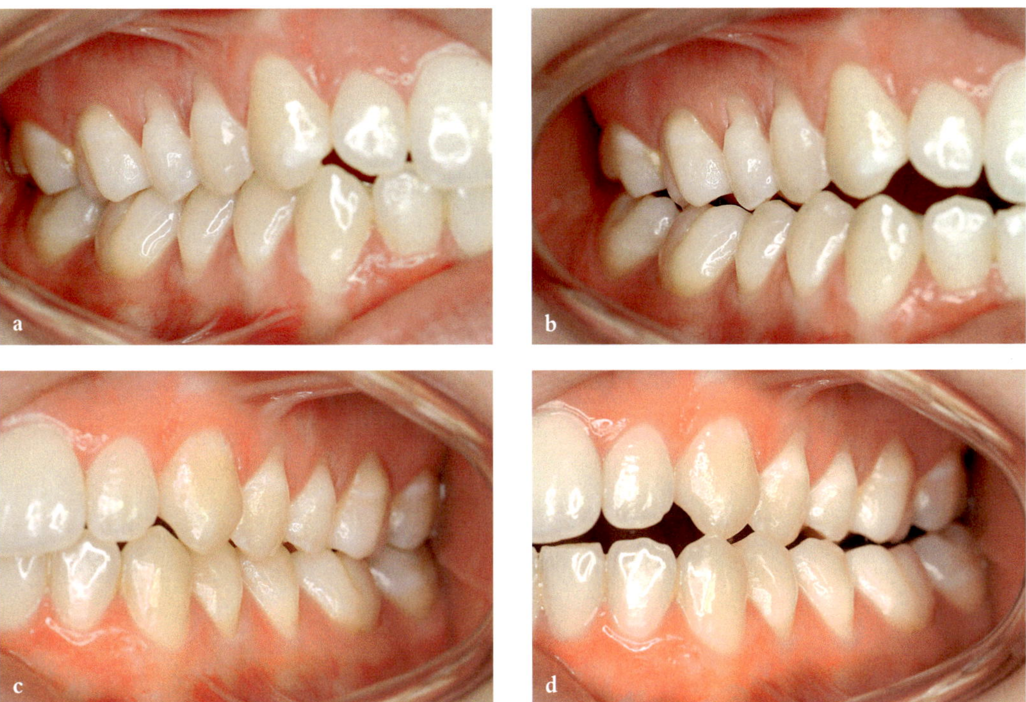

Fig 12-10 **(a)** Non-bruxer with non-carious cervical lesions (NCCLs) in her right maxillary premolars. **(b)** Group function occurs during right lateral movement, which may account for NCCLs. **(c)** Gingival recess is seen on the left side; NCCLs are starting to develop in maxillary premolars. **(d)** Group function during left lateral movement.

stress" – is the tooth flexure caused by occlusal forces. They also suggest that with ideal occlusion, mastication and bruxism forces are exerted and dissipated along the dental axis. In contrast, when there is malocclusion, lateral forces are produced which concentrate on the cervical region and cause enamel's hydroxyapatite crystals to break and become more susceptible to the action of acids and abrasion from tooth brushing, which will lead to the development of cervical lesions.[50] Later, Grippo[57] coined the term "abfraction" to describe this type of tooth substance loss. This author supports a multifactorial etiology for NCCLs (for him, abfractions), the precipitating cause of which is occlusal stress acting in combination with the effects of acids and abrasion from toothbrushing and toothpaste; he calls this process "stress corrosion".[58] A series of finite-element studies supporting these theories has been published; providing evidence that there is occlusal force concentration at the level of the cervical region.[33,59–61] However, others have not been able to demonstrate force concentration at the cervical level.[62] Litonjua and co-workers[63] conducted a thorough review of the finite-element studies and photoelasticity studies on which the abfraction theory is based. These authors claim that, although these studies demonstrate that force concentration occurs in the cementoenamel junction area, they fail to explicitly prove that enamel and dentin fractures occur. They challenge abfraction theoreticians to experimentally and clinically prove that occlusal stress concentration in the cervical region is the precipitating cause of wedge-shaped lesions. An in-vitro trial in which premolars extracted for orthodontics reasons were subject to hard tooth brushing and occlusal loads failed to demonstrate a significant role of such loads in the progress of cervical lesions.[64]

Several studies have related bruxism to NCCLs; these lesions are more prevalent in bruxers than in non-bruxers.[55,65] Some of these studies have reported an association with occlusal facets.[66–69] Others found an association between NCCLs, group function presence, and teeth not showing increased periodontal mobility.[34] Also, the fact that NCCLs should occur in mobile teeth has been considered to be an oddity; on the contrary, they frequently coexist with occlusal facets and occur in mouths where there is no canine disocclusion.[48] NCCLs are six times more common in subjects with a group-function occlusal scheme than in subjects with canine disocclusion.[70] The case presented in Figure 12-10 may be used as a model of this theory.

Nevertheless, a study from the articulated casts of dental students failed to prove a correlation between occlusal wear and cervical lesions[71] (Fig 12-11). In contrast, in a longitudinal study conducted over a period of 14 years, Pintado and coworkers[72] demonstrated a significant correlation between NCCL progress and increased occlusal wear in the same tooth belonging to a young bruxer. Their study is very illustrative and it aims at supporting the occlusal theory; however, its scientific value is relative, since only one patient participated. An important piece of information provided by these authors is that an originally dish-shaped lesion turned into a wedge-shaped lesion over time.

It may be concluded that the studies supporting the abfraction theory are mainly based on finite-element studies and laboratory studies and there is scarce clinical proof of this theory. In the future, perhaps the precursors of this theory will be able to develop an in-situ model that confirms the results of these computerized developments.

*Chemical erosion*

Members of the "Australian school" have called the occlusal-force theory into question; the theory of an erosive mechanism being the primary NCCL etiology is passionately advocated by them.[28] They have demonstrated that 96% of NCCLs develop in teeth showing attrition or erosion, on both occlusal and incisal surfaces. The authors found significant correlation between the occurrence of cervical lesions and occlusal wear of the erosive type at the level of premolars and molars – in the latter case, especially in the mandibular teeth (Fig 12-12), which has been ascribed to increased salivary protection at the level of the upper teeth. In their opinion, tooth-brushing corrosion and abrasion play the supplementary role of further aggravating the lesions, since hard tissues are softened by the action of acid.

Later, a longitudinal prospective research study showed that subjects individuals with a reduced buffering capacity are at increased risk for the development of cervical lesions.[73] However, in an in-vitro study, 8% of the teeth developed NCCLs when subjected to occlusal forces while submerged in a medium of sulfuric acid at 10% concentration; another group of teeth also submerged in the same medium but not subjected to loads did not develop lesions.[74] Grippo and Masi[75] conducted an in-vitro trial and showed how the combined activity occurring in teeth stressed by simulated occlusal loads in an erosive citric-acid medium accelerated the loss of tooth substance. Erosion from acid intake is said to soften dental hard tissues, causing them to become vulnerable to the abrasive effect of immediate tooth brushing.[76]

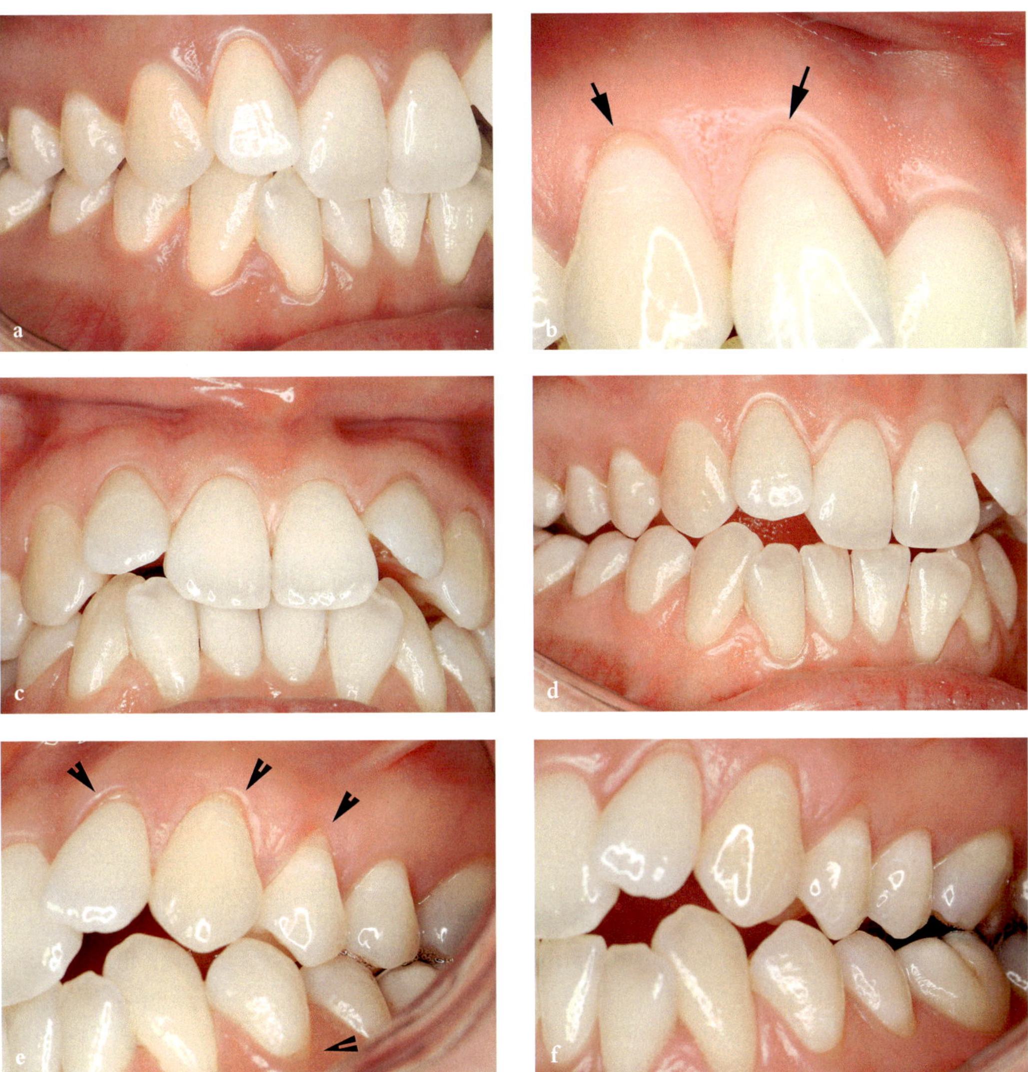

Fig 12-11 **(a)** Non-bruxer with a fresh non-carious cervical lesion (NCCL) in her right maxillary lateral incisor. **(b)** NCCLs (arrows) in the canine and right maxillary lateral incisor. **(c)** However, this tooth has no contact with its antagonists. The fact that its mamelons are intact proves this. **(d)** During lateral movement with canine protection, there is no contact either. **(e)** There are NCCLs on the left side as well. **(f)** During lateral movement, contact is present in the canine only.

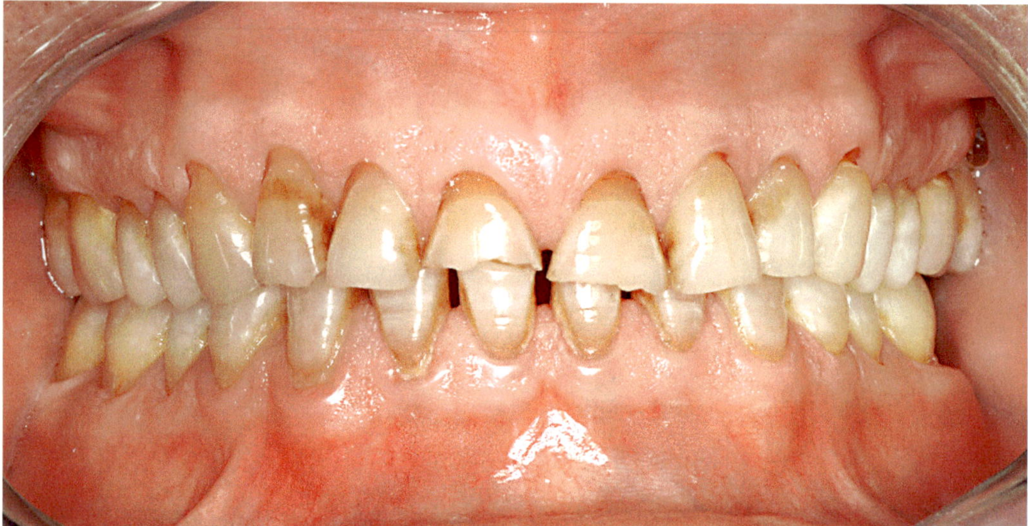

Fig 12-12 Non-carious cervical lesions (NCCLs) can be seen in almost all the teeth of this bruxer, who had a habit of sucking several lemons every day.

*Comment*
The conclusion to be drawn from the literature review is that the etiology of NCCLs is very complex and no specific mechanism can account for all the occurrences of these lesions. Obviously it is a multifactorial process, and the combined action of some or all of the factors we have mentioned leads to NCCL onset and progress.[32,58,67,77] Which of such factors plays the most decisive role remains a mystery. It is also possible that some factors might potentiate other(s), and that the predominance of some factors over the rest in each individual can account for the great morphologic variety these lesions present clinically. Thus, we suggest doing a thorough physical examination of those patients who present with NCCLs, in order to identify all the potential etiologic factors involved in the development and progress of these anomalies. Since most NCCLs present in young individuals, early diagnosis at a young age is very important.[36] The clinician should look for signs of acid in the oral cavity, test the quantity and quality of the saliva, control the methods of hygiene, and control bruxism. As for bruxism control, it is vital that canine guidance be restored, in order to avoid potential horizontal interference between the cusps of the posterior teeth; also a splint should be made for use during sleeping.

The terms "abrasion", "erosion", and "abfraction" each describe a specific etiologic mechanism to which NCCLs cannot be fully ascribed, so these lesions should still be called "NCCLs" until their true originating mechanism is accurately identified.

## Effects on Soft Tissues

### *Lingual Scalloping and Buccal Mucosa Ridging, or "Linea alba"*

Some authors consider that a scalloped tongue (one showing indentations on its lateral edge: Fig 12-13) and the presence of a jugal mucosa ridging or "linea alba" (Fig 12-14) are clear signs of bruxism.[78–82] They are even considered to be the two most reliable clinical signs of active bruxism, and they are caused by the force exerted by soft tissues against the surfaces of the teeth. These signs are said to regress once the parafunction stops.[83]

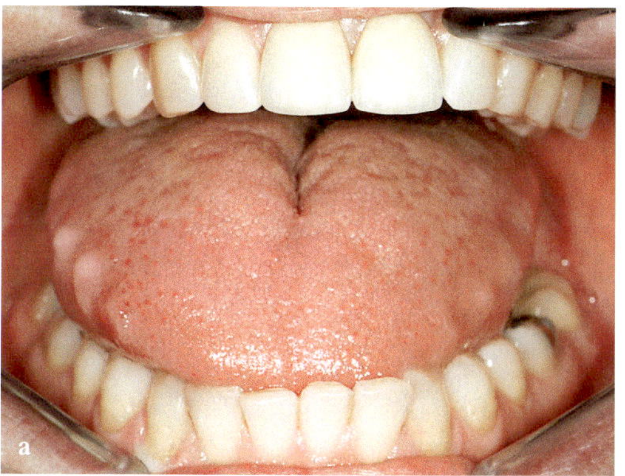
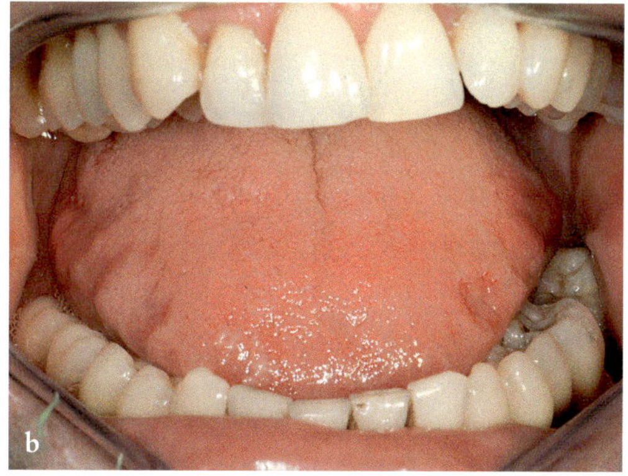

Fig 12-13 **(a and b)** Bruxers showing lingual scalloping.

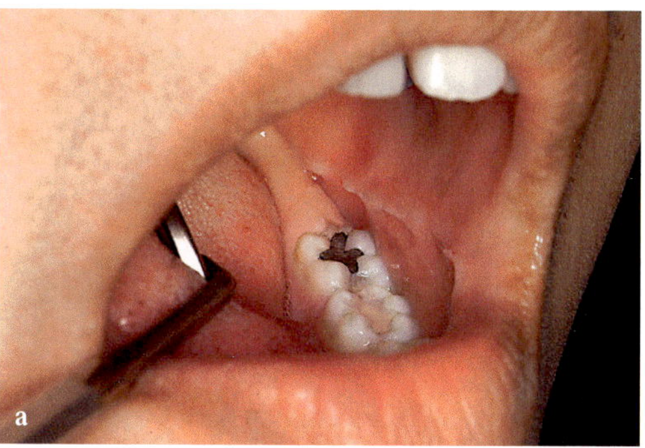
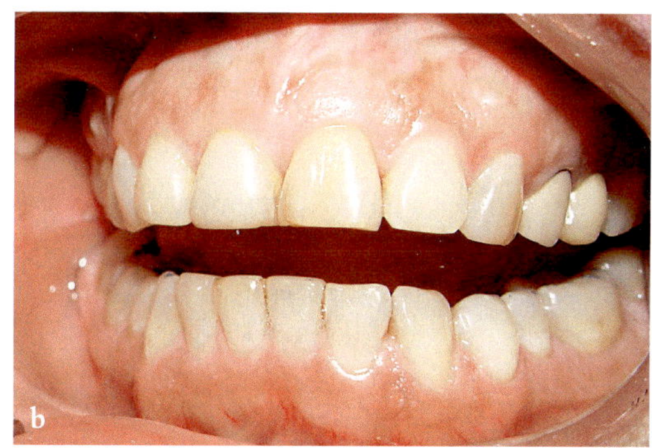

Fig 12-14 **(a and b)** Jugal mucosa ridging or "linea alba".

*Prevalence*

Tongue indentations (TI) have a prevalence of 75%; this value was obtained from a population of patients with periodontal disease. A sensitivity of 77% and a specificity of 75% were reported after correlating TIs with three indicators of tooth clenching (X-ray evidence of periodontal trauma, tooth mobility, and tooth-clenching awareness).[78] A study of a sample of individuals with a history of at least 5 years of active bruxism reported a linea alba prevalence of 58.6% and a TI prevalence of 41.4 %.[80]

It has also been suggested that lingual scalloping is likely to be caused by a vacuum effect created between the tongue and the palate during sustained tooth clenching. The author of this theory[81] claims that it is essential that lips be sealed in order for a vacuum to exist; from this, he infers that without such a vacuum, no tooth clenching would be possible. He suggests the use of a very simple device he developed himself. Such a device breaks the vacuum, thus preventing tooth clenching. Although this shows a powerful talent for invention, it has not been scientifically validated so far. Besides, the author suggests that this device be used during sleep, although it is known that tooth-clenching bruxism is typical of wakefulness and it represents only 11.4% of the total sleep bruxism.[84]

The study of a population of Japanese bank employees conducted in 1999 failed to prove the hypothesis that these two clinical signs are related to bruxism. The authors reported linea alba prevalence of 61.5% and TI prevalence of 51.2%.[85]

*Linea alba*

Linea alba is a whitish ridging or line which is parallel to the dental occlusion plane. It consists of hyperkeratinization of the jugal mucosal epithelium, and it will usually occur bilaterally.[86,87] As mentioned previously, some authors have related it to the pressure exerted by the cheek on the buccal surfaces of posterior teeth during bruxism; however, this mechanism has not been reliably demonstrated by research studies so far. With the aim of proving this hypothesis, Takagi and Sakurai[87] compared the pressure exerted by the cheeks of two groups of subjects with a full complement of teeth. One group included subjects with linea alba; the other group included subjects without linea alba (control group). The same levels of pressure were recorded for both groups during the 10-second maximum voluntary contraction of the teeth. However, the group of subjects with linea alba showed significant pressure increase during deglutition. These forces were higher than the ones recorded during maximum tooth clenching, and were not observed in the members of the control group. Based on these results, the authors ascribe linea alba formation to the forces exerted during deglutition, and not to tooth clenching.

*Tongue indentations*

TI affect both the upper and lower portions of the circumferential edge of the tongue.[88] In order to observe them, the patient is requested to open their mouth slightly and keep their tongue in a rest posture; otherwise, tongue protrusion would make the tongue increase in size, thus preventing TI visualization.

Some authors have ascribed the development of TIs to bruxism.[78,80,82,83] Others have suggested that TIs are caused by macroglossia secondary to systemic amyloid disease.[89,90] With the aim of solving this mystery, Yanagisawa and co-workers[88] studied a group of individuals with TIs and another group of individuals without TIs. In order to clarify the physiologic mechanism involved in TI development, they used a small sensor to measure the pressure exerted by the tongue during deglutition, during maximum voluntary contraction (MVC), during 10% MVC and, finally, for 10 minutes in the rest posture. They also obtained casts of both dental arches and the tongue, in order to obtain the tongue/arch width ratio. Both groups were found to exert the same pressures in all the tests conducted. A higher tongue/arch width ratio was found in the group of individuals with TIs. The authors rule out a potential relationship between lingual pressure and TI development, though they consider tongue size to be a factor in the development of indentations. Although their study is a great step forward in the search for evidence, to a certain extent it may be said to lack methodologic order. Since no data about the potential presence of bruxism in both study populations were obtained, the results of the study cannot be related to a potential parafunctional etiology, all the more so because the tongue is composed of muscle tissue, and thus the macroglossia observed in the group of subjects with TIs may result from tongue hypertrophy caused by tooth clenching. If this is the case, then TIs would be associated with bruxism. However, this is just mere speculation, since no data about the presence of bruxism were obtained in the study. Future research studies should consider the importance of obtaining such data in order to identify the (so far controversial) origin of TIs.

## Effects on Bone

### *Torus and Exostosis*

Torus and exostosis are asymptomatic bony outgrowths that occur in both jaws and consist of compact and cancellous bone. Their etiology remains highly controversial, bruxism being one of the factors under discussion. They have different names depending on their anatomic location inside the oral cavity, the most common ones being torus mandibularis (TM) and torus palatinus (TP).

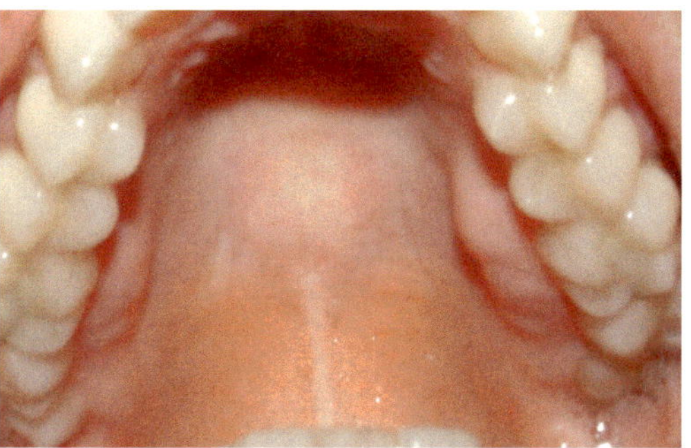

Fig 12-15 Palatal exostosis.

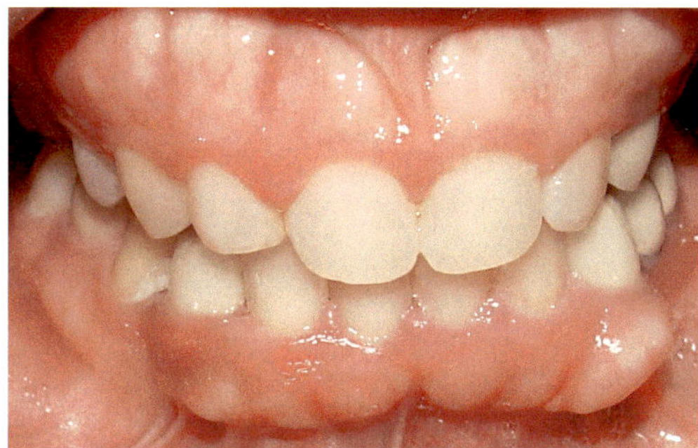

Fig 12-16 Bruxer showing vestibular exostosis maxillary and mandibular.

Mandibular tori occur in the lingual surface of the mandible, above the mylohyoid line and at the level of canines and premolars; palatal tori occur along the midline of the hard palate. Tori are variable in shape; they can be flat, spindle-shaped, lobulated, or nodular.[91] Flat tori are more common in the palate, while nodular tori prevail in the mandible.[92–96]

Though less common, so-called exostosis may be present. Exostoses consist of multiple bony-tissue nodules on the vestibular face of both jawbones (vestibular exostosis) or on the palatal face of the maxilla (palatal exostosis). Torus and exostosis have a similar histology.[97] They are composed of mature cancellous and compact bone and they both represent a benign hyperplasic process, which progresses slowly and gradually and is self-limiting.[98]

Usually, the fact that this process is asymptomatic causes patients to be unaware of its presence; however, tori may sometimes interfere with speech or mastication, and, when they are big, they may cause people with removable complete or partial dentures to experience settling problems and irritation. In these cases, torus removal is indicated. Although slow postoperative recurrence may occur, no malignant change has been reported as of now. Palatal exostoses may lead to periodontal surgery complications, because they interfere with mucoperiosteal flap repositioning.[99]

*Prevalence*

Torus and exostosis prevalence varies with age, race, and ethnicity, and the identification method used. The studies conducted directly on skeletal elements report higher prevalence than those conducted on patients. These differences have been ascribed to the fact that some outgrowths that are not very large may be masked by the fibromucosa covering, which renders their clinical identification difficult.[100] Haugen[101] claims that the lack of consensus on the use of the term "torus" in research studies is one of the reasons behind such discrepancies in prevalence.

For the sake of analysis of prevalence, it is essential to recognize that exostoses and tori are separate entities, and should be considered independently. Besides, palatal exostoses must be differentiated from vestibular exostoses, and mandibular tori must be differentiated from palatal tori.

*Palatal exostoses*

Palatal exostoses are frequently located at the level of the maxillary molars (Fig 12-15); prevalence has been reported to range between 8.1% and 56%.[99,100,102–104] The scant research studies conducted on patients have shown prevalence to be higher in men,[99,100,102] while other studies have failed to report on gender-related differences in prevalence owing

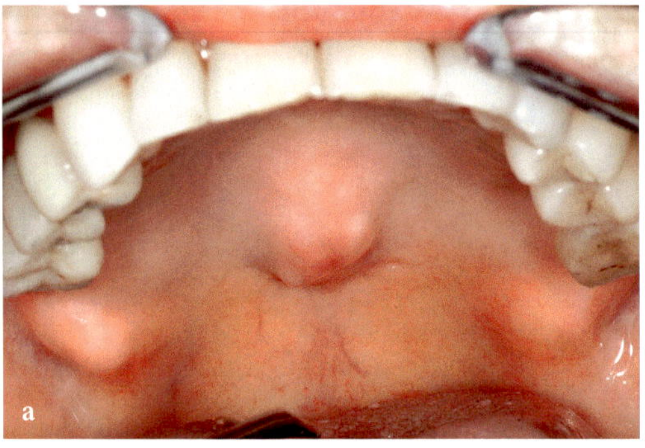


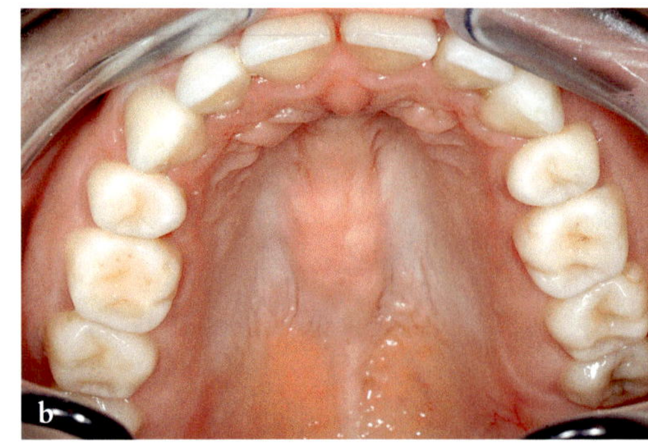


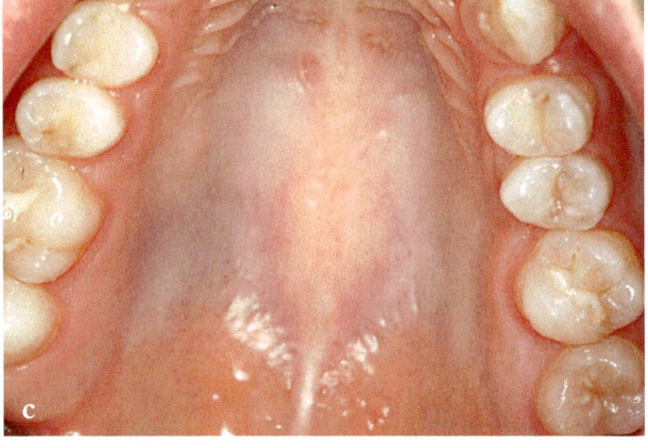


Fig 12-17 Torus palatinus: **(a)** nodular-shaped; **(b)** flat; **(c)** spindle-shaped.

to their having been conducted on specimens.[103,104] Small, nodular-shaped palatal exostoses have been reported to be the most common.[104]

*Vestibular exostoses*

Vestibular exostoses are nodular-type outgrowths occurring on the vestibular aspect of the maxilla and the mandible (Fig 12-16). They have been related to the presence of powerful masseters, excessive masticatory forces, and dental facets from bruxism.[105] Prevalence, which is higher in men than in women, has been reported to range between 0.09% and 18.8%,[100,106,107] and prevalence increases in direct proportion to age; also, they are more common in the maxilla than in the mandible.[100]

*Torus palatinus*

Woo[108] described the torus palatinus as a widening of the palatal midline and of the corresponding portion of the nasal floor (Fig 12-17) composed of cancellous bone covered by a layer of compact bone. Prevalence ranges between 0.4% and 66.5%.[92,94,99,101,108–118]

Though most of the studies report a higher prevalence in women,[94,99,101,111,112,115,117,119–123] other studies have reported a higher prevalence in men.[99,109,118]

*Torus mandibularis*

Mandibular tori are outgrowths on the lingual aspect of the mandible and are usually symmetric rather than unilateral (Fig 12-18).[101,111,115,122] Like palatal tori, they have a wide ranging prevalence – between 0.5% and 63.4%.[94,99,101,109,111,113–115,117,118,123] Some publications agree that the most common type of mandibular torus is the nodular single torus.[97,101,111,115] Most research studies agree that they are more common in men;[101,109,115,117,121,122,124,125] however, they have also been reported to be more common in women.[126] Other authors have found them to occur equally in people of either sex.[92,96,111,127]

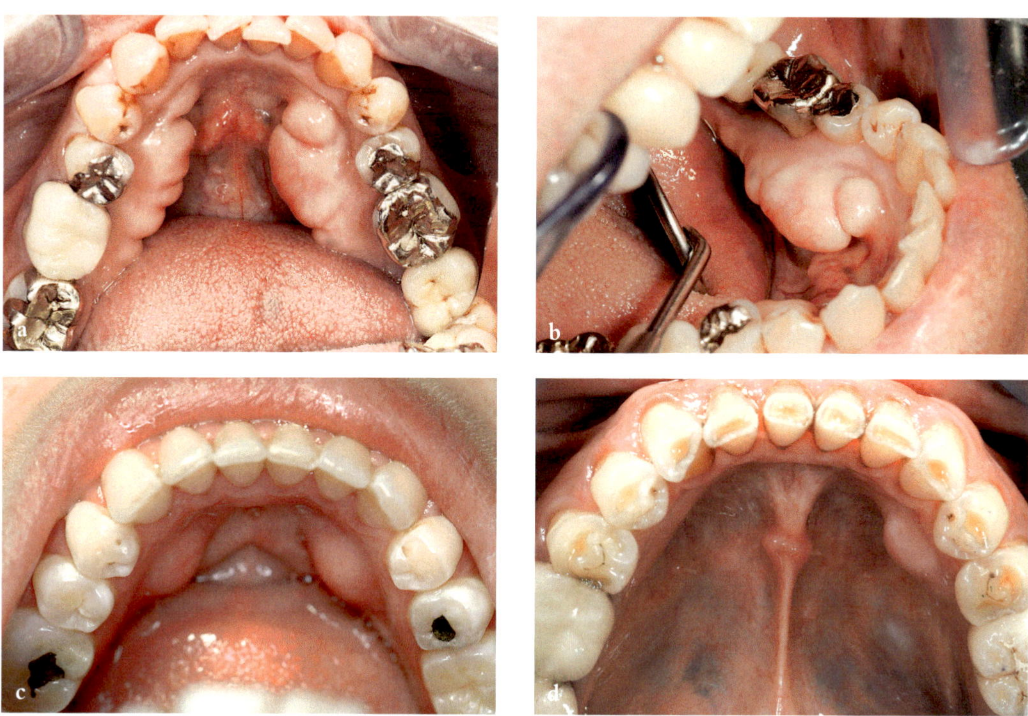

Fig 12-18 Torus mandibularis: **(a and b)** bilateral, nodular; **(c)** bilateral, lobulated; **(d)** unilateral, lobulated.

Race seems to be a factor which determines torus prevalence significantly; the highest prevalence is found in Eskimos and Asians.[108,113–115,117,128]

The presence of tori in children is considered to be an oddity,[108,123] since they occur in patients around the age of 30.[111,112,120]

Although palatal and mandibular tori may coexist in some patients, this is rare.[101,111,119] Also, some case reports describe subjects with both tori and exostoses.[95,100,129,130] Some authors have suggested that these cases should be considered to be a "multiple exostoses syndrome".[100,104]

*Etiology*

Several hypotheses have been proposed with the aim of determining the potential cause of exostoses. Genetics,[131,132] the environment,[124,125] and masticatory stress have been suggested.[125,132–134] Some authors agree to ascribe exostoses to an interplay of these factors combined with a threshold susceptibility existing in certain individuals.[101,119] That these bony outgrowths are not congenital, are very rare in children,[108] and age at presentation is around 30 years suggests that certain environmental factors (masticatory function and parafunction) may be involved in the etiology of exostoses. In the Eskimos, a powerful jaw with highly developed muscles, combined with a high prevalence of tori, reflect a strong association with functional demands, since Eskimos chew very tough food (e.g., skins, bones, dried meat). Also, the important role of functional forces in the development of mandibular tori has been shown; these tori are more common in individuals with a greater number of teeth, and when the number of teeth decreases in old age, the number of tori decreases too.[134] However, Reichart and co-workers[115] have reported the presence of tori in patients without any teeth and patients with some remaining teeth.

Suzuki and Sakai[131] suggested that a hereditary factor may potentially be involved in exostosis, since one or both parents of 85% of children with palatal tori will show the same problem. Haugen[101] considers tori to be a dynamic process resulting from genetic factors, environmental factors, and functional factors (masticatory stress particularly) acting in combination throughout life.

Even more significant than masticatory forces are parafunctional forces, since they may double the MVC force. A study of two populations (one of bruxers and another of non-bruxers) by using a quasi-continual mathematical model showed a potential relationship between tori and bruxism. The report concludes that genetic factors account for 30% and occlusal stress for 70% of TM's etiology.[132] The author suggests that in order for tori to remain throughout time, teeth should be present. In tune with this theory, mandibular tori have been reported to have disappeared 5–7 months after the extraction of teeth.[135] A phenomenon similar to tori sometimes is seen in edentulous areas of the mouth, under the pontics: the so-called "subpontic hyperostosis".[136] Subpontic hyperostoses will usually occur in the posterior sector of the mandible, and they will spontaneously regress after bridge removal. Although the etiology of subpontic hyperostosis has not been scientifically identified, one hypothesis suggests that it results from the increased functional stress exerted on the bone through the pillars.[137] Evidently, this factor is similar to one of the factors considered to be involved in the development of tori.[134]

A study conducted in Thailand found a strong relationship between presence of mandibular tori and tooth clenching and/or grinding. Besides, the authors of this study agree with other authors[101,119] that tori may have a multifactorial etiology: genetic and environmental factors plus bruxism and certain diets may contribute to torus development in those patients with a predisposing threshold level.[117] Matthews[105] found a significant association between tooth wear and torus occurrence. This association has also been reported by other authors.[115,117,122] Jainkittivong and Langlais[100] mention that the association between exostosis and dental attrition is on the rise, and they suggest that there is a chance that occlusal hyperfunction might boost the occurrence of exostosis in subjects with a genetic predisposition.

However, other researchers have failed to prove an association with bruxism. A study reported no significant correlation between occlusal load signs (attrition and periodontal widening) and the presence of vestibular exostosis.[107] On comparing a group of patients with TMD with a control group, other authors found bruxism and mandibular torus prevalence to be higher among the members of the first group; however, palatal torus prevalence was similar in both groups.[93] In accordance with this last research study, a significant increase in the occurrence of mandibular tori in patients with TMD has also been reported.[126] However, TMD are not synonymous with bruxism, since not all patients with TMD develop bruxism, and vice versa.

Once more, the lack of consensus among the different research studies suggests the multifactorial nature of the etiology of tori and exostoses. Undoubtedly, bruxism is one of the most important factors. Lastly, it should be remembered that tori are not to be considered strict signs of bruxism; their presence should be considered as a warning signal that further research of signs and symptoms should be undertaken in order to identify parafunction.[117]

### Coronoid Process Elongation

Primary bilateral coronoid process hyperplasia (CPH) is a rare condition characterized by an abnormal bony elongation that will gradually and progressively cause mouth-opening restrictions. Such restrictions occur because the coronoid process impinges on the inner aspect of the zygomatic arch. Fewer than 100 cases, most of them bilateral and occurring in males, have been reported in the literature. A survey of 2,000 panoramic radiographs reported a prevalence of 0.5%.[138] Nevertheless, higher values were reported by Isberg and co-workers,[139] who studied a sample of consecutive patients with jaw-movement restrictions and found that 5% of them suffered from CPH.

Initial presentation generally occurs at the beginning of puberty, the typical symptom being the painless limitation of jaw movements. The professional may attempt to force the movement with his or her fingers, but to no avail; the feeling that there is a rigid stop can be perceived. CPH can be unilateral or bilateral; unilateral CPH usually is a sequel of trauma, TMJ ankylosis, osteochondroma, or exostosis, and it is usually associated with facial asymmetry. In a review of the literature, Nickerson and co-workers[140] found that 15 out of 19 unilateral CPH cases corresponded to osteochondromas and exostoses.

Surgical excision of coronoid processes is the first-line treatment; histologically, such coronoid processes are characterized by an overgrowth of normal mature bone, with an occasional osteosclerotic or fibrocartilaginous component – which should not be considered to be a sign of neoplastic growth.[141]

Several theories on pathogenesis have been proposed; for example, persistence of the epiphyseal plate,[142] genetic inheritance,[143] mandibular hypomobility,[144] TMJ dysfunction,[139] hormonal factors,[145] and temporalis muscle hyperactivity.[146] Owing to its relationship with bruxism, we will analyze temporalis muscle hyperactivity in detail. The temporalis-muscle hyperactivity hypothesis was first proposed in 1951 by Sarnat and Engel,[147] who ascribed such hyperactivity to temporalis muscle traction; this hypothesis was later supported by others.[139,146,148,149] According to Isberg and Elliasson,[150] it is important to differentiate between a congenital form and an acquired form; the latter is characterized by a mandibular hypomobility period related to the TMJ pathology. These researchers suggest that a hypomobility period combined with the traction exerted by the temporalis muscle – which would lead to reactive bone hyperplasia – will result in CPH. This hypothesis is based on experiments with monkeys; these animals showed coronoid-process elongation secondary to TMJ ankylosis.[151] An example of this is provided in Figure 12-19: a child with congenital TMJ ankylosis shows significant CPH on the ipsilateral side.

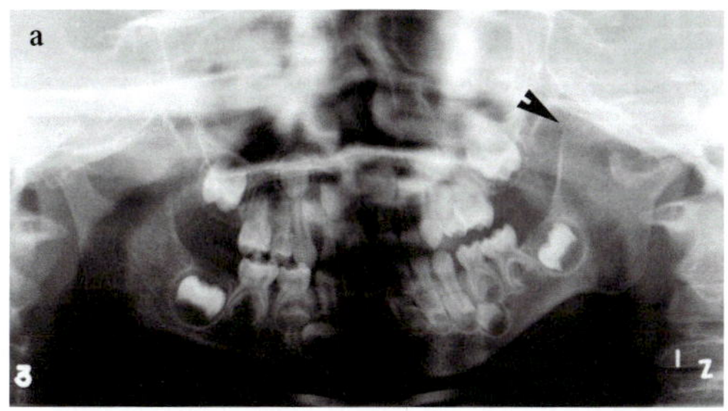

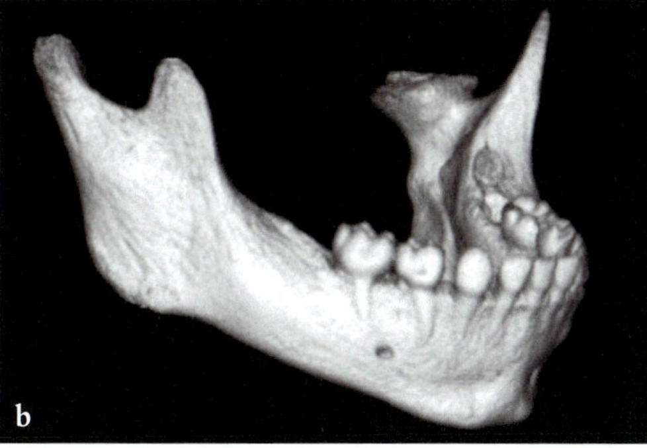

Fig 12-19 **(a)** Panoramic radiograph of a child with left temporomandibular joint disorder (TMJ) ankylosis. There is marked elongation of the coronoid process (arrow). **(b)** Computed tomography showing the elongation of the coronoid process in more detail.

Hohl and co-workers' experiments[151] were later replicated by another group of researchers, who experimentally induced mandibular hypomobility in monkeys. Such hypomobility resulted in elongation of the coronoid process and bone deposition in the gonial angle region.[144] In this study, the authors suggest that the continuous traction

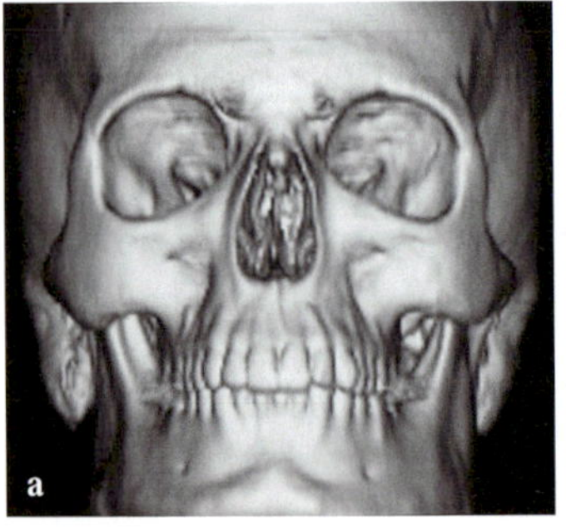


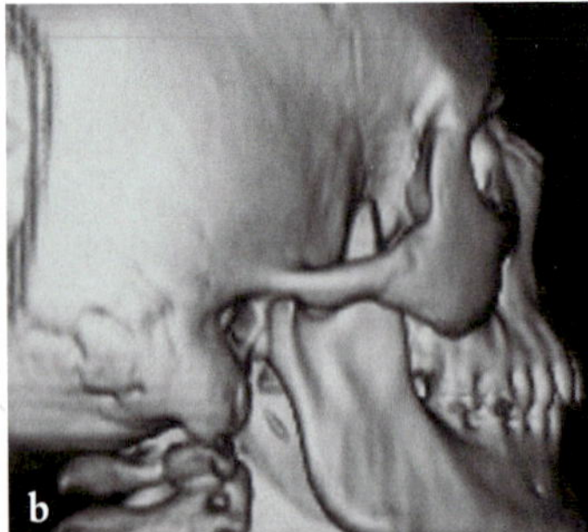


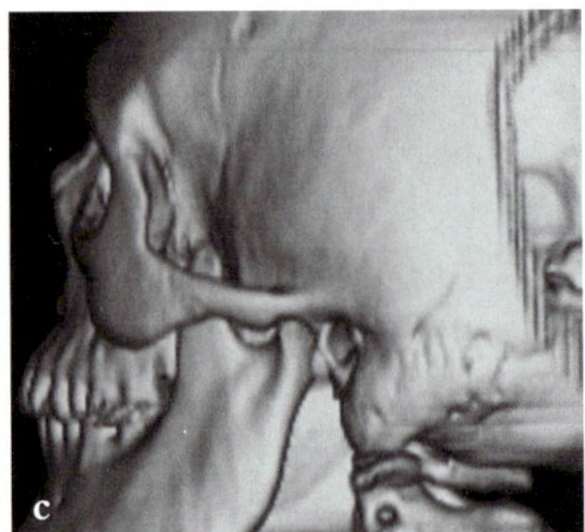


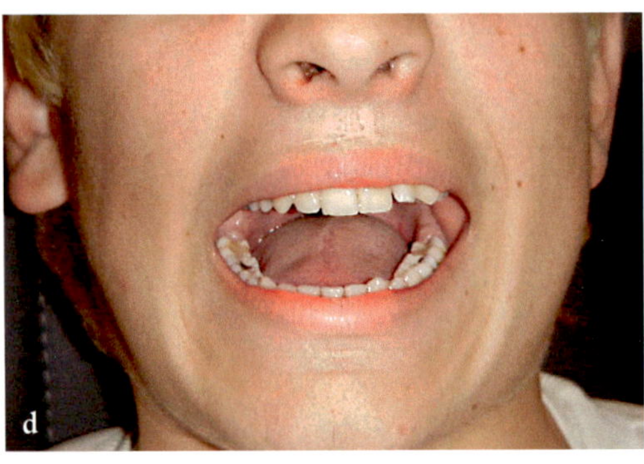


Fig 12-20 **(a)** Computed tomography showing a bruxer's square jaw. **(b and c)** Elongation of both coronoid processes. **(d)** Mouth-opening limitation as a result of coronoid-process impingement on the zygomatic arch.

exerted by the temporalis muscle is likely to alter blood flow in the area of the tendinous insertion in the coronoid process, which will result in a degenerative process, with subsequent calcium deposition in the tendon and development of reactive bone hyperplasia.

Later, Murakami and co-workers[149] suggested that patients with CPH associated with square jaw morphology should be included in a different subgroup. After studying a series of patients with a long history of hypomobility, coronoid process, and mandibular angle hyperplasia, and masseter and temporalis muscle contracture (Fig 12-20), the authors suggest that coronoid process and mandibular angle overgrowth is likely to result from a significant, prolonged masseter and temporalis muscle contraction. They disagree with Isberg and Elliasson's suggestion from 1990,[150] since they do not consider CPH to result from hypomobility secondary to sustained contracture of the levator muscles. Despite their different opinions, the reports of all these authors have two points in common: (a) patients with square jaw morphology, and (b) coronoid process overgrowth due to temporalis muscle overcontraction. Thus, since both (a) and (b) can easily be ascribable to bruxism, diagnostic considerations should include bruxism.

Nevertheless, the low prevalence of CPH associated with tooth-clenching bruxism puts the fact that the latter can be a potential CPH etiology factor into doubt. However, the possibility that other factors associated with tooth-clenching bruxism may be involved should not be dismissed. Most publications agree that the likelihood of CPH recurrence after surgical removal is high. This may suggest certain genetic predisposition in some subjects. The fact that CPH was found in two pairs of siblings led some authors to consider genetic inheritance to be an etiology factor.[143,152] Recurrence, however, may be prevented by following a mouth-opening elongation and parafunction-control exercise program.[149]

Future controlled research studies should elucidate the role of sustained tooth clenching in the development of CPH.

## References


1. Richardson ME. Late lower arch crowding in relation to skeletal and dental morphology and growth changes. Br J Orthod 1996;23:249–254.
2. Richardson ME. The aetiology of late lower arch crowding alternative to mesially directed forces: a review. Am J Orthod 1994;105:592–597.
3. Brunsvold MA. Pathologic tooth migration. J Periodontol 2005;76:859–866.
4. Carranza FA. Occlusal trauma. In: Carranza FA (ed). Glickman's Clinical Periodontology. Philadelphia: WB Saunders, 1990:284–306.
5. Martinez-Canut P, Carrasquer A, Magan R, Lorca A. A study on factors associated with pathologic tooth migration. J Clin Periodontol 1997;24:492–497.
6. Hirschfeld L, Greiger A. Etiologic factors of tooth malposition. In: Hirschfeld L, Geiger A (eds). Minor Tooth Movement in General Practice. St Louis, MO: CV Mosby, 1974:78–139.
7. Marks M, Levit HL. Etiology of adult tooth malposition. In: Marks MH, Corn H (eds). Atlas of Adult Orthodontics. Philadelphia: Lea & Febiger, 1989:57–58.
8. Southard TE, Southard KA, Tolley EA. Periodontal force: a potential cause of relapse. Am J Orthod 1992;101: 221–227.
9. Abboud M, Grüner M, Koeck B. Anterior crowding: just an esthetic problem. J Orofac Orthop 2002;63:264–273.
10. Osborn JW. An investigation into the interdental forces occurring between the teeth of the same arch during clenching of the jaws. Arch Oral Biol 1961;5:202–211.
11. Picton DCA. Tilting movements of teeth during biting. Arch Oral Biol 1962;7:151–159.
12. Southard TE, Beherents RG, Tolley EA. The anterior component of occlusal force. 1: Measurement and distribution. Am J Orthod 1989;96:493–500.
13. Southard TE, Southard KA, Stiles RN. Factors influencing the anterior component of occlusal force. J Biomech 1990;23:1199–1207.
14. Oh SH, Nakano M, Bando E, Shigemoto S, Kori M. Evaluation of proximal tooth contact tightness at rest and during clenching. J Oral Rehabil 2004;31:538–545.
15. Klatzky M. Masticatory stresses and their relation to dental caries. J Dent Res 1942;21:387–390.
16. Nishigawa K, Bando E, Nakano M. Quantitative study of bite force during sleep associated bruxism. J Oral Rehabil 2001;28:485–491.
17. Southard TE, Beherents RG, Tolley EA. The anterior component of occlusal force. 2: Relationship with dental malalignment. Am J Orthod 1990;97:41–44.
18. Acar A, Alcan T, Erverdi N. Evaluation of the relationship between the anterior component of occlusal force and postretention crowding. Am J Orthod 2002;122:336–370.
19. Picton DCA. Distortion of the jaws during biting. Arch Oral Biol 1962;7:573–580.
20. Koriot TWP, Hannam AG. Deformation of the human mandible during simulated tooth clenching. J Dent Res 1994;73:56–66.
21. Gates GN, Nicholls JI. Evaluation of mandibular arch width change. J Prosthet Dent 1981;46:385–392.
22. Dörfer CE, von Bethlenfalvy ER, Staehle HJ, Pioch T. Factors influencing proximal dental contact strengths. Eur J Oral Sci 2000;108:368–377.
23. Jiang T, Ai M. In-vivo mandibular elastic deformation during clenching on pivots. J Oral Rehabil 2002;29: 201–208.
24. Hidaka O, Iwasaki M, Saito M, Morimoto T. Influence of clenching intensity on bite force balance, occlusal contact area, and average bite pressure. J Dent Res 1999;78: 1336–1344.
25. Kikuchi M, Korioth TWP, Hannam AG. The association among occlusal contacts, clenching effort, and bite force distribution in man. J Dent Res 1997;76:1316–1325.
26. Young WG, Khan F. Sites of dental erosion are salivary dependent. J Oral Rehabil 2002;29:35–43.
27. Bevenius J, L'Estrange P, Karlsson S, Carlsson GE. Idiopathic cervical lesions: in vivo investigation by oral microendoscopy and scanning electron microscopy. A pilot study. J Oral Rehabil 1993;20:1–9.
28. Khan F, Young WG, Shahabi S, Daley TJ. Dental cervical lesions associated with occlusal erosion and attrition. Aust Dent J 1999;44:176–186.
29. Brady JM, Woody RD. Scanning microscopy of cervical erosion. J Am Dent Assoc 1977;94:726–729.
30. Absi E, Addy M, Adams D. Dentine hypersensitivity. The development and evaluation of a replica technique to study sensitive and non-sensitive cervical dentine. J Clin Periodontol 1989;16:190–195.
31. Bergström J, Lavstedt S. An epidemiologic approach to toothbrushing and dental abrasion. Community Dent Oral Epidemiol 1979;7:57–64.
32. Levitch LC, Bader JD, Shugars DA, Heymann HO. Non-carious cervical lesions. J Dent 1994;22:195–207.
33. Piotrowski BT, Gillette WB, Hancock EB. Examining the prevalence and characteristics of abfractionlike cervical lesions in a population of US veterans. J Am Dent Assoc 2001;132:1694–1701.
34. Aw TC, Lepe X, Johnson GH, Mancl L. Characteristics of noncarious cervical lesions: a clinical investigation. J Am Dent Assoc 2002;133:725–733.
35. Oginni AO, Olusile AO, Udoye CI. Non-carious cervical lesions in a Nigerian population: abrasion or abfraction? Int Dent J 2003;53:275–279.
36. Borcic J, Anic I, Urek MM, Ferreri S. The prevalence of non-carious cervical lesions in permanent dentition. J Oral Rehabil 2004;31:117–123.

37. Bernhardt O, Gesch D, Schwahn C et al. Epidemiological evaluation of the multifactorial aetiology of abfractions. J Oral Rehabil 2006;33:17–25.
38. Padbury AD, Ash MM. Abrasion caused by three methods of toothbrushing. J Periodontol 1974;45:434–438.
39. Sangnes G, Gjermo P. Prevalence of oral soft and hard tissue lesions related to mechanical toothcleansing procedures. Community Dent Oral Epidemiol 1976;4:77–83.
40. Lussi A, Schaffner M, Hotz P, Suster P. Epidemiology and risk factors of wedge-shaped defects in a Swiss population. Schweiz Monatsschr Zahnmed 1993;103:276–280.
41. Meister F, Braun RJ, Gerstein H. Endodontic involvement resulting from dental abrasion or erosion. J Am Dent Assoc 1980;101:651–653.
42. Dyer D, Addy M, Newcombe RG. Studies in vitro of abrasion by different manual toothbrush heads and standard toothpaste. J Clin Periodontol 2000;27:99–103.
43. Litonjua LA, Andreana S, Bush PJ, Tobias TS, Cohen RE. Wedged cervical lesions produced by toothbrushing. Am J Dent 2004;17:237–240.
44. Radentz WH, Barnes GP, Cutright DE. A survey of factors possibly associated with cervical abrasion of tooth surfaces. J Periodontol 1976;47:148–154.
45. Saxton CA, Cowell CR. Clinical investigation of the effects of dentifrices on dentin wear at the cementoenamel junction. J Am Dent Assoc 1981;102:38–43.
46. Svinnseth PN, Gjerdet NR, Lie T. Abrasivity of toothpastes. An in-vitro study of toothpastes marketed in Norway. Acta Odontol Scand 1987;45:195–202.
47. Joiner A, Pickles MJ, Tanner C, Weader E, Doyle P. An in-situ model to study the toothpaste abrasion of enamel. J Clin Periodontol 2004;31:434–438.
48. Miller N, Penaud J, Ambrosini P, Bisson-Boutelliez C, Briancon S. Analysis of etiologic factors and periodontal conditions involved with 309 abfractions. J Clin Periodontol 2003;30:828–832.
49. Bergström J, Eliasson S. Cervical abrasion in relation to toothbrushing and periodontal health. Scand J Dent Res 1988;96:405–411.
50. Lee WC, Eakle WS. Possible role of tensile stress in the etiology of cervical erosive lesions of the teeth. J Prosthet Dent 1984;52:374–380.
51. Stroner WF. Cervical erosion involving the lingual surface of a mandibular canine and adjacent premolars. J Am Dent Assoc 1983;107:256–260.
52. Braem M, Lambrechts P, Vanherle G. Stress-induced cervical lesions. J Prosthet Dent 1992;67:718–722.
53. Burke FJ, Whitehead SA, McCaughey AD. Contemporary concepts in the pathogenesis of the class V noncarious lesion. Dent Update 1995;22:28–32.
54. Ott RW, Proschel P. Etiology of wedge-shaped defects: a function-analytical, epidemiologic and experimental study. Dtsch Zahnarztl Z 1985;40:1223–1227.
55. Xonga FA. Bruxism and its effect on the teeth. J Oral Rehabil 1977;4:65–76.
56. McCoy G. The etiology of gingival erosion. J Oral Implantol 1982;10:361–362.
57. Grippo JO. Abfractions: a new classification of hard tissue lesions of teeth. J Esthet Dent 1991;3:14–19.
58. Grippo JO, Simring M. Dental erosion revisited. J Am Dent Assoc 1995;126:619–630.
59. Rees JS, Hammadeh M, Jagger DC. Abfraction lesion formation in maxillary incisors, canines and premolars: a finite element study. Eur J Oral Sci 2003;111:149–154.
60. Rees JS, Hammadeh M. Undermining of enamel as a mechanism of abfraction lesion formation: a finite element study. Eur J Oral Sci 2004;112:347–352.
61. Rees JS. The role of cuspal flexure in the development of abfraction lesions: a finite element study. Eur J Oral Sci 1998;106:1028–1032.
62. Geramy A, Sharafoddin F. Abfraction: 3D analysis by means of the finite element method. Quintessence Int 2003;34:526–533.
63. Litonjua LA, Andreana S, Patra AK, Cohen RE. An assessment of stress analyses in the theory of abfraction. Biomed Mater Eng 2004;14:311–321.
64. Litonjua LA, Bush PJ, Andreana S, Tobias TS. Effects of occlusal load on cervical lesions. J Oral Rehabil 2004;31: 225–232.
65. Heymann HO, Sturdevant JR, Bayne S et al. Examining tooth flexure effects on cervical restorations: a two-year clinical study. J Am Dent Assoc 1991;122:41–47.
66. Schiller R, Marquardt E, Albers HK. Connection between the polished occlusal facets and pathological findings in the masticatory system of young adults. ZWR 1985;94: 228–232.
67. Bader JD, McClure F, Scurria MS, Shugars DA, Heymann HO. Case-control study of non-carious cervical lesions. Community Dent Oral Epidemiol 1996;24:286–291.
68. Mayhew RB, Jessee SA, Martin RE. Association of occlusal, periodontal, and dietary factors with the presence of noncarious cervical dental lesions. Am J Dent 1998;11:29–32.
69. Telles D, Pegoraro LF, Pereira JC. Prevalence of noncarious cervical lesions and their relation to occlusal aspects: a clinical study. J Esthet Dent 2000;12:10–15.
70. Heymann HO. Future restorative needs in the light of tooth biodynamics. In: First International ESPE Dental Symposium. Munich, 1998.
71. Estafan A, Furnari PC, Goldstein G, Hittelman EL. In-vivo correlation of noncarious cervical lesions and occlusal wear. J Prosthet Dent 2005;93:221–226.
72. Pintado MR, DeLong R, Ko C, Sakaguchi RL, Douglas WH. Correlation of noncarious cervical lesion size and occlusal wear in a single adult over a 14-year time span. J Prosthet Dent 2000;84:436–443.
73. Lussi A, Schaffner M. Progression and risk factors for dental erosion and wedge-shaped defects over a 6-year period. Caries Res 2000;34:182–187.
74. Whitehead SA, Wilson NH, Watts DC. Development of noncarious cervical notch lesions in vitro. J Esthet Dent 1999;11:332–337.

75. Grippo JO, Masi JV. Role of biodental engineering factors (BEF) in the etiology of root caries. J Esthet Dent 1991;3:71–76.
76. Kelly MP, Smith BGH. The effect of remineralizing solutions on tooth wear in vitro. J Dent 1988;16:147–149.
77. Spranger H. Investigation into the genesis of angular lesions at the cervical region of the teeth. Quintessence Int 1995;26:149–154.
78. Sapiro SM. Tongue indentations as an indicator of clenching. Clin Prev Dent 1992;14:21–24.
79. Crispian S, Stephen RF, Stephen RP. Oral Diseases, ed 2. Singapore Toppan Printing Co.: 1966:217.
80. Kampe T, Tagdae T, Bader G, Edman G, Karlsson S. Reported symptoms and clinical findings in a group of subjects with longstanding bruxing behavior. J Oral Rehabil 1997;24:581–587.
81. Long JH. A device to prevent jaw clenching. J Prosthet Dent 1998;79:353–354.
82. Miller VJ, Yoeli Z, Barnea E, Zeltser C. The effect of parafunction on condylar asymmetry in patients with temporomandibular disorders. J Oral Rehabil 1998;25: 721–724.
83. Gray RJM, Davies SJ, Quayle AA. A clinical approach to temporomandibular disorders. 3: Examination of the articulatory system: the muscles. Br Dent J 1994;177: 25–28.
84. Lavigne GJ, Rompre PH, Montplaisir JY. Sleep bruxism: validity of clinical research diagnosis criteria in a controlled polysomnographic study. J Dent Res 1996;75: 546–552.
85. Piquero K, Ando T, Sakurai K. Buccal mucosa ridging and tongue indentation: incidence and associated factors. Bull Tokyo Dent Coll 1999;40:71–78.
86. Gary CC, John FN. Principles of Oral Diagnosis. MO: Mosby–Yearbook, 1993:64.
87. Takagi I, Sakurai K. Investigation of the factors related to the formation of the buccal ridging. J Oral Rehabil 2003;30:565–572.
88. Yanagisawa K, Takagi I, Sakurai K. Influence of tongue pressure and width on tongue indentation formation. J Oral Rehabil 2007;34:827–834.
89. Falk RH, Comenzo RL, Skinner M. The systemic amyloidoses. N Engl J Med 1997;337:898–909.
90. Rogers AJ, Bruce AJ. The tongue in clinical diagnosis. J Eur Acad Dermatol Venereol 2004;18:254–259.
91. Thoma KH. Oral Pathology, ed 3. St Louis: CV Mosby, 1950:1336.
92. Gorsky M, Raviv M, Kfir E, Moskona D. Prevalence of torus palatinus in a population of young and adult Israelis. Arch Oral Biol 1996;41:623–625.
93. Sirirungrojying S, Kerdpon D. Relationship between oral tori and temporomandibular disorders. Int Dent J 1999; 49:101–104.
94. Austin JE, Radford GH, Banks SO. Palatal and mandibular tori in the Negro. N Y State Dent J 1965;31:187–191.
95. Antoniades DZ, Delazi M, Papanayiotou P. Concurrence of torus palatinus with palatal and buccal exostosis: a case report and review of the literature. Oral Surg Oral Med Oral Pathol Oral Radiol Endod 1998;85:552–557.
96. Al Quran FA, Al-Dwairi ZN. Torus palatinus and torus mandibularis in edentulous patients. J Contemp Dent Pract 2006;7:112–119.
97. Neville BW, Damm DD, Allen CM, Bouquot JE (eds). Oral and Maxillofacial Pathology. Philadelphia: WB Saunders, 1995:17–20.
98. Regezi JA, Sciubba JJ. Oral pathology: clinico-pathologic correlations. Philadelphia: WB Saunders, 1989:386–387.
99. Sonnier KE, Horning GM, Cohen ME. Palatal tubercles, palatal tori, and mandibular tori: prevalence and anatomical features in a U.S. population. J Periodontol 1999;70: 329–336.
100. Jainkittivong A, Langlais RP. Buccal and palatal exostoses: prevalence and concurrence with tori. Oral Surg Oral Med Oral Pathol 2000;90:48–53.
101. Haugen LK. Palatine and mandibular tori: a morphologic study in the current Norwegian population. Acta Odontol Scand 1992;50:65–77.
102. Touyz LZ, Tau S. Frequency and distribution of palatal osseous alveolar marginal exostoses-POAMES. J Dent Assoc S Afr 1991;46:471–473.
103. Larato DC. Palatal exostoses of the posterior maxillary alveolar process. J Periodontol 1972;43:486–489.
104. Nery EB, Corn H, Eisenstein IL. Palatal exostosis in the molar region. J Periodontol 1977;48:663–666.
105. Matthews GP. Mandibular and palatine tori and their etiology. J Dent Res 1933;13:245 (abstract).
106. Bouquot JE, Gundlach KKH, Morgantown W. Oral exophytic lesions in 23,616 white Americans over 35 years of age. Oral Surg Oral Med Oral Pathol 1986;62:284–291.
107. Horning G, Cohen ME, Neils TA. Buccal alveolar exostoses: prevalence, characteristics, and evidence for buttressing bona formation. J Periodontol 2000;71: 1032–1042.
108. Woo JK. Torus palatinus. Am J Phys Anthropol 1950;8: 81–111.
109. Hrdlicka A. Mandibular and maxillary hyperostoses. Am J Phys Anthropol 1940;27:1–67.
110. Miller SC, Roth H. Torus palatinus: a statistical study. J Am Dent Assoc 1940;27:1950–1957.
111. Kolas S, Halperin V, Jefferis K, Huddleston S, Robinson HBG. The occurrence of torus palatinus and torus mandibularis in 2,478 dental patients. Oral Surg Oral Med Oral Pathol 1953;6:1134–1141.
112. King DR, Moore GE. The prevalence of torus palatinus. J Oral Med 1971;26:113–115.
113. Yaacob H, Tirmzi H, Ismail K. The prevalence of oral tori in Malaysians. J Oral Med 1983;38:40–42.
114. Chew CL, Tan PH. Torus palatinus: a clinical study. Aust Dent J 1984;29:245–248.
115. Reichart PA, Neuhaus F, Sookasem M. Prevalence of torus palatinus and torus mandibularis in Germans and Thai. Community Dent Oral Epidemiol 1988;16:61–64.

116. Naidich TP, Valente M, Abrams K, Spreitzer JJ, Doundoulakis SH. Torus palatinus. Int J Neuroradiol 1997;3:229–243.
117. Kerdpon D, Sirirungrojying S. A clinical study of oral tori in southern Thailand: prevalence and the relation to parafunctional activity. Eur J Oral Sci 1999;107:9–13.
118. Bernaba JM. Morphology and incidence of torus palatinus and mandibularis in Brazilian Indians. J Dent Res 1977;56:499–501.
119. Eggen S, Natvig B. Concurrence of torus mandibularis and torus palatinus. Scand J Dent Res 1994;102:60–63.
120. Vidic B. Incidence of torus palatinus in Yugoslav skulls. J Dent Res 1966;45:1511–1515.
121. Jainkittivong A, Apinhasmit W, Swasdison S. Prevalence and clinical characteristics of oral tori in 1520 Chulalongkorn University dental school patients. Surg Radiol Anat 2007;29:125–131.
122. Apinhasmit W, Jainkittivong A, Swasdison S. Torus palatinus and torus mandibularis in a Thai population. Sc Asia 2002;28:105–111.
123. Shah DS, Sanghavi SJ, Chawda JD, Shah RM. Prevalence of torus palatinus and torus mandibularis in 1000 patients. Indian J Dent Res 1992;3:107–110.
124. Eggen S, Natvig B. Variation in torus mandibularis prevalence in Norway: a statistical analysis using logistic regression. Community Dent Oral Epidemiol 1991;19:32–35.
125. Ossenberg NS. Mandibular torus: a synthesis of new and previously reported data and discussion of its cause. In: Cybulski JS (ed). Contributions to Physical Anthropology 1978–1980. Otawa: National Museum of Canada, 1981: 1–52.
126. Clifford T, Lamey PJ, Fartash L. Mandibular tori, migraine and temporomandibular disorders. Br Dent J 1996;180:382–384.
127. Belsky JL, Hamer JS, Hubert JE, Isogna K, Johns W. Torus palatinus: a new anatomical correlation with bone density in postmenopausal women. J Clin Endocrinol Metab 2003;88:2081–2086.
128. Moorrees CFA, Osborne RH, Wilde E. Torus mandibularis: its occurrence in Aleut children and its genetic determinants. Am J Phys Anthropol 1952;10:319–329.
129. Blackemore JR, Eller DJ, Tomaro AJ. Maxillary exostoses: surgical management of an unusual case. Oral Surg Oral Med Oral Pathol Oral Radiol Endod 1975;40:200–204.
130. Topazian DS, Mullen FR. Continued growth of a torus palatinus. J Oral Surg 1977;35:845–846.
131. Suzuki M, Sakai T. A familial study of torus palatinus and torus mandibularis. Am J Phys Anthropol 1960;18:263–272.
132. Eggen S. Torus mandibularis: an estimation of the degree of genetic determination. Acta Odontol Scand 1989;47: 409–415.
133. Ramfjord S, Ash MM. Occlusion, ed 3. Philadelphia: WB Saunders, 1983:180–183.
134. Eggen S, Natvig B. Relationship between torus mandibularis and number of present teeth. Scand J Dent Res 1986;94:233–240.
135. Johnson OM. The tori and masticatory stress. J Prosthet Dent 1959;9:975–977.
136. Cailleteau JG. Subpontic hyperostosis. J Endod 1996;22: 147–149.
137. Appleby DC. Investigating incidental remission of subpontic hyperostosis. J Am Dent Assoc 1991;122:61–62.
138. Hönig JF, Merten HA, Korth OE, Halling F. Coronoid process enlargement. Dentomaxillofac Radiol 1994;23: 108–110.
139. Isberg A, Isacsson G, Nah KS. Mandibular coronoid process locking: a prospective study of frequency and association with internal derangement of the temporomandibular joint. Oral Surg Oral Med Oral Pathol 1987; 63:275–279.
140. Nickerson JW, Grafft ML, Sazima HJ. Bilateral coronoid process enlargement: report of case. J Oral Surg 1969;27: 885–890.
141. Gerbino G, Bianchi SD, Bernardi M, Berrone S. Hyperplasia of the mandibular coronoid process: long-term follow-up after coronoidotomy. J Craniomaxillofac Surg 1997;25:169–173.
142. Shira R, Lister R. Limited mandibular movements due to enlargement of the coronoid process. J Oral Surg 1958;16: 183–191.
143. Van Hoof R, Besling W. Coronoid process enlargement. Br J Oral Surg 1973;10:339–348.
144. Isberg AM, McNamara JA, Carlson DS, Isacsson G. Coronoid process elongation in Rhesus monkeys (macaca mulata) after experimentally induced mandibular hypomobility: a cephalometric and histologic study. Oral Surg Oral Med Oral Pathol 1990;70:704–710.
145. Rowe NL. Bilateral developmental hyperplasia of the mandibular coronoid process. Br J Oral Surg 1963;1:90–104.
146. Lyon LZ, Sarnat BG. Limited opening of the mouth caused by enlarged coronoid processes: report of case. J Am Dent Assoc 1963;67:644–650.
147. Sarnat BG, Engel MB. A serial study of mandibular growth after removal of the condyle in the Macaca rhesus monkey. Plast Reconstr Surg 1951;7:364–380.
148. Kai S, Hijiya T, Yamane K, Higuchi Y. Open-mouth locking caused by unilateral elongated coronoid process: report of case. J Oral Maxillofac Surg 1997;55:1305–1308.
149. Murakami K, Yokoe Y, Yasuda S, Tsuboi Y, Iizuka T. Prolonged mandibular hypomobility patient with "square mandible" configuration with coronoid process and angle hyperplasia. J Craniomandibular Pract 2000;18:113–119.
150. Isberg AM, Elliasson S. A cephalometric analysis of patients with coronoid process enlargement and locking. Am J Orthod Dentofacial Orthop 1990;97:35–40.
151. Hohl TH, Shapiro PA, Moffett BC, Ross A. Experimentally induced ankylosis and facial asymmetry in the macaque monkey. J Maxillofac Surg 1981;9:199–210.
152. York BV, Cockerham S. Bilateral hyperplasia of the coronoid processes in siblings. Oral Surg Oral Med Oral Pathol 1983;56:584–585.

Chapter 13

# Effects of Bruxism on Teeth and Its Relationship with Endodontics

*Fernando Goldberg*

## Introduction

Only a few endodontics research studies and publications associate the diseases affecting the masticatory (stomatognathic) system dynamics with pulp, radicular, and peri-radicular alterations.[1–9] However, the masticatory system is a working machine whose parts are closely related to each other. This chapter will discuss such relationships from several points of view. It considers teeth affected by bruxism or by daily or work-related habits, in two main sections:

- the relationship with *pulp and peri-radicular alterations*
- the relationship with *alterations in crown and root structure integrity*.

## Pulp and Peri-radicular Alterations

### *Diagnosis*

In certain circumstances, patients suffering from occlusal alterations, bruxism, or mild but continuous trauma in some teeth will present with degenerative or inflammatory processes that affect pulp health. In this sense, among local traumas Morse[10] includes a wide range of daily or work-related habits that may cause attrition, erosion, abrasion and/or abfraction and may result in pulp and/or periodontal diseases. Daily habits include pipe smoking, nail biting, opening hair slides with the teeth, etc. (Fig 13-1). With regard to work-related habits, seamstresses hold pins and shoemakers and carpenters hold nails between their teeth, musicians play wind instruments, students and office workers bite on pens or pencils, etc. (Fig 13-2).

Degenerative processes caused by local or general occlusal traumas include pulp atrophy and pulp dystrophic calcifications; the latter can be nodule-shaped or diffuse (Fig 13-3). Landay and Seltzer[5] and Cooper and co-workers[4] mention that excessive occlusal forces maintained for a long time may cause pulp alterations, which are nothing but irrefutable proof of tissue aging as a result of the constant traumatic stimulus. In many cases,

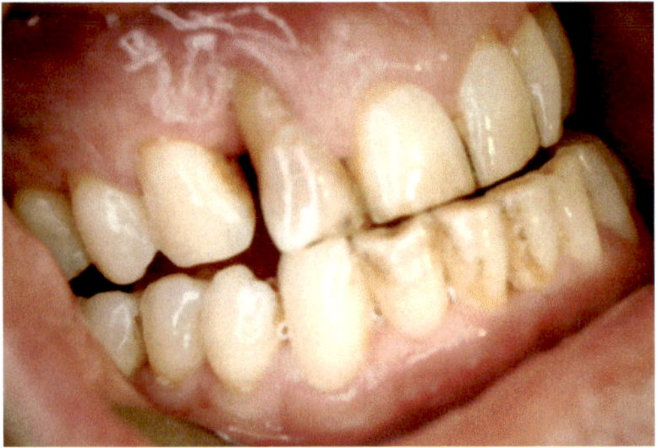

Fig 13-1 A pipe smoker. He would rest the pipe on the right maxillary lateral incisor area, where significant gingival recession can be observed. The incisor showed significant mobility and bone loss.

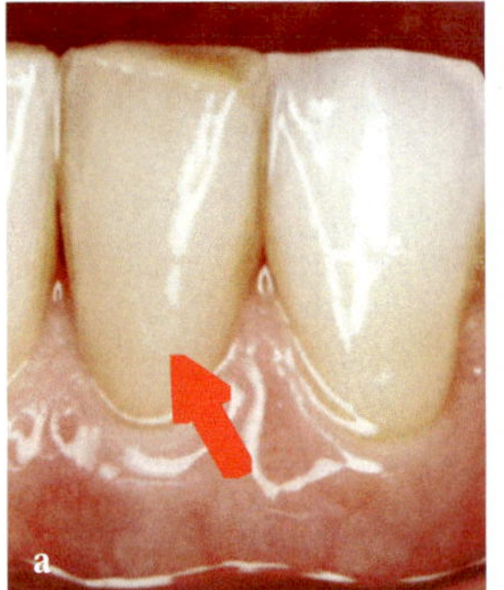

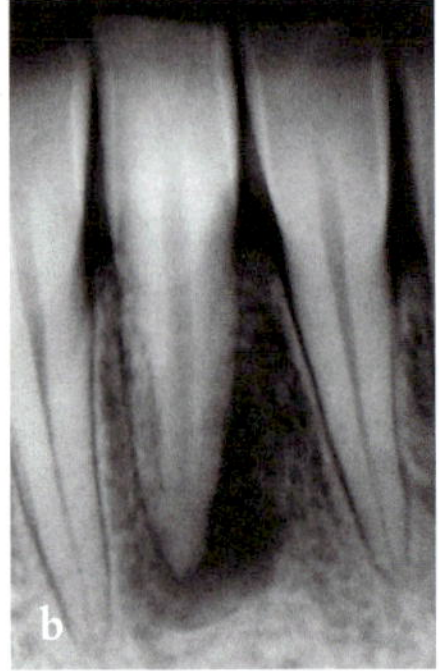

Fig 13-2 Office worker who had a habit of strongly biting the pen at the level of the lateral incisors on the right side of the mouth. **(a)** Right mandibular incisor, where incisal wear and change in crown color can be seen (arrow). **(b)** Incisor radiograph: marked peri-radicular radiolucency.

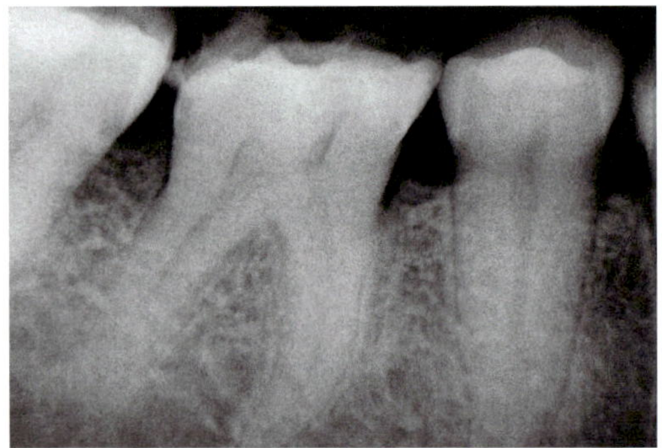

Fig 13-3 Radiograph of a mandibular molar showing occlusal wear from intense bruxing. Note the significant pulp chamber calcification.

these pulp alterations are accompanied by loss of small enamel structures on friction surfaces; this causes dentin to become exposed to the oral environment (Fig 13-4). Quite frequently, this enamel loss affecting mastication surfaces (attrition) coexists with enamel and cement loss in the cervical region (abfraction). In this case, the pulp defends itself by increasing the mineralization of its own structure, which is known as "sclerotic dentin".[11,12] This results in partial or total calcification of dentinal tubule lumen size (Fig 13-5).

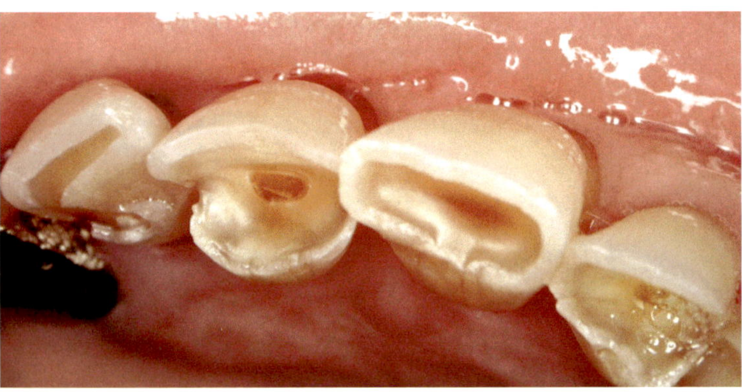

Fig 13-4 Bruxer's anterior–superior dental segment, showing incisal-edge wear by attrition plus acid erosion, with enamel loss and exposure of the underlying dentin.

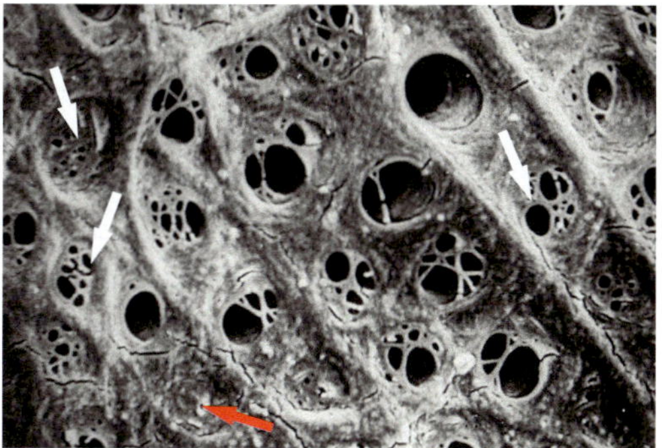
Fig 13-5 A large number of dentinal tubules can be seen in the partial (white arrow) or total (red arrow) obliteration phase. Scanning electron microscopic view.

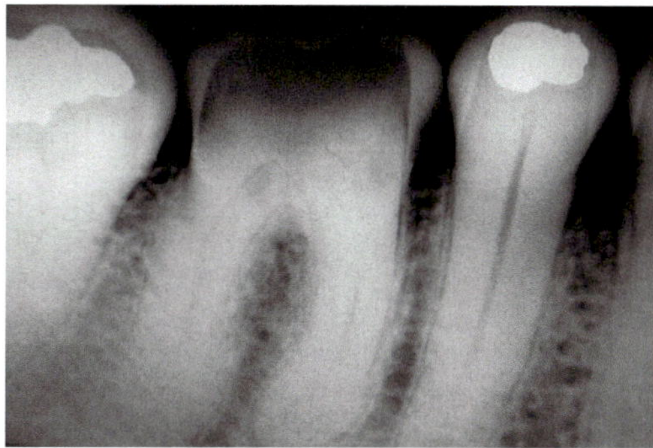
Fig 13-6 Radiograph of a mandibular molar showing significant attrition on the occlusal surface and severe pulp chamber calcification.

Frequently, mineralization of the underlying pulp structure occurs too, with formation of secondary, reparative or reactional dentin.[3,4,6,7,11,13] Thus, due to the lack of space, pulp tissue decreases in size and pulp vitality starts to diminish (Fig 13-6). Clinically, apart from enamel loss, a change of color on the exposed dentin surface in the worn area may be observed; in slow-evolution cases, such change of color is accompanied by reduced pulp sensitivity. In contrast, when wear progresses quickly, the pulp has no time to react and defend itself; this will result in a pulp inflammatory state with increased sensitivity, which in some circumstances may require pulpectomy.

Groves Cooke[14] reports the case of a patient who presented with moderate pulp pain in the area of the maxillary incisors; he was diagnosed with occlusal trauma from protrusive bruxism. A night guard was made for the patient, and within a year pulpal symptoms had disappeared and pulp vitality was normal.

Yu[15] describes two clinical cases where occlusal trauma resulted in the onset of pulp and peri-radicular alterations. In observations of rats, Kvinnsland and co-workers[16] found that occlusal trauma might generate pulpal blood flow alterations.

It is important to remember that dentin and pulp are a single organ, since dentin is formed by the pulp, and its mass contains the odontoblastic prolongations. On the surface of dentin there are approximately 20,000 dentinal tubules per square millimeter, the diameter of which is approximately 1 μm per dentinal tubule.[12] Multiplying these numbers by the exposed surface area allows us to fully appreciate the extent of the damage.

In slow wear processes there is usually a balance between the loss of superficial mineralized tissue and pulpal defense mechanisms. While the aggressor approaches pulp tissue, the pulp creates a barrier that keeps it apart from such aggressor. If possible, and provided that the area involved does not interfere with occlusion, protection of the exposed dentin with appropriate restorative materials can be attempted. However, if the defense mechanisms are overwhelmed by the aggression, if the pulpal defense reaction causes the pulp to become exhausted or exposed, or if bacteria and their products penetrate deeply, then pulp inflammation, or necrosis, will occur. In these circumstances, there is no choice but to proceed with the appropriate endodontic treatment (as described later).

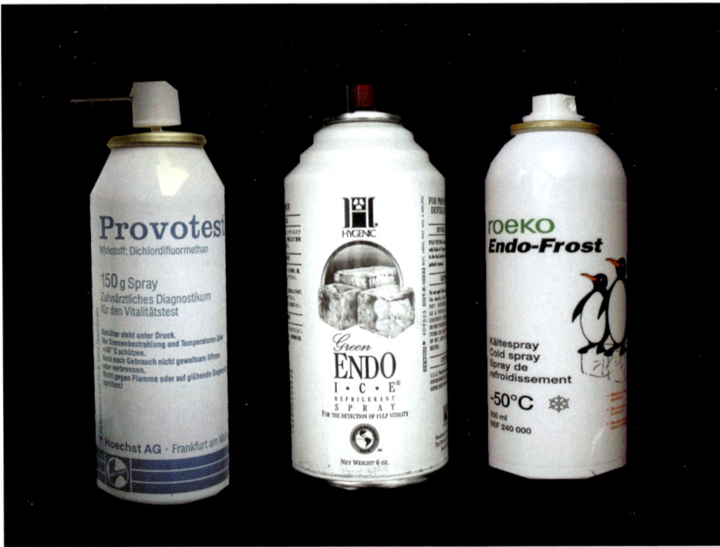


Fig 13-7 Three cold-spray products for pulp vitality testing: Provotest, EndoIce, and Endo-Frost.

Tronstad and Langeland[3] conducted a histologic evaluation of 45 human permanent teeth with attrition; odontoblastic layer alterations were observed in all of them: pulp inflammation in 29 teeth, extensive degenerative changes in 13 teeth, and pulp necrosis in 3 teeth. Sivasithamparam and co-workers[17] studied 448 patients with dental wear; in 52 of them (11.6%) pulp almost reached the dental surface or was completely exposed. The palatal surface of anterior–superior teeth and the incisal surface of anterior–inferior teeth were the most affected.

On many occasions, the symptoms may be rather unclear. In the first stage (pulp inflammation), patients will present with pain caused by thermal changes; patients cannot always accurately localize the cause of such pain, since when masticatory system alterations are present, many teeth may be affected by this problem. In order to avoid misdiagnosis, thermal stimuli tests must be conducted: cold (small ice bar) and heat (piece of heated gutta-percha) must be applied to the suspected tooth and the adjacent teeth. On other occasions, resolution of symptoms occurs, and the patient feels well for a few days. After a brief period, the patient starts experiencing localized pain on mastication and sensitivity to percussion – usually symptoms of dental pulp necrosis and onset of periradicular involvement. In these cases, the results of thermal-change pulp-sensitivity tests may be quite erratic, especially if the teeth have multiple roots. The reason for this is that pulp necrosis does not always occur in all root canals at the same time, so some sensitivity may still be present.

Thus, in order to test pulp sensitivity to thermal changes, the use of products that generate intense cold, like EndoIce (Hygenic, USA), Endo-Frost (Roeko, Germany), Provotest (Hoechst AG, Germany), or other similar products, is recommended (Fig 13-7). These tests are commercially available in the form of sprays. A small cotton pellet is sprayed with the product and softly placed on the tooth surface, to see if any reaction or symptom occurs. It is essential that the cotton pellet be

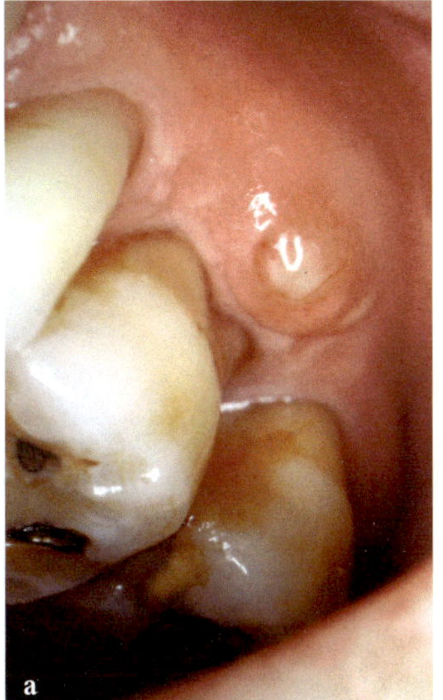


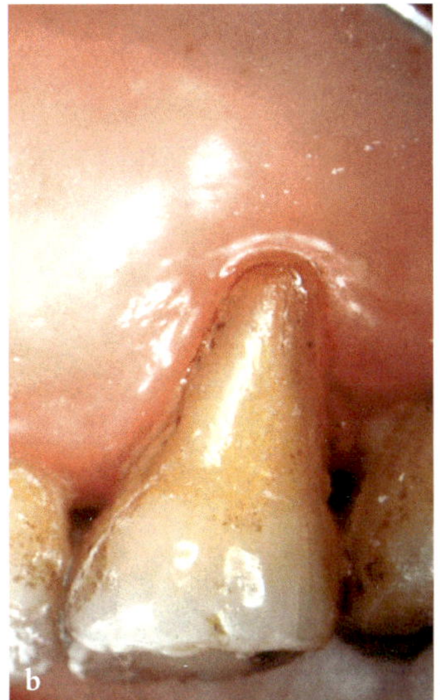


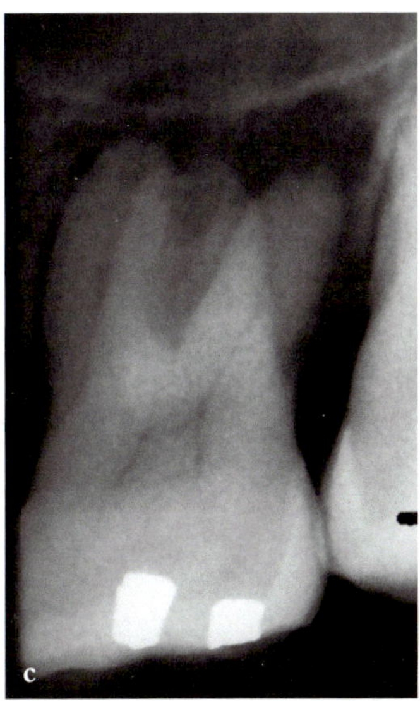


Fig 13-8 **(a)** Vestibular surface of a bruxer's maxillary molar; gingival recession and a vestibular fistula of endodontic origin can be seen. **(b)** Palatal view of the same molar; significant gingival retraction at the level of the palatal root can be seen. **(c)** Severe pulp chamber calcification can be seen on the radiograph, with peri-radicular radiolucent areas at the apical level of the three tooth roots – signs of pulp necrosis. The crown structure of the tooth is unimpaired, with just two superficial amalgam restorations.

placed on the tooth in a very gentle way, in order to prevent the patient from suffering intense pain in case of positive vitality. The above-mentioned products are usually more reliable than battery-powered pulp testers.[18]

In the early stages of pulp necrosis, X-ray evaluation is not useful for diagnosis, since no radiolucency changes will be observed in the peri-radicular area. Radiologically, only a pulp chamber that has decreased in size due to the presence of calcifications can be seen. If things are left like this, within a few days the patient will likely experience acute spontaneous pain that is radiologically demonstrated by periodontal widening or by a well-defined peri-radicular lesion (Fig 13-8). In these cases, root canal treatment is indicated (see below).

At the Second International Conference on Endodontics, in 1958, the following conclusion was drawn: "Though it is unlikely, there is a chance that bruxism might cause dental pulp necrosis." In this respect, Ingle,[1] and Natkin and Ingle[2] claim that such possibility is not so unlikely; the fact that the symptoms will commonly go unnoticed prevents correct diagnosis.

### *Treatment of Teeth with Pulp and Peri-radicular Alterations*

As has already been described, in teeth affected by a mild, persistent occlusal trauma, either local or involving several teeth, a change in pulp size occurs due to the formation of nodule-shaped or diffuse calcifications. This interferes with the localization of the pulp chamber and makes reaching the root canals difficult during endodontic treatment.

Before starting with the root canal treatment, the clinician should conduct a thorough clinical examination of the tooth involved in order to accurately evaluate its external anatomy. Usually the internal anatomy of the pulp chamber will be similar to its external anatomy, thus, the latter may be indicative of the internal situation the professional will have to deal with. Also, when canals are difficult to reach, it is advisable not to use rubber

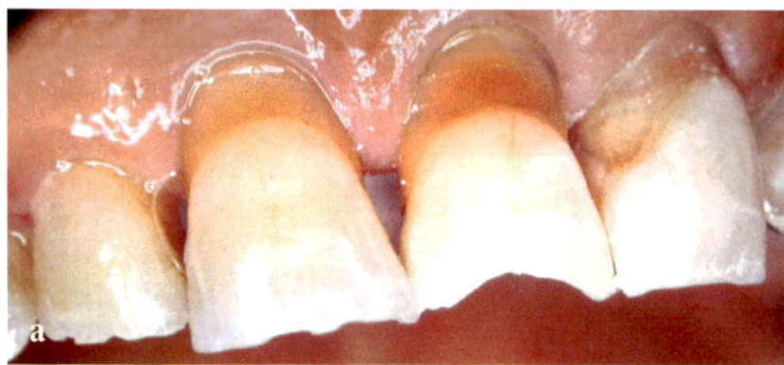

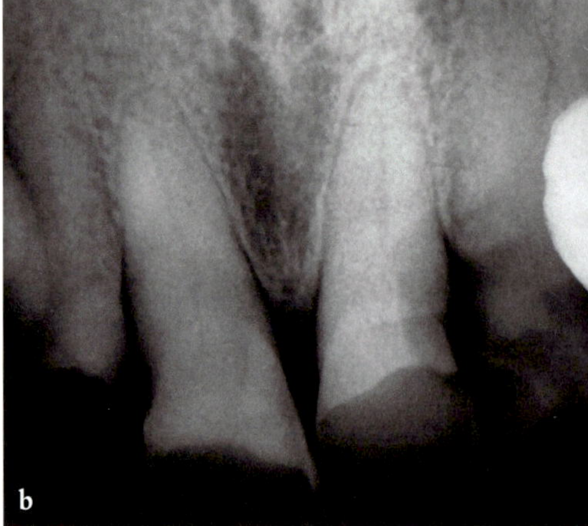

Fig 13-9 Bruxer's anterior–superior dental area. **(a)** There is incisal-edge loss due to attrition plus erosion, with marked gingival retraction and abfraction at the level of the tooth neck of the two central incisors and one lateral incisor. **(b)** Radiograph of the described area, where incisal-surface wear and calcification of the root canals of both central incisors at the cervical level can be seen.

dam during the first steps of the opening; this will allow the clinician to fully appreciate the external anatomy of the tooth and use it as a guide during the procedure. After locating the entrance to the canal(s), rubber dam is placed in order to continue with the procedure. For didactic purposes, and owing to some interesting differences that are useful to emphasize, we will divide treatments into single-rooted and multiple-rooted tooth management.

## *Single-rooted teeth*

### *X-ray study*

In patients with masticatory system diseases, pulp calcification will usually involve just the cervical third of the root canal (Fig 13-9). Thus, when such a tooth needs endodontic treatment, access to the chamber and root-canal entrance localization are difficult. If the radiograph is well-proportioned and is not elongated, it is possible to measure from the incisal edge to the point where the canal becomes visible on the radiograph. By having this measure in mind while trying to localize the canal, accidental perforation will be avoided, since such a measure provides a good estimate of the preparation limit.

### *Clinical aspects*

In these patients, anterior teeth, both of the maxilla and the mandible, will usually show wear on the incisal edges, which turn into true incisal surfaces (see Fig 13-9). Although, in this dental segment, conventional endodontic openings are made on the palatal or lingual surface of the tooth, in certain cases it is advisable to make the opening on the worn incisal surface, in order to preserve more of the dental tissue and to access the root canal directly (Fig 13-10). On many occasions, in the center of this area the dentin will be darker in color; this represents reactional dentin, which the pulp has formed in order to defend itself. This trail will usually lead to the entrance of the root canal. In bruxers, incisal wear is usually accompanied by gingival recession, which causes the cervical third of the affected tooth root to become visible. Thus, if our above-mentioned recommendation is followed and the rubber dam is not used at this stage, it will be possible to make the opening by having the cervical third of the root constantly visible and serving as a guide. In these cases, care is needed to make sure that, while drilling the tooth, the bur follows the root's longitudinal axis line and penetrates in the center of the mesiodistal thickness (Fig 13-11).

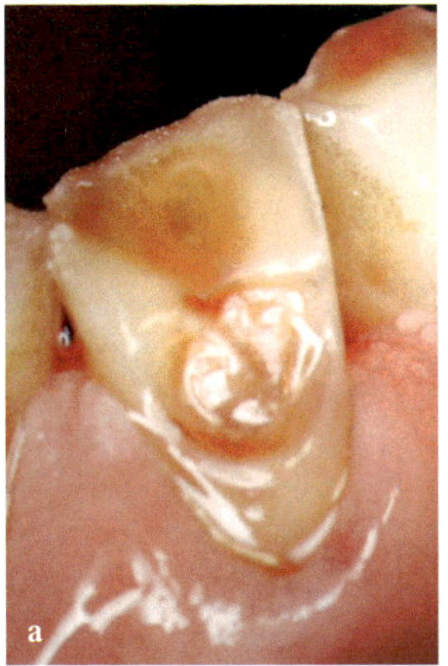

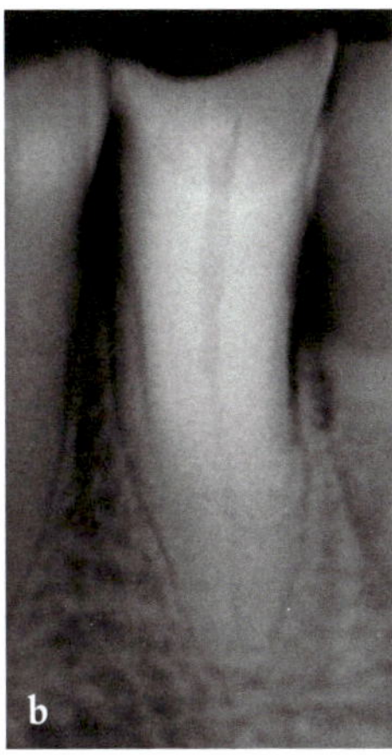

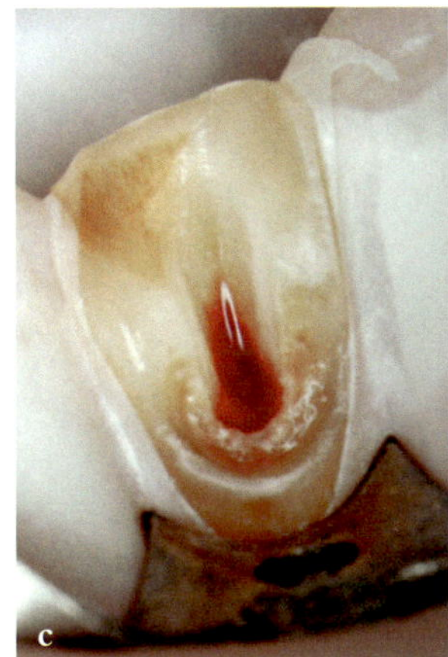

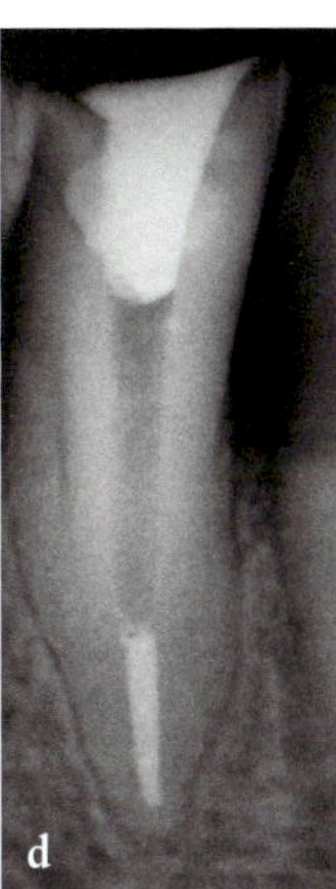


Fig 13-10 **(a)** Bruxer's canine showing severe wear by attrition softened by erosion, on the incisal and buccal surfaces. **(b)** Preoperative radiograph. **(c)** Picture taken after the endodontic opening was made on the worn surface. **(d)** Postoperative radiograph following endodontic treatment; it shows prosthetic anchorage preparation.

On making the opening, it is advisable to control every step visually and radiologically in order to prevent accidents from happening. Using a straight endodontic explorer may be useful while conducting the visual inspection.

*Multiple-rooted teeth*

*X-ray study*

When calcification of part of the pulp chamber of premolars and molars occurs, it affects the pulp chamber's roof, floor, and walls, which become markedly convex. Thus, the pulp chamber decreases in size and has an ill-defined radiographic appearance. In this respect, it must be remembered that the radiograph will show an overlapping of planes in the buccolingual direction; because of this, only the mesiodistal width of the pulp chamber will be visible, while buccolingual depth will not. In fact, the pulp chamber is always wider than what is seen on a radiograph. Radiographs are just the two-dimensional representation of a three-dimensional reality.

If a restoration is present in the tooth to be treated, it is advisable to radiologically verify the proximity of such restoration to the pulp chamber. This should be kept in mind as a reference point while making the opening.

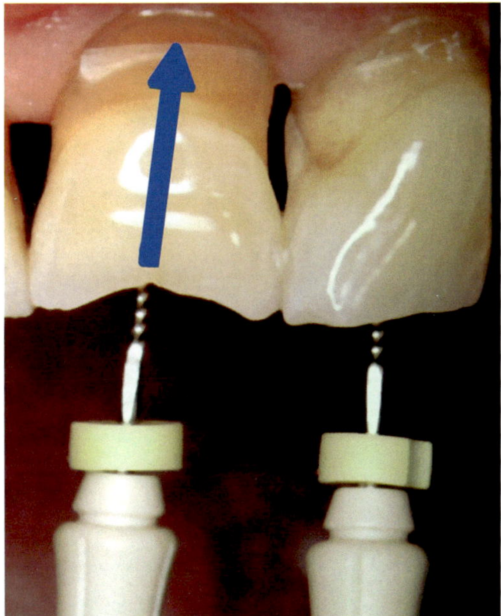

Fig 13-11 The same patient as in Figure 13-9. Since localizing the root canal was difficult, localization is being attempted before placement of the rubber dam. For this purpose, the orientation of the cervical area of the root, clearly visible due to gingival recession (arrow), serves as a guide.

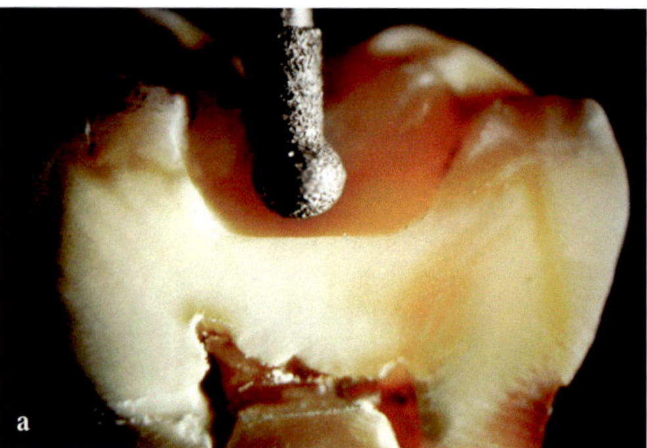

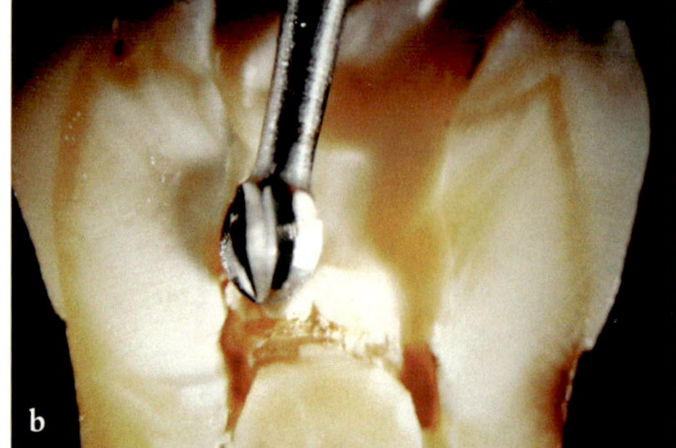

**Fig 13-12** **(a)** Enamel and dentin removal in vitro in a molar whose pulp chamber has reduced in size due to pulp calcification. **(b)** Layer-by-layer dentin removal using round tungsten-carbide burs operated at low speed until pulp exposure is achieved.

*Clinical aspects*

What we have mentioned for the anterior segment also applies to the posterior segments: it is also extremely important to perform a thorough visual inspection of the external anatomy of the crown of the tooth. Molars with a broad, quadrangular occlusal surface are suggestive of a square or trapezoidal pulp chamber, with widely spaced root-canal openings and a high likelihood of the presence of four well-defined canals. Molars with a triangular occlusal surface are suggestive of a small chamber floor, root-canal entrances that are close to each other, and root canals that are aligned like a scalene triangle. It should be remembered that, although maxillary molars usually have three roots, in fact they will almost always have four canals – i.e., two canals in the mesiobuccal root. The mesiobuccal canal is usually located under the mesiobuccal cusp; the mesiopalatal canal is located slightly mesial of the line which connects the entrances to the mesiobuccal and palatal canals. With regard to mandibular molars, it should be remembered that, though they usually have two roots, sometimes they may have four canals owing to the division of the distal canal.

As for the anterior segment, also in these cases gingival recession will allow the clinician to make out the shape and direction of the exposed roots and use these references as a guide while making the opening. Thus, when locating the pulp chamber becomes a problem, it is advisable to make the opening without using rubber dam until the root canals have been located. Once part of the mineralized tissue has been removed through the occlusal surface and when near to the pulp chamber roof, it is advisable to remove the dentin layer by layer by using a spherical bur at low speed (Fig 13-12). Checking the floor thus prepared is essential, and this should be carried out by means of visual inspection with the aid of a straight endodontic explorer. When the explorer penetrates deeply, it is a good sign that access is being gained to the pulp chamber. The roof chamber should be drilled very carefully and it should be fully removed in order to expose the pulp chamber (see Fig 13-12). Once access to the chamber has been achieved, it is essential that rubber dam be placed in order to fully isolate the surgical area.

When calcifications are present in the pulp chamber and the entrance to the canals, they must be thoroughly removed in order to have full and proper access to the endodontic anatomy.

It should be remembered that the calcifications on the chamber walls hide the entrance to root canals; thus, such calcifications should be removed in order to have direct access to the canals. Removal is performed by using a tapered-fissure bur or a cylindrical bur without a cutting edge so as to avoid damaging the chamber floor. The Batt bur is the perfect tool for doing this (Fig 13-13). By operating the bur on the chamber walls to be rectified, the "dentinal shelf" which interferes with direct entry is removed. Pulp stones may be removed by using a spoon excavator for pulp or dentin or ultrasonics with special inserts (Fig 13-14). It is advisable to avoid accidents by not using burs on the pulp chamber floor.

Once the calcifications have been removed from the pulp chamber and nothing interferes with root-canal access, root-canal exploration is performed by using a file of the proper size according to the size of the canal. Exploration files are intended for reconaissance purposes. The use of a #08 or #10 file for narrow canals and a #15 or #20 file for wider canals is recommended. The file will help determine the level of accessibility, the

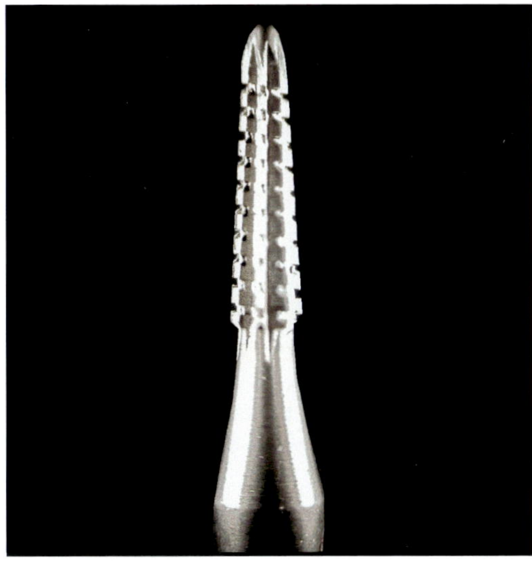

Fig 13-13 Batt bur whose rounded end is inactive in order to prevent pulp-chamber floor wear.

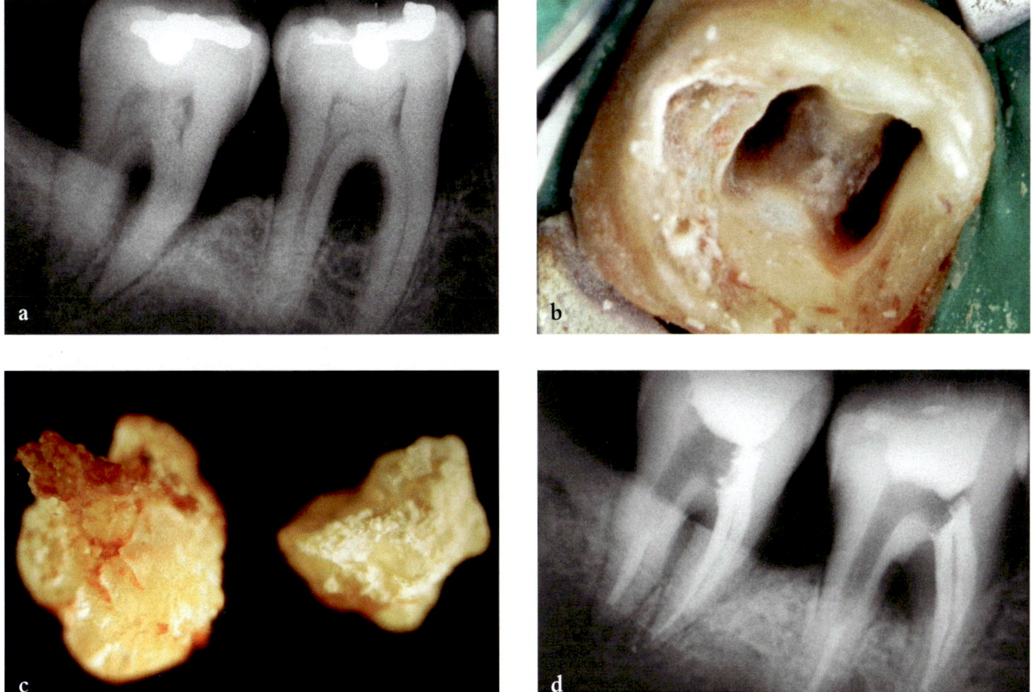


Fig 13-14 **(a)** Radiograph of mandibular molar area, with marked pulp chamber calcification in both teeth. **(b)** Pulp chamber of one of the molars once calcification has been removed, and walls and root-canal openings have been prepared. **(c)** Pulp calcifications removed from both molars. **(d)** Postoperative radiographs following endodontic treatment (the distal canals were prepared for prosthetic anchorage).

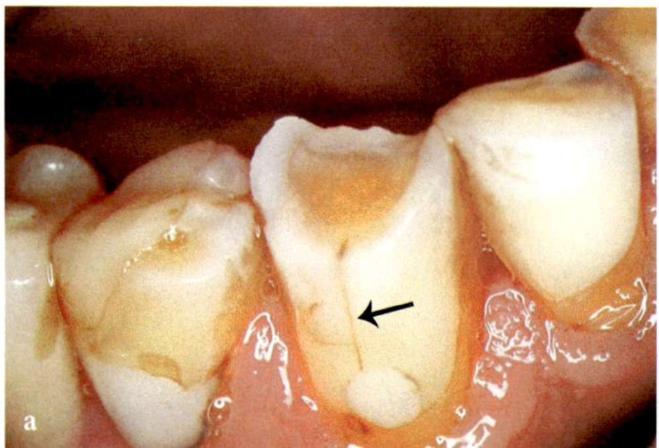
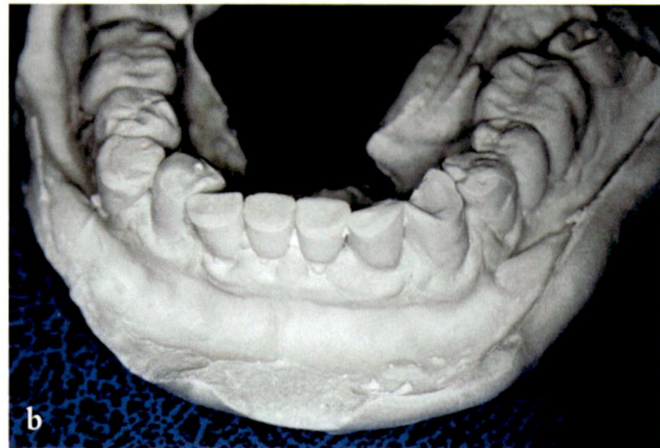

Fig 13-15 **(a)** Right lateral mandibular area of a bruxer's dental arch. Severe attrition aggravated by erosion can be seen on the incisal and occlusal surfaces. A darker line (arrow) consistent with a crack in the crown can be seen in the canine. **(b)** Plaster cast of the mandibular arch: severe wear of occlusal surfaces can be seen.

possible presence of calcifications, the number of canals, canal curvature, etc. Before inserting the exploration file, it is advisable to bend its end slightly in order to make penetration easier.

Once the exploration has been done, the rest of the procedure is the same as in any regular endodontic treatment.

### *Implications in Post-endodontic Repair*

We must consider two issues: the immediate post-operative scenario, and long-term prognosis. Following endodontic treatment, patients will usually present with mild periodontitis typically caused by the surgical trauma. These symptoms are usually more prominent and persistent in those patients whose teeth are subject to excessive occlusal work. In these cases, it is advisable to slightly relieve the treated tooth of occlusion.

With regard to the long-term prognosis, Ingle,[1] Seltzer,[19] and Rosenberg[7] consider that excessive local occlusal trauma may be a contributing factor in endodontic treatment failure. Harn and co-workers[9] report on two clinical cases in which excessive occlusal trauma contributed to the failure of an endodontic treatment and of an apical surgical resection respectively. These authors report that repair occurred in both cases after occlusal adjustment.

It should also be mentioned that, despite reconstruction, the tooth becomes weaker with the endodontic treatment. That is the reason why these patients are more susceptible to tooth cracks and fractures.

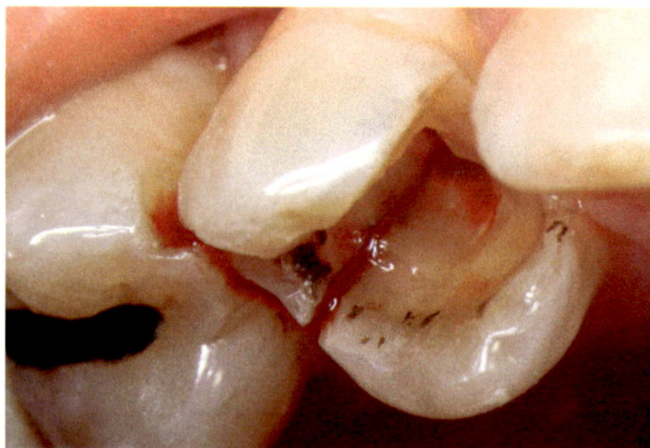

Fig 13-16 Picture of a maxillary premolar showing a dental fracture in the distal wall.

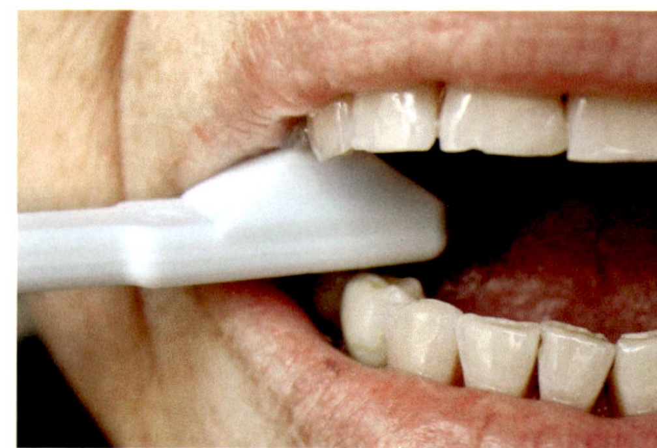

Fig 13-17 This patient is biting on a Tooth Slooth so as to detect a potential dental crack or fracture.

***Teeth that Maintain Pulp Vitality and Will Support Individual or Group Fixed Prostheses***

Sometimes, pulp and dentin structural alterations will occur in teeth for the above-mentioned traumatic reasons (bruxism, local trauma, work-related habits, etc.); then they will need to undergo extensive preparation for prosthetic reconstruction purposes. At this point, it is essential to make a very sound evaluation. The absence of symptoms should not be considered to be suggestive of a normal, healthy, dental pulp.[7] When the pulp is affected by degenerative changes from excessive work, it is biologically exhausted and has little chance of defending itself against new trauma caused by crown preparation. The pulp may not withstand the aggression, and eventually, following prosthetic restoration, such symptoms may occur as to make endodontic treatment necessary – but now under unfavorable access conditions.

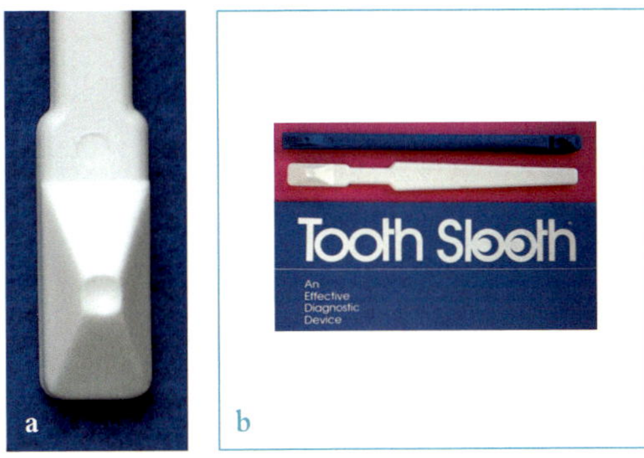


Fig 13-18 **(a and b)** Two versions of the Tooth Slooth.

## Alterations in Crown and Root Structural Integrity

### *Diagnosis*

*Teeth without prosthetic reconstruction, and their relationhip to tooth cracks and fractures*

The presence of cracks or fractures in the teeth of patients with occlusal disorders – either general (bruxism) or local (daily or work-related habits) – is relatively common. Sometimes, such cracks or fractures will affect the crown of the tooth only, but on other occasions (the most severe ones) they will affect both the crown and the root (Figs 13-15 and 13-16). Patients will commonly complain of acute pain when a hard piece of food comes between the occlusal surface of the affected tooth and the antagonist tooth. If the pulp is still vital, these symptoms are associated with thermal-change-related pain.

On visual inspection, sometimes a sinuous line showing a slight change in color may be observed. Radiologically, such lines will go unnoticed owing to the overlapping of radiopaque structures. In these cases, as a method for diagnosis it is advisable to place a flat piece of wood or plastic on the occlusal surface of the tooth under observation and have the patient bite on it. This way, an attempt to reproduce the pain described by the patient is made (Figs 13-17 and 13-18). Also, the use of dye detectors in the diagnosis of crown cracks (Fig 13-19) can be very helpful.

Radiologically, on certain occasions cracks are accompanied by horizontal or vertical bone loss (depending on the crack depth) which may resemble periodontal disease. Such radiographical appearance may be associated with a localized, narrow gingival pocket. Many times, cracks are present in teeth with large restorations, but they can also be present in teeth with small restorations (Figs 13-20 and 13-21). In patients with highly developed masseter muscles, strong masticatory muscles and a tendency to bruxism, dental cracks and fractures can be seen in teeth with no restorations.

*Teeth with intraradicular anchorage, and their relationship to tooth cracks and fractures*

When intraradicular anchorage is present in the tooth, there is a greater likelihood of dental crack or fracture.[20] This is especially common in bruxers or patients suffering from some kind of occlusal trauma. However, in a study of 227 cases, Cohen

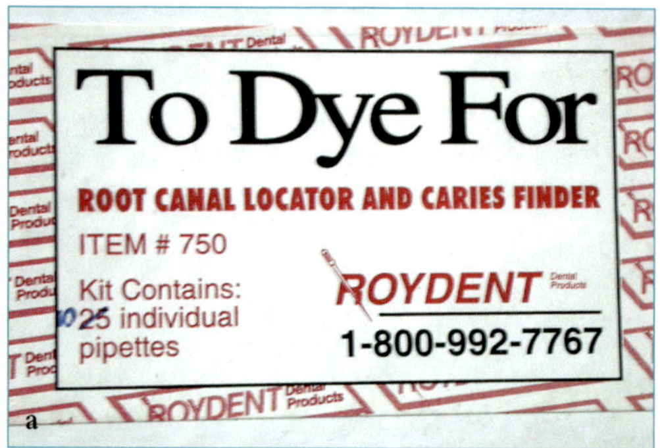


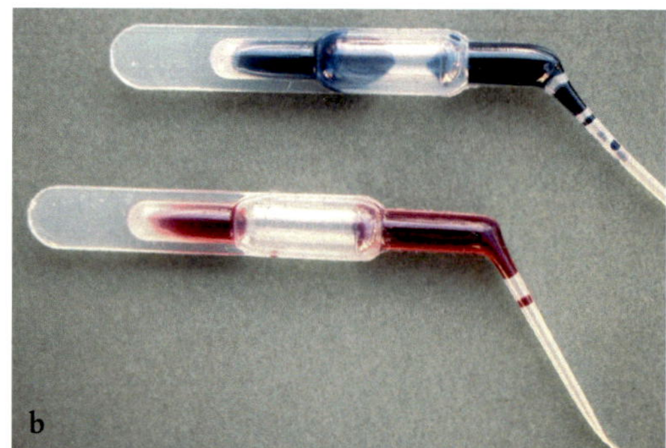

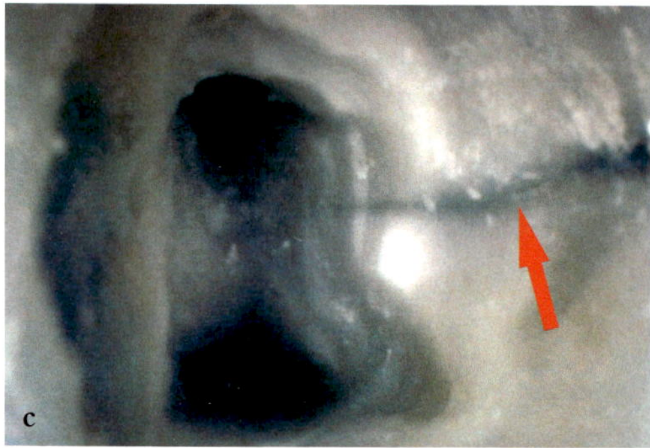

Fig 13-19 **(a and b)** The Roydent detector. **(c)** Pulp chamber of a mandibular molar, where a crack highlighted by a dye detector is visible (arrow).

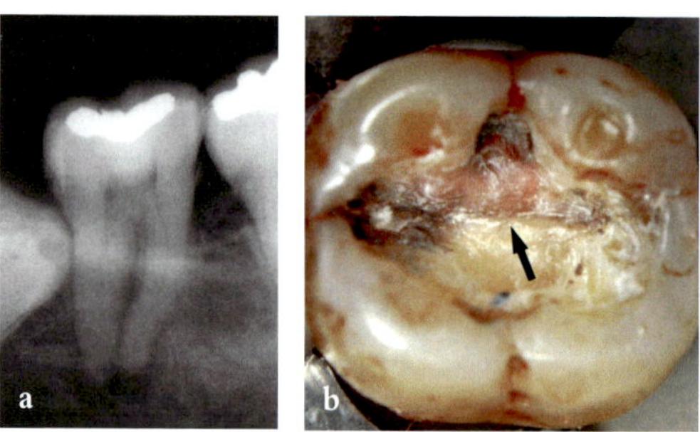

Fig 13-20 **(a)** Radiograph of the mandibular second molar of a patient suffering from occlusal stress; a medium-sized crown restoration can be seen. The pulp chamber has reduced in size due to the presence of calcifications; a radiolucency, sign of pulp necrosis, is visible in the apical area. **(b)** A crown crack line is clearly visible on the occlusal surface (arrow).

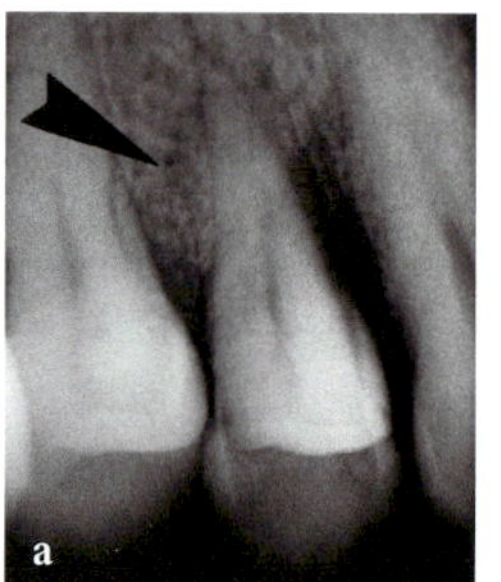

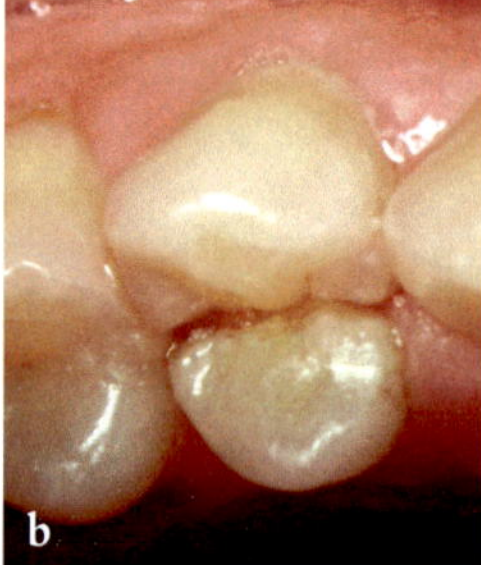

Fig 13-21 **(a)** Radiograph of the maxillary first premolar of a heavy bruxer who was referred describing acute pain in the right maxillary area. **(b)** The same premolar: a fracture can be observed.

and co-workers[21] found no evidence that bruxism had been a significant factor in root fracture incidence. Usually, when root fracture occurs in teeth with intraradicular anchorage, a localized or elongated wide periodontal radiolucency at the level of the apical end of the anchorage will be seen. That is where the fulcrum of the lever which produces the anchorage is set, especially if no splint or cervical ferrule attach the anchorage to the tooth (ferrule effect) (Figs 13-22 and 13-23).

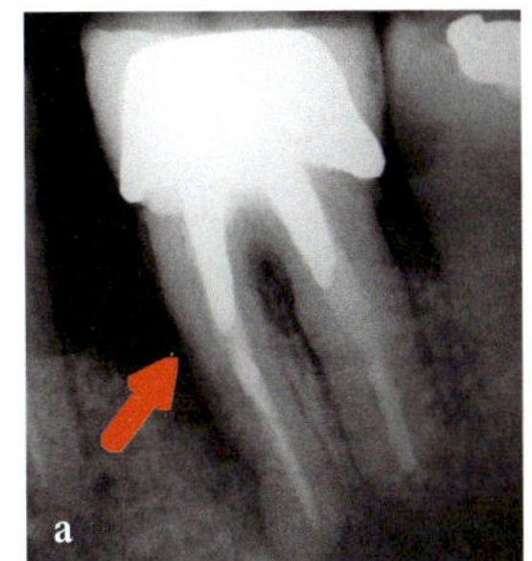

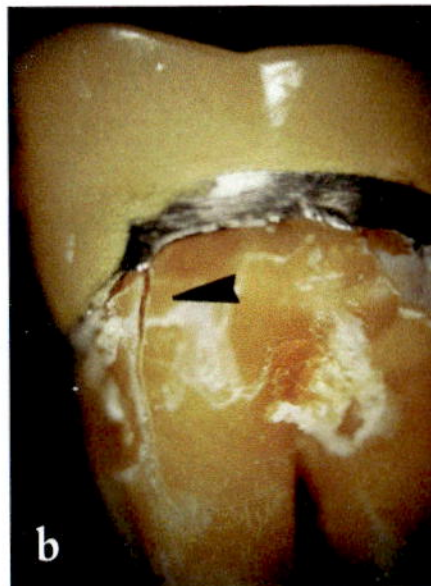

Fig 13-22 **(a)** Radiograph of a mandibular molar with intraradicular anchorage, where deep bone loss adjacent to the molar's mesial root can be seen (arrow). **(b)** The molar after extraction; the fracture line stands out (arrow).

When an individual restoration (without attachment to other teeth in the arch) is present in the tooth in question, tooth mobility associated with pain on mastication may occur. On certain occasions, a fistula may be seen next to the gingival margin. For diagnostic purposes, a gutta-percha cone should be placed in the fistula opening and deeply introduced into the fistula's path. Then an X-ray study is done to determine the point reached by the cone. When cracks or fractures are present, the cone will reach the external surface of the root at the level of the crevice. If the cone can be traced to the apical area of the tooth exactly, a purely endodontic problem should be considered. When no gingival fistula is present, diagnosis is more difficult to make.

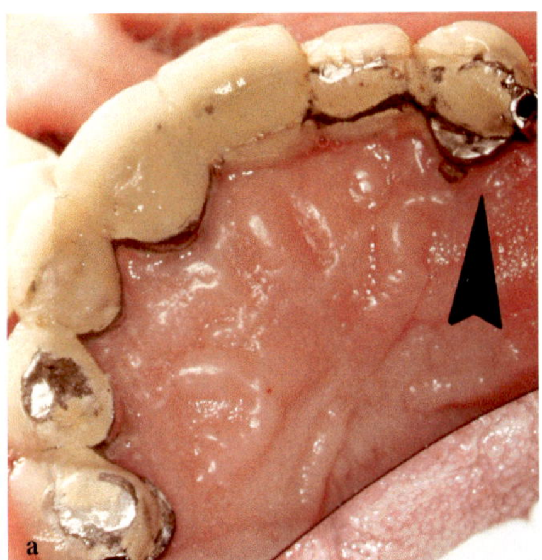

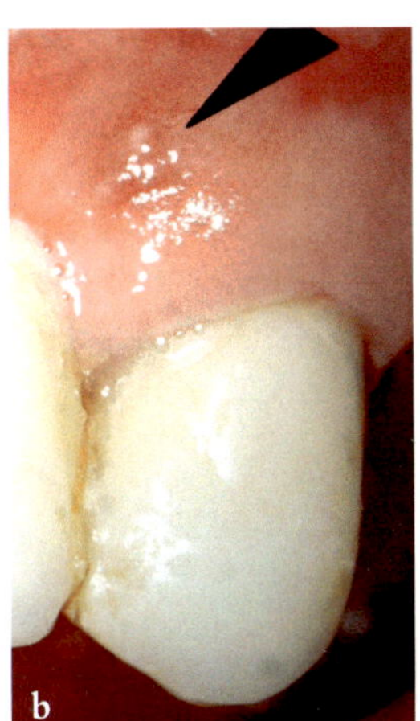

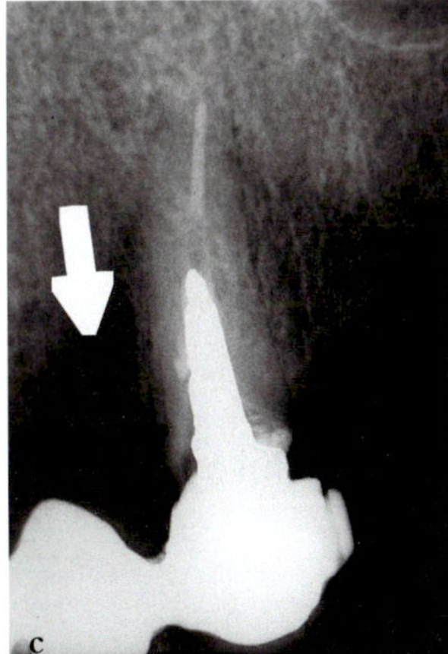

Fig 13-23 **(a)** A patient's anterior–superior maxillary region; note porcelain loss on the palatal surfaces of the fixed prosthesis due to severe bruxism. The arrow points to the left maxillary canine. **(b)** The left maxillary canine showing a gingival fistula (arrow). **(c)** Radiograph of the same canine. A dislodged intraradicular anchorage and deep lateral bone loss (arrow) are present – signs of the existing root fracture.

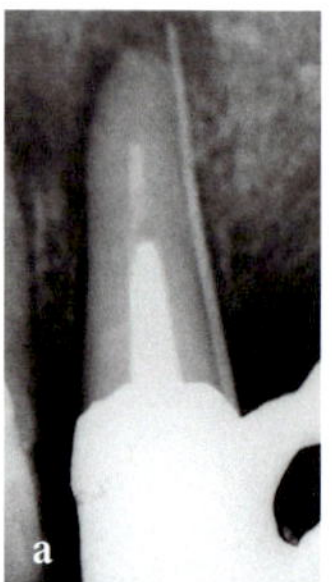

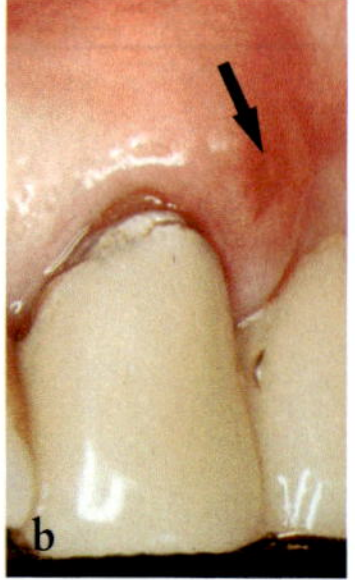

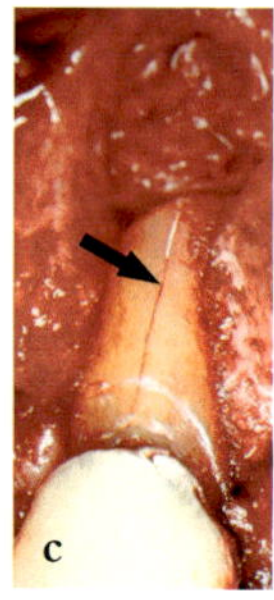


Fig 13-24 **(a)** Radiograph of a lateral maxillary incisor with intraradicular anchorage and fixed prosthesis; bone loss limited to the dental root can be observed. A gutta-percha cone inserted into the gingival fistula shows the fistula's path. **(b)** The incisor with the fistula (arrow). **(c)** The root fracture (arrow) can be clearly seen with the aid of an exploratory flap.

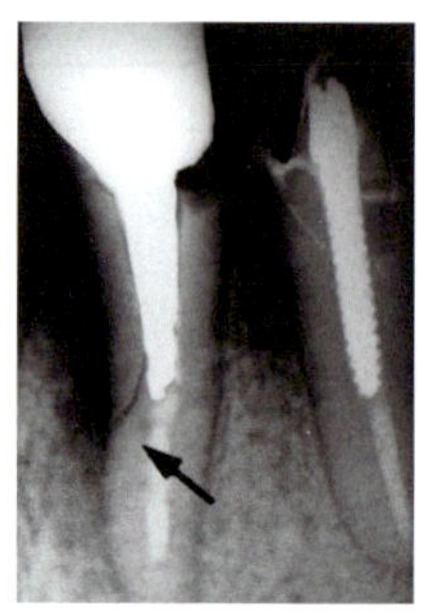

Fig 13.25 Radiograph of a mandibular canine. There is a root fracture at the level of the most apical area of the post (arrow).

The condition may have an endodontic etiology (failed endodontic treatment), a periodontal etiology (periodontal disease), or it may be secondary to the presence of a dental crack or fracture. As a general rule, when there is an endodontic etiology, damage is limited to a specific tooth, and the radiolucent X-ray image corresponds to the apical area, though it may also correspond to the lateral area when a lateral canal is present. Endodontic etiology is usually related to a poor endodontic treatment. When there is a periodontal etiology, the condition will commonly be generalized and several teeth will be affected. In this case, the periodontal pocket surrounds the entire tooth circumference. Frequently, there is gingival involvement and plaque and calculus adherent to the external surface of the root. When root cracks or fractures are implicated in the etiology, the radiolucent image appears laterally in the radiographs, the pocket is clinically narrow, deep and limited to one or two points of the tooth circumference. If in doubt, a definitive diagnosis can be attained by an exploratory flap (Fig 13-24).

When prosthetic restorations join several teeth, diagnosis is usually more difficult. Patients present with clinical symptoms that are not specific to a particular tooth. X-ray studies are very useful for accurate diagnosis. When a gingival fistula is present, fistula exploration – already described – is indicated. Sometimes, the fracture line is clearly visible on the radiograph, which facilitates diagnosis (Fig 13-25). On certain occasions, when no clinical or radiographic changes are detected that may be useful for diagnosis, a time interval should elapse until things can be sorted out. Do not intervene if the cause of the problem is unclear.

Sometimes, patients with intraradicular anchorage and who have these occlusal habits will present with fractured posts or screws inside the root canal (Figs 13-26 and 13-27). In such cases, it is important to verify that no root crack or fracture is present, and X-ray studies should be done to determine the depth and size of the remaining anchorage. This allows evaluation of the advisability of keeping the affected tooth in the mouth, and action will be taken accordingly (see Fig 13-27).

In bruxers and patients affected by daily or work-related habits, or in patients who have prosthetic restorations with intraradicular anchorages, fracture of intraradicular posts or screws is relatively frequent. Practitioners should be on the alert, since such fractures are a potential prelude to root fracture. For this reason, once the fractured anchorage has been removed, and before or just following the new prosthetic restoration, a treatment plan addressing alterations of the masticatory dynamics should be considered. Moule and Kahler[22] provide a detailed list of clinical symptoms and radiographic signs that facilitate root fracture diagnosis. One symptom may be present, or several at the same time.

- *Clinical symptoms:* A long history of mild or moderate pain, generally associated with chronic infection; pain on mastication; isolated, deep and narrow periodontal pocket on one of the root surfaces; intraradicular anchorage often decemented.
- *X-ray alterations:* Root fragment separation; radiolucent line along the root or the endodontic obturation; radiolucent space on the sides of the intraradicular anchorage; double images of the external surface of the root; bone loss adjacent to the dental furcation; widened periodontal space; radiolucent halo around the root surface; step-like bony defects; individual horizontal bone loss in the molar area; diffuse V-shaped bone resorption in the molar area; bone resorption along the fracture line; in apicectomy cases, apical retrograde obturation dislocation; endodontic failure after initial success; direct visualization of the fracture.

Owing to the variety of symptoms, diagnosing a vertical fracture may sometimes be difficult. In a study by Tamse and co-workers,[23] general practitioners were able to correctly diagnose vertical fractures only in one-third of 92 teeth with root fractures.

*Relationship with root resorption*

Rosenberg[7] considers abnormal occlusal stress to be the potential cause of internal and external dental resorptions. Though its incidence is very low, bruxism has been proposed by Hethersay[8] as one of the predisposing factors to invasive cervical resorption. He studied 222 patients with 257 teeth

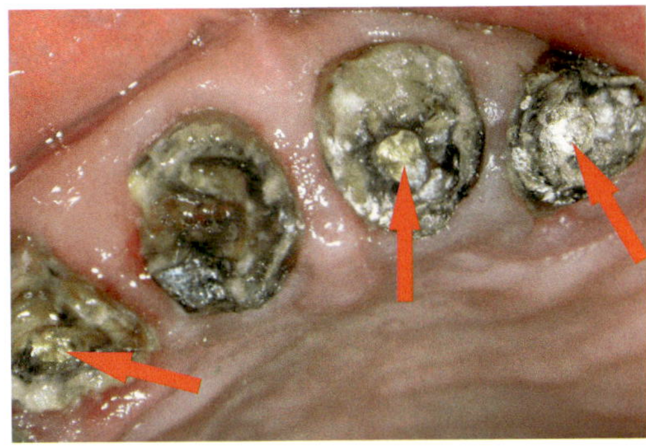

Fig 13-26 A heavy bruxer's anterior–superior area, where three fractured posts can be seen inside their respective root canals (arrows).

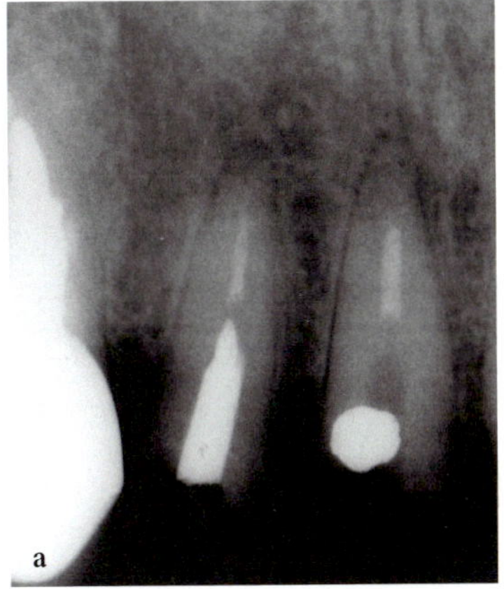


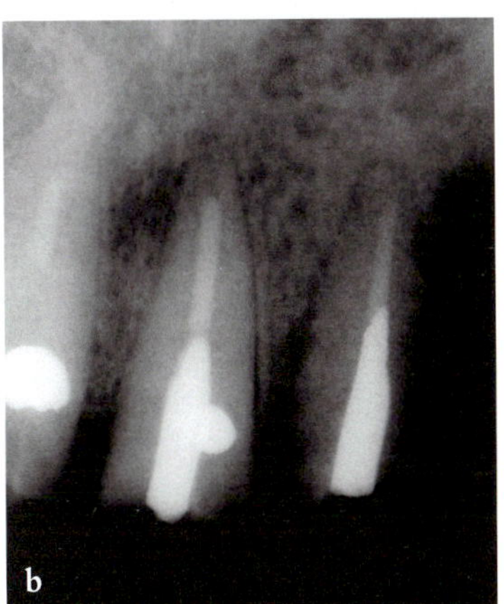


Fig 13-27 **(a and b)** Radiographs of the patient in Figure 13-26, showing the three fractured posts.

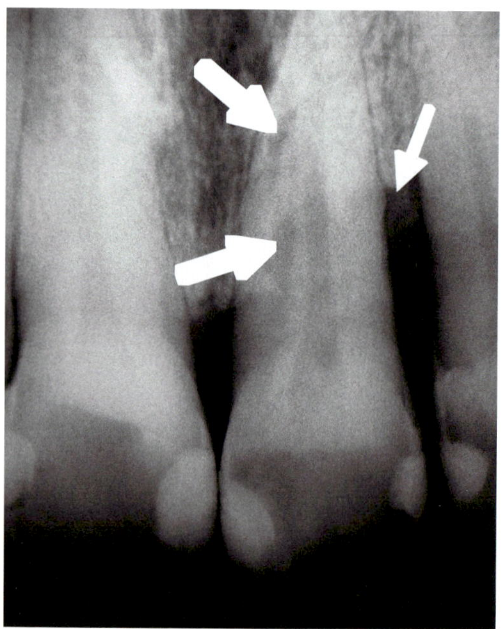

Fig 13-28 Radiograph of a musician's maxillary central incisor. The patient played a wind instrument, and he would constantly rest the instrument's mouthpiece on that tooth. Note the significant dental wear in the crown area. There is also bone loss adjacent to the distal area of the root (thin arrow) and a radiolucency on its mesial surface consistent with a possible root resorption (thick arrows).

showing variable degrees of invasive cervical resorption. This pathology was associated with bruxism in just six patients. Although occlusal stress accounts for a low percentage of dental resorption cases, its incidence cannot be dismissed. Rawlinson[24] reports on a mandibular first premolar affected by a severe occlusal trauma from bruxism showing severe apical and bone root resorption. Bone repair was achieved and root resorption stopped by means of endodontic treatment, occlusal adjustment, and the aid of a bite guard.

Figure 13-28 depicts the case of a male musician who plays a wind instrument; he presented describing sensitivity to percussion in the maxillary central incisor. This tooth was subject to localized, continuous trauma, since it supported the mouthpiece of the instrument. The pulp was vital, and some time was allowed to elapse before any treatment was undertaken. A recall radiograph showed possible root resorption. Figure 13-29 depicts the case of a male patient showing symptoms of bruxism. The patient presented with pulp symptoms in the left maxillary canine, and a radiograph demonstrated clear subgingival cervical root resorption.

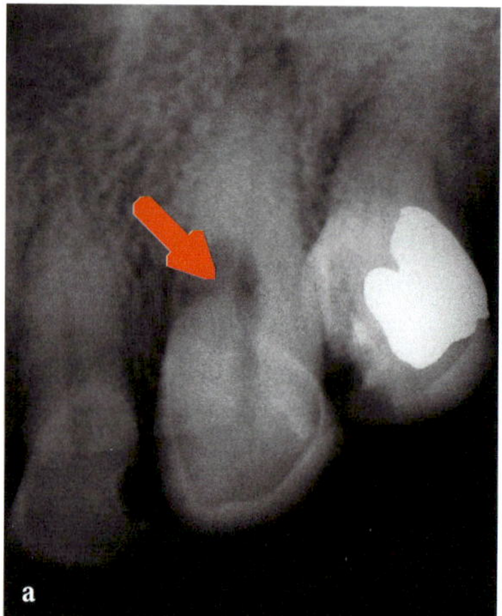


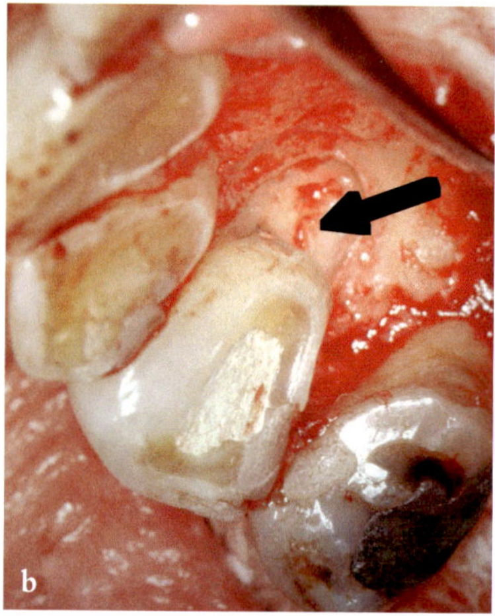


Fig 13-29 **(a)** Radiograph of a maxillary canine showing cervical root resorption (arrow). **(b)** Severe attrition from bruxism can be seen on the palatal surface of the canine. On raising the flap, the cervical root resorption area (arrow) is clearly visible.

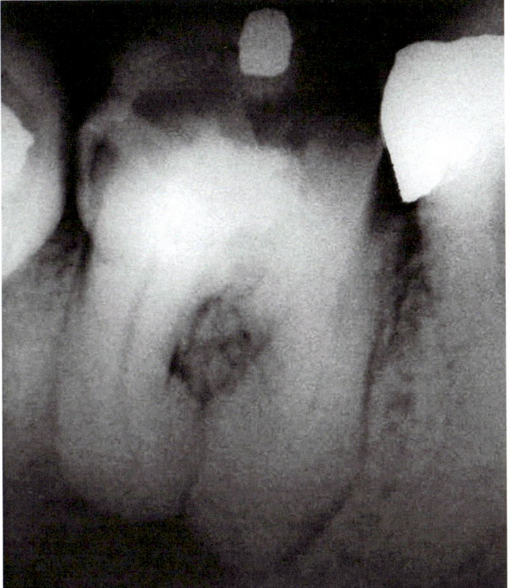

Fig 13-30 Radiograph of a bruxer's mandibular molar, with apical hypercementosis in both roots.

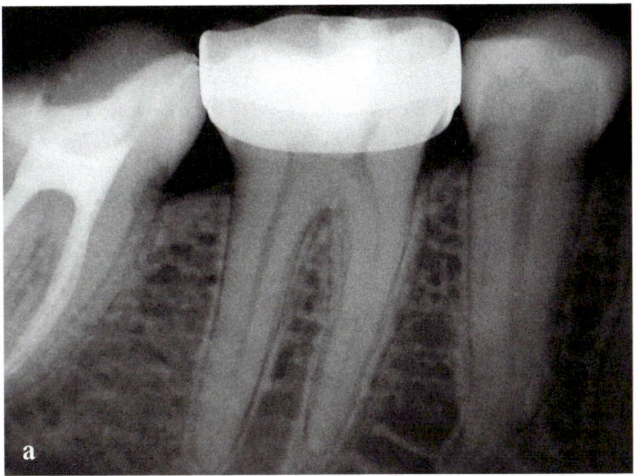

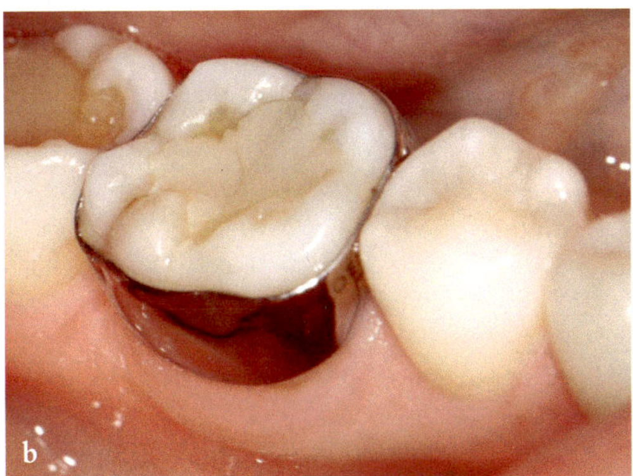

Fig 13-31 **(a)** Radiograph of a mandibular first molar to which an orthodontic band has temporarily been attached as protection, owing to the presence of an incomplete crown crack. **(b)** The molar with the orthodontic band.

*Relationship with apical dystrophic calcifications*

Rarely, the action of excessive occlusal forces over long periods may cause apical dystrophic calcifications to develop (hypercementosis)[7] (Fig 13-30). Determining the cause of these calcifications is very difficult because, although teeth are subjected to excessive forces on many an occasion, calcifications do not always develop.

### Treatment

*Crown cracks without pulpal and/or peri-radicular symptoms*

When there is a crack affecting just the crown and no pulpal symptoms are present, no endodontic treatment is indicated and only preventive therapy is required (e.g., if there is a cavity, enhancing the strength of crown walls by means of adhesive techniques, and/or cementing a band to the crown peripherally, so that the band can serve as support for some time – Fig 13-31). In such cases, placing intraradicular anchorage is not advisable, since it will only cause fracture to occur sooner and the tooth to split into parts. Treat occlusal misadjustments and carry out periodical clinical and radiographic follow-up. Patients should be warned of potential treatment failure.

When a crack is present, try to maintain pulp vitality whenever possible: pulp is the best defense against bacterial penetration. Always prefer prevention over therapeutics!

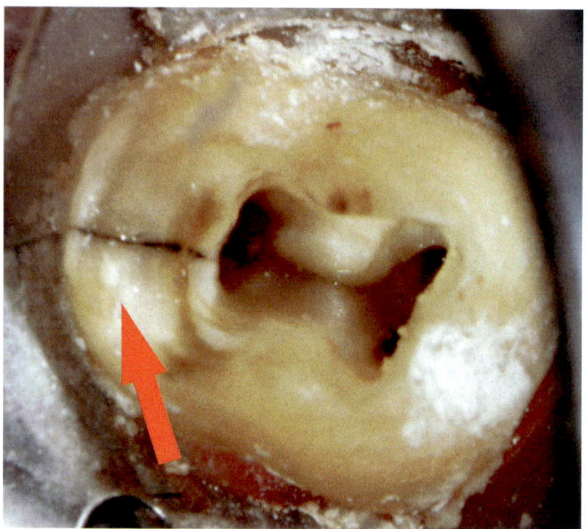

Fig 13-32 Picture of a mandibular molar, with the prepared endodontic cavity where a distal crack (arrow) can be seen.

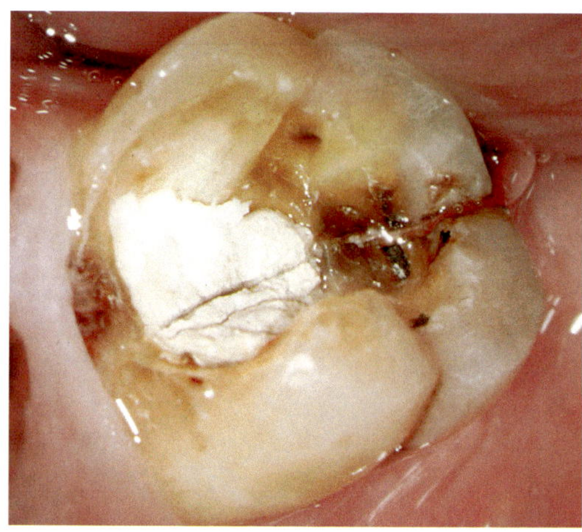

Fig 13-33 Mandibular molar showing a complete mesiodistal crack (arrow).

*Crown cracks or fractures with pulp and/or peri-radicular symptoms*

When a patient presents with irreversible pulpal symptoms, severe and spontaneous pain, or pulp necrosis with or without a peri-radicular lesion, there is no alternative but to perform endodontic treatment. The occlusal opening should be done with extreme care in order to preserve as much crown structure as possible. Crown restoration should be performed by following the procedure described above for cases in which there is pulp vitality: use of adhesive techniques and crown surface protection by means of a support band. Always treat occlusal maladjustments. If the crack extends along the axial walls of the pulp chamber without affecting the chamber floor, there is increased likelihood of success[25] (Figs 13-32 and 13-33). In this case, Gutmann and Rakusin[25] suggest obturating the fracture area with glass ionomer cement. Carry out periodical clinical and radiographic follow-up. If a crown fracture is seen with clear separation of both parts, removal of the crown portion is carried out in order to perform a prosthetic restoration of the tooth from the root remainder. If the fracture extends below the free border of the gum, and for the sake of restoration if needed, orthodontic root extrusion can be performed. In both cases, endodontic treatment is indicated.

*Crown–root cracks or fractures*

When a crown-root crack is present, prognosis is poor, and the only choice is to attempt to retain the tooth for a longer period (Figs 13-34 and 13-35). The patient should be made aware of the need to resort to this solution so that he or she can fully agree to it. If no endodontic treatment has been carried out, it should be performed. If fractures are present, the possibility of removing one of the parts should be considered, provided that the remaining part keeps its functional and esthetic value (Fig 13-36). When prosthetic restorations with intraradicular anchorage are present and a root crack or fracture is diagnosed, prognosis is very poor. Several treatment options have been suggested, all of them having a low success rate.[22]

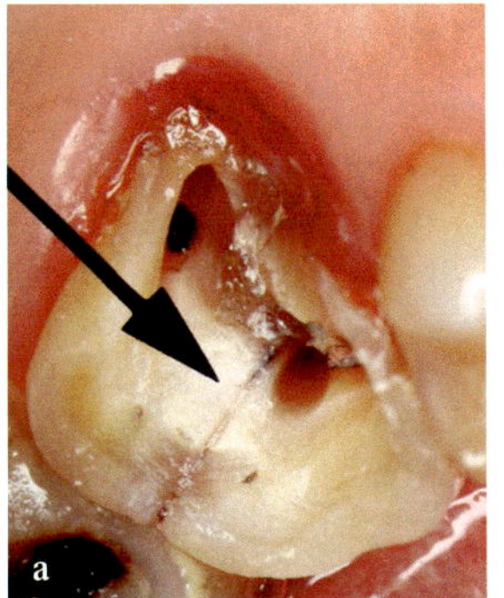
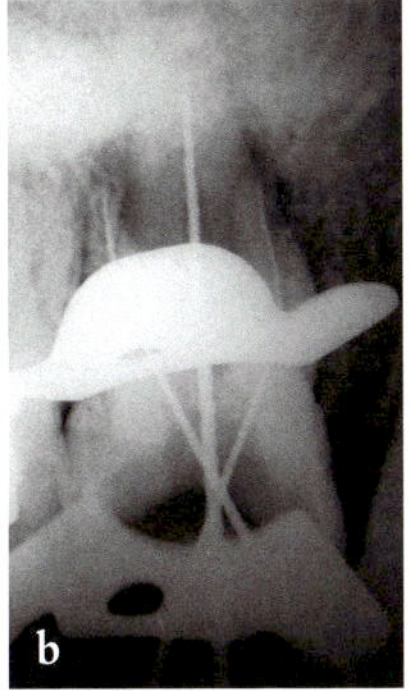

Fig 13-34 **(a)** A maxillary first molar where a crack can be seen on the pulp chamber floor in the mesiodistal direction (arrow). **(b)** Working length radiograph from which radiolucent peri-radicular images can be seen in both buccal roots.

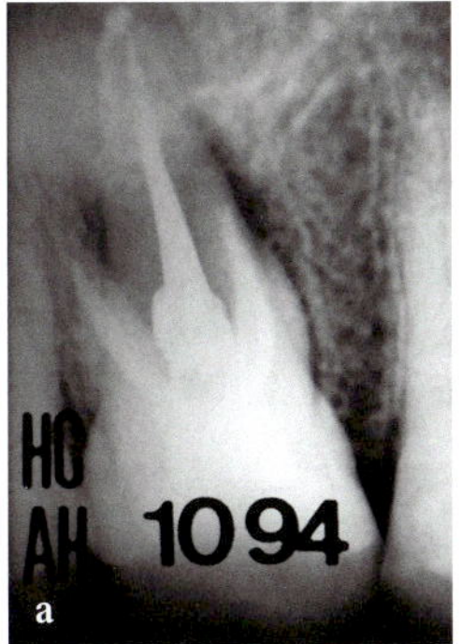

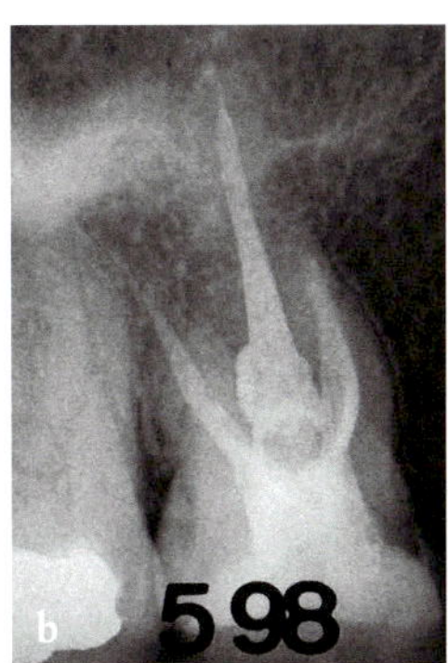


Fig 13-35 **(a)** Immediate postoperative radiograph and **(b)** recall radiograph (3 years and 7 months after the endodontic treatment) of the patient in Fig 13-34. Peri-radicular normality and bone repair of the area affected by the lesion can be observed. The pulp chamber was fully obturated with glass ionomer cement.

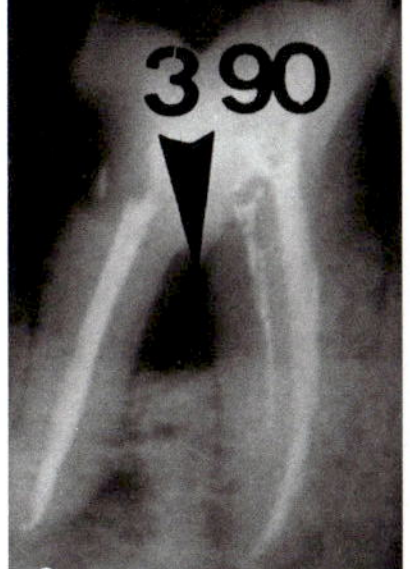

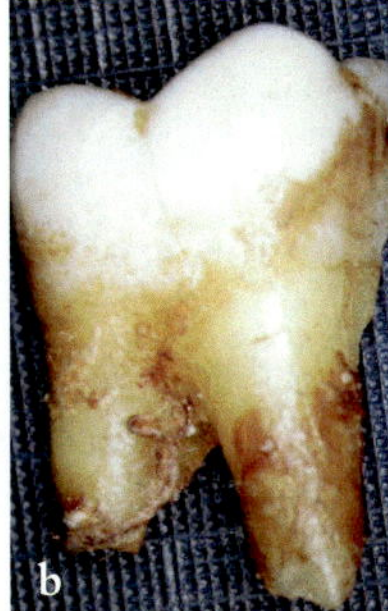
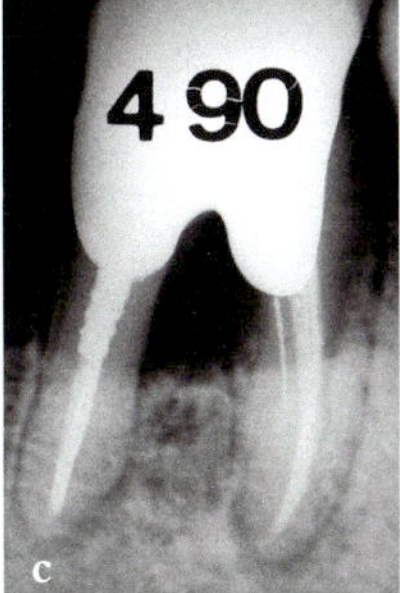

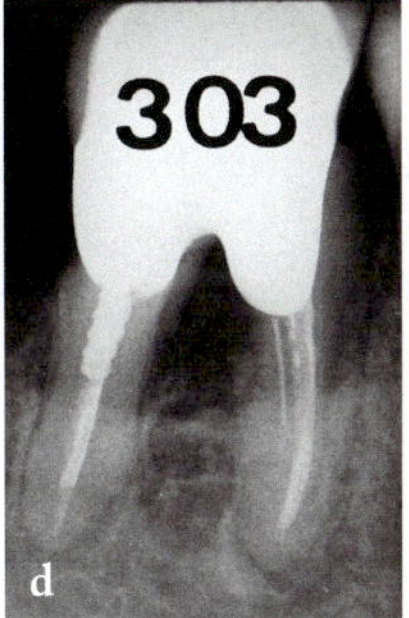

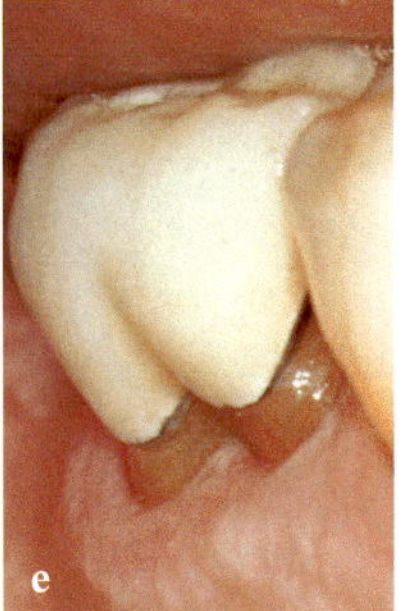

Fig 13-36 **(a)** Radiograph of a mandibular molar where a radiolucent image representing a crown–root fracture (arrow) is visible in the area of the furcation. **(b)** Extracted fragment involved in the fracture of the molar. **(c)** Immediate postoperative image following intraradicular anchorage placement and prosthetic restoration. **(d)** Follow-up radiograph nearly 13 years later. **(e)** The molar, where normal gingival can be appreciated in the furcation area.

*Fractures in posts or screws inside the root canal not affecting the dental root*

When there is a broken post inside the root canal, several procedures can be resorted to in order to attempt its removal. The patient should be warned that the maneuver is difficult and that root fracture or root-wall perforation or weakening may occur.

Removal maneuvers should be performed under a bright light to clearly distinguish the post or screw structure. Removal of fiberglass posts, zirconium posts, etc. is more complicated. It is also difficult to remove posts that are twisted around the dentin wall structure. The first maneuver consists of carving a slot around the post with the aid of a small round bur. LN burs (Dentsply-Maillefer, Ballaigues, Switzerland) are very useful for this procedure, since their long, thin neck does not interfere with vision (Fig 13-37).

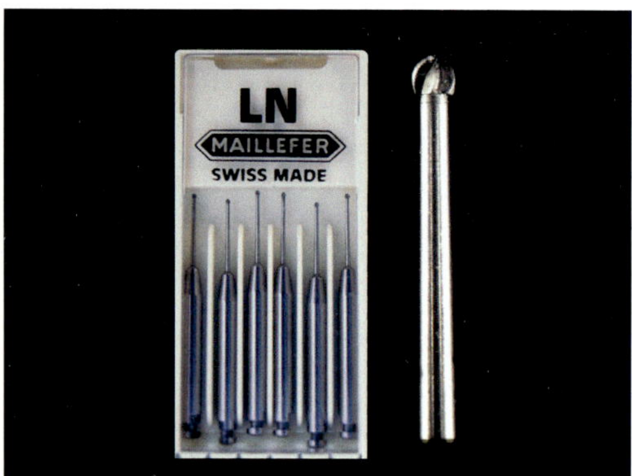


**Fig 13-37** Box containing LN burs, and a magnified view of the tip of one of them.

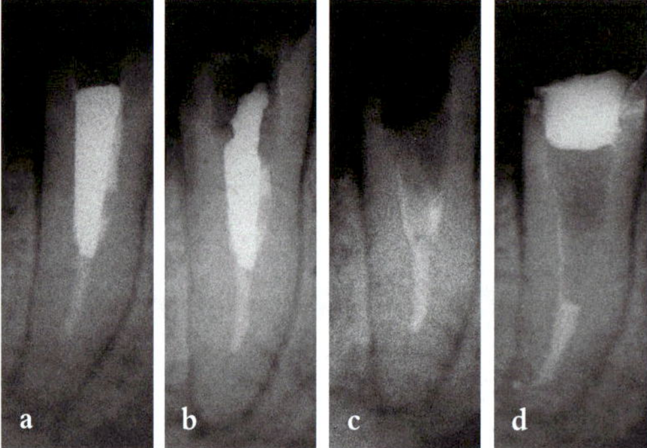

**Fig 13-38** **(a)** Mandibular premolar radiograph showing a fractured post inside the root canal. The canal was poorly treated, and a radiolucent peri-radicular image can be seen. **(b)** A groove was made around the post with an LN bur, to apply lateral ultrasound vibration over the fractured post. **(c)** Post removed from the root canal. **(d)** Immediate postoperative image following the endodontic retreatment.

When the slot has been carved, it is possible to work on the post laterally with the aid of ultrasound, in order to crack the cement of the tooth–post interface (Fig 13-38). An ultrasound insert of the proper size should be used so that it can fit the slot carved between the post and the tooth wall. Ultrasound irrigation should always be used so as to avoid tooth and bone overheating.

Special removal systems are available, such as the Thomas extractor (France) and the Ruddle post-removal system (SybronEndo, USA) (Fig 13-39). They feature trephines for making a groove around the post. The kit includes trephines of several sizes to match the size of the post to be removed. Then, a tubular insert of the same size as the trephine and having a small handle is screwed on to the fractured post. The insert must be screwed on to the post end in a clockwise direction (Thomas system) or in a counterclockwise direction (Ruddle system).

When the insert has been correctly screwed to the post, extraction pliers with two branches are used: one of them adjusts to the surface of the tooth and the other one adjusts to the handle of the insert. One of the branches is slowly opened by means of a threaded system; in this way, traction is exerted on the fractured post, which will then be removed (Fig 13-40). Removing a fractured post is complicated; it demands time, experience, wit, and good luck.

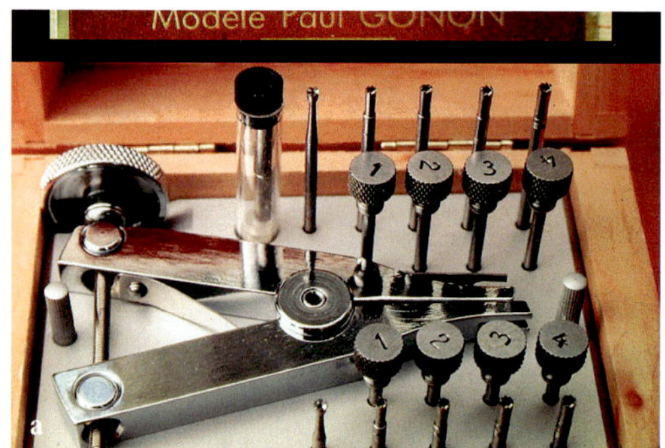


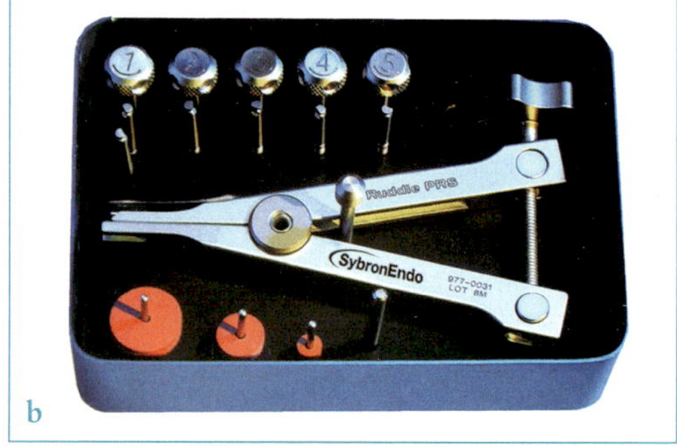


**Fig 13-39** Post removal systems: **(a)** Thomas extractor system, and **(b)** Ruddle post removal system.

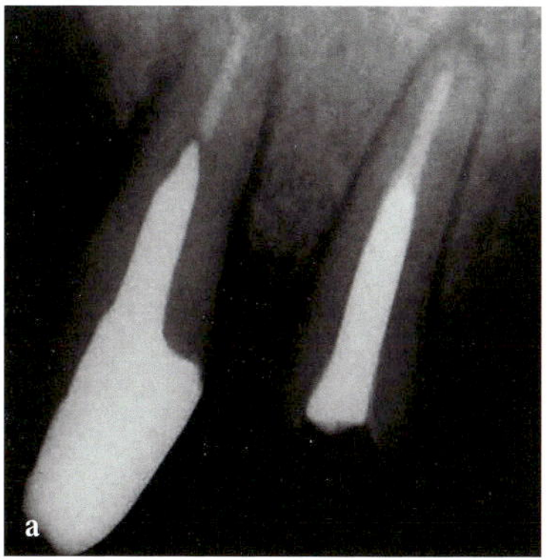

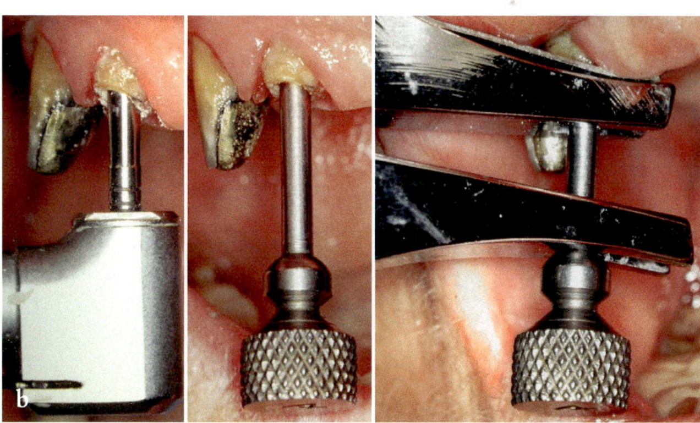

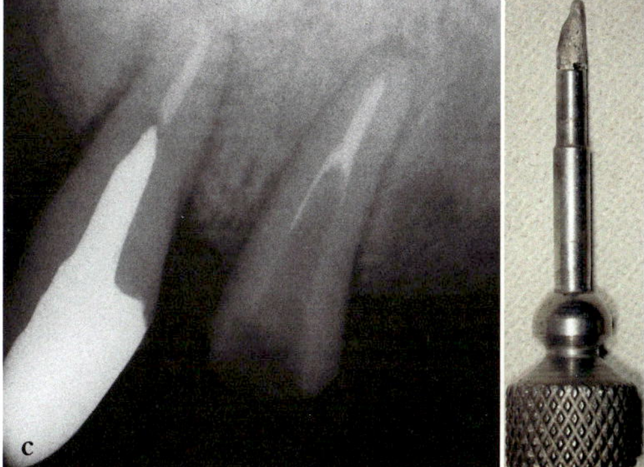

**Fig 13-40** **(a)** Radiograph of a maxillary lateral incisor showing a fractured post inside the root canal. **(b)** Left: Trephine being used to make a slot around the fractured post. Middle: Tubular insert of the same size as the trephine, already screwed on to the post. Right: Extraction pliers with a scissor mechanism exerting traction over the post. The fixed branch rests on the dental root; the other branch exerts traction on the insert screwed on to the fractured post. **(c)** Postoperative radiograph, and the extracted post.

*Root resorption*

In case of internal root resorption, pulpectomy is the treatment of choice. In external root resorption, the prognosis will depend on the extent and the degree of bone involvement their treatment entails. When endodontic treatment is indicated, temporary calcium hydroxide therapy may be used to offset external resorption effects. In other circumstances, when the dental structure is extensively damaged, endodontic treatment should be supplemented by surgical treatment whether the pulp is vital or necrosed.

First, endodontic treatment should be carried out, and then the corresponding surgery. Once the flap is made and the resorption area reached, the resorption cavity should be thoroughly curretted to remove the existing granulation tissue. Then the cavity should be obturated. The obturation material will be chosen according to the extent of resorption and the degree of esthetic involvement. Examples of the materials used for this are: amalgam, resin–glass ionomer cements (Vitremer, 3M, USA), SuperEBA (Bosworth Co., USA), and ProRoot MTA (Dentsply Tulsa Dental, USA) (Fig 13-41).

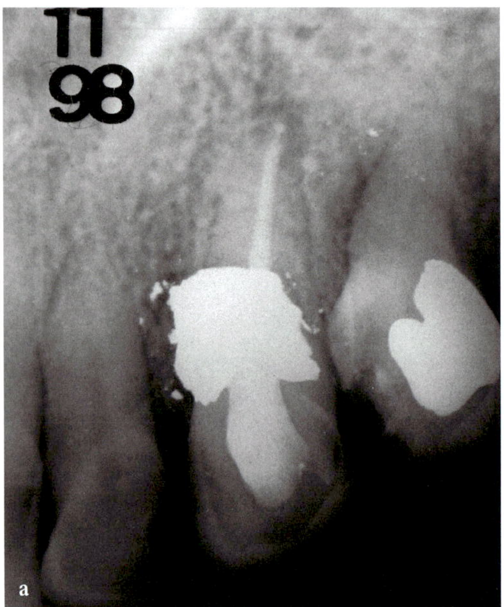


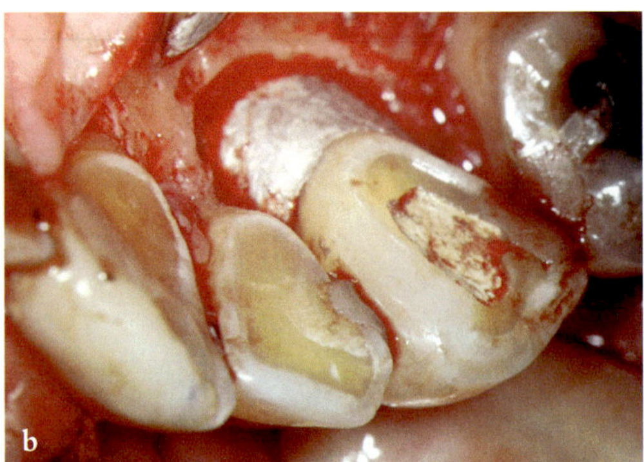

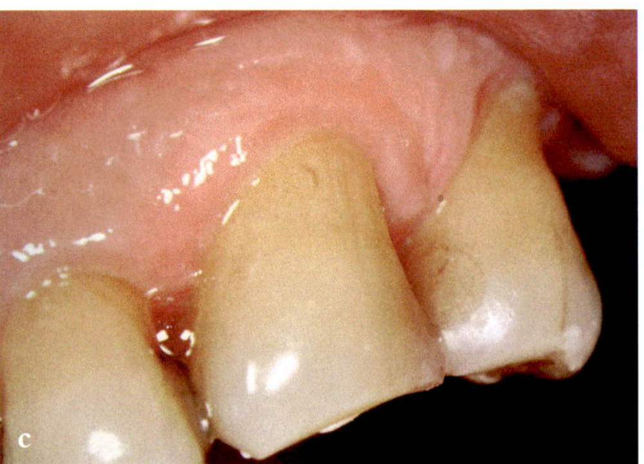

Fig 13-41 **(a)** Postoperative radiograph of the patient in Fig 13-29. The root canal was treated and cervical root resorption was obturated with amalgam. **(b)** Intraoperative picture after obturating the resorption with amalgam. **(c)** Vestibular view one week after suture removal.

*Apical dystrophic calcifications*

These calcifications should not be considered to be pathologic. They therefore require no treatment, though follow-up should be done in order to monitor their progress clinically and radiologically.

*Comment*

Treatment of the underlying cause – that is, control of the masticatory system alterations causing the condition – should be included in the therapy indicated for each of the above-described situations.

## References


1. Ingle JI. Alveolar osteoporosis and pulpal death associated with compulsive bruxism. Oral Surg Oral Med Oral Pathol 1960;13:1371–1381.
2. Natkin E, Ingle JI. A further report on alveolar osteoporosis and pulpal death associated with compulsive bruxism. J Am Soc Periodontics 1963;1:260–263.
3. Tronstad L, Langeland K. Effect of attrition on subjacent dentin and pulp. J Dent Res 1971;50:17–30.
4. Cooper MB, Landay MA, Seltzer S. The effects of excessive occlusal force on the pulp. II: Heavier and longer term forces. J Periodontol 1971;42:353–359.
5. Landay MA, Seltzer S. The effects of excessive occlusal force on the pulp. Oral Surg Oral Med Oral Pathol 1971;32:623–638.
6. Haugen E, Mjör IA. Pulpal reactions to attrition. J Endod 1975;1:12–14.
7. Rosenberg PA. Occlusion, the dental pulp, and endodontic treatment. Dent Clin North Am 1981;25:423–437.
8. Hethersay GS. Invasive cervical resorption: an analysis of potential predisposing factors. Quintessence Int 1999;30: 83–95.

9. Harn WM, Chen MC, Chen YHM, Liu JW, Chung CH. Effect of occlusal trauma on healing of periapical pathoses: report of two cases. Int Endod J 2001;34:554–561.
10. Morse DR. Clinical Endodontology: A Comprehensive Guide to Diagnosis, Treatment and Prevention. Springfield: Charles C. Thomas, 1974.
11. Stanley HR, Pereira J, Spiegel E, Broom C, Schultz M. The detection and prevalence of reactive and physiologic sclerotic dentin, reparative dentin and dead tracts beneath various types of dental lesions according to tooth surface and age. J Oral Pathol 1983;12:257–289.
12. Ten Cate AR. Histología. Desarrollo, estructura y función oral, ed 2. Buenos Aires: Ed Med Panamericana, 1986.
13. Canalda Sahli C, Brau Aguadé E. Endodoncia. Técnicas clínicas y bases científicas Barcelona. Masson, 2001.
14. Groves Cooke H. Reversible pulpitis with etiology of bruxism. J Endod 1982;8:280–281.
15. Yu CY. Role of occlusion in endodontic management: report of two cases. Aust Endod J 2004;30:110–115.
16. Kvinnsland S, Kristiansen AB, Kvinnsland I, Heveraas KJ. Effect of experimental traumatic occlusion on periodontal and pulpal blood flow. Acta Odontol Scand 1992;50: 211–219.
17. Sivasithamparam K, Harbrow D, Vinczer E, Young WG. Endodontic sequelae of dental erosion. Aust Dent J 2003; 48:97–101.
18. Petersson K, Söderström C, Kiani-Anaraki M, Lévy G. Evaluation of the ability of thermal and electrical tests to register pulp vitality. Endod Dent Traumatol 1999;15: 127–131.
19. Seltzer S. Endodontology: Biologic Considerations in Endodontic Procedures. New York: McGraw-Hill, 1971.
20. Fuss Z, Lustig J, Katz A, Tamse A. An evaluation of endodontically treated vertical root fractured teeth: impact of operative procedures. J Endod 2001;27:46–48.
21. Cohen S, Berman LH, Blanco L, Bakland L. A demographic analysis of vertical root fractures. J Endod 2006;32:1160–1163.
22. Moule AJ, Kahler B. Diagnosis and management of teeth with vertical root fractures. Aust Dent J 1999;44:75–87.
23. Tamse A, Fuss Z, Lustig J, Kaplavi J. An evaluation of endodontically treated vertically fractured teeth. J Endod 1999;25:506–508.
24. Rawlinson A. Treatment of root and alveolar bone resorption associated with bruxism. Br Dent J 1991;22: 445–447.
25. Gutmann JL, Rakusin H. Endodontic and restorative management of incompletely fractured molar teeth. Int Endod J 1994;27:343–348.

Chapter 14

# Influence of Trauma from Occlusion on the Periodontium

*Guillermo Schinini and Andres R. Sanchez*

## Introduction

The relationship between occlusal force and the onset and progress of periodontal disease has been a controversial topic for more than a century. The primary goal of this chapter is to evaluate the scientific evidence available to date, with a special interest in the interpretation of various lines of research on this topic.

At the beginning of the 20th century, Karolyi[1] asserted that a relationship exists between excessive occlusal forces and periodontal destruction. Subsequently, Stillman[2] in 1917 and Box[3] in 1935 suggested that excessive occlusal forces were the primary cause of periodontal disease. They recommended occlusal therapy to control tissue breakdown caused by periodontal disease.

Historically, trauma from occlusion has been defined as a submicroscopic or microscopic periodontal-membrane injury causing reversible pathologic mobility.[4] In 1962, Glickman and Smulow[5] carried out a monkey-model study and reported a close relationship between excessive occlusal forces and the course of inflammation. Microscope observations revealed that artificially created excessive occlusal pressure changed the pathway of inflammation from the gingiva into the underlying tissues (specifically, periodontal ligament); but, in the absence of such excessive forces, inflammation followed the course of the blood vessels.[6] Another interesting finding from this study was that particularly excessive pressure, but not excessive tension, could change the alignment of the transeptal fibers, and produce angular bone resorption and infrabony pockets.

In an earlier study in 1954, Macapanpan and Weinmann[7] reported that both excessive pressure and tension produced alterations in the periodontal ligament, and that inflammation passed into that altered area. On the other hand, the authors considered that, provided that such force was so severe as to cause necrosis of the periodontal ligament, this necrotic tissue would act as a barrier preventing the inflammation from extending into the underlying periodontal tissues.[8,9]

Later on, in a study of human autopsy material, these authors corroborated the relationship between excessive occlusal forces and the course of gingival inflammation.[10] They also stated that excessive occlusal forces do not change the vascular and cellular features of gingival inflammation, but they do change the environment around the inflammation and consequently lead to changes in its direction. Finally they postulated that, when inflammation spreads beyond the marginal gingiva and combines with occlusal trauma, they become interrelated co-destructive factors in periodontitis.

In contrast, Stahl,[11] who also studied autopsy material, did not find such an association. Histologically, he found that the inflammatory process spread into the crestal septum instead of spreading into the periodontal ligament space, and further suggested that "periodontal tissues may have adaptive capabilities to withstand abnormal occlusal forces which also limit inflammatory infiltration into the periodontal spaces from the marginal gingiva".

Waerhaug[12,13] studied 48 teeth that had been extracted owing to advanced destructive periodontal disease. The goal of this investigation was to find out to what extent traumatic occlusal forces and subgingival plaque were involved in the pathogenesis of infrabony pockets. Before extracting the teeth, the author recorded premature contacts, mobility, and cuspal interferences. In opposition to Glickman's theory, he found a close relationship between subgingival plaque front and the remaining attachment fibers, as well as between downgrowth of subgingival plaque and bone loss architecture. Therefore, based on these findings, Waerhaug postulated that there was no evidence suggestive of the involvement of trauma from occlusion in the pathogenesis of infrabony pockets.

More recently, several authors have reviewed the literature on this topic and agreed that there is not enough information available on the relationship between the progression of periodontal disease and trauma from occlusion.[14–17] However, it is important to mention that other authors disagree, since they consider such occlusal discrepancies to be a risk factor for periodontitis.[18,19]

## Periodontal Lesions

In the normal periodontium, the apical cells of the junctional epithelium are located at the cement–enamel junction, and correspond with the coronal level of connective tissue attachment. In the diseased periodontium (periodontitis), the termination of the junctional epithelium is located on the cementum surface, because of the apical downgrowth of junctional epithelium. The distance from the cement–enamel junction to the apical cells of the junctional epithelium reflects the loss of connective tissue attachment caused by the process of the disease.

In addition, this loss of connective tissue attachment is accompanied by loss of crestal alveolar bone, formation of a long junctional epithelium, and a gingival pocket.

Periodontitis has a multifactorial etiology. However, all different forms of periodontitis appear to have a common series of underlying events leading to tissue breakdown and tooth attachment loss.[20]

## Occlusal Trauma Lesions

The American Academy of Periodontology defines "occlusal trauma" as an injury to the attachment or tooth as a result of excessive occlusal forces. In other words, occlusal trauma refers to a response or effect on the periodontium.[21] In addition, depending on the size of forces and the status of the supporting tissues, occlusal trauma can be classified as primary or secondary (Fig 14-1).

- *Primary occlusal trauma* is an injury resulting in tissue changes from excessive occlusal forces applied to a tooth with normal support.

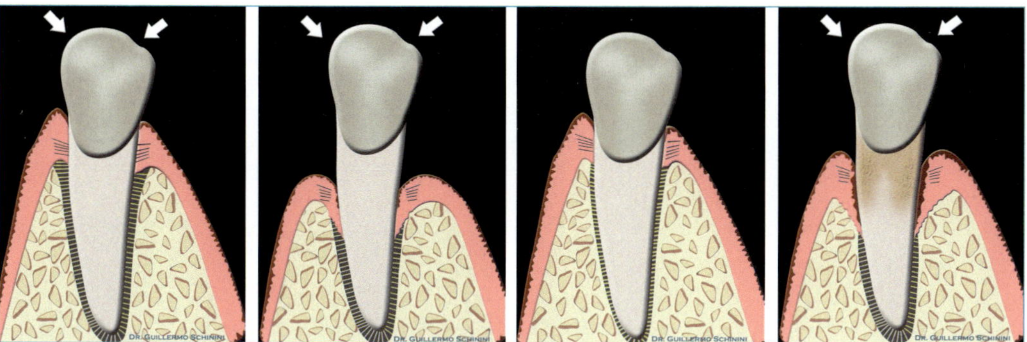

Fig 14-1 **(a)** Primary occlusal trauma: normal bone level with normal attachment level and excessive occlusal force. **(b)** Secondary occlusal trauma: reduced bone support and reduced attachment level with normal/excessive occlusal force. **(c)** Healing response of occlusal trauma lesion after eliminating excessive forces. **(d)** Combined periodontal/occlusal trauma lesion demonstrating downgrowth of the junctional epithelium in a plaque-associated lesion.

- *Secondary occlusal trauma* is an injury resulting in tissue changes from normal or excessive occlusal forces applied to a tooth with reduced support.[22]

Clinically, all the following signs and symptoms can be detected in patients with occlusal trauma: tooth mobility, fremitus, premature occlusal contacts, wear facets, pathologic tooth migration, fractured teeth, and thermal hypersensitivity. Several case studies are presented in Figures 14-2 to 14-9.

Radiographically, widening of the periodontal ligament (PDL) space, vertical or circumferential bone loss, and root resorption have been demonstrated. Histologically, studies report increased width of the periodontal ligament, and increased numbers of blood vessels and leukocytes. In addition, there is a larger number of osteoclastic cells, and a decrease in the percentage and number of collagen fibers inserted in the cementum and alveolar bone.[23,24]

The chapter will now focus on the published scientific evidence regarding the relationship between occlusal trauma and healthy or diseased periodontal tissues.

## Effect of Occlusal Trauma on the Healthy Periodontium

Svamberg and Lindhe[25,26] studied a series of Beagle dogs and demonstrated that excessive occlusal forces in the healthy or inflamed periodontium resulted in increased tooth mobility, vascularization, and bone resorption. These forces, however, did not cause apical migration of the epithelial attachment or inflammatory changes in the supracrestal component. The authors concluded that trauma from occlusion does not induce gingival inflammation or infiltration of round cells in the supra-alveolar connective tissue of healthy gingiva. It also does not aggravate an established gingival inflammation or facilitate the spread of the inflammation or round cell infiltration into the periodontal ligament.

Subsequently, in 1976, Polson et al[27] used the squirrel monkey model to evaluate the periodontal response to jiggling forces applied to second and third mandibular bicuspids in the mesiodistal direction. They reported that, 2 weeks after receiving jiggling forces, the appearance of the alveolar bone and the periodontal ligament showed considerable abnormal changes without loss of connective tissue attachment. Ten weeks later, the histological appearance was significantly

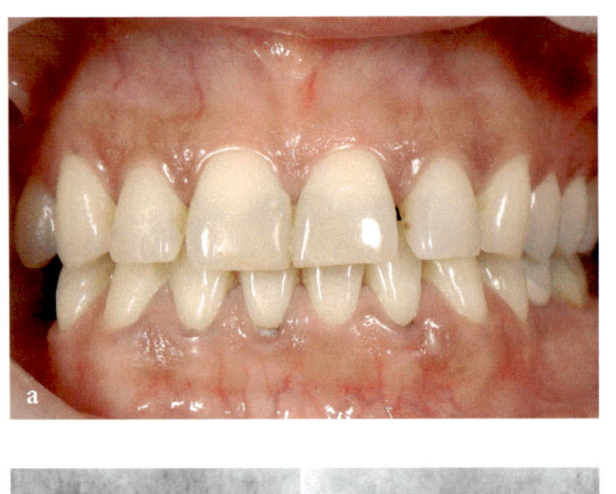
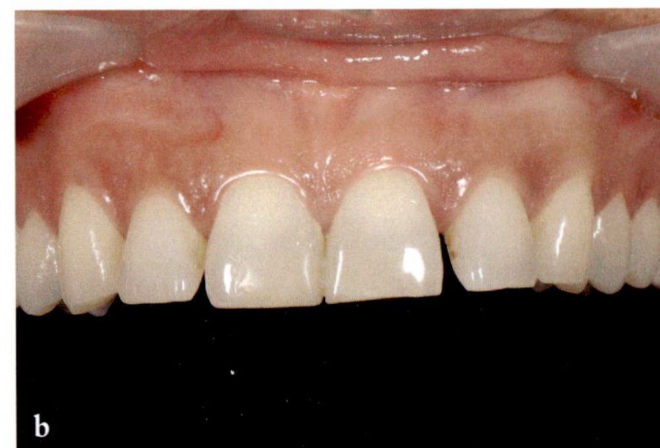
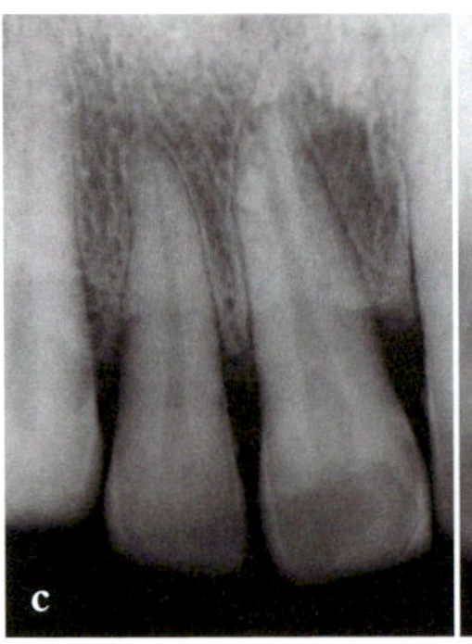
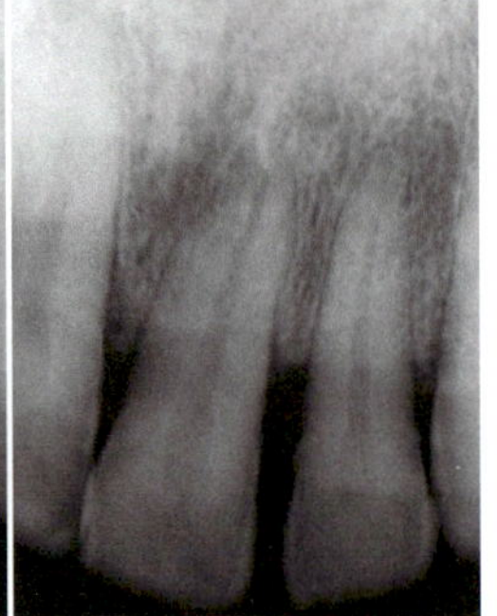
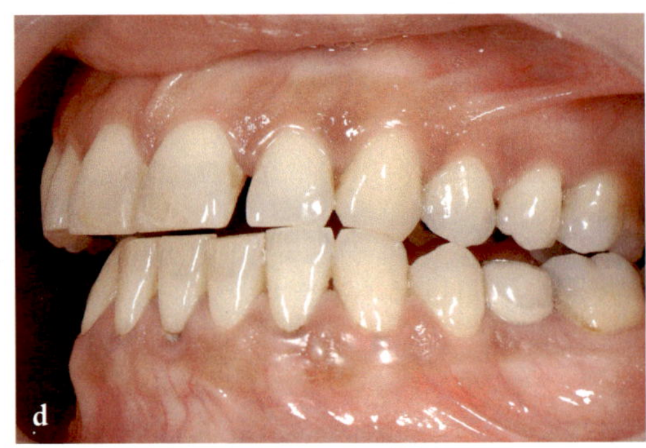
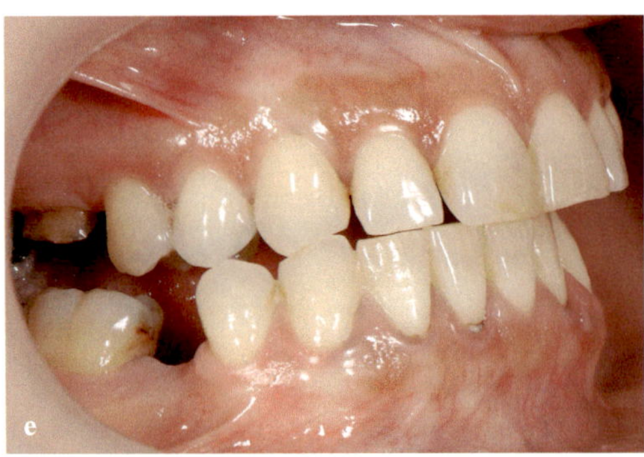

Fig 14-2 **(a)** Chronic generalized periodontitis in a young female smoker. Note the presence of supra- and subgingival calculus despite the patient presenting with adequate oral hygiene. **(b)** Front view of maxillary incisors. Note how pathologic migration of lateral incisors is generating diastemas. **(c)** Radiographic evidence of trauma from occlusion in the same patient, showing bone loss and widening of the periodontal ligament space. **(d)** Lateral right excursion of the mandible showing group function involving lateral incisors due to excessive incisal wear. **(e)** Lateral left excursion of the mandible in the same patient.

different, with the presence of fewer osteoclasts, which suggested that osseous resorption was not occurring during this phase. These findings would probably represent periodontium adaptation to excessive occlusal forces. Clinically, tooth mobility occurred in all directions (buccal–lingual, mesiodistal, and vertical). The authors concluded that jiggling trauma caused loss of crestal bone height as well as a considerable loss of alveolar bone volume.

The evidence suggests that occlusal trauma affecting a healthy periodontium,[27] an inflamed periodontium,[25] or a reduced but healthy periodontium[28,29] will not cause loss of connective tissue attachment or periodontal pocket formation.

On the other hand, in the absence of inflammation, the abnormal changes in alveolar bone as a result of occlusal trauma can be reverted when excessive forces are discontinued. Histologically, these studies showed that when occlusal trauma was eliminated, the lesion healed, with new bone deposition and PDL fibers showing normal orientation and cellular activity. In addition, the vascularity of the widened PDL membrane was re-established and bone resorptive activity discontinued. Therefore, initially, the periodontal supporting structures will undergo physiologic adaptation with widened PDL, loss of alveolar bone height and volume, and increased tooth mobility. In a subsequent phase, the periodontium will try to repair or regenerate the affected tissues.[30,31]

In conclusion, these research studies suggest that trauma from occlusion *per se* will not initiate gingivitis or periodontitis, and once the causative factors are removed the lesion will heal.

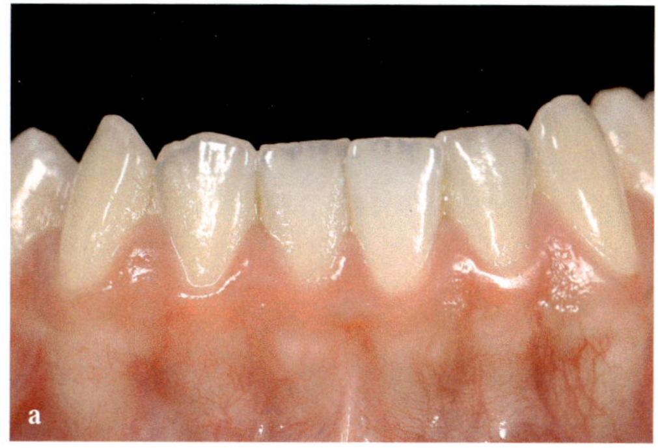

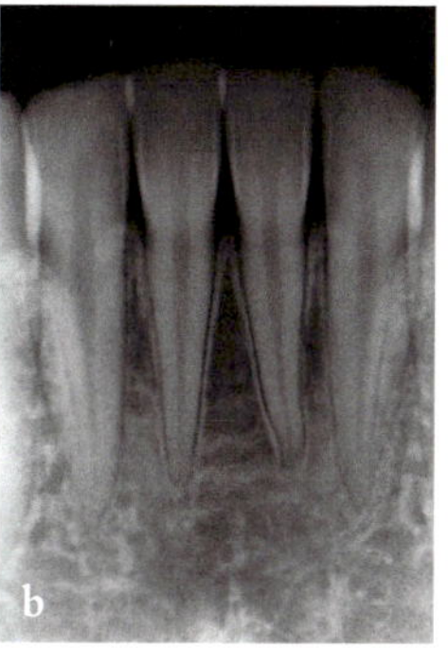

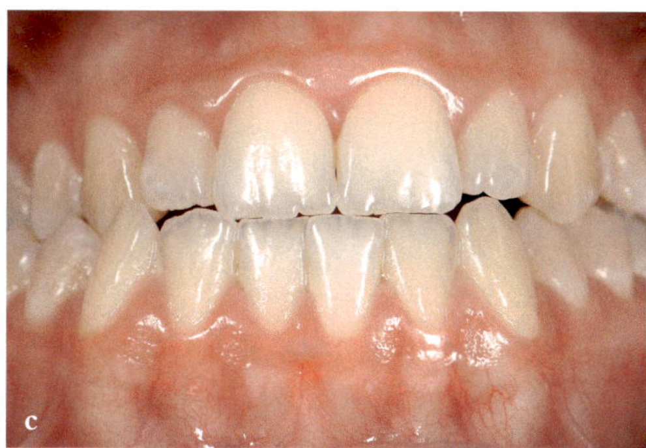

Fig 14-3 **(a)** Mandible incisors in a young healthy patient with persistent pain in central incisors. **(b)** Radiographically, there is a normal bone level and increased periodontal ligament space. **(c)** Increased occlusal forces on the two central mandibular incisors due to malocclusion and unilateral crossbite.

## Effect of Occlusal Trauma on the Diseased Periodontium

Using the Beagle dog model, Lindhe and Svamberg[32] induced experimental periodontitis on the mesial aspect of the fourth premolar through a combination of surgery and plaque retention model. Several weeks later, the authors installed a device in the maxillary arch to allow occlusal contact with the distal surface of the antagonist fourth premolar. A second device was installed in the mandible consisting of a lingual spring attached to a lingual bar, thus allowing the tooth to return to its original position. Jiggling forces were applied for a period of six months; after this time, the radiographic analysis showed a marked difference in the osseous morphology. Besides, the authors reported the presence of angular defects, infrabony pockets on the pressure side, and a widening of the PDL space in experimental sites when compared to control sites. Histometric analysis demonstrated an increased amount of attachment loss in the experimental sites subjected to a combination of periodontal disease and occlusal trauma when compared to control sites subjected only to periodontal disease. The authors concluded that trauma from occlusion in the dog model seems to accelerate the progression of experimental periodontitis.[32-34]

Meitner et al[35] conducted other animal experiments and studied the effect of trauma from occlusion on marginal periodontitis. The authors used the squirrel monkey model, and compared periodontitis lesions alone for 20 weeks and jiggling forces superimposed on the periodontitis lesions for the last 10 weeks. The radiographic analysis of the groups showed an increased loss of alveolar crest height in the test group when compared to the control group. The histomorphometric analysis of the interproximal areas failed to demonstrate marked differences in attachment loss in three of the four pairs of interproximal surfaces.

This study conflicts with Glickman's proposed theory of co-destruction, since it suggests that it is highly improbable that occlusal trauma superimposed to periodontitis will increase the progression of attachment loss. Drawing conclusions or comparing the results of both studies is difficult, because the animal models used, the methods through which periodontal disease was induced, and the jiggling forces applied were different.[36] No controversy exists, though, about the fact that trauma from occlusion increases the amount of alveolar bone loss.

However, from a strict treatment planning viewpoint, it is important to know when and how to indicate a sequence of therapy in situations where both periodontal disease and occlusal trauma exist.

A group of researchers from the University of Rochester (NY) carried out several studies and evaluated periodontal response after selectively removing either inflammation or trauma, or both at the same time. After experimentally inducing periodontitis and trauma in monkeys, only jiggling forces were discontinued.[31] After 10 weeks' of discontinued occlusal trauma, the histological examinations revealed that there was no decrease in tooth mobility and no evidence of bone regeneration.

Kantor et al[37] used the same experimental model and eliminated both factors. They found that new bone formation was apparent, but somehow it had not increased the height of the alveolar bone, probably owing to some irreversible crestal bone loss. Later on in subsequent studies,[38,39] when inflammation was eliminated in the presence of continued jiggling forces, there was a reduction in tooth hypermobility, but no difference in the level of connective tissue attachment or location of crestal alveolar bone between control and experimental sites. However, the authors stated that "bone regeneration may occur in the presence of active continued hypermobility after resolution of inflammation".

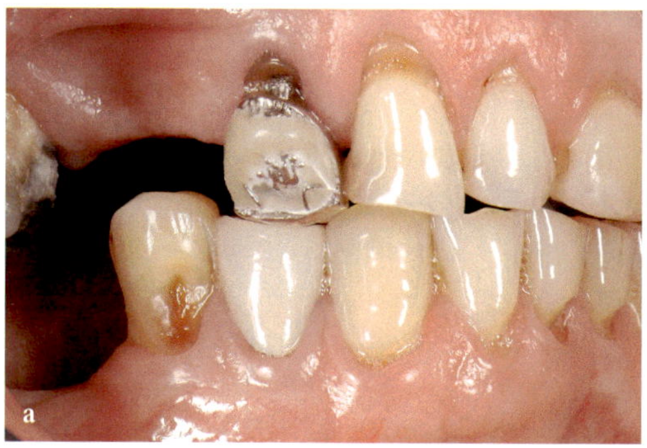
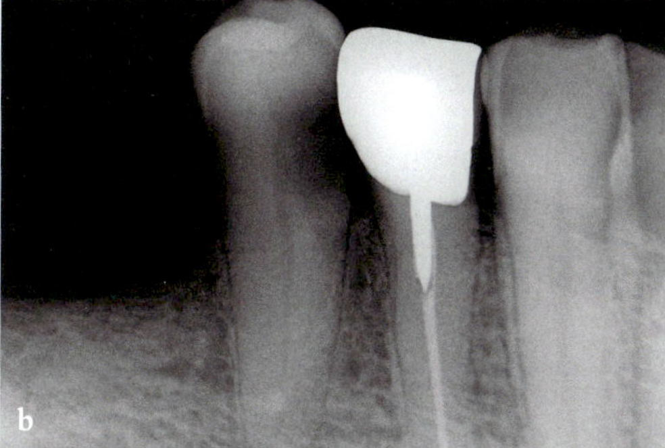

**Fig 14-4** **(a)** Adult patient with bruxism presenting dental abfractions, defective restorations, and poor plaque control. **(b)** Radiographically, there is no vertical bone loss or widening of the periodontal ligament space despite coexistent parafunctional habits.

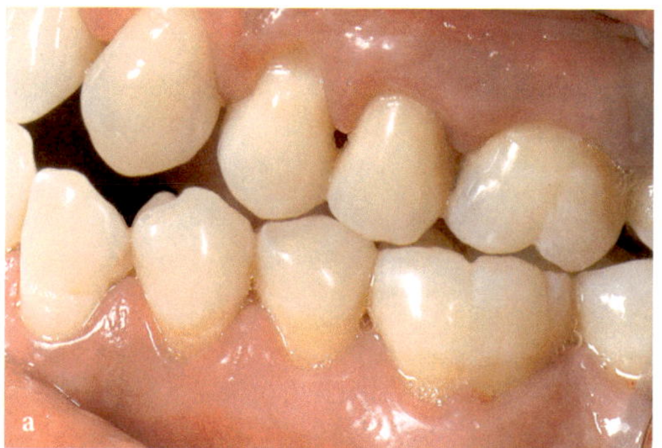
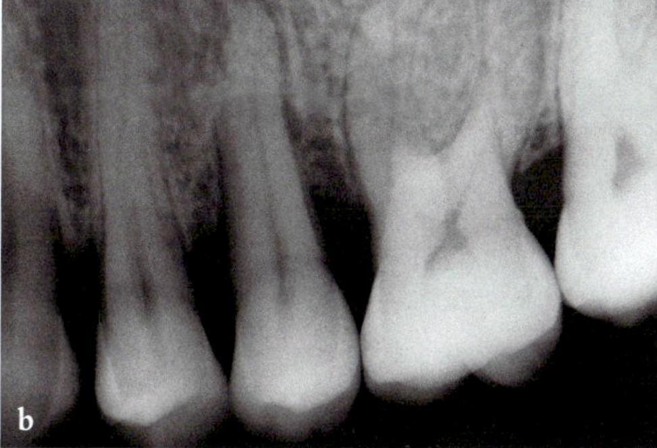

**Fig 14-5** **(a)** Secondary occlusal trauma in a 38-year-old male with chronic periodontitis. Note cuspal interference on the working side. **(b)** Angular funnel-shaped defect on the second premolar and loss of bone levels on the adjacent teeth.

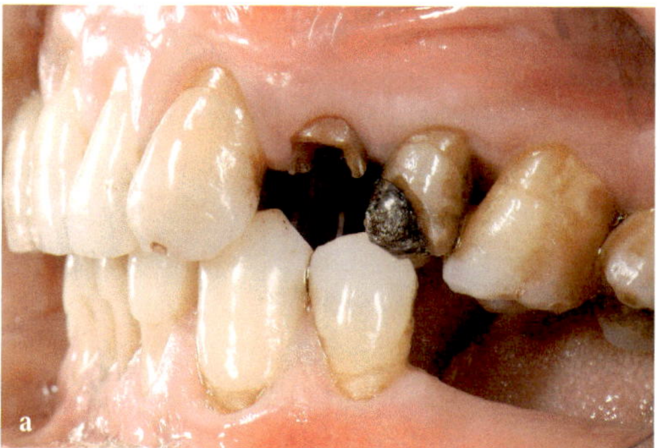
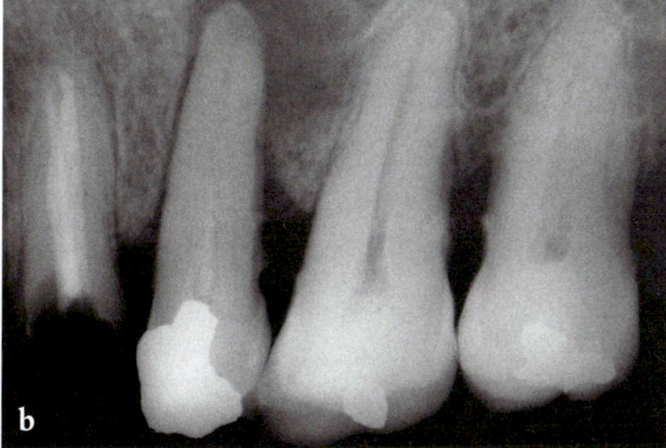

**Fig 14-6** **(a)** Severe chronic periodontitis in a 60-year-old patient with posterior bite collapse and increased mobility in the maxillary premolar area due to jiggling forces. Note the crown fracture in the first premolar and an enamel cuspal fracture in the second premolar. **(b)** Angular bone defect, subgingival calculus, and increased periodontal ligament space around the second premolar.

## Human Clinical Evidence

One of the clinical parameters or signs suggestive of the presence of trauma from occlusion is *tooth hypermobility*, even though this parameter alone cannot prove the existence of trauma from occlusion. Loss of alveolar bone height is considered to be associated with an increase in tooth mobility; however, in teeth subjected to trauma from occlusion, the adaptation process to the trauma as well as the response of the supporting tissues will also clinically manifest as increased tooth mobility.[40]

In the diagnosis of trauma from occlusion, clinicians should consider the presence of persistent pain, increased tooth mobility (measurements at different time intervals), and radiographic evidence of bone loss. The presence of a widened periodontal ligament could suggest that the tooth is being affected by occlusal trauma or is undergoing a process of physiologic adaptation.

According to Ramfjord and Ash,[40] the relationship between periodontal disease and trauma from occlusion is controversial in part owing to the lack of specific criteria to identify occlusal trauma.

Jin and Cao[41] established a new occlusal analysis to account for the presence or absence of premature contacts in centric relation, as well as during lateral and protrusive movements. At the same time, the authors indicated that different parameters could be used in combination as diagnostic indices of trauma from occlusion; they called these clinical indices *trauma from occlusion index* and *adaptability index*. The former index comprises the presence of functional mobility (also known as "fremitus") and radiographic widening of the PDL; the adaptability index involves the presence of tooth wear facets and radiographic thickening of the lamina dura.

Yuodelis and Mann[42] indicated that teeth with contacts on the non-working side (balancing side) had significantly deeper pocket depth, more alveolar bone loss, and greater mobility. On the other hand, Shefter and McFall[43] were not able to find any association between several patterns of occlusal contacts and the severity of periodontal disease. In addition, Pihlstrom et al[44] evaluated the association between occlusal trauma signs, periodontitis severity, and radiographic bone loss in the maxillary first molars of 300 patients. The authors concluded that, compared to teeth without premature occlusal contact, teeth with premature occlusal contacts in centric, balanced, non-balanced, and protrusive excursions showed no increased periodontal disease severity. In addition, they found that teeth demonstrating fremitus and widened PDL had deeper probing depths, more attachment loss, and less percentage of radiographic bone support.

Hanamura et al[45] investigated the relationship between periodontal status and bruxism in two groups of patients (periodontal and bruxism) using measurements of alveolar bone height, clinical attachment level, mobility, and occlusal wear. The authors reported that both disease entities are in general not closely associated.

Jin and Cao[41] attempted to correlate the signs of trauma from occlusion with the severity of periodontal disease in 32 patients with moderate to severe chronic periodontitis. This study demonstrated no differences regarding probing depths, clinical attachment level, and osseous support between teeth that presented premature occlusal contacts and those that did not. However, posterior teeth with premature contacts in centric occlusion or on the non-working side demonstrated widening of the PDL. In addition, the authors showed that given the same amount of attachment loss, teeth with occlusal trauma showed less osseous support than teeth without trauma, and this difference in alveolar bone support was more pronounced with an increase in attachment loss. These findings suggest that trauma from occlusion positively correlates with alveolar bone loss in patients with moderate to severe chronic periodontitis.

Burgett et al[46] carried out a randomized clinical trial on the influence of occlusal adjustment

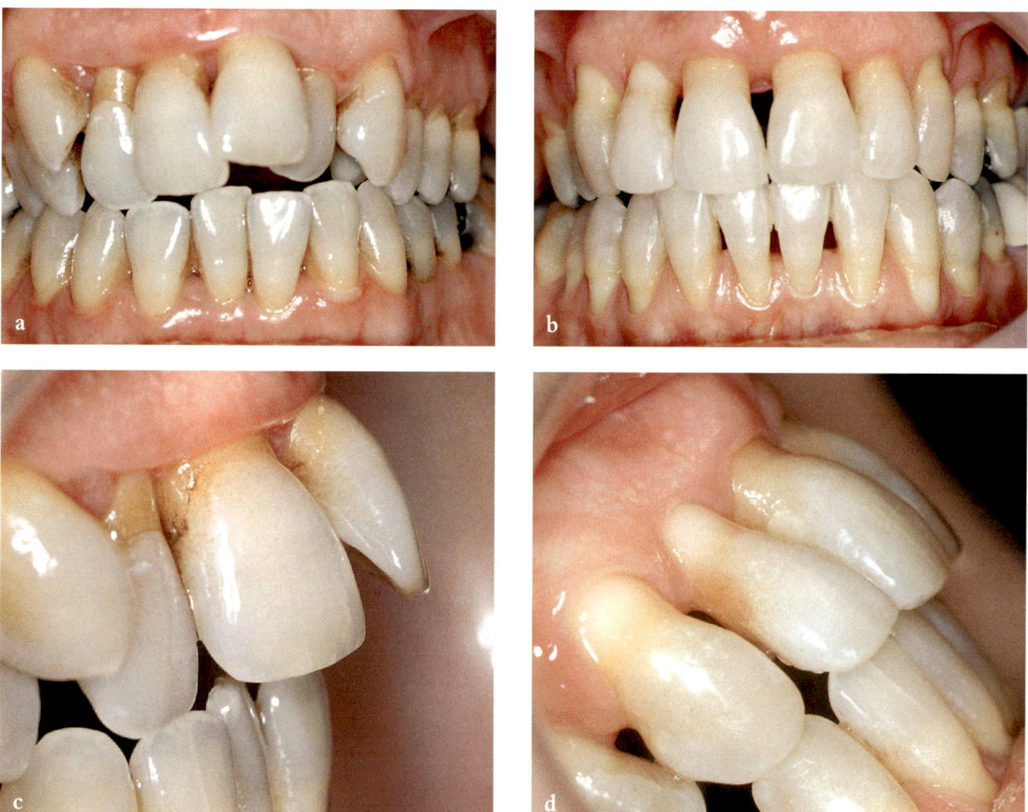


Fig 14-7 **(a)** Dental chaos associated with generalized periodontal disease in a 42-year-old patient. Note premature contact on the lateral right maxillary incisor. **(b)** Clinical presentation 3 years after completing periodontal–orthodontic therapy. **(c)** Lateral view before treatment. **(d)** Lateral view after periodontal–orthodontic therapy.

therapy in patients undergoing periodontal treatment. They evaluated these patients for tooth mobility, probing depths, and clinical attachment levels for a period of 2 years. After receiving nonsurgical periodontal treatment, the patients were randomized to two groups; the experimental group received occlusal therapy, and the control group did not receive any occlusal therapy. Afterwards, a split-mouth design was used; patients received a modified Widman flap in one quadrant, and scaling and root planing in the contralateral quadrant. The results demonstrated that teeth receiving occlusal therapy gained an average of 0.4 mm clinical attachment when compared to teeth that had not received occlusal therapy. The authors also reported no differences between both groups in terms of probing depths and mobility index. The clinical attachment gain in patients subject to occlusal therapy was statistically significant but clinically insignificant.

Nunn and Harrel[47] investigated the effect of different occlusal discrepancies on periodontitis progress in 89 private-practice patients. The authors gathered information from periodontal examinations that included a detailed occlusal analysis (discrepancies between initial contact in

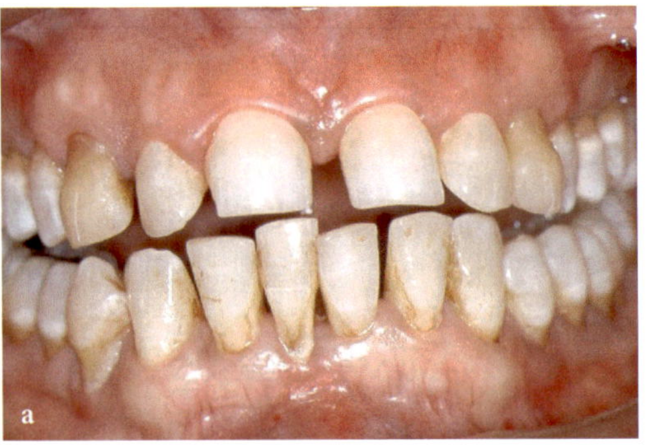

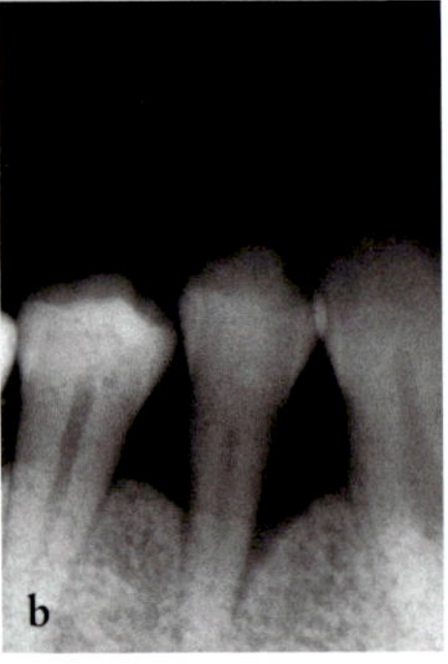

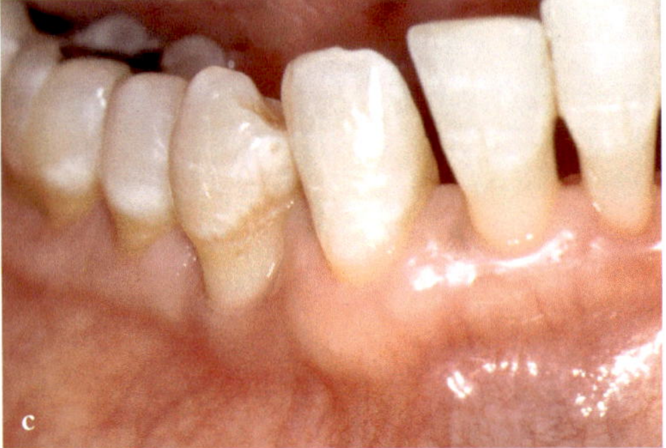

Fig 14-8 **(a)** Pathologic migration of several teeth in a 55-year-old woman with chronic periodontitis. **(b)** Vertical bone defects and light extrusion of the first mandibular premolar. **(c)** Buccal displacement of the first premolar due to jiggling forces in this periodontally treated patient.

centric relation and maximum intercuspation; working, non-working side in lateral and protrusive movements) at baseline and after 12 months. In this study, the subjects were divided into three different groups according to the periodontal treatment status. One group received periodontal surgical treatment, another group received periodontal non-surgical treatment only, and the third group received no periodontal treatment. The authors demonstrated that subjects presenting occlusal discrepancies had deeper probing depths, increased mobility, and worse periodontal prognosis when compared to patients having no occlusal discrepancies. Therefore, the authors concluded that occlusal factors are a risk factor of periodontitis progress in patients with pre-existing periodontal disease.[47,48] Later, another study by the same authors evaluated the effect of occlusal factors on the gingival width. They did not find any association between premature occlusal contacts and changes in the width of the gingival keratinized tissue.[49]

A recent cross-sectional epidemiologic study investigated the potential associations between dynamic occlusal interferences and periodontitis in 2,980 subjects from north-eastern Germany.[50] The authors evaluated different periodontal clinical parameters (probing depths, clinical attachment levels, plaque index), and occlusal parameters (premature occlusal contacts on working and non-working sides, and contacts in protrusion in premolars and molars). The results showed a negative influence of premature contacts on the non-working side on the probing depths (–0.13 mm) and clinical attachment levels (–0.14 mm). The authors stated that the impact of occlusal variables on periodontal parameters was proven to be statistically significant, but should be considered very small in magnitude. Therefore, data from this study show evidence of a statistically significant association but weak clinical significance.

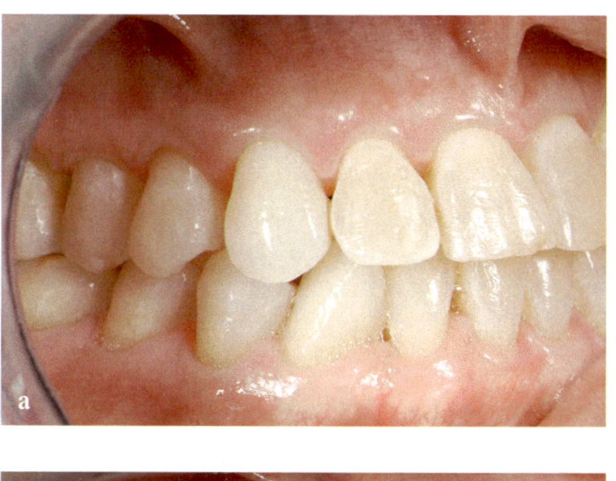


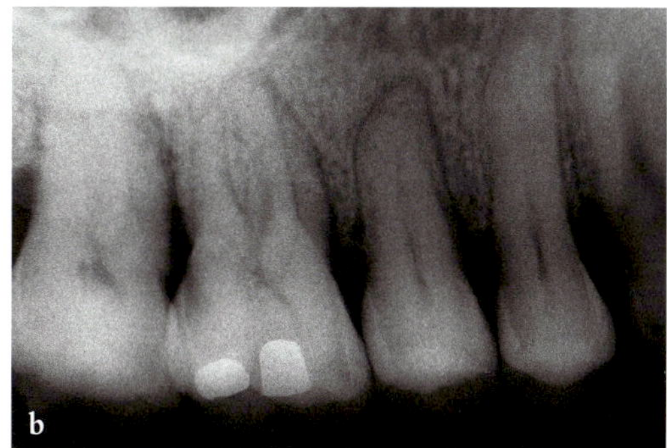


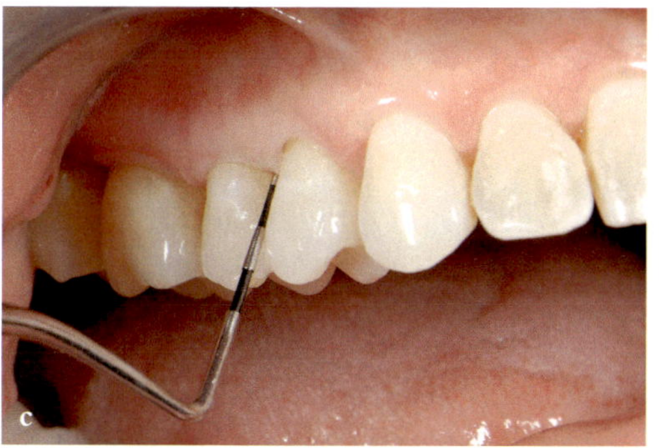


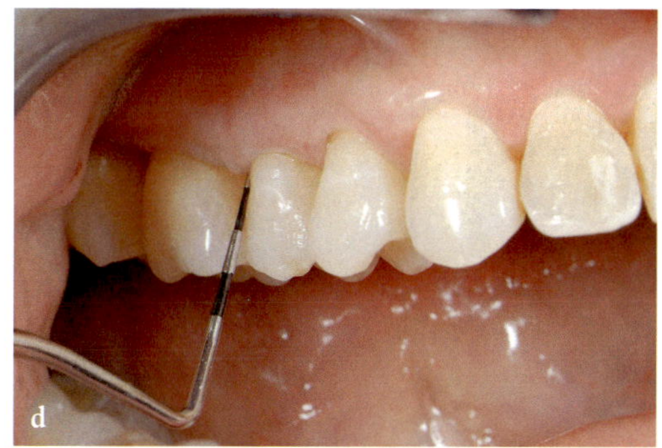


Fig 14-9 **(a)** A 50-year-old patient whose oral hygiene is adequate. The patient presented with parafunctional habits and increased mobility of the second premolar and first maxillary molar. **(b)** Radiographically, there was increased periodontal ligament space around the second premolar and bone loss around the first and second molars. **(c)** Probing pocket depth was less than 3 mm on the mesial surface of the second maxillary premolar. **(d)** Probing pocket depth was less than 3 mm on the distal surface of the second maxillary premolar.

## Conclusion

Although excessive occlusal forces can produce alterations in the periodontal tissues, temporomandibular joint, masticatory muscles, dental surfaces, and pulpal tissues, the objective of this chapter has been to focus on the effect of occlusal trauma on periodontal tissues.

The scientific evidence published to date clearly suggests that trauma from occlusion *per se* will not lead to periodontal disease or cause gingivitis to progress to periodontitis. Besides, the sequelae of the lesion caused by trauma can be reverted in teeth without pre-existing periodontitis. However, the role of occlusal trauma as a co-destructive factor in teeth with pre-existing periodontitis is still controversial.[51]

Even though animal and human autopsy studies have shown a considerable negative effect on the tooth attachment apparatus, the clinical significance of these findings in humans is currently unknown owing to the absence of appropriate clinical data on the issue. On the other hand, several studies have demonstrated the detrimental impact of occlusal trauma and tooth mobility on the healing of periodontal tissues.[52,53]

Although it is generally recognized that nonprogressive tooth mobility does not influence the development of periodontal disease, the healing response of the mobile teeth is less favorable than for teeth with no mobility. These data seem to indicate the need for occlusal adjustments along with an appropriate treatment approach to solve the inflammatory and infectious components of periodontal disease.

## References


1. Karolyi M. Beobachtungen über pyorrhea alveolaris. Öst Ung Vierteeljschr Zahnheilk 1901;17:279–283.
2. Stillman PR. The management of pyorrhea. Dent Cosmos 1917;59:405–414.
3. Box HK. Experimental traumatogenic occlusion in sheep. Oral Health 1935;29:9–15.
4. Mühlemann HR, Herzog H, Vogl A. Occlusal trauma and tooth modility. Schweiz Mdschr Zahnheilkd 1956;66:527.
5. Glickman I, Smulow JB. Alterations in the pathway of gingival inflammation into the underlying tissues induced by excessive occlusal forces. J Periodontol 1962;33:7–13.
6. Weinmann JP. Progress of gingival inflammation into the supporting structures of the teeth. J Periodontol 1941;12: 71–82.
7. Macapanpan IC, Weinmann JP. The influence of injury to the periodontal membrane on the spread of gingival inflammation. J Dent Res 1954;33:263–272.
8. Glickman I, Smulow JB. Further observations on the effects of trauma from occlusion. J Periodontol 1967;38: 280–293.
9. Glickman I. Role of occlusion in the etiology and treatment of periodontal disease. J Dent Res 1971(Suppl 2); 50(2):199–204.
10. Glickman I, Smulow JB. Effect of excessive occlusal forces upon the pathway of gingival inflammation in humans. J Periodontol 1965;36:141–147.
11. Stahl SS. The responses of the periodontium to combined gingival inflammation and occluso-functional stresses in four human surgical specimens. Periodontics 1968;6:14–22.
12. Waerhaug J. The infrabony pocket and its relationship to trauma from occlusion and subgingival plaque. J Periodontol 1979;50:355–365.
13. Waerhaug J. The angular bone defect and its relationship to trauma from occlusion and down growth of the subgingival plaque. J Clin Periodontol 1976;3:110–122.
14. Svanberg GK, King GJ, Gibbs CH. Occlusal considerations in periodontology. Periodontol 2000 1995;9:106–117.
15. Gher ME. Non-surgical Pocket Therapy: dental occlusion. Ann Periodontol 1996;1:567–580.
16. Gher ME. Changing concepts: the effect of occlusion on periodontitis. Dent Clin North Am 1998;42:285–297.
17. Deas DE, Mealey BL. Is there association between occlusion and periodontal destruction? J Am Dent Assoc 2006;137:1381–1389.
18. Harrel SK. Occlusal forces as a risk factor for periodontal disease. Periodontol 2000 2003;32:111–117.
19. Hallmon WW, Harrel SK. Occlusal analysis, diagnosis and management in the practice of periodontics. Periodontol 2000 2004;34:151–164.
20. Page RC, Kornman KS. The pathogenesis of human periodontitis: an introduction. Periodontol 2000 1997;14:9–11.
21. Hallmon WW. Occlusal trauma: effect and impact on the periodontium. Ann Periodontol 1999;4:102–108.
22. American Academy of Periodontology. Parameter on occlusal traumatism in patients with chronic periodontitis. Parameters of care supplement. J Periodontol 2000; 71:873–875.
23. Biancu S, Ericsson I, Lindhe J. Periodontal ligament tissue reactions to trauma and gingival inflammation: an experimental study in the beagle dog. J Clin Periodontol 1995;22:772–779.
24. Svanberg GK, Lindhe J. Vascular reactions in the periodontal ligament incident to trauma from occlusion. J Clin Periodontol 1974;1:58–69.
25. Svamberg G. Influence from trauma from occlusion on the periodontium of dogs with normal or inflamed gingival. Odontol Revy 1974;25:165–178.
26. Svamberg G, Lindhe J. Experimental tooth hypermobility in the dog: a methodological study. Odontol Revy 1973;24:269–282.
27. Polson AM, Meitner SW, Zander HA. Trauma and progression of marginal periodontitis in squirrel monkeys. III: Adaption of interproximal alveolar bone to repetitive injury. J Periodontal Res 1976;11:279–289.
28. Lindhe J, Ericsson I. The influence of trauma from occlusion on reduced but healthy periodontal tissues in dogs. J Clin Periodontol 1976;3:110–122.
29. Ericsson I, Lindhe J. Lack of effect of trauma from occlusion on the recurrence of experimental periodontitis. J Clin Periodontol 1977;4:115–127.
30. Budtz-Jorgensen E. Bruxism and trauma from occlusion: an experimental model in macaca monkeys. J Clin Periodontol 1980;7:149–162.
31. Polson AM, Meitner SW, Zander HA. Trauma and progression of marginal periodontitis in squirrel monkeys. IV: Reversibility of bone loss due to trauma alone and trauma superimposed upon periodontitis. J Periodontal Res 1976;11:290–298.
32. Lindhe J, Svamberg G. Influence of trauma from occlusion on the progression of experimental periodontitis in the beagle dog. J Clin Periodontol 1974;1:3–14.
33. Nyman S, Lindhe J, Ericsson I. The effect of progressive tooth mobility on destructive periodontitis in the dog. J Clin Periodontol 1978;5:213–225.
34. Ericsson I, Lindhe J. Effect of longstanding jiggling on experimental marginal periodontitis in the beagle dog. J Clin Periodontol 1982;9:497–503.
35. Meitner S. Co-destructive factors of marginal periodontitis and repetitive mechanical injury. J Dent Res 1975 (Special issue c);54:78–85.

36. Polson AM, Zander HA. Effect of periodontal trauma upon intrabony pockets. J Periodontol 1983;54:586–591.
37. Kantor M, Polson AM, Zander HA. Alveolar bone regeneration after removal of inflammatory and traumatic factors. J Periodontol 1976;47:687–695.
38. Lindhe J, Ericsson I. The effect of elimination of jiggling forces on periodontally exposed teeth in the dog. J Periodontol 1982;53:562–567.
39. Polson AM, Adams RA, Zander HA. Osseous repair in the presence of active tooth hypermobility. J Clin Periodontol 1983;10:370–379.
40. Ramfjord SP, Ash MM. Significance of occlusion in the etiology and treatment of early, moderate and advanced periodontitis. J Periodontol 1981;52:511–517.
41. Jin LJ, Cao CF. Clinical diagnosis of trauma from occlusion and its relation with severity of periodontitis. J Clin Periodontol 1992;19:92–97.
42. Yuodelis RA, Mann WV. The prevalence and possible role of nonworking contacts in periodontal disease. Periodontics 1965;3:219–223.
43. Shefter GJ, McFall WT. Occlusal relations and periodontal status in human adults. J Periodontol 1984;55:368–374.
44. Pihlstrom B, Anderson KA, Aeppli D, Schaffer EM. Association between signs of trauma from occlusion and periodontitis. J Periodontol 1986;57:1–6.
45. Hanamura H, Houston F, Rylander H et al. Periodontal status and Bruxism: a comparative study of patients with periodontal disease and occlusal parafunctions. J Periodontol 1987;58:173–176.
46. Burgett FG, Ramfjord SP, Nissle RR et al. A randomized trial of occlusal adjustment in the treatment of periodontitis patients. J Clin Periodontol 1992;19:381–387.
47. Nunn M, Harrel SK. The effect of occlusal discrepancies on periodontitis. I: Relationship of initial occlusal discrepancies to initial clinical parameters. J Periodontol 2001;72:485–494.
48. Harrel SK, Nunn M. The effect of occlusal discrepancies on treated and untreated periodontitis. II: Relationship of occlusal treatment to the progression of periodontal disease. J Periodontol 2001;72:495–505.
49. Harrel SK, Nunn M. The effect of occlusal discrepancies on gingival width. J Periodontol 2004;75:98–105.
50. Bernhardt O, Gesch D, Look JO et al. The influence of dynamic occlusal interferences on probing depth and attachment level: results of the study of health in Pomerania (SHIP). J Periodontol 2006;77:506–516.
51. Zander HA, Polson AM. Present status of occlusion and oclusal therapy in periodontics. J Periodontol 1977;48:540–544.
52. Fleszar TJ, Knowles JW, Morrison EC et al. Tooth mobility and periodontal therapy. J Clin Periodontol 1980;7:495–505.
53. Neiderud AM, Ericsson I, Lindhe J. Probing pocket depth at mobile/nonmobile teeth. J Clin Periodontol 1992;19:754–759.

# Chapter 15

# Effects of Bruxism on Muscles

*Arturo E. Manns Freese*

## Introduction

Pathophysiologic disorders of jaw muscles and associated musculature (neck and hyoid muscles), in combination with the signs and symptoms encountered by patients (temporomandibular pain and functional disturbance) specifically associated with parafunctional etiologic causes (such as bruxism), are grouped into a broad diagnostic category of temporomandibular disorders known as *muscular disorders*. In patients seeking treatment, muscular disturbances have a high prevalence and they are the most frequent reason for the consultation.[1,2] In terms of muscular pain encountered by patients, only odontogenic pain or odontalgia is more frequent.

In order to understand muscular disorders we should think first of muscles in a healthy condition and functioning normally. In this state of the stomatognathic musculature with its nerve supply, it is possible to identify the following functional features:

- free movement or three-dimensional mandibular displacement within the limits set by joint ligaments
- lack of pain and jaw fatigue during normal functioning or at rest
- normal muscular tone with lack of muscular hypertonicity.

Normal muscular function may be interrupted or altered by certain etiologic factors such as bruxism. When the physiologic mechanisms of adaptation and tissue resistance are overstretched, it is possible to trigger a state of muscular pathophysiology involving muscular disorders. The patient will basically manifest:

- *functional disturbance of jaw dynamics*, characterized by either hypermetria in the maximal jaw opening along with frequent lateral deviation (towards right or left) at the end of maximal opening – this deviation is also known as jaw deflection;[3] or *hypometria* or limitation of jaw opening
- *pain* during jaw movement and/or at rest – *subjective* (stated by the patient) as well as *objective* (through muscular palpation), frequently accompanied by jaw muscle fatigue in the morning and/or at daytime

- *hypertonicity* or *muscle hyperactivity*, characterized by a state of abnormal or involuntary muscular contraction in all or part of the jaw fibers (myospasm).

It is only possible to understand the development of a muscular pathophysiologic condition as a sequel of a repetitive bruxism activity after understanding basic physiologic mechanisms related to the contractile process of the skeletal musculature (to which the stomatognathic muscles belong).

## Principles of Skeletal Muscle Physiology

A skeletal muscle is made up of hundreds to thousands of muscular fibers. Each muscular fiber is an individual multinuclear cell, representing the contractile element of the muscle. Muscular fibers are separated in bunches or bundles by connective tissue which also penetrates into the bundle or bunch of fibers, surrounding, at the end, every fiber individually: epimysium, perimysium, and endomysium. These tissues provide a viscoelastic structure in parallel with the individual muscular fibers, and they also offer a passage to the nerves and lymphatic blood vessels which run along the inner part of the muscle and surround the muscular fibers.

At the end of the muscle the connective tissue is condensed into a tendon on which muscular fibers are fixed. At the same time, the tendon is fixed to the bone or fascia (Fig 15-1). In this way, the contractile force of the muscle is transmitted through the tendon to the bone or other place of insertion. Connective tissues, placed in parallel or in series, give the muscles viscoelastic properties which contribute to the muscular mechanics.

### *Mechanics of Muscular Contraction*

The specific function of the skeletal muscle, to which the stomatognathic musculature belongs, is to contract and thus carry out mechanical work: force development and/or movement generation.[4-7] Muscular contraction, as will be described below, includes the shortening of the contractile elements of the muscle (muscle fibers) through the mechanism of displacement of both thick and thin myofilaments which form it ultrastructurally. This is related to the active process by which force is generated in the muscle. Every human movement involves rotation of body segments around their joint axes. In a physical sense, muscular work is produced, with an angular movement of two bones around a joint. This mechanical action is produced by the interaction of forces associated with external load (represented by the body segment plus the additional external load) and the muscular activity (the necessary contraction to produce the angular movement). The ability of a force to produce rotation is physically referred to as a *torque* or *force moment*. Expressed in other terms, the torque represents either the rotational effect of a force with respect to an axis, or the tendency of a force to produce rotation. Torque **(T)** is a vector, represented by its magnitude and direction or orientation, and it is quantified as the product of a force **(F)** and the moment arm **(r)**:

$$T = F \times r$$

The force of a contracting muscle over a unit area of an object is known as *muscular tension*. It is represented by the *muscular torque*. In contrast, the force exerted by the weight of an object over the contracting muscle is known as "load", represented by the *load torque*. The muscular torque and the load torque have, in consequence, opposite force components.

Taking into account these biomechanical facts it is possible to divide muscular contractions into groups.

- *Isometric contractions* (*iso* = equal, similar: *metric* = total muscular length between both insertions). These are muscular contractions without any significant change in the muscular length due to viscoelastic elements placed in series with respect to the muscular contractile elements. Under this muscular contractile condition the load torque is equal in magnitude to the muscular torque but opposite with regards to direction. Although there is no change in the total muscular length, the muscular fibers do shorten. This means that there is no bone movement but there is a great development of muscular tension. An example is contraction of jaw elevator muscles during teeth clenching. During long isometric contraction, usually with great muscular tension, the muscle undergoes fatigue more quickly due to a significant reduction of blood and energy supply – as will be explained later.

- *Anisometric contractions.* These are non-isometric contractions; that is, contractions with variations in the total muscular length. This contractile condition is present when a muscle is activated and its muscular torque is different from the load torque. This term includes either concentric or isotonic contractions and eccentric contractions, which determine shortening or lengthening of the muscle length, respectively.
- *Concentric or isotonic contractions* (*iso* = equal, similar; *tonic* = muscular tension). These are muscular contractions in which the muscular torque is greater than the load torque and, as a result, the muscle gets shorter. Under this contractile condition there will be movement in the bone in which it is inserted. In a physical context work has been performed (shortening) in accordance with the angular movement of two bones surrounding a joint. An example is the isotonic contraction of the jaw elevator muscles causing the jaw to elevate.
- *Eccentric contractions.* These are muscular contractions in which the load torque is greater than the muscular torque, so the muscle gets longer. For example, in cases of protrusive bruxism associated with grinding or jaw sliding between centric and eccentric positions, the lateral pterygoid muscle suffers a contraction under muscular lengthening during the slow condylar retrusion into the joint cavity. The same happens with the elevator muscles during laterotrusive bruxism (from right to left) or protrusive (forward and backward) under grinding or jaw sliding between centric and eccentric positions. During this eccentric muscular work, the muscle develops

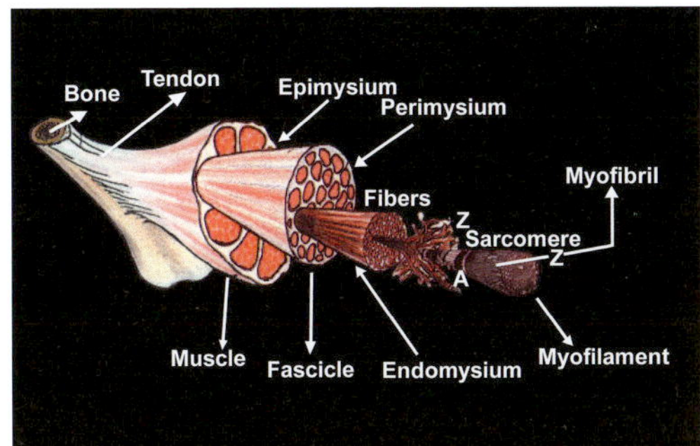


**Fig 15-1** Structural composition of skeletal muscle.

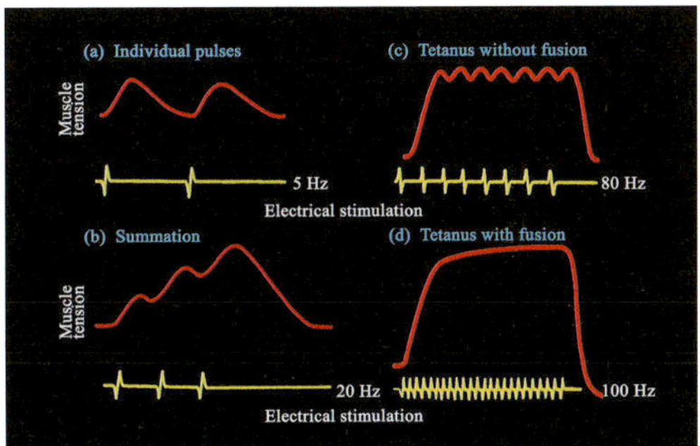


**Fig 15-2** Muscular active tension varies with the frequency of stimulation of the muscle through its nerves. **(a)** With successive low-frequency triggering there are isolated unique muscular contractions or twitches. **(b)** Higher frequency stimulation produces a summation of contractions with an increment of the developed tensional force. **(c)** An even higher frequency of stimulation produces a higher force but some differentiated waves are seen. This corresponds to short relaxation phases after each stimulus. **(d)** With a higher frequency of stimulation each stimulus does not produce force waves and the resulting tensional force is higher than during tetanic contraction without fusion. (Adapted from Kandel et al.[6])

different magnitudes of muscular tension (depending on the load torque) as it becomes larger. This is the position in which there may be greater probability of muscular damage. This is especially significant when the muscle is near its optimal muscular length. In this length there may exist maximal overlapping of thick and thin filaments, associated with a maximum of myosin bridges connected to the active sites of actin (sarcomeric length: 2.0–2.5 µm).
- *Tetanic contractions.* These may be caused by a quick and repetitive stimulation of the muscle (high stimulation frequency, 20–100 Hz). The contractile mechanism activation is repetitive before total relaxation, as a result of fusion of contractions (Fig 15-2). It is a critical phenomenon, especially during repetitive clenching (bruxism), which is basically the final result of repetitive rhythmic contractions (isometric type) of the jaw muscles. Tension developed by these repetitive and fusioned contractions is considered higher (two or three times) than that developed during an individual muscular contraction or twitch response caused by a sole stimulus. Remember that the twitch response is the basic muscular response to an individual stimulus, which consists of a short period of contraction followed by a longer period of relaxation (Fig 15-2).

In order to explain the reason for this it is necessary to remember that the muscle has not only fibers but also fibrous elastic connective tissue in parallel with the contractile elements (mainly epimysium, perimysium, and endomysium) and tendons. They transfer viscoelastic properties to the muscle, contributing to the muscular mechanical response (Fig 15-1). During a contraction the element or contractile muscular unit (represented by the muscular fiber and its sarcomeres) is shortened and produces effects in the muscle ends. However, connective tissues (and their viscoelastic properties) produce a force opposed to the shortening of the contractile element. In other words, they are intended to recover their original form by resisting the force or muscular tension. With a single stimulus, the condition of spring of the viscoelastic connective elements (especially those arranged in series) absorbs first the tension developed during the beginning of the contractile element activity, in such a way that only one part of the contractile tension is manifested externally in the muscle ends. On the other hand, during high-frequency stimulation the contractile element is activated during a period of time so that it is possible to oppose inertia or resistance of the connective elements. As a result, all the muscular contractile tension is manifested in the ends of the muscle.

### Masticatory Force

When the jaw elevator muscles are isometrically contracted, an intermaxillary force is generated. This is known as the *masticatory force* or force of mastication, having an identical direction to that of a line joining muscular insertions (muscular axis).[4] However, masticatory force is generated from different muscles with different muscular axes, so they act as a whole with a force direction resulting from the parallelogram of forces.

The main emphasis of experimental research on measuring masticatory force in human beings has been on recording habitual masticatory force and the maximal voluntary masticatory force by means of a gnathodynamometer. The force during normal mastication generally ranges between 20 and 25 kgf, but the maximal functional masticatory force exerted is 60–70 kgf. This means that there is a 3:1 relationship between the maximal masticatory force developed between both dental arches and that effectively used when chewing.

Various factors influence the magnitude of the masticatory force in humans.
- *Gender and age.* Masticatory force increases with age to a total development at the age of

15–20 years. There is no clear difference between men and women.

- *Type of food.* Quality and consistency of food affects the masticatory force. Primitive peoples, who chew hard food and even use their teeth as working tools, have higher values of masticatory force. It has been observed that in individuals with habitual unilateral mastication the masticatory force is double on the active side compared with the passive side.
- *Dental groups.* It has been proven that the maximal functional masticatory force is greater at the first molar level and less at anterior teeth level. This is because the molars have a greater periodontal area and also a more favorable biomechanical position as regards the insertion of the elevator muscles.
- *Jaw position in the vertical plane.* Every muscle has an optimal length of contraction at which there is the greatest number of cross-bridges between the myofilaments of actin and myosin in their sarcomeres (optimal sarcomere length). In jaw elevator muscles this length is in relation to a vertical dimension, corresponding to an interocclusal separation of 13–21 mm measured at interincisal level. In this optimal vertical dimension, the jaw elevator muscles have the ability to exert the greatest masticatory force with the least electromyographic activity.
- *Jaw position in the horizontal plane.* The force generated in the intercuspal position is much greater than that generated when the jaw is displaced by a few millimeters to a more lateral position. In this same way the force generated in the protrusive position is half in relation to that in the intercuspal position. This is so because the muscular and joint proprioceptors, and the periodontal mechanoreceptors of the contacting teeth, limit earlier the contraction of jaw muscles in eccentric positions.
- *State of the teeth.* Pathologic dental conditions such as pulpitis, periodontal disease or caries lessen the masticatory force with the aim of reducing pain in the compromised area.
- *Temporomandibular disorders.* Temporomandibular pain (either myogenic or atrogenic) or functional discomfort in any components of the stomatognathic system may disturb the muscular function and decrease masticatory force.
- *Craniofacial skeletal characteristics.* Clinical research has shown that when the jaw has an anterior rotational growth direction and the gonial angle is lower, the optimal vertical dimension is nearer the vertical occlusal dimension. But, when the jaw has a posterior rotational growth direction and the gonial angle is higher, the optimal vertical dimension is further than the vertical occlusal dimension. This affects directly development of the masticatory force capacity.

The factors described above demonstrate that the recorded values are not directly correlated with the maximal muscular power developed by the jaw elevator muscles. There are important nervous regulation processes limiting the recorded values of the maximal masticatory force measured between both dental arches, represented not only by the dental mechanosensitive periodontal sensation but also by the pressure sensations evoked at temporomandibular, muscle, and tendon levels. Any further increase in jaw force may cause pain and, therefore, cause lesions of some components of the stomatognathic system. This inhibitory nervous regulation over the elevator muscles is governed by sensory neuromuscular mechanisms preventing clenching beyond a certain threshold of critical force, so protecting the morphofunctional system integrity.

## Ultrastructure of Skeletal Muscle

Every muscular fiber covered by the cellular membrane (called sarcolemma) has a group of subunits, also cylindrical shaped, like the muscle fiber, but

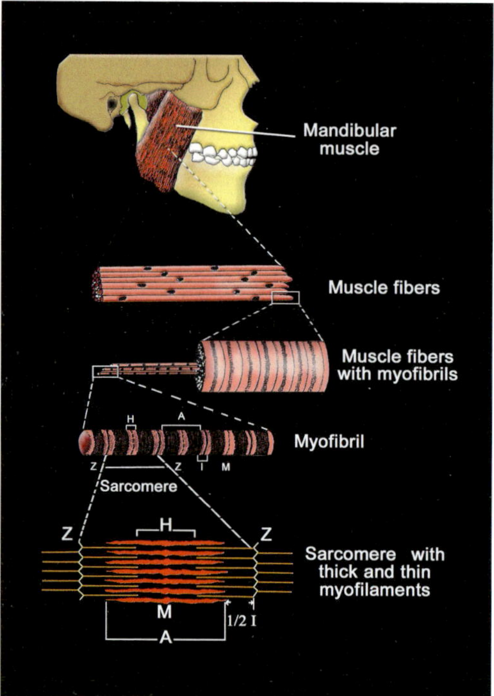


Fig 15-3 Ultrastructure of the jaw muscle. (From Manns and Díaz.[4])

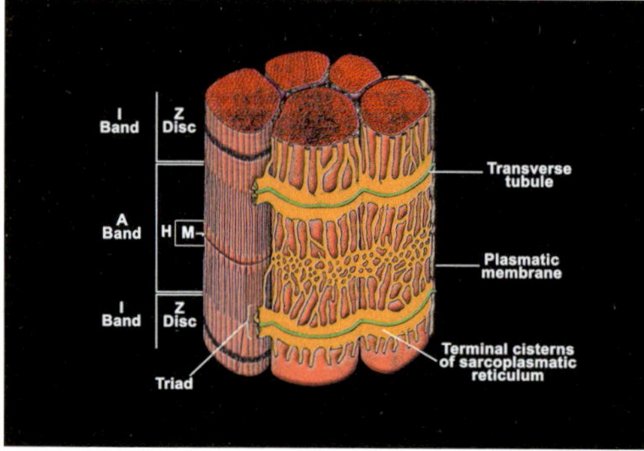


Fig 15-4 Schematic of the structure of a muscle fiber, with the sarcotubular system surrounding the myofibrils. (Adapted from Ganong.[5])

with much smaller diameter; these are called myofibrils (Fig 15-3). They do not have any covering. The space between them is occupied by the cytoplasm of the muscular fiber (called sarcoplasm), which contains the nucleus and mitochondria, along which there is a tubular membranous net that has an important role in the process of muscular excitation (contraction), called the sarcotubular system (Fig 15-4). This system is made up of transverse tubules and the sarcoplasmic reticulum. Transverse tubules, which represent invaginations of the sarcolemma turned inward, are involved in transmitting the muscular action potential (electrical discharge associated with contraction) towards the myofibrils to the inner part of the muscular fiber. On the other hand, the sarcoplasmic reticulum has a relationship with calcium movement and muscular cellular metabolism.

Transverse striations, typical of skeletal muscle, are the product of a succession of dark transverse bands (A-bands) and pale bands (I-bands) along the myofibrils. This is due to the fact that the myofibrils are made up of myofilaments of contractile proteins: thin myofilaments (made up of actin, tropiomysin, and troponin proteins) and the thick filaments (myosin protein). Pale I-bands have only thin myofilaments. A-bands have both thin and thick myofilaments (Fig 15-5). Each myofibril is composed of repetitive units arranged in series, known as sarcomeres, representing the morphofunctional unit of the muscle. It is the part of the myofibril in between two Z-discs, dividing the I-bands into two halves (see Fig 15-3).

Under normal circumstances, skeletal muscle contraction occurs as a result of motor nerve impulses traveling from the central nervous system through motoneurons, called alpha motoneurons. In the specific case of the jaw musculature they are grouped together, forming the motor nucleus of the *trigeminal nerve*. That is why skeletal muscle is also known as voluntary muscle, because it is generally, but not always, under the voluntary control of the skeletal motor system. Each alpha motoneuron innervates a certain number of muscular fibers through a branched axon. This group is called a motor unit. In the case of the masseter and temporal muscles, there are 600–900 muscular fibers for each trigeminal motoneuron (Fig 15-6).

Muscular contraction originates from the displacement of thick and thin myofilaments as a result of the formation and breaking of cross-bridges between the filaments of myosin and actin (Fig 15-7). The energy necessary to move these cross-bridges (specifically represented by the interaction of the heads of myosin molecules with the reactive sites of actin) is offered by the conversion of adenotriphosphate (ATP) to adenodiphosphate (ADP). The myosin activated by its joining with actin (in the presence of calcium ions, liberated by muscular action potential and inhibiting the regulating troponin–tropomyosin proteins) is the catalyst for the hydrolysis from ATP to ADP.

The greater the muscle force, the greater is the amount of ATP. Adenotriphosphate must be considered, therefore, as a "specialized fuel", enabling muscular mechanical work.

Taking into account these facts about the structure and basic functions of the skeletal muscle, it is possible to explain briefly the process of excitation–contraction muscular coupling.

Excitation–contraction coupling is related to the sequence of events beginning with the depolarization of the sarcolemma or muscular action potential

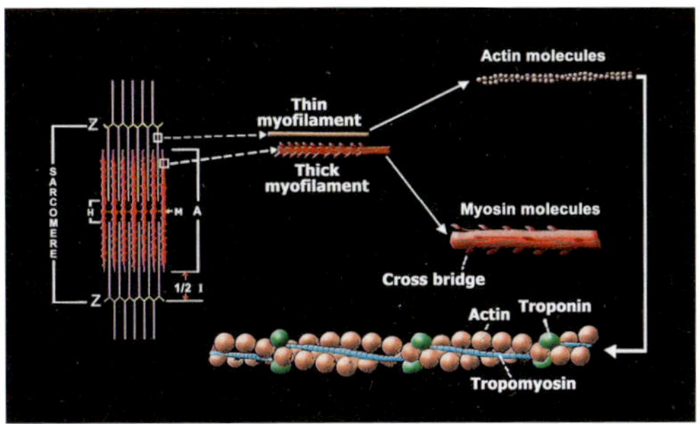


Fig 15-5 Ultrastructure of a sarcomere, showing the thin and thick myofilaments with their constituent contractile proteins. (From Manns and Díaz.[4])

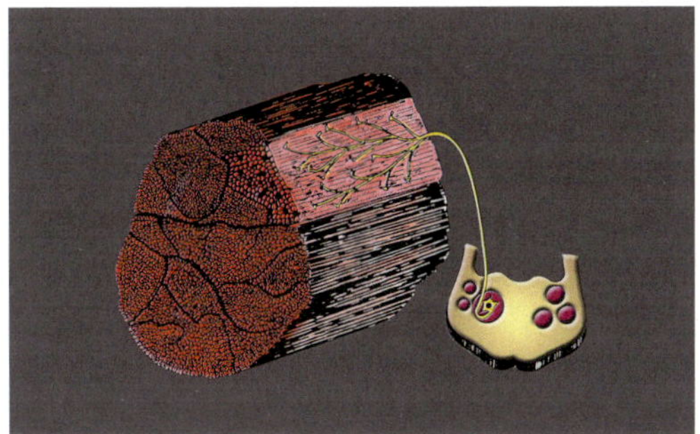

Fig 15-6 Trigeminal motor unit consisting of an alpha motoneuron placed in the trigeminal motor nucleus, the ramified axon, plus skeletal muscular fibers. (From Manns and Díaz.[4])

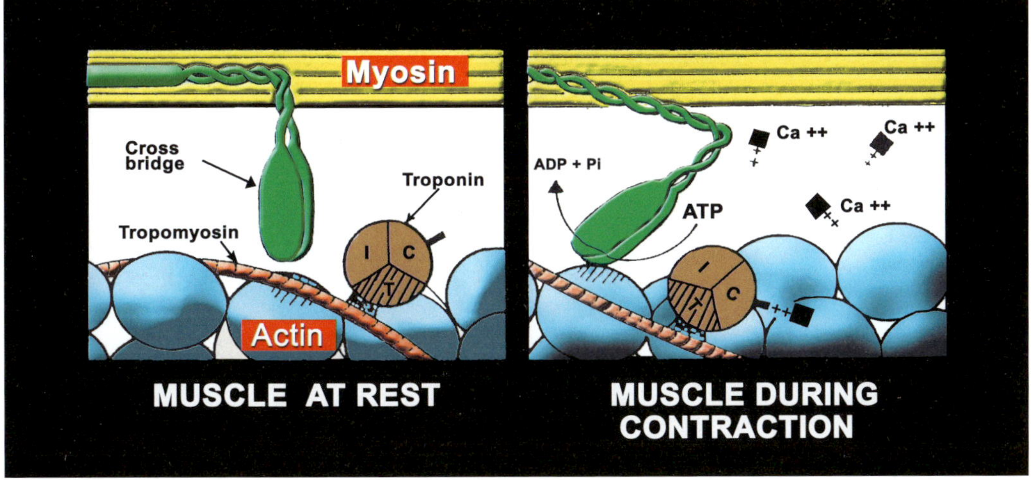


Fig 15-7 Beginning of a muscular contraction by ionic calcium and interaction between thick and thin myofilaments (actin, tropomyosin, and troponin). The sarcomeric shortening occurs when the myosin cross-bridges of the thick myofilaments interact with the actin reactive sites of the thin myofilaments. (Adapted from Ganong.[5])

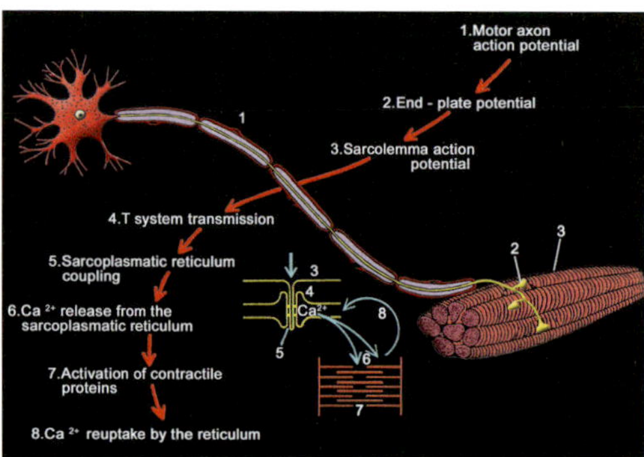


**Fig 15-8** Sequence of events of the excitation–contraction coupling of skeletal muscle.

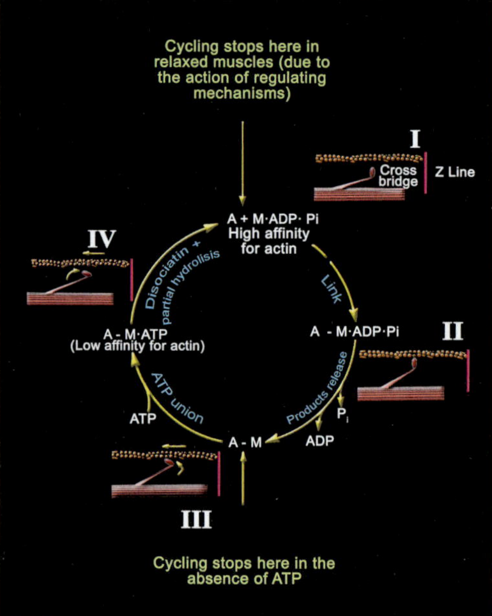


**Fig 15-9** Movement cycle of myosin bridges during the process of muscular contraction.

and finishing with activation of the contractile elements, producing muscular contraction. Calcium ions are the mediators between the processes of excitation and contraction (Figs 15-8 and 15-9).

It is possible to derive from analysis of the physiologic mechanisms of muscular contraction that the immediate energy source used by the contractile unit (represented by the sarcomeres) is ATP. This means that as soon as the ADP is formed, it must be again and quickly phosphorylated into ATP. As the amount of ATP available in the muscular fiber is reduced, the muscle has to replace it during and after contraction.

The muscle uses the same energy-generating mechanisms as those in every nucleated cell, although the relative importance of these different mechanisms varies with the different cell types.

*Direct phosphorylation*

Phosphocreatine (PCr) is a compound with energy-rich phosphate bonds. The adenotriphosphate is formed by the transference of a phosphate group of PCr to adenodiphosphate catalyzed by the enzyme creatine kinase. Therefore, PCr represents an immediate deposit for the regeneration of sarcoplasmic ATP and constitutes an extremely fast process of chemical reaction. As ATP and PCr represent the energy that a muscle is able to use immediately, either of them may supply the contractile muscular energy. However, due to the low muscle fiber cytoplasmatic and sarcoplasmic concentration (ATP: 3–5 micromoles per gram of wet muscular tissue, and PCr: 20 micromoles per gram) they can provide energy only for a few seconds during hard muscular exercise. Therefore, as ATP and PCr are rapidly exhausted, the energy source reloading the muscle with ATP must come from more complex mechanisms; these are discussed below.

*Anaerobic glycolysis*

If the provision of cell oxygen is not sufficient, the glucose or glycogen degraded to pyruvic acid does not enter the cycle of citric acid but is reduced to lactic acid. This is a very fast energy generating process and quickly satisfies the demands of ATP and PCr, even in fast muscle cells. So it is important not only in this type of fiber but also in any muscular fiber when the oxygen supply is not sufficient. However, this mechanism has a net production of only 16,000 calories and two molecules of ATP for each glucose molecule (or three if the

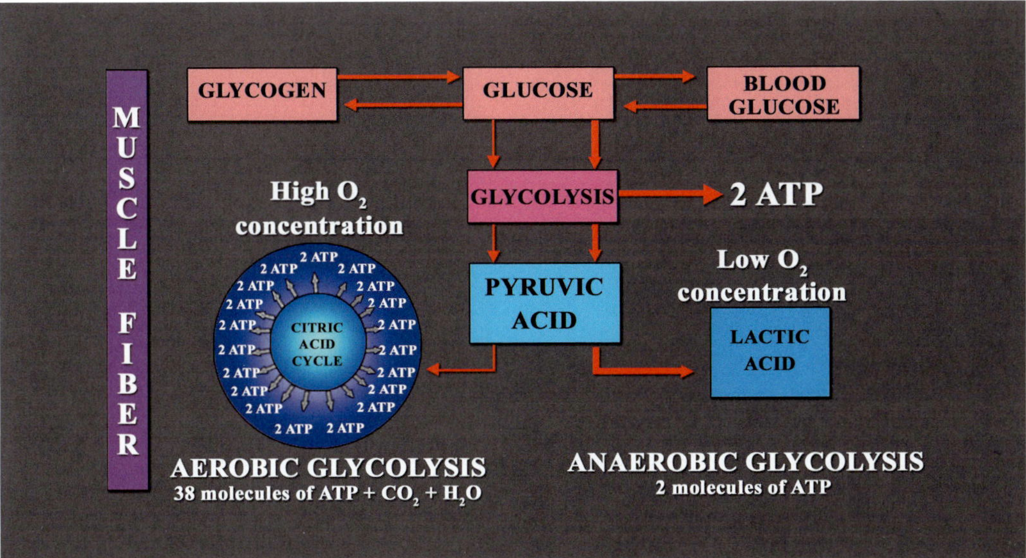


**Fig 15-10** Biochemical mechanism of aerobic and anaerobic glycolysis in the production of ATP.

glucose is derived from glucogen of the muscular cell). Therefore, it is a much more inefficient glycolysis mechanism from the energy point of view, compared to the oxidative phosphorylation of aerobic glycolysis. Also, as a metabolic result, it produces lactic acid, which in spite of having a rapid diffusion towards the bloodstream is accumulated in an important amount within the muscle during long isometric contractions.

This fact explains, partly, the diminution of isometric muscular tension during muscular fatigue, which is simultaneous with the depleting levels of glycogen and PCr associated with the production of lactic acid. This means that, in the extreme, exhaustation of ATP implies contractile inability (Fig 15-10).

*Oxidative phosphorylation*

This type of cellular energy-generating mechanism is much slower than the previous types. Nevertheless, aerobic glycolysis and the oxidation of acetyl-CoA (derived from pyruvic acid in the cycle of citric acid with the oxidative phosphorylation associated with the respiratory chain) provides the necessary energy to efficiently regenerate the highly energy union of ATP and PCr. This is important especially during the recovery of the muscle, after a period of higher demand contraction or during exercise or muscular work of low or medium intensity.

The main part of the energy for resynthesis of ATP and PCr by oxidative phosphorylation comes from the degradation of glucose in the interior of the muscular fiber with proper oxygenation, known as aerobic glycolysis. Glucose, as with anaerobic glycolysis, comes from the blood or from a glucose polymer stored within the muscle, known as glycogen.

During aerobic glycolysis, glucose is degraded to pyruvic acid and is metabolized through the cycle and the so-called tract of the respiratory enzymes (cytochrome-oxidase) to $CO_2$ and $H_2O$. The aerobic metabolism of the glucose to $CO_2$ and $H_2O$ liberates enough energy to form large amounts of ATP from ADP: 38 ATP and 686,000 calories from one glucose molecule. The final products – $CO_2$ and $H_2O$ – are quickly and easily diffused to the bloodstream.

*Oxidation of free fatty acids*
Oxidation of free fatty acids coming from the white fat of the body constitutes another source for the formation of ATP and PCr, mainly during low-intensity muscular exercise. The free fatty acids are oxidated in the mitochondria to acetyl-CoA, which then enters into the cycle of citric acid. Amino acids, as alamine, may enter this cycle after deamination. However, the oxidation of proteins usually plays a limited role as an energy source during the contractile process.

*Summary*
To sum up, oxidative phosphorylation, compared to anaerobic glycolysis, is highly efficient as a generator of energy, but it can operate continually only if the muscular circulation is good enough. Even so, it is a slow process – it may not match the magnitude and speed of the maximal consumption of ATP by the skeletal muscle fibers during quick contraction. Neither may it match that occurring during intensive isometric contractions; the main part of muscular fibers contain mitochondria too close to the capillaries.

Finally, according to this analysis of the cellular muscular energy-generating mechanisms it is important to note that in aerobic conditions the ATP is rephosphorylated during oxidative phosphorylation by the mitochondria, using glycogen, glucose, and free fatty acids as fuel. It is a slow mechanism, but highly efficient and a generator of great amounts of ATP. If the contractile process is anaerobic, the ADP is rephosphorylated by PCr, at the cost of the anaerobic glycolysis, with the production of lactate as a metabolic product. In spite of being a faster mechanism of energy generation it is far less efficient. So, in absence of good oxygenation, skeletal muscles may work only for short periods because the total energy available is very limited compared with the situation of aerobic muscular work.

## Comparing Normal Function and Parafunction

To understand the meaning and influence of parafunctional activities in the development of temporomandibular disorders (especially at the stomatognathic muscle level) it is important to compare normal functional activity and parafunctional activity (mainly, bruxism) of the stomatognathic system (Table 15-1).

With regard to the first two factors in the table, it is easily seen that the magnitude and frequency of dental contacts during parafunctional activity will affect the structures of the stomatognathic system to a greater extent than during functional activity. If we consider that the maximal masticatory force is about 60–70 kgf,[4] it is possible to deduce that during chewing and swallowing only a part of the maximal jaw force is used (about 30%). But during bruxism a force slightly less than or similar to the maximal force is developed. Also, bruxists contract their stomatognathic musculature, specifically their jaw elevator group, for longer periods than normal individuals.

With regard to the duration of bruxism events, Baba and co-workers[14] have demonstrated that bruxism events in patients with chronic bruxism were longer (27 seconds per hour) compared with normal (7.4 seconds).

The main part of the functional activity (chewing, swallowing, and phono-articulation) consists of a rhythmic pattern of alternating isotonic and isometric contractions, with relaxation pauses. This physiologic activity permits a good supply of oxygen to the muscles by aerobic glycolysis. Parafunctional activities, in contrast, consisting of eccentric contractions and, above all, long and intense isometric contractions, hinder the normal blood flow to the muscle with a reduction of oxygen supply. The consequence is slow energy production by anaerobic glycolysis. We shall see later how this has a pathophysiologic impact on the muscle.

*Table 15-1*

**Comparison between normofunction and parafunction.**

| Factors | Normal function | Parafunction (bruxism) |
|---|---|---|
| Intensity of dental contact | Mastication: 20.7–26.6 kgf<br>Swallowing: 25.0–30.2 kgf<br>(Gibbs et al[8]) | 42.3 kgf (15.6–81.2 kgf)<br>(Nishigawa et al[9]) |
| Frequency of dental contacts | 17.5 min during 24 h<br>(Graf[10] and Glickman[11]) | 30–170 min in 8 h of sleeping<br>(Brewer and Hudson[12])<br>38.7–162 min per night of sleeping<br>(Trenouth[13]) |
| Duration of bruxism events | 7.4 s per hour<br>(Baba et al[14]) | 27 s per hour<br>(Baba et al[14]) |
| Type of elevator muscular contraction | Isotonic and isometric<br>(physiologic) | Isometric or eccentric<br>(non-physiologic) |
| Source of contractile energy | Aerobic glycolysis (great amount of ATP + $CO_2$ and $H_2O$) | Anaerobic glycolysis (scarce amount of ATP + lactic acid) |
| Jaw position | Intercuspal position<br>(relatively stable) | Eccentric occlusal position<br>(relatively unstable) |
| Direction of occlusal forces | Vertical (well tolerated) | Horizontal (not well tolerated) |
| Influence of protection reflexes | Present | Reduced |

With regard to jaw position, most functional activities are carried out in the intercuspal position. This means occlusal stability and the distribution of functional forces over several teeth, minimizing the potential harm to an individual tooth.[3] In contrast, parafunctional activities are mainly carried out with the jaw in eccentric positions,[15] in which there are few dental contacts and the condyles are displaced from the stable musculoskeletal position or stable centric relations. Powerful parafunctional forces are established over a few teeth and in an unstable condylar position, creating a high probability of pathologic effects on the muscles, teeth, and joints.

During mastication and swallowing there is a predominance of vertical jaw movements. Vertical occlusal forces are well supported by the tooth periodontium, but during parafunctional (mainly eccentric) activity occlusal forces are developed horizontally and laterally over the teeth, increasing the probability of damage in the supporting structures.

Finally, with regard to the influence of protective reflexes, these neuromuscular reflexes are present during functional activities, protecting the stomatognathic structures against potentially harmful forces. During parafunctional activities the protective neuromuscular reflexes seem to be reduced because of an increase in excitation thresholds of some receptors (adaptation mechanisms), and they have a less important effect on inhibition of jaw muscle activity.[16,17] This permits the development of greater jaw forces during parafunctional activities, increasing the probability of damage in the stomatognathic structures.

## Pathophysiology of Muscular Disorders and Related Pain

Muscular disorders are pathophysiologic conditions of muscular pain or myalgia developed in the stomatognathic musculature, and are associated with jaw functional disorders. Muscular pain and myalgia are the most frequent problem reported by patients. Myofascial pain is a somatic deep musculoskeletal pain reported by patients (localized in the jaw, temple, or preauricular area) or detected on muscular palpation, originating in the skeletal muscles, muscular fascia, or tendons. Myofacial pain is mainly due to excitation (mechanically and by chemical agents) of free nerve endings within the muscles or in the fascia, by local mediators of the inflammation or neurogenic inflammation (peripheral sensitization), frequently combined with changes in the central neurons (central sensitization) caused by longstanding injured tissue.[18]

Dworkin and Le Resche[19] and De Laat[18] classify muscular disorders within group I according to the diagnostic criteria of axis I (physical disorders) of temporomandibular disorders.

- Group I – Muscular disorders: myofascial pain; and myofascial pain with limited opening
- Group II – Disc displacement: with reduction; without reduction with limited opening; without reduction without limited opening
- Group III – Arthalgia, arthritis and arthrosis.

Myofascial pain (Ia) is of muscular origin and includes various painful conditions, as well as the pain associated with localized painful areas on palpation, with the following clinical characteristics:

- reported pain in the jaw, temples, face, and preauricular area or within the ear at rest or during movement
- pain during palpation reported by the patient in three or more of the following 20 examined sites (right and left sides are considered separate sites for each muscle): anterior, medium, and posterior temporal; origin, body, and insertion of the superficial masseter; deep masseter; medial pterygoid; temporal tendon.

Myofascial pain with limited opening (Ib) is a functional limitation of the movement and rigidity of muscle resistance to stretching, combined with myofascial pain. Clinical characteristics are:

- myofascial pain as described in (Ia)
- unassisted maximum jaw opening of less than 35–40 mm
- maximum passive opening (assisted) of more than 3 mm compared to the unassisted opening.

By using this classification of group I we deliberately exclude other less common muscular conditions that are not the subject of exact diagnostic criteria: muscular spasms (continual muscular contractions), myositis (generalized pain in a specific muscle, associated with inflammation or infection), and contractures (limitation of mobility range, with consequent resistance to passive stretching). These muscular conditions have less specific diagnostic criteria owing to the lack of standardized research.

Myofascial pain is different from cutaneous pain in the sense that it is a deep somatic pain that is dull and poorly localized, and frequently irradiated to other deep regions (muscles, joints, fascia, and tendons) or to superficial areas. This is because the second-order sensitive neurons that transmit muscular pain have an important convergence of cutaneous, dental, muscular, and joint afferents, and because they are exposed to more significant descendent central inhibition than the neurons that transmit cutaneous pain.[20] Some researchers agree that muscular hyperactivity or hyperfunction developed during parafunctioning (the psychophysiologic theory, or theory of neurogenic hyperactivity of central origin) plays an important role in pathogenesis of jaw musculature and associated musculature (the weak link theory): the physiologic tolerance and adaptative capacity of the muscular link may be exceeded. This last statement is supported by research on patients in which it was possible to reproduce muscular pain, muscular fatigue, and cephalgia by means of parafunctional simulation of low and high intensity, but over an extended period.[20–26] In addition, it is clear that etiologic predisposing factors (occlusal or psychologic or behavioral factors) have a great influence on muscular pathogenesis.

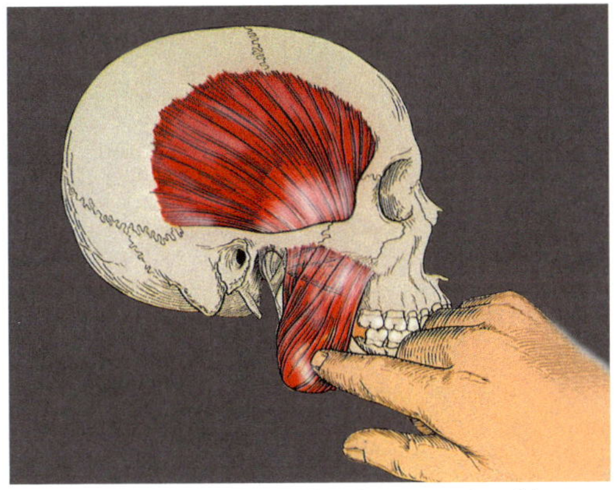

Fig 15-11 Palpation of a myofascial trigger point of the masseter muscle. (Adapted from Netter's Head and Neck Anatomy for Dentistry.)

## Types of Muscular Pain

Myofascial pain or localized muscular pain of short duration is a kind of acute pain caused by the stimulation of muscular nociceptors, perceived in the injured area. The most frequent cause is brief trauma (contusion, stretching, and contractures). The pain caused by stretching is mainly important in eccentric muscular contractions, corresponding to contraction under muscular elongation – for example during eccentric bruxism (protrusive, laterotrusive, or lateroprotrusive).

The other type of pain caused by an injury or muscular damage of longer duration (long-lasting muscular hyperactivity, ischemia, and inflammation) can be categorized as chronic. Clinically, pain may be considered chronic after a 3-month period. In this painful muscular situation, nociceptors are sensitized and the pain is no longer restricted to the injury. It radiates to other deep and superficial areas and is perceived in areas lacking nociceptive stimulation – this is "referred pain".

Frequently with this type of pain there are so-called "myofascial trigger points" (Fig 15-11). These are localized hypersensitive areas that are painful during compression and which may result in referred pain or spasm of other muscles but not necessarily in the areas where the trigger points are located.

Myospasm is a state of abnormal and involuntary contraction characterized by an increment of muscular activity of all or some of the fibers. It is not accompanied by a CNS disorder. A muscle in spasm is unable to relax voluntarily, is shortened and has resistance to stretching, and is hard and tense during palpation. Myospasm of a certain magnitude may definitely cause pain.

There is a relationship between the spasm intensity and the pain. However, it is not the muscular pain that generates the spasm. The pain associated with the involuntary contraction is probably due to a muscular *ischemia* that leads to the liberation of alogenic substances.

Clinically, we have the following. The myofascial trigger points give rise to not only muscular pain but also referred pain and, frequently, a state of spasm of the muscles pertaining to the same muscular group. For example, the trigger point in the masseter muscle may produce spasm in other elevator muscles. Nevertheless, the same muscle with a myofascial trigger point does not present spasm. Muscles with myospasm tend to be hyperfunctional or with a hypervalency condition in relation to those with lesser functional requirements (e.g., its antagonist muscle), resulting in a state of jaw muscle incoordination.

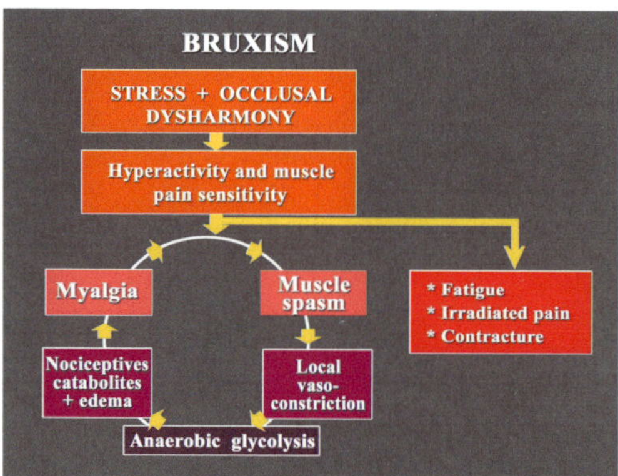


Fig 15-12 Vicious-circle model of spasm – muscular pain – spasm.

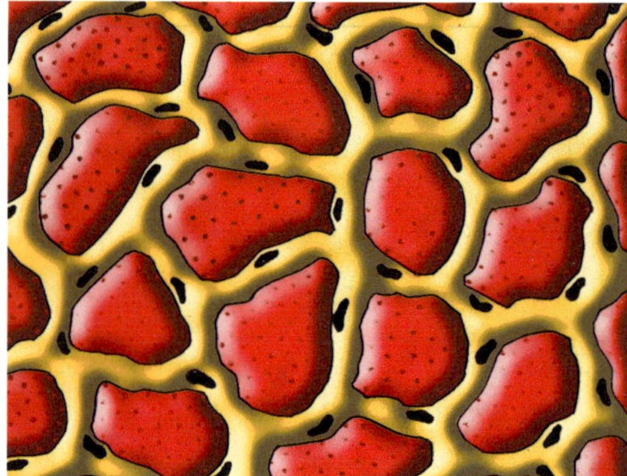

Fig 15-13 Cross-section of skeletal muscle showing the relationships of blood capillaries and muscular fibers.

Incoordination is produced by a disruption of the jaw dynamics, which in the first stages is characterized by mouth hypermetria (50–60 mm opening measured between the incisal edges of maxillary and mandibular canines). Hypermetria is a state of hypermobility of the jaw accompanied by exaggerated translational movements of the condyles. It is basically a product of muscular incoordination, with functional prevalence of the protrusive musculature, especially of the lower heads of the lateral pterygoid muscle.[15] Hypermetria, associated with the shortening of jaw muscles through myospasm, is frequently accompanied by deviation of the jaw in its final opening (uncorrected jaw deviation or deflection). In cases of spasm or long-term chronic muscular hyperactivity, a series of muscular pathophysiologic disturbances may occur that finally may affect connective tissues and produce a limitation of mouth opening (hypometria).

In addition, spasm in one or more jaw muscles produces a slight change in the jaw position so that the teeth do not close together properly. For example, spasm in the lower head of the lateral pterygoid produces a constant contraction of this muscle, resulting in a slight disclusion of the posterior teeth on the same side (ipsilateral), and early contact of the anterior teeth on the opposite side (contralateral). Occlusal alterations resulting from spasm of the jaw elevator muscles are clinically less detectable. Patients usually refer to a sense of not being able to close their teeth properly or comfortably (occlusal instability).[3]

In the past there was a concept of a "spasm – pain – spasm" vicious circle (Fig 15-12), but this cannot be supported through a critical analysis of the literature. EMG studies have demonstrated that a muscle in pain and with a myofascial trigger point has no increase in its EMG activity, even though it is sensitive on palpation. Experiments with animals have demonstrated that alpha motoneurons that innervate muscle with a tissue lesion and pain are frequently inhibited rather than excited. Further, it is not accepted nowadays that a long-term muscle lesion with concomitant pain might excite its gamma motoneurons, which might increase the fusal discharge and activation of alpha motoneurons that innervate the affected muscle. The inhibitory effect of gamma and alpha motoneurons on a muscle in long-term pain might represent a physiologic protection with the aim of limiting the contractile forces operating over the injured muscle. This last statement is supported by studies that measured maximal functional masticatory force in patients with muscular disorders, who had a reduction of the

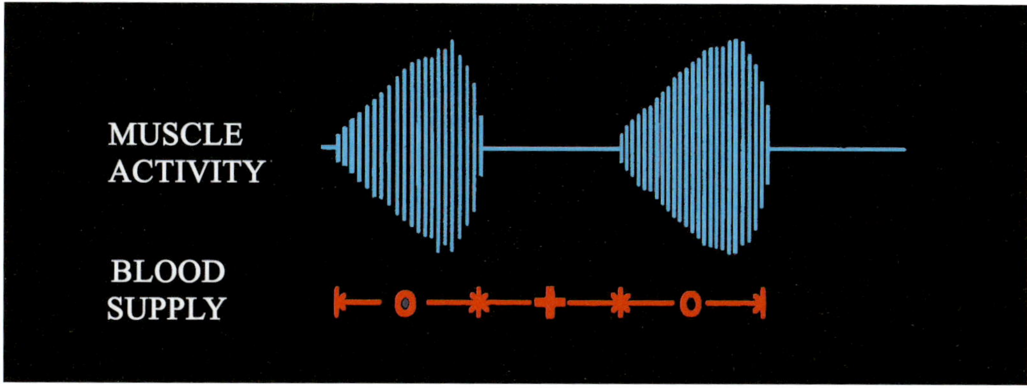


Fig 15-14 Time course of the blood supply to the jaw elevator muscles during chewing. During jaw closing and the occlusal phase the blood supply diminishes drastically. It increases during jaw opening.

maximal voluntary contraction and the masticatory force.[4]

The muscular pain manifested during muscular disorders may be explained through the pathophysiologic mechanisms that trigger it.

- *Muscular ischemia* depends on the force or isometric tension developed during parafunction, as well as its frequency and duration. The pain caused by this mechanism is brief, because the ischemic phase produced by the isometric contraction then disappears and is followed by a reactive hyperemia.
- *Muscular lesions* are caused by repetitive microtrauma or parafunctions. They consist of tiny lesions of the muscular tissue: myofibrils, sarcolemma, and connective tissues. These lesions appear during eccentric contractions, developed not only by eccentric bruxism but also during mouth opening with myospasm of the elevator muscles or with protective cocontraction of elevators and depressors (the splinting reflex). Microlesions cause inflammation and a consequent sensitization of nociceptors. They have a greater propensity than the ischemia mechanism to produce long-term pain.

The following subsections cover in more detail both these pathophysiologic mechanisms generating muscular pain.

### Muscular Ischemia

Skeletal muscles have a rich blood supply, consisting of an intricate capillary network. Capillaries are distributed in such a way that each muscular fiber is in connection with four or five capillaries (Fig 15-13).

The oxygen supply to the muscle is a function only of the inward blood flow. During inactive contractile muscular periods, only some muscular capillaries are open. With functional muscular activity (rhythmic alternation of isotonic and isometric contractions with relaxation periods), blood vessels dilate after the muscular contraction and the blood flow increases, so the supply of available oxygen also increases (Fig 15-14). To a certain extent, the increment in oxygen consumption is proportional to the released energy, and every energy need is offered by the process of anaerobic glycolysis. In addition, during the interchange of fluids through the capillary walls the amount of fluid getting out of the capillaries is usually higher than the amount entering them. The excess fluid is caught by the lymphatic system and eventually drained to the venous system. This process enables

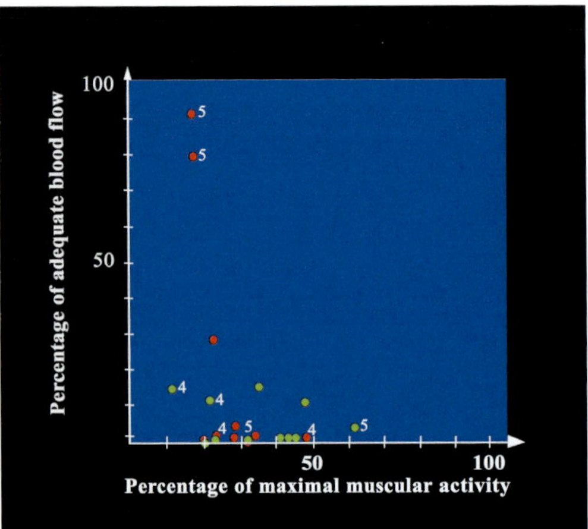


Fig 15-15 Relationship between blood flow and the magnitude of contractile muscular activity in two subjects (4, masseter; 5, temporalis).

**Intense and long parafunctional contractions**

Muscular ischemia and vessel constriction with less supply of $O_2$

▼

Less pyruvic acid enters the citric acid cycle, and gradual predominance of anaerobic glycolysis with less ATP and lactic acid as final products

▼

Increment in intramuscular pressure blocks lymphatic or venous drainage

▼

Lactic acid accumulation (acidosis or pH); metabolic products ($K^+$, ATP, no oxidized products; free radicals $O_2^-$) and vessel neuroactive substances (local mediators and neuropeptides) caused by the tissue lesion. They generate a hyperosmolarity area, accumulation of intersticial liquid and muscular edema with an increase of hydrostatic pressure: MYOSITIS

▼

Muscular pain: MYALGIA, caused by stimulation of nociceptive terminals

* Acidosis
* Increase in hydrostatic pressure
* Local mediators of pain and inflammation
* Neuropeptides
* ATP, K+ and free radicals $O_2^-$

▼

Inhibition of the enzymatic energy action of the muscle, generating:
MUSCULAR FATIGUE (diminution of the muscular contractile ability) and
CONTRACTURE (continual muscular contraction, even without motor nervous stimulation)

Fig 15-16 Theoretical model of the sequence of events from the pathophysiologic mechanism of muscular ischemia to muscle pain, myositis, fatigue, and contracture.

a constant pressure of the interstitial liquid, as well as a constant interchange of tissue liquids.[27]

In contrast, when the muscle is isometrically contracted there is an increase in the intramuscular pressure, which in some cases may exceed the systolic blood pressure – this may produce a compression of blood vessels, impeding normal blood flow. A reduction in blood flow is produced also to a lesser extent by the compression and occlusion of arteries and veins entering the muscle.[28] The higher the intensity of the isometric contraction, the more severe is the reduction of this blood supply.

It has been demonstrated[28] that, in jaw muscles clenching for 90 seconds in the intercuspal position and with a contractile power equivalent to 25% of the effort of maximal vertical clenching, there is a blockage or significant reduction of the blood supply. Even during clenching corresponding to 10% of the maximal vertical clenching there may be a severe reduction of blood flow in some patients (Fig 15-15).

During repetitive and long-lasting isometric contractions (as is frequent during bruxism), the blood flow is blocked and the concentration of oxygen decreases to a very low level (muscular hypoxia). As previously mentioned, chronic myospasm also contributes to this blood flow disorder.

Research has demonstrated that the masseter muscle has a higher density of capillaries than the muscles of extremities.[29] From a functional point of view, this means a higher demand for blood supply of the jaw muscle. In addition, on the basis of hemoglobin content, the research demonstrated a higher density of capillaries in men's masseter muscle than in women's (1.1 to 2.0 times higher). This fact might be related not to the type of muscular fibers but to the smaller transverse section area of muscular fibers in women.

Figure 15-16 shows a theoretical model of the sequence of events that can lead from the pathophysiologic mechanism of muscular ischemia to muscle pain, myositis, fatigue, and muscular contracture.

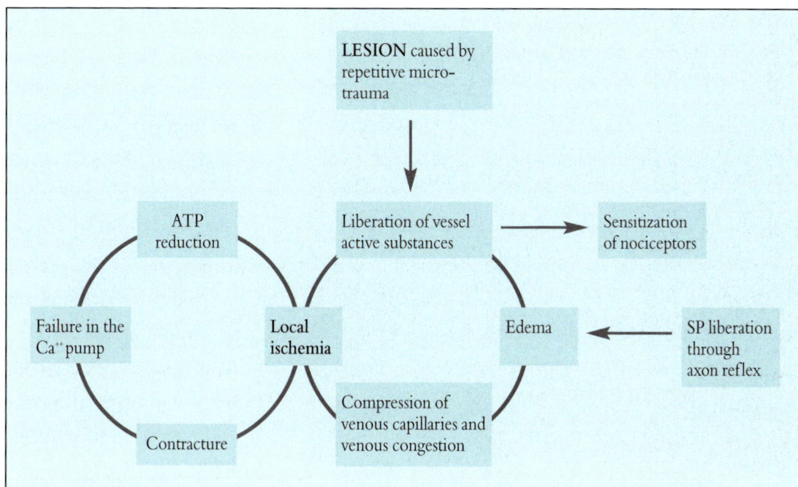


Fig 15-17 Theoretical model of contracture. SP, substance P.

### *Muscular Lesions Caused by Repetitive Microtrauma*

After a lesion occurs there follows the liberation of local mediators of inflammation and pain, such as serotonin (5-HT) and vasoactive substances such as bradykinins, prostaglandins and histamines, which produce vasodilation and an increase in the capillary permeability, which result in a localized edema. These substances have additional neuroactive activity as they concomitantly sensitize the nociceptors near the lesion. This peripheral sensitization of nociceptors affects the liberation of neuropeptides (substance P and calcitonin gene-related peptide) not only in situ but also, by means of the axon reflex, in neighboring areas close to the lesion (by antidromic transmission) through the non-activated ramifications of some of the sensitized nociceptive nerve fibers. This leads to the appearance of new receptive fields, which means that these free terminals may respond to a completely normal mechanical stimulus, such as a local light pressure, subjectively referred to as pain (allodynia). All these processes, which involve so-called peripheral sensitization, represent at the same time a mechanism that explains the hyperalgesia in injured muscles.

In most patients the edema and peripheral nociceptive sensitization represent the last stage in a series; then the lesion heals and muscular pain (spontaneous or excited by palpation) lessens. In less favorable cases, due to a reduction in muscular physiologic tolerance and/or an increase of parafunctional overcharge in the form of repetitive microtrauma, the edema may worsen and produce compression of venous capillaries as well as venous congestion, which leads finally to a localized ischemia liberating more bradykinin. In this way a vicious circle is set up between the edema and the sensitization of nociceptors. Without proper therapy the pain can continue for a long time.

In addition, the ischemia affects physiologic muscular processes because it causes a lack of energy (ATP). This fact leads not only to a $Ca^{++}$ pump failure (necessary for calcium uptake by the sarcoplasmic reticulum and muscular relaxation), but also to the addition of ATP molecules to the myosin heads, which leaves these joined to the active sites of actin. This triggers a local contracture (i.e., maintaining the contractile ability without the necessity of muscular action potentials). It is as yet unknown whether contractures might constitute one of the main mechanisms for the generation of myofascial trigger points. This theoretical model is explained in Fig 15-17.

We shall now look at four recent publications related to the described pathophysiologic mechanism. In two of them, microlesions producing morphologic changes (biochemical) generated during contractile activity under muscular over-effort are mentioned. Friden[30] demonstrated, after exercise with muscular over-exertion, a disorganization of the sarcomeric myofilaments of muscle fibers and a tearing in the muscle structures particularly localized in Z-discs, and sarcoplasmic reticulum with liberation of ATP. Bani and co-workers[31] observed the following morphologic and chemical changes in the masseter muscle of a rat, induced by occlusal wearing: (1) higher concentration of sarcoplasmic $Ca^{++}$; (2) interstitial edema and fibrosis of muscular fibers in different grades; (3) muscle fiber injury: myofibril disorganization and broken sarcolemma; (4) reduction of lumen in blood capillaries and signs of endothelial lesion. These changes were restricted to I-type muscular fibers than on the whole muscle.

The next two publications studied the effect of local mediators of pain and inflammation, histamine, and serotonin, in relation to muscular pain. In the first one Watanabe and co-workers[32] arrived at the following conclusions:

- Histamine might be involved in inducing pain, and possibly in muscular fatigue, accompanied by muscular disorders.
- In mice under electric masseteric stimulation (2 mA for 10 minutes) there was an increase in concentration of muscular histamine three hours after the stimulation, reaching a maximum six or eight hours later and then gradually decreasing.
- There was a 74% decrease in muscular pain in humans using an antihistamine compared with 48% when using an anti-inflammatory analgesic.

In the other publication Emberg and co-workers[33] found that the muscular pain (local myalgia) studied in patients with muscular disorders was significantly associated with the serum concentration of serotonin. They found an association between the low level of concentration of serum 5-HT and local allodynia in jaw muscles of the patients under study.

Finally, it is important to state that longer term pain produces a change in the process and central modulation of pain (i.e., changes in the neuroplasticity of the second-order nociceptive neurons), called "central sensitization". One of the most significant changes is hyperexcitability and spontaneous hyperactivity (deep hyperalgia) of these nociceptive neurons, as a result of a great flow of nociceptive discharges transmitted to them from the peripheral nociceptors. This hyperexcitability and spontaneous pain are probably due (as demonstrated with experimental myositis) to co-activation of NK-1 (neuroquinine-1) receptors because of the action of substance P, and also mainly of the *N*-methyl-D-aspartic acid (NMDA) receptors because of the action of glutamate.[20] These results may suggest the following application and clinical understanding: blockage, especially of NK-1 receptors, or, in a more limited way, of NMDA receptors, might reduce hyperalgesia and spontaneous pain. At the same time, as the mechanisms of central sensitization make the second-order nociceptive neurons last, even when the peripheral lesion has healed and does not represent any nociceptive source, the blockage of the mentioned receptors might also have a major therapeutic impact over the chronic and long-lasting pain. In addition, the deep hyperalgesia related to the sensitization of second-order neurons of the trigeminal caudal subnucleus may also occur in association with a disorder or diminution of efficacy of systems or mechanisms of descending inhibitory endogenous control of pain, which may lead to a more generalized hyperalgesia and somatic sensorial disorders. We should not forget that there are only endorphin receptors in the trigeminal caudal subnucleus. For this reason, the inhibitory descending systems stimulate interneurons only at this

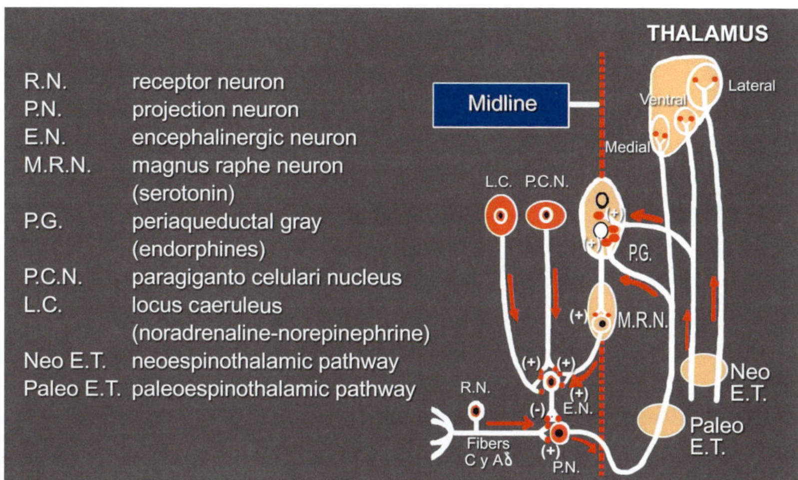


Fig 15-18 Systems of descending inhibitory endogenous control of pain.

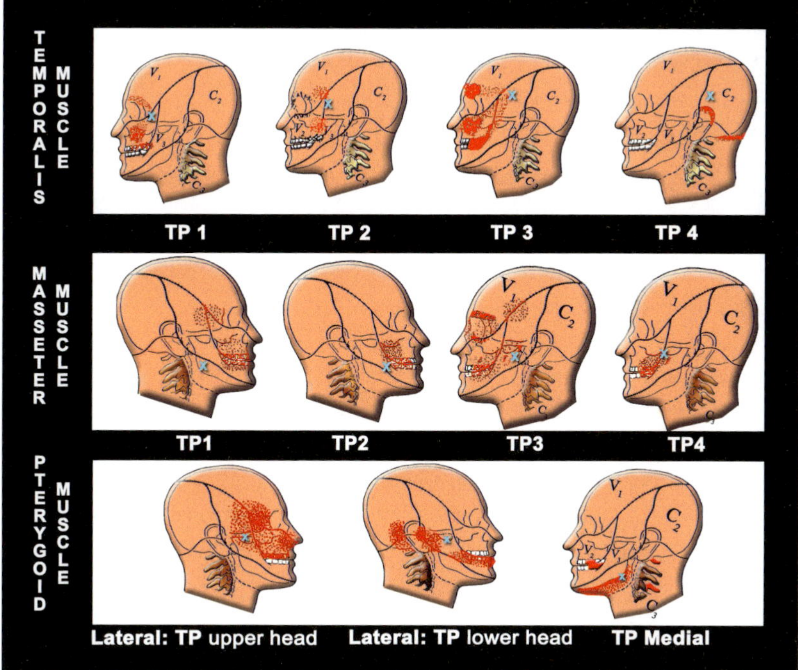


Fig 15-19 Referred pain schemes (in red) of elevator and pterygoid muscles. X (in cyan) indicates the myofascial trigger points (TP) in the area corresponding to each muscle.

level (Fig. 15-18). This last mechanism is very important in long-lasting pain. We should remember that second-order nociceptive neurons localized in the trigeminal caudal subnucleus are submitted to a central inhibition more significant than cutaneous nociceptive neurons.

With regard to the additional symptomatology of muscular pain, muscular fatigue (of which the person is aware) may appear at various times – when the person wakes up (morning muscular fatigue) or throughout the day, mainly when chewing hard food or when speaking. Muscular

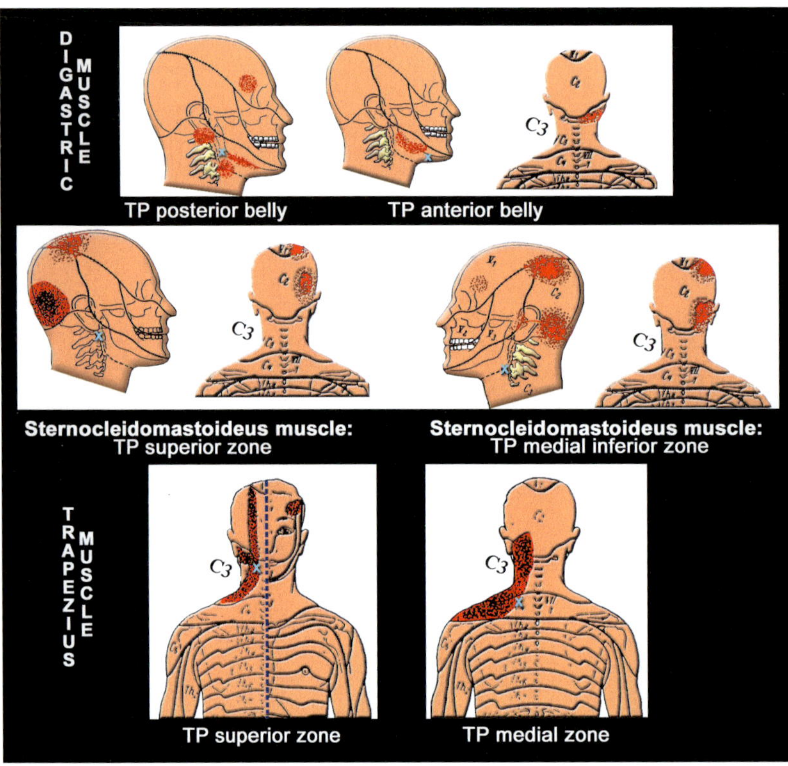


**Fig 15-20** Referred pain schemes (in red) of digastric and neck muscles. X (in cyan) indicates the myofascial trigger points (TP) in the area corresponding to each muscle.

fatigue is frequently accompanied by a partial but constant state of contraction lasting some minutes, even without muscular action or stimulation via the conventional nervous path – called contracture. Contracture is mainly due to a lack of ATP, so the myosin bridges stay joined to the active sites of actin and it is favored by a blockage of calcium reuptake at sarcoplasmic reticulum level. In this state the muscle has lost its viscoelastic ability and the ability to elongate passively, even in the absence of active contraction. Clinically it is characterized by nodules of variable size in the muscular mass; they are painful on palpation and are nowadays recognized to be a consequence of an isolated contracture of a group of muscular fibers.

Referred pain from stomatognathic muscles is not unusual and every muscle has an established pattern of pain reference which is useful during diagnosis.[34,35] For example, the myofascial trigger points of the temporal muscle may refer the pain of the lateral or anterior part of the skull and the maxilla (Figs 15-19 and 15-20). Instead, the sternocleidomastoid muscle may refer the pain to the TMJ area and inner ear, as well as the posterior, superciliary area, and anterior part of the skull (Figs 15-21 and 15-22).

As already stated, myofascial trigger points correspond to a localized area circumscribed to the spasm of the skeletal muscle fibers which transform into a hypersensible area, sending painful stimuli to the central nervous system. Referred pain may be defined in two different ways:

- as a pathophysiologic mechanism by which pain impulses coming from particular areas of the body (especially deep structures of viscera or muscles) originate localized pain in other (mainly superficial) areas; or

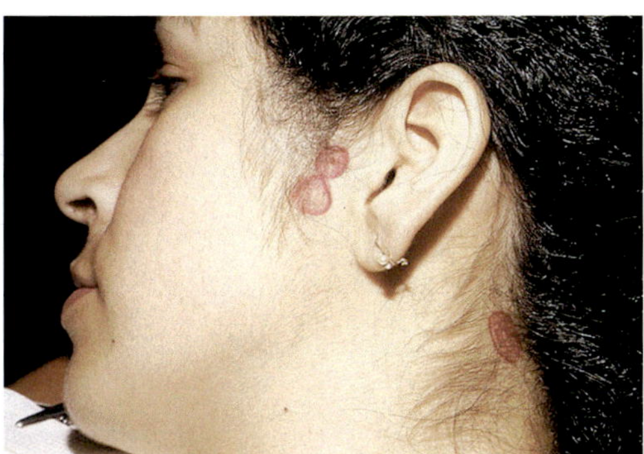

Fig 15-21 Lateral view of a patient with a localized myofascial trigger point in the upper zone of the sternocleidomastoid muscle and referred pain in the temporomandibular joint and pre-auricular zones.

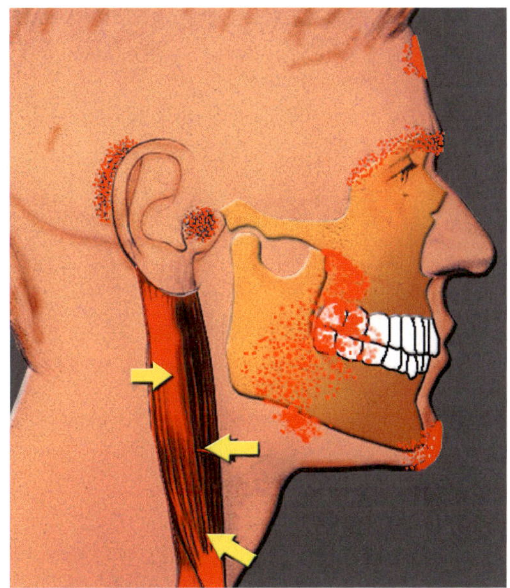

Fig 15-22 Scheme of myofascial trigger points of the sternocleidomastoid muscle in the upper, medial and lower portions with their referred pain.

- as a deep and long-lasting somatic pain that triggers pain in other rather superficial places, owing to the generation of a sensory nociceptive input which may vary the processing at central level of the second-order neurons of the nociceptive pathways.

The action mechanism of referred pain is not completely clear, but basically it depends on:

- convergence of nociceptive afferent information to common central neurons of the myofascial trigger point and the reference site as well (Fig 15-23)
- central summation and excitatory facilitation of the second-order nociceptive neurons, caused by a condition of pathways divergence (Fig 15-24).

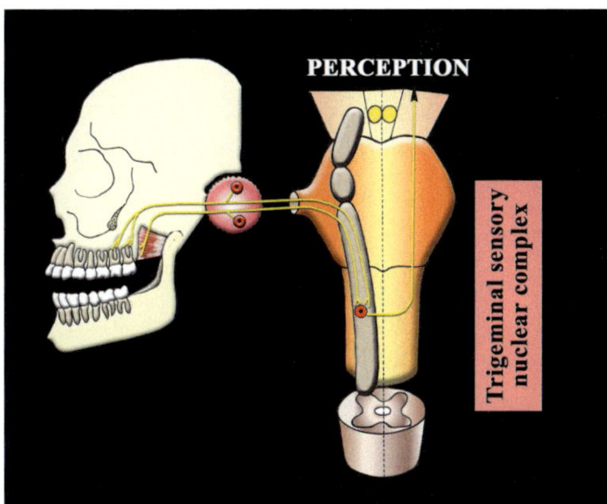


Fig 15-23 Scheme of the mechanism of referred pain. Observe the convergence of the information afferents to a common central neuron of the trigeminal caudal subnucleus, coming from the trigger point (lower head of the lateral pterygoid muscle) and the reference site of pain (maxillary posterior teeth). The upper arrow indicates the thalamocortical pathway of perception.

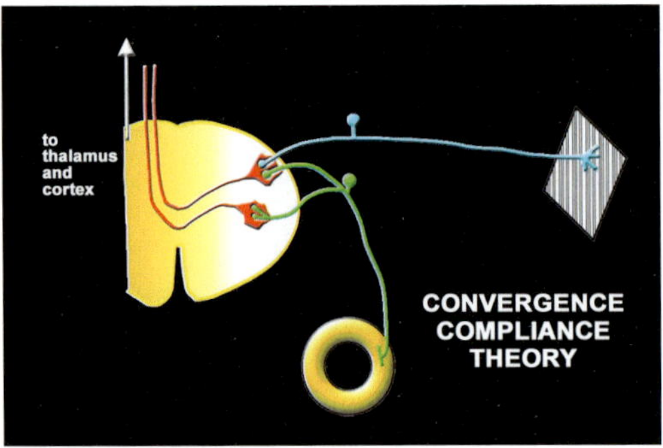


Fig 15-24 Central summation and excitatory facilitation of the second-order nociceptive neuron.

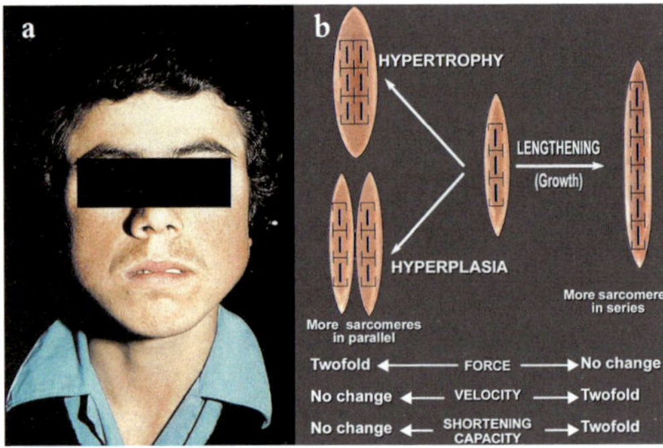


Fig 15-25 **(a and b)** Patient with bilateral masseteric hypertrophy and the sarcomeric structural adaptation scheme.

Muscular referred pain of the stomatognathic musculature is a consequence of a more chronic and long-lasting muscular disorder, different from myalgia, which is a localized, acute and more recent pain.

In addition, longer-lasting muscular disorders may trigger an inflammatory reaction of tendon tissues, because of an overcharging of the muscular tendons. This pathologic state is called "tendonitis", which is relatively frequent in muscular disorder conditions. Tendons get very sensitive on palpation and during chewing of hard food.

Also, edema and an increase in muscle interstitial hydrostatic pressure may, in certain cases, cause necrosis and destruction of their contractile elements. Then these elements are repaired by the connective tissue, producing a condition known as "myofibrosis". In a certain percentage of clinical cases, the muscular over-effort may produce damage of blood vessels within the muscle, resulting in extravasation which, in conjunction with the edema and myositis, may stimulate a scarring process in the connective tissue component of the muscle. This formation of fibrous, inelastic, connective scarring tissue within the muscle is usually associated with hypometria or persistent trismus after the elimination of pain and spasm of the jaw muscles.

The fact that training causes an increase of muscular performance is well known. Continual training causes growth of the muscular mass, known as *hypertrophy*. The same effect occurs during parafunctional activity, in which certain muscles or muscular groups exhibit isometric contraction over long periods of time. Hypertrophy means an increase in the size of individual muscular fibers and it is attributed to an increment in the number of individual muscular myofibrils owing to an increase in the number of in-parallel sarcomeres.[28] Muscular hypertrophy, therefore, constitutes an adaptation state of the muscle in the presence of functional over-effort (Fig 15-25).

The muscular disturbances described above are not restricted to the jaw musculature. Owing to an increased parafunctional activity, frequently there is a disorder in the muscular cranial–cervical balance. Thus, the neck musculature may also present symptoms of fatigue and spasm, referred to by patients as pain and/or tension in the neck and shoulders. Ehrlich and co-workers[36] recorded EMG activity of sternocleidomastoid, trapezium, and paravertebral muscles and rectus abdominis in 10 university students at rest and during strong clenching, in supine and sitting positions. They concluded that, in both positions, teeth clenching produced:

*Table 15-2*

**Classical diagnostic classification of muscular disorders.**

**Protective co-contraction or splinting reflex (trismus)**
*Definition:* muscular stiffness reflex induced as preventing pain during movements
*Diagnostic criteria:* frequent pain; pain on palpation; limited jaw dynamics; stiffness; jaw stiffness on manipulation

**Myofascial pain (myalgia – with or without trigger point)**
*Definition:* regional pain associated with painful sensitiveness in firm bands of muscles and tendons
*Diagnostic criteria:* continual pain, usually hard in one or more muscles; painful localized palpation; sensitive points

**Myositis (tendomyositis – inflammatory myalgia)**
*Definition:* generalized painful inflammation, usually of the whole muscle
*Diagnostic criteria:* acute muscular pain; painful palpation over the whole muscle; possible growth in volume; limited jaw dynamics

**Myospasm (acute trismus)**
*Definition:* abnormal and involuntary contraction of the muscle, characterized by a muscular hyperactivity in all or part of the muscular fibers; muscle unable to relax voluntarily, having resistance to stretching
*Diagnostic criteria:* acute pain; limited jaw dynamics; continual muscular contractions (fasciculations); increased EMG activity, even at rest

**Muscular contraction (chronic trismus)**
*Definition:* chronic resistance of the muscle to passive stretching
*Diagnostic criteria:* generally not painful; limited jaw range; muscular firmness when passive stretching

**Hypertrophy**
*Definition:* abnormal thickness of the muscle
*Diagnostic criteria:* not painful; great increase in volume; limited jaw range (occasionally)

- an increment of neck muscular activity to between 7.6 and 33 times the activity at rest
- an increment of the trunk muscles to between 1.4 and 3.3 times the activity at rest.

With regard to otologic symptoms (tinnitus, hypoacusia, otic fullness sensation) and balance symptoms (vertigo), which frequently accompany temporomandibular disorders, Myrhaug[37] demonstrated, clinically and electromyographically, that they are due to a myospasm of the tensor tympani muscle; and according to Phillip and co-workers[38] and Düker and co-workers[39] there are disturbances in the active opening of the Eustachian tube by the dilator tubae eustachii or tensor veli palatini muscle. Both muscles are also innervated by the trigeminal nerve.

Finally, another common symptom associated with muscular disorders is cephalgia. This is a pathologic condition with a variety of symptoms and different hypotheses about its etiology. Nevertheless, a significant percentage of cephalgias are related to jaw muscular hyperactivity developed during bruxism. This makes it possible to establish a potential correlation between muscular hyperactivity and the presence of cephalgia.

## Conclusion

Muscular disorders have been described, including them in Dworkin and Le Resche's group I diagnostic classification and dividing them into two categories: myofascial pain, and myofascial pain with limited opening. Types of muscular pain have been analyzed as the main manifestation of muscular disorders, dividing them into two categories: (a) more chronic and (b) long-lasting pain, not restricted to the same place as the lesion but that frequently radiates and is perceived in deeper or superficial areas ("referred pain").

However, there exists a more classical diagnostic classification of muscular disorders that divides them into the categories listed in Table 15-2. Even though these pathophysiologic classifications may be present in patients with muscular disorders, diagnosis may be difficult and confusing; which is why it is important to emphasize that a diagnostic classification of real categories, like Dworkin and Le Resche's, is more useful for scientific research and clinical therapy because it is based on a limited number of categories.

## References


1. Rauhala K, Oikarimer K, Raustia A. Role of temporomandibular disorders in facial pain: occlusion, muscle and TMJ pain. J Craniomandibular Pract 1999;17:254–261.
2. Manns A, Scharager D, Martínez B. Estudio de la correlación entre sintomatología disfuncional y parafunciones en una población de pacientes con trastornos temporomandibulares (in press).
3. Okeson JP. Tratamiento y Afecciones Temporomandibulares, ed 5. Madrid: Elsevier S.A., 2003.
4. Manns A, Díaz G. Sistema Estomatognático. Santiago: Facultad de Odontología, Universidad de Chile, 1995.
5. Ganong WF. Fisiología Médica, ed 15. Mexico: El Manual Moderno S.A., 1996.
6. Kandel ER, Schwartz JH, Jessell TM. Principios de Neurociencia, ed 4. Spain: McGraw-Hill and Interamericana de España S.A.U., 2001.
7. Enoka RM. Neuromechanics of Human Movement, ed 3. USA: Human Kinetics, 2002.
8. Gibbs CH, Mahan PE, Lundeen HC et al. Occlusal forces during chewing and swallowing as measured by sound transmission. J Prosthet Dent 1981;46:443–449.
9. Nishigawa K, Bando E, Nakano M. Quantitative study of bite force during sleep-associated bruxism. J Oral Rehabil 2001;28:485–491.
10. Graf H. Bruxism. Dent Clin North Am 1969;13:659–665.
11. Glickman I. Clinical Periodontology, ed 4. Philadelphia: Saunders, 1972.
12. Brewer AA, Hudson PC. Application of miniature electronic devices for the study of tooth contact in complete dentures. J Prosthet Dent 1961;11:62–68.
13. Trenouth MJ. The relationship between bruxism and temporomandibular joint dysfunction as shown by computer analysis of nocturnal tooth contact patterns. J Oral Rehabil 1979;6:81–87.
14. Baba K, Clark GT, Watanabe T, Ohiyama T. Bruxism force detection by a piezoelectric film-based recording device in sleeping humans. J Orofac Pain 2003;17:58–64.
15. Schulte W. Die exzentrische Okklusion. Berlin: Quintessenz Verlags, 1983.
16. Miralles R, Carvajal E, Manns A, Rossi E. Estudio comparativo de umbrales presorreceptivos en dientes con normofunción vs. hiperfunción o trauma oclusal. Rev Dent Chile 1980;11:3–7.
17. Mühlbradt L, Jenz KP, Lukas D. Die Berührungschwelle bei gesunden und erkrankten Parodontien. Dtsch Zahnärztl Z 1976;31:306–312.
18. De Laat A. Scientific basis of masticatory disorders. In: Linden RWA (ed). The Scientific Basis of Eating. Basel: Karger, 1998.
19. Dworkin SF, Le Resche L. Research diagnostic criteria. J Craniomandib Disord 1992;6:301–355.
20. Mense S. Fundamentos fisiopatológicos del dolor muscular. In: Sandro Pala (ed). Mioartropatías del Sistema Masticatorio y Dolores Orofaciales. Milan: RC Libri, 2003.
21. Christensen LV. Facial pain and internal pressure of masseter muscle in experimental bruxism in man. Arch Oral Biol 1971;16:1021–1031.
22. Christensen LV. Influence of muscle pain tolerance on muscle pain threshold in experimental tooth clenching in man. J Oral Rehabil 1979;6:211–217.
23. Scott DS, Lundeen TF. Myofascial pain involving the masticatory muscles: an experimental model. Pain 1980;8: 207–215.
24. Villarosa GA, Moss RA. Oral behavioral patterns as factors contributing to the development of head and facial pain. J Prosthet Dent 1985;54:427–430.
25. Glaros AG, Tabaccachi K, Glass EG. Effect of parafunctional clenching on temporomandibular disorder pain. J Orofac Pain 1998;12:145–152.
26. Glaros AG, Forbes M, Shanker J, Glass EG. Effect of parafunctional clenching on temporomandibular disorder pain and propioceptive awareness. J Craniomandibular Pract 2000;18:198–204.
27. Silvestri A, Cohen S, Connolly R. Muscle physiology during funcional activities and parafunctional habits. J Prosthet Dent 1980;44:64–67.

28. Möller E. Neuromuskuläre Aspekte der normalen und der gestörten Funktion des mastikatorischen Systems. In: Drücke W, Klemt B (eds). Kiefergelenk und Okklusion. Berlín: Quintessenz Verlags, 1980.
29. Suyisaki M, Misawa A, Ikai A, Kim Young-Sung, Tanabe H. Sex differences in the hemoglobin oxygenation state of the resting healthy human masseter muscle. J Orofac Pain 2001;15:320–328.
30. Friden J. Muscle soreness after exercise: implications of morphological changes. Int J Sports Med 1984;5:57–66.
31. Bani D, Bani T, Berllamini M. Morphologic and biochemical changes of the masseter muscle induced by occlusal wear: studies in a rat model. J Dent Res 1999;78: 1735–1744.
32. Watanabe M, Tabata T, Huh JI et al. Possible involvement of histamina in muscular fatigue in temporomandibular disorders: animal and human studies. J Dent Res 1999;78: 769–775.
33. Emberg M, Hedenberg-Magnusson B, Alstergren P, Lundeberg T, Kopp S. Pain, allodynia, and aerum aerotonin level in orofacial pain of muscular origin. J Orofac Pain 1999;13:56–62.
34. Travel J. Tempromandibular joint pain referred from the muscles of the head and neck. J Prosthet Dent 1960;4: 745–752.
35. Schimek JJ, Schimek F. The temporomandibular joint pain dysfunction syndrome and the orofacial pain. J Gnathol 1988;7:19-30.
36. Ehrlich R, Garlick D, Minio M. The effects of jaw clenching on the electromyographic activities of two neck and two trunk muscles. Orofac Pain 1999;13: 115–120.
37. Myrhaug H. Parafunktionen im Kauapparat als Ursache eines otodentalen Syndroms, Vols 6 and 7. Berlin: Quintessenz Verlag, 1969.
38. Phillip V, Munker G, Kamposch G. Die Funktion der Tuba Eustachii bei Patienten mit Kiefergelenkerkrankungen. Dtsch Zahnärztl Z 1972;27:806–810.
39. Düker J, Philipp V, Fiebelkorn W. Sensorische Störungen bei Kiefergelenkerkrankungen. Dtsch Zahnärztl Z 1972; 27:811–818.

Chapter 16

# Temporomandibular Joint Dysfunction and Bruxism

*Xiomara Restrepo-Jaramillo, Ross H. Tallents, and Stephanos Kyrkanides*

## Introduction

Temporomandibular disorders (TMD) are a collective entity embracing a number of clinical problems that involve the masticatory musculature and temporomandibular joints (TMJs) and associated structures, or both.[1] It is characterized as unilateral or bilateral pain in the TMJ and its associated craniofacial musculature. Other symptoms include tinnitus, ear fullness, and various joint sounds.[2] The most common symptoms are pain on palpation of the joint and/or muscles of mastication, reduced mouth opening, restriction in excursive jaw movement (right, left, and protrusion), and clicking or grating sounds in the joint on movement of the mandible.[3] Historically there are several classifications, and this can create confusion. One of the most comprehensive classifications is the Research Diagnostic Criteria (RDC/TMD). This system classifies TMD along two axes.

- Axis I refers to the clinical evaluation of TMD conditions. Three diagnostic groups can thus be distinguished: (1) muscle disorders, (2) internal derangement (ID), and (3) degenerative joint disease (DJD) (arthritis).
- Axis II rates pain-related disability and psychologic status in association with TMD.[4]

## Definitions

Internal derangement of the TMJ (disc displacement, DD) has been defined as an abnormal relationship of the articular disc relative to the mandibular condyle, fossa, and articular eminence. Two conditions can be distinguished.

- Disc displacement *with* reduction (DDR) is where the disc is displaced anteriorly, medially, laterally (or mixed) in the closed jaw position. In the open jaw position the posterior band of the disc is on the superior aspect of the condyle (Fig 16-1). This condition is usually associated with clicking.[5]
- Disc displacement *without* reduction (DDNR) is where the disc does not reduce to a normal relationship. The disc is located anteriorly to the condyle and articular eminence. This

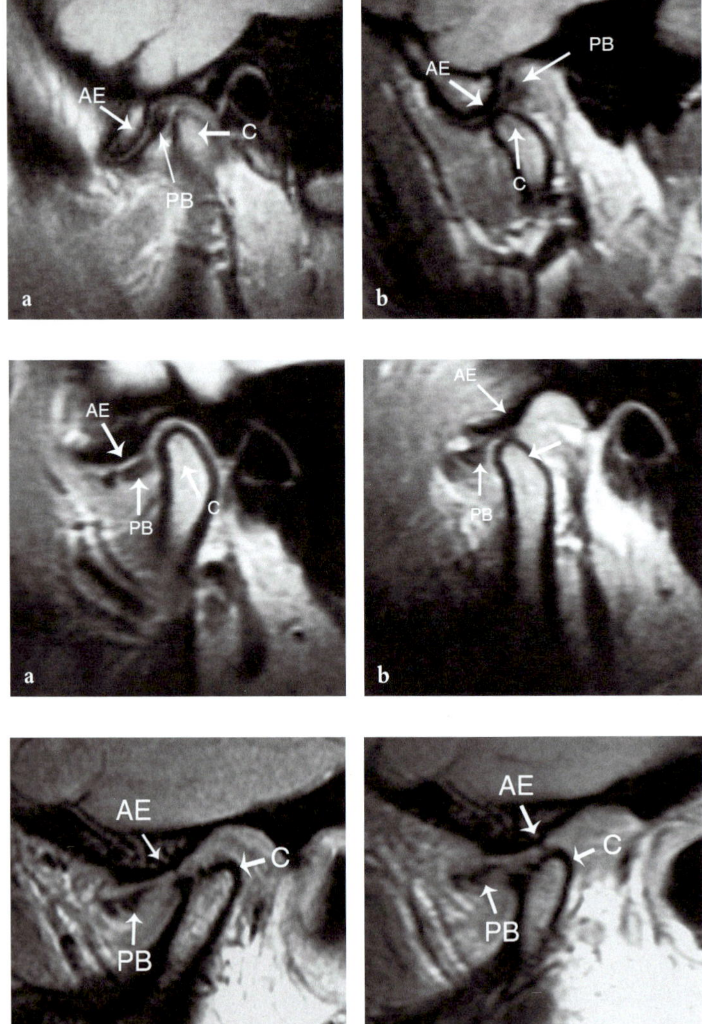


**Fig 16-1** Magnetic resonance image of a patient with disc displacement with reduction. **(a)** Closed jaw position: the posterior band (PB) of the disc is anterior to the condylar head (C) and inferior to the articular eminence (AE). **(b)** In the open jaw position the disc is reduced.

**Fig 16-2** Magnetic resonance image of a patient with disc displacement without reduction. **(a)** Closed jaw position: the posterior band of the disc (PB) is anterior to the condylar head (C). **(b)** Open jaw position: the PB remains anterior.

**Fig 16-3** Magnetic resonance image of a patient with degenerative joint disease. **(a)** Closed jaw position: the disc is displaced anteriorly, is deformed, and has lost its normal morphology. The articular eminence (AE) is sclerotic and flattened. There is also an osteophyte and the condylar head (C) is flattened. **(b)** In this case the disc remains anterior in the open jaw position.

condition may be associated with limitation of jaw opening and pain (Fig 16-2).[6–10]

Degenerative joint disease (osteoarthritis, OA) is defined as a complex of interactive degradative and repair processes in cartilage, bone, and synovium, with secondary components of inflammation.[11] In the temporomandibular joints with DD, OA may be present with or without pain, muscle tenderness, headaches, limitation of jaw movements, clicking, or crepitus (Fig 16-3).

## Prevalence Studies

Epidemiologic studies have evaluated the prevalence of TMJ disease in adults, adolescents, and children. Autopsy studies in both young and mature adults showed the prevalence of internal

derangement of the TMJ to be 10–32% in the general population.[12,13] Many studies found prevalence of disc displacement in the asymptomatic general population ranging from 15% to 34%.[14–19] Studies of symptom-free populations (asymptomatic volunteers) suggest that internal derangement of the TMJ occurs in asymptomatic subjects with a prevalence ranging from 10% to 33%.[16–20] The high prevalence of DD in asymptomatic volunteers is not unique to the TMJ. Magnetic resonance imaging (MRI) studies of asymptomatic subjects in which the knee, cervical spine, and lumbar spine were evaluated indicate a similar prevalence in asymptomatic subjects.[21–27] These studies demonstrate that disc displacement in TMJ, cervical, and lumbar herniations, and meniscal and cruciate tears can be present in patients without clinical signs and symptoms. There is also a high prevalence (34%) of TMJ internal derangement in asymptomatic children and young adult volunteers, suggesting that disc displacement is present at a young age.[16,20] In fact, the prevalence of DD in symptomatic children and young adults is 80–85%,[16] similar to that in adult symptomatic subjects. These results may suggest that soft tissue changes may begin early in childhood and that disc displacement of the TMJ may be considered as a pre-existing condition, which may be a risk factor when found with other predisposing, initiating, and perpetuating factors.[12,16,17,28–31] The prevalence of degenerative joint disease in a pediatric symptom-free population is approximately 1–2% and in symptomatic children is 15%. In symptomatic children and young adults the prevalence rages from 26% to 37%.[16,17,29]

In fact, adult subjects with TMJ disease present with other joint problems. The prevalence of other joint problems (cervical spine, lumbar spine, and knees) in asymptomatic subjects is 10% and in symptomatic subjects is 31–40%.[20] In fact, the prevalence of herniations and meniscal tears (C-spine, L-spine, and knees) ranges from 16% to 52% in asymptomatic subjects.[21–27] This may represent a comorbid condition in patients with TMD, similar to fibromyalgia, irritable bowel, chronic muscle soreness, and multiple allegies.[32,33]

## Etiology

TMJ disease is generally believed to be multifactorial in nature.[34,35] Currently, it is generally accepted that the etiology of TMD includes predisposing, initiating, and/or perpetuating factors.[36] Predisposing factors increase the risk of TMD and may include gender, systemic conditions, and psychological and structural factors. It is well known that chronic TMJ dysfunction is more prevalent in females of reproductive age, being as high as 80%.[37]

The discrepancy between the genders is not clearly understood, although theories suggest a hormonal influence as shown by differences in the pain signaling process by the activation of cytokine production via estrogen receptors in the TMJs.[38–42] Also, the fact that women seek healthcare for pain more frequently than men must also be considered.[43]

TMD may coexist with many systemic conditions such as joint laxity, chronic fatigue syndrome, fibromyalgia, irritable bowel syndrome, chronic tension-type headache, multiple chemical sensitivities, post-concussive syndrome, chronic pelvic pain, chronic low back pain, and interstitial cystitis.[32] Interestingly, it has been found that many of these unexplained clinical conditions share demographic, clinical, and psychosocial features, as well as objective findings such as myalgia, fatigue, and sleep disturbances. Inadequate information is available on the cause, pathophysiology, natural history, prognosis, and medical management of these syndromes, which suggests directions for future research.[32,33,44]

Psychological factors (demographics, emotion, personality, and behavior) may have a direct or indirect role in pain disorders and are considered to be major issues in the onset, exacerbation, or perpetuation of pain. In some cases they have an influence on the predictability of treatment outcomes. It is known that chronic pain is associated with psychologic factors such as stress and depression, and it is common to find TMD as a comorbid condition in TMD patients.[45–48]

The interest in occlusal and other structural factors was started by Costen's hypothesis.[49] Although the original hypothesis was later refuted, the occlusal–structural model of TMD causation has been extremely popular for decades – along with the belief that unfavorable occlusal features, such as occlusal interferences, differences between the retruded-contact position (RCP) and the intercuspal position (ICP) slide length, bruxism, extensive overbite and overjet, unilateral posterior crossbite, incisor dental midline discrepancy, number of unreplaced missing posterior teeth, etc., can lead to neuromuscular disturbances, pain, dysfunction, and arthritic changes in the TMJ.[50–54] However, the role of occlusion in the pathogenesis of TMD is still controversial. Studies of nonpatient populations do not provide sufficient evidence of an association between TMD and occlusal factors.[55] In recent years, the etiologic significance of occlusal factors has been increasingly questioned and there is no universal agreement supporting the presence of occlusal interferences and the induction of TMJ disease. Epidemiologic studies have demonstrated only a weak or nonexistent relationship.[56–62]

Initiating factors include trauma, parafunctional habits, and adverse loading or overloading of the TMJ. Injuries of the TMJ might be direct or indirect trauma and micro- or macrotrauma. These include whiplash injury, scuba diving, endotracheal intubation, playing some musical instruments, and third molar extraction.[63] Parafunctional habits such as chewing gum, biting nails and pencils, and grinding teeth are believed to be a source of microtrauma. Perpetuating or sustaining factors include mechanical and muscular stress, and metabolic problems. There may also be behavioral, social, and emotional conditions. Clinicians often suggest that bruxism is an initiating and perpetuating factor and that this would lead to morphologic alterations (disc displacement, degenerative joint disease) in the TMJ.[1–3,64]

## Pathways to Joint Degeneration

It is believed that there are two possible pathways leading to joint degeneration: degeneration of tissue, and physical forces. The first involves degeneration of cartilage, disc, synovial tissue, and bone even with normal functions of the joint.[11]

TMJ disease has been noted with increased frequency in individuals with mitral valve prolapse, indicating a possible etiologic association with altered collagen metabolism. Altered collagen metabolism may be important in joint laxity. Higher ratios of collagen type III to type II + I have been reported in patients with internal derangement and systemic joint laxity compared to control subjects.[65–67] Genetic predisposition to altered collagen metabolism may result in a morphologic abnormality of any joint including the TMJ. Morrow and co-workers[20] have suggested that there is a 3–4 times increase in other joint problems compared to asymptomatic controls.

The second pathway involves the role of physical forces causing damage to the normal articular cartilage matrix, by inducing elaborating proinflammatory cytokines (interleukin [IL]-1, IL-6), metalloproteinases, nitric oxide, and Cox-2, and inappropriate repair responses.[11] With physiologic loading, there is a balance between synthesis and breakdown within the tissue (catabolic and anabolic activity). When loading exceeds these physiologic limits, protective and compensatory mechanisms are recruited to prevent, limit, or support repair of damage (e.g., missing molars).[54–58,68,69] Tissues with decreased loading decrease anabolic activity (i.e., insufficient matrix is produced). In contrast, overloading initially induces adaptive responses (such as hypertrophy and hyperplasia), but when the adaptive capacity is exceeded, damage to the cells may result, leading to cell necrosis (apoptosis). When the capacity of the complex load-absorbing system (fibrocartilage, synovial membrane, subchondral bone, capsular ligaments, masticatory muscles) is exceeded or reduced (meaning first or second pathways), the tissue may become damaged.[70,71] In fact, a recent study in somatic mosaic mice overexpressing IL-1β suggests that cytokines may induce osteoarthritic changes in the TMJ associated with increases in Cox-2, nitric oxide, and matrix metalloproteinases. This suggests that an abnormal expression of cytokines may produce catabolic changes.[72]

Sacapino has demonstrated that anterior disc position may induce changes, particularly in retrodiscal tissues.[73] Retrospective studies support the notion that internal derangement is likely to progress to osteoarthritis in 25% of symptomatic subjects.[9,74–77] However, studies have reported that DDR may persist for decades, and this progression to DJD may not be a general rule in patients without DD 18% of the time.[78] Osteoarthritis and disc displacement appear to be strongly associated but may also represent mutually independent temporomandibular disorders.[70,79] The initiation and sequence of disc degeneration is not well understood. It has been suggested to occur by enzymatic breakdown of the extracellular matrix and possibly from local inflammation.[80] Lavage studies in TMD have strongly demonstrated the role of chemical mediators of pain and inflammation, degradative enzymes, cytokines (IL-1, tumor necrosis factor), growth factors (transforming growth factor), and free radicals, in the enzymatic breakdown of cartilage, considered to be a key factor in degenerative progression.[81–84] A recent study of somatic mosaic mice suggested IL-1β may induce similar pro-inflammatory cytokines and degeneration as suggested by lavage studies.[72]

## The Role of Bruxism

Bruxism has been suggested as an initiating and/or perpetuating factor in certain subgroups of temporomandibular disorders, but the exact role of bruxism in the etiology remains unclear.[85] Clinicians universally believe that bruxism leads to signs and symptoms characteristic of TMD, but the prevalence of bruxism and clenching are the same across diagnostic groups.[86] The assumption is that chronic joint loading produces microtrauma that leads to TMJ dysfunction. Some suggest that bruxism represents a comorbid condition in association with TMD. This section will explore the potential causal relationship between bruxism and internal derangement of the TMJ.

The American Sleep Disorders Association (ASDA) has defined bruxism as a "diurnal or nocturnal stereotyped movement disorder characterized by grinding, clenching, bracing, gnashing of the teeth".[87] This involuntary activity of the jaw musculature is characterized, in awake individuals, by jaw clenching (so-called awake bruxism) and, on rare occasions, by tooth gnashing and/or grinding. During sleep bruxism (SB), both clenching and tooth grinding are observed. Awake bruxism can occur alone or concomitantly with sleep bruxism.[88] The prevalence of awake bruxism in the general population is approximately 20%, while the prevalence of sleep bruxism is about 8%.[89,90] There is a 69% prevalence of sleep bruxism in children aged 3–13 years, and a progressive decrease with age during childhood and preadolescence has been suggested.[91–93] Lavigne and Montplaisir have reported a progressive decrease in the prevalence of bruxism from young adulthood to old age.[90]

The diagnosis of sleep bruxism is based on a report of tooth grinding or clenching in combination with at least one of the following signs: abnormal tooth wear, sounds associated with bruxism, and jaw muscle discomfort.[87] But the predictive value of these signs has been questioned.[94,95] Oral parafunctions, especially bruxism, may cause tooth wear. However, in an epidemiologic study of tooth wear, only about 40% of possible etiologic factors could be identified, and bruxism explained only 3% of clinically recorded tooth wear.[96] The highest explanatory value for tooth wear was a reduced number of teeth. A probable interpretation is that, in dentitions with missing teeth, there may be an increased risk of wear. Gradual attrition of the occlusal surfaces of the teeth is a physiologic process, but there are many factors that can influence the type and rate of wear.[97] It is now well established that the etiology of tooth wear is multifactorial.[98,99] Erosion has, in recent years, been emphasized as a more important factor for tooth surface loss and wear than was previously assumed.[100]

Preventive measures, after a careful differential diagnosis, are the first choice in the management of tooth wear. Restoration of an excessively worn dentition, especially one with a reduced number of teeth, is defensible only for esthetic reasons and to avoid further damage to the remaining dentition. Restoring a worn dentition either to treat or to prevent bruxism has no scientific basis.[101]

Tooth wear is a manifestation of loss of tooth structure due to non-carious processes such as attrition, erosion, and abrasion.[99] The exact prevalence of tooth wear is unclear primarily owing to different assessment criteria or definitions of the condition, but it has been reported to range from 13% to 98%.[102,103] Tooth wear is considered to be an age-related process,[104] and it too has a multifactorial etiology that includes the presence of parafunctional habits, occlusal characteristics, diet, and salivary function and composition.[105] Tooth wear is commonly considered to be a proxy of bruxism, and it has been used in research as a predictor of patients' bruxism level in an effort to investigate the relationship between bruxism and TMD. Tooth wear clearly provides information about a history of forceful tooth-to-tooth contact, but it does not validate current ongoing bruxism, nor can it indicate whether a subject has clenching activity. Therefore, any conclusions about the relationship between bruxism and TMD symptoms based on tooth wear must be carefully interpreted.[95] The clinician must be able to distinguish between physiologic and normal tooth wear and pathologic and abnormal tooth wear. Occlusal wear that occurs in response to normal loading cannot be regarded as normal. In addition, occlusal wear that occurs at a rate faster than compensatory physiologic mechanisms is not physiologic. Labeling of tooth wear must be viewed also in the context of the cultural environment under which it has occurred.[106]

The diagnosis of sleep bruxism is based also on the report of jaw muscle discomfort.[87] For years, musculoskeletal craniofacial pain has been considered a dogma because many of the traditional theories used to explain the clinical phenomenon of musculoskeletal pain involved unclear descriptions, such as muscle hyperactivity, spasm, or overworking.[107,108] Even though many studies involving craniofacial muscle treatments are based on the rationale of correcting these features and show remarkably high success rates (70–90%),[109–114] observable clinical success cannot be used in support of the validity of the "hyperactivity – muscle spasm – overwork" theory.[115]

Abnormal muscle function leading to muscle overwork and fatigue has long been regarded as a cause of pain.[116–119] The theory of the vicious cycle (also referred to as the "pain – spasm – pain theory") was proposed to explain the role for the persistence of pain through a mutually reinforcing, vicious link between pain and muscle hyperactivity. Muscle hyperactivity has been suggested for decades to be the cause of chronic pain conditions, such as tension-type headache, myofascial pain, and TMD.[120] The pain model for TMD was, therefore, based on two premises: that muscle hyperactivity can lead to pain, and pain leads to tonic hyperactivity. The first premise would appear to be true – when the muscles are voluntarily contracted for longer periods, the muscle fibers start to present fatigue; the second premise is questionable.

The pain-adaptation model formulated by Lund and co-workers in 1991 was supposed to account for all known changes of motor function in situations of pain. This model is based on the following postulates. Persistent pain has a general effect on the motor system, including changes in facial expression and body position, and avoidance of physical work. Activation of the nociceptors in one part of the body inhibits the agonist motor neurons and facilitates the antagonists. The nociceptors of the skin, teeth, connective tissue, muscles, and joints have a similar effect on the motor system. The conclusion is that motor effects are independent of the type of tissue in which pain arises. These changes related to pain are considered adaptive, to prevent future damage and to allow tissue repair.[121,122] The spatial pain distribution, pain intensity, temporal aspects of pain, and mood are factors that likely affect motor function.[123]

Camparis and Siqueira in 2006[124] did not show statistically significant differences for bruxism between patients with pain and without pain, even though patients without pain presented 20% more bruxism episodes than those with pain. The influence of pain on the bruxism pattern has been studied in patients with non-myofascial pain, compared with subjects without any facial pain, and it has been observed that patients with pain presented with 40% fewer bruxism episodes, suggesting that pain decreases the number of bruxism episodes.[125] Questions persist about the belief that the presence or absence of facial pain may be associated with higher or lower frequency and amplitude, and with the type of muscle contraction of sleep bruxism episodes.

Studies have examined the association between bruxism and TMD symptoms, and often these have corroborated the paradigm that TMD is caused by parafunctional activities such as bruxism.[126–129] However, the findings are not conclusive. There have been methodologic differences. In studies in which the possible role of bruxism is examined, divergent techniques have been used for the identification of this motor phenomenon. Sometimes, patients' self-reporting is used.[129,130] However, it is important to realize that self-reports of any behavior run the risk of bias towards either over- or under-reporting.[85] Instruments have been used to establish a more reliable diagnosis of bruxism – polysomnography (PSG), audio-visual recordings in a sleep laboratory,[74,131] electromyography (EMG), and piezoelectric film-based recording[132] – but it is still unknown whether these recording techniques yield comparable outcomes. Also, most studies use different criteria (e.g., different cut-off thresholds) to decide whether or not a diagnosis of bruxism can be established.[133,134] In addition, sleep bruxism is believed to be highly variable over time, sometimes even on a day-to-day basis, with subjects showing no activity during some nights and intense activity during others.[135]

It has been suggested that bruxism is a risk factor for masticatory muscle and/or TMJ pain. However, the pain associated with bruxism is not a universal finding: many subjects who appear to brux nightly have no pain. This implies that the degree of specificity of the bruxism–TMD association is low, which reduces the probability of establishing a valid causal relationship.[85,130] In fact, it has been shown that no statistically significant differences exist for bruxism and sleep variables between groups of bruxism subjects with TMD and bruxism subjects without TMD.[124]

Bruxism and/or oral parafunctions have been described as increasing loading forces in the TMJ that can contribute to dysfunction and pathology. Many different hypotheses have tried to explain the possible mechanism. The "TMJ osteoarthrosis concept" is that abnormal joint loading may change the equilibrium between cartilage degradation and synthesis, exceeding the functional adaptive capacity of the tissues in the joint. Excessive joint loading can lead to proteoglycan degradation, alterations in the synovium, inflammation, changes in the synovial fluid leading to impaired lubrication and nutrition of chondrocytes, and ultimately cartilage degradation.[136–138]

The "oxidative stress and degenerative TMJ hypothesis" has been proposed as a model for the molecular pathogenesis of degenerative TMJ disease. Abnormal mechanical stresses on the TMJ may lead to the generation of free radicals through hypoxia reperfusion injury, microbleeding leading to hemoglobin deposition in intra-articular tissues, phospholipid catabolism, and other mechanisms. This accumulation of free radicals in the joint may lead to cartilage matrix degradation and the elaboration of an inflammatory response, ultimately affecting the biomechanical properties of the articular tissues.[139,140]

Despite all attempts to establish a mechanism of how parafunctional masticatory activity, such as clenching and bruxism, acts as a major factor in TMJ pathology, studies that show morphologic articular changes that can be related to joint overloading are lacking and the question is still unresolved.

Experimental bruxism studies done in healthy subjects have shown that bruxism may be able to induce acute pain in temporal regions, cheeks, supraorbital regions, TMJs, and teeth.[141–143] However, it is still unclear why some patients with sleep bruxism develop chronic pain while others do not. Some bruxing patients without any facial pain reported morning fatigue or pain, but did not develop chronic pain. Persistent and chronic pain conditions are associated with prolonged functional changes in the nervous system, commonly referred to as "central sensitization".[144] Thus, in chronic pain patients, factors such as central sensitization, neuroplasticity, dysfunction of the inhibitory neural descending system, and psychosocial abnormalities may be present. Diffusion and amplification of persistent deep pain, such as TMD, may also be the result of an increase in endogenous descending facilitation.[145]

## Conclusion

To strengthen the case for causal relationships between TMD, bruxism, and stress, data need to be collected at multiple time points that are associated with the conditions under examination. PSG seems most appropriate to use for studies, because it enables discrimination between bruxism and other orofacial motor activities. However, PSG is costly and time-consuming. Ambulatory EMG might be a good alternative for use in longitudinal studies.[85] It has been suggested, though, that these entities could coexist with bruxism without there being any causal relationships.[146]

## References

1. Okesson JP. Orofacial Pain: Guidelines for Assessment, Diagnosis and Management. Carol Stream, IL: Quintessence, 1996:116.
2. Harris M, Feinmann C, Wise M, Treasure F. Temporomandibular joint and orofacial pain: clinical and medicolegal management problems. Br Dent J 1993;174:129–136.
3. Drangsholt M, Le Resche L. Temporomandibular disorder pain. In: Crombien IK (ed). Epidemiology of Pain. Seattle: IASP Press, 1999:203–233.
4. Dworkin SF, Le Resche L. Research diagnostic criteria for temporomandibular disorders: review, criteria, examinations and specifications. J Orofac Pain 1992;6:301–355.
5. Roberts CA, Tallents RH, Katzberg RW et al. Clinical and arthrographic evaluation of temporomandibular joint sounds. Oral Surg Oral Med Oral Pathol Oral Radiol Endod 1986;62:373–376.
6. Katzberg RW, Dolwick MF, Bales DJ, Helms CA. Arthrotomography of the temporomandibular joint: new technique and preliminary observations. AJR Am J Roentgenol 1979;132:949–955.
7. Rasmussen OC. Clinical findings during the course of temporomandibular arthropathy. Scand J Dent Res 1981; 89:283–288.
8. Magnusson T. Five-year longitudinal study of signs and symptoms of mandibular dysfunction in adolescents. Cranio 1986;4:338–344.
9. Kurita K, Westesson PL, Yuasa H et al. Natural course of untreated symptomatic temporomandibular joint disc displacement without reduction. J Dent Res 1998;77:361–365.
10. Magnusson T, Egarmarki I, Carlsson GE. A prospective investigation over two decades on signs and symptoms of temporomandibular disorder and associated variables: a final summary. Acta Odontol Scand 2005;63:99–109.

11. Pelletier JP, Martel-Pelletier J, Howell DS. Etiopathogenesis of osteoarthritis. In: Arthritis and Allied Conditions: A textbook of Rheumatology. 13th edition. Koopman, WJ, (ed). Baltimore: Williams and Wilkins, 1997:1969–1984.
12. Oberg Y, Carlsson GE, Fajers CM. The temporomandibular joint: a morphometric study on a human autopsy material. Acta Odontol Scand 1971;29:349.
13. Solberg WK, Hansson TL, Nordstrom B. The temporomandibular joint in young adults at autopsy: a morphologic classification and evaluation. J Oral Rehabil 1985; 12: 303–321.
14. Westesson PL, Eriksson L, Kurita K. Reliability of a negative clinical temporomandibular joint examination: prevalence of disk displacement in asymptomatic temporomandibular joint. Oral Surg Oral Med Oral Pathol 1989;68:551–554.
15. Tallents RH, Hatala M, Katzberg RW, Westesson PL. Temporomandibular joint sounds in asymptomatic volunteers. J Prosthet Dent 1993;69:298–304.
16. Ribeiro RF, Tallents RH, Katzberg RW et al. The prevalence of disk displacement in symptomatic and asymptomatic volunteers aged 6 to 25 years. J Orofac Pain 1997;11:37–46.
17. Tallents RH, Katzberg RW, Murphy W, Proskin H. Magnetic resonance imaging findings in asymptomatic volunteers and symptomatic patients with temporomandibular disorders. J Prosthet Dent 1996;75:529–533.
18. Katzberg RW, Westesson PL, Tallents RH, Drake CM. Orthodontics and temporomandibular joint internal derangement. Am J Orthod Dentofacial Orthop 1996; 109:515–520.
19. Kircos LT, Ortendhal DA, Mark A, Arakawa M. Magnetic resonance imaging of the TMJ disk in asymptomatic volunteers. J Oral Maxillofac Surg 1987;45:852–854.
20. Morrow D, Tallents RH, Katzberg RW, Murphy WC, Hart TC. Relationship of other joint problems and anterior disk displacement in symptomatic TMD patients and in asymptomatic volunteers. J Orofac Pain 1996;10:15–20.
21. Nagendak WG, Fernandez FR, Halburn LK, Teitge RA. Magnetic resonance imaging of meniscal degeneration in asymptomatic knees. J Orthop Res 1990;8:311–312.
22. Kornick J, Trefelner ME, McCarty S et al. Meniscal abnormalities in the asymptomatic population in MR imaging. Radiology 1990;177:463–465.
23. Boden SD, Davis DO, Dina TS et al. A prospective and blinded investigation of magnetic resonance imaging of the knee: abnormal findings in asymptomatic subjects. Clin Orthop 1992;282:177–185.
24. Shellock FG, Morris E, Deutsch AL et al. Hematopoietic marrow hyperplasia: high prevalence on MR images of the knee in asymptomatic marathon runners. AJR Am J Roentgenol 1992;158:335–338.
25. Boden SD, McCowin PR, Davis DO et al. Abnormal magnetic resonance scans of the cervical spine in asymptomatic subjects. J Bone Joint Surg 1990;72: 1174–1184.
26. Boden SD, Davis DO, Dina TS, Patronas NJ, Wiesel SW. Abnormal magnetic resonance scans of the lumbar spine in asymptomatic subjects: a prospective investigation. J Bone Joint Surg 1990;72:403–408.
27. Brunner MC, Flower SP, Evancho AM et al. MRI of the athletic knee: findings in asymptomatic professional basketball and collegiate football players. Invest Radiol 1989;24:72–75.
28. Paesani D, Westensson PL, Hatala M, Tallents RH, Kurita K. Prevalence of temporomandibular joint internal derangement in patients with craniomandibular disorders. Am J Orthod Dentofacial Orthop 1992;101: 41–47.
29. Sanchez-Woodworth R, Katzberf R, Tallents RH et al. Radiographic assessment of temporomandibular joint pain and dysfunction in the pediatric age group. J Dent Child 1988;55:278–281.
30. Nebbe B, Major PW. Prevalence of TMJ disk displacement in a pre-orthodontic adolescent sample. Angle Orthod 2000;7:454–463.
31. Katzberg R, Tallents RH, Hayakawa K et al. Internal derangements of the temporomandibular joint: findings in the pediatric age group. Radiology 1985;154:125–127.
32. Aaron L, Buchwald D. A review of the evidence for overlap among unexplained clinical conditions. Ann Intern Med 2001;134:868–881.
33. Aaron LA, Burke MM, Buchwald D. Overlapping conditions among patients with chronic fatigue syndrome, fibromyalgia, and temporomandibular disorder. Arch Intern Med 2000;160:221–227.
34. Dibbets JMH, Van der Weele LT. Prevalence of TMJ symptoms and x-ray findings. Eur J Orthod 1989;11: 31–36.
35. Yemm R. A neurophysiological approach to the pathology and aetiology of temporomandibular dysfunction. J Oral Rehabil 1985;12:343–353.
36. McNeill (ed). Craniomandibular Disorders: Guidelines for Evaluation, Diagnosis and Management. Chicago, IL: Quintessence, 1990.
37. Warren MP, Fried JL. Temporomandibular disorder and hormones in women. Cells Tissues Organs 2001;169: 187–192.
38. LeResche L, Sauders K, Von Korff MR, Barlow W, Dworkin SF. Uses of exogenous hormones and risk of temporomandibular disorder pain. Pain 1997;69:153–160.
39. Macfarlane TV, Blinkhorn AS, Davies RM, Kincey J, Worthington HV. Association between female hormonal factors and oro-facial pain: study in the community. Pain 2002;27:5–10.
40. Pehillips JM, Gatchel RJ, Wesley AL, Ellis E. Clinical implications of sex in acute temporomandibular disorders. J Am Dent Assoc 2001;132:49–57.
41. Le Resche L, Sherman JJ, Huggins K et al. Musculoskeletal orofacial pain and other signs and symptoms of temporomandibular disorders during pregnancy: a prospective study. J Orofac Pain 2005;19:193–201.

42. Bradbury J. Why do men and women feel and react to pain differently? Research suggests men and women may not process pain signals the same way. Lancet 2003;361:2052–2053.
43. Le Resche L. Gender, cultural and environmental aspects of pain. In: Loeser JD (ed). Bonica's Management of Pain. Philadelphia: Lipincott Williams & Wilkins, 2001:191–195.
44. Perrini F, Tallents RH, Katzberg RW et al. Generalized joint laxity and temporomandibular disorders. J Orofac Pain 1997;11:215–221.
45. Fricton JR, Olsen T. Predictors of outcome for treatment of temporomandibular disorders. J Orofac Pain 1996;10:54–65.
46. Feinmann C, Harrison S. Liaison psychiatry and psychology in dentistry. J Psychosom Res 1997;43:467–476.
47. John MT, Miglioretti DL, Le Resch L, Von Korff M, Critchlow CW. Widespread pain as a risk factor for dysfunctional temporomandibular disorders. Pain 2003;102:257–263.
48. Phillips JM, Gatchel RJ, Wesley AL, Ellis R. Clinical implications of sex in acute temporomandibular disorders. J Am Dent Assoc 2001;132:49–57.
49. Costen JB. A syndrome of ear and sinus symptoms dependent upon disturbed function of the temporomandibular joint. Ann Otol Rhinol Laryngol 1934;43:1–15.
50. Kirveskari P, Alanen P, Jamasa T. Association between craniomandibular disorders and occlusal interferences in children. J Prosthet Dent 1992;67:692–696.
51. Pullinger AG, Seligman DA. Overbite and overjet characteristics of refined diagnostic groups of temporomandibular disorder patients. Am J Orthod Dentofacial Orthop 1991;100:401–415.
52. Pullinger AG, Seligman DA, Gornbein JA. A multiple logistic regression analysis of the risk and relative odds of temporomandibular disorders. J Dent Res 1993;72:968–979.
53. Seligman DA, Pullinger AG. Temporomandibular joint derangements and osteoarthritis subgroups differentiated according to active range of mandibular motion. J Craniomandib Disord 1988;2:35–40.
54. Seligman DA, Pullinger AG. The role of functional occlusal relationships in temporomandibular disorders. J Craniomandib Disord 1991;5:265–279.
55. Tallents RH, Macher DJ, Kyrkanides S, Katzberg RW, Moss ME. Prevalence of missing posterior teeth and intraarticular temporomandibular disorders. J Prosthet Dent 2002;87:45–50.
56. Kahn J, Tallents RH, Katzberg RW, Moss ME, Murphy WC. Prevalence of dental occlusal variables and intraarticular temporomandibular disorders: molar relationship, lateral guidance, and nonworking side contacts. J Prosthet Dent 1999;82:410–415.
57. Kahn J, Tallents RH, Katzberg RW, Moss ME, Murphy WC. Association between dental occlusal variables and intraarticular temporomandibular joint disorders: horizontal and vertical overlap. J Prosthet Dent 1998;79:658–662.
58. Roberts CA, Tallents RH, Katzberg WR et al. Comparison of internal derangements of the TMJ with occlusal findings. Oral Surg Oral Med Oral Pathol 1987;63:645–650 .
59. Mohl ND, Ohrbach R. The dilemma of scientific knowledge versus clinical management of temporomandibular disorders. J Prosthet Dent 1992;67:113–120.
60. De Boever JA, Carlsson GE, Klineberg IJ. Need for occlusal therapy and prosthodontic treatment in the management of temporomandibular disorders. I: Occlusal interferences and occlusal adjustment. J Oral Rehabil 2000;27:367–379.
61. Seligman DA, Pullinger AG. Association of occlusal variables among refined TM patient diagnostic groups. J Craniomandib Disord 1989;3:227–236.
62. Clark GT, Tsukiyama Y, Baba K, Watanabe T. Sixty-eight years of experimental occlusal interference studies: What have we learned? J Prosthet Dent 1999;82:704–713.
63. Goldman JR. Soft tissue trauma. In: Kaplan AS, Assael LA (eds). Temporomandibular Disorders: Diagnosis and Treatment. Philadelphia: WB Saunders, 1991:190–223.
64. Dawson P. Evaluation, Diagnosis and Treatment of Occlusal Problems. St Louis, MO: CV Mosby, 1974.
65. Westling L. Temporomandibular joint dysfunction and systemic joint laxity. Swed Dent J 1992;16(Suppl 81):1–79.
66. Kuivaniemi H, Tromp G, Prockop DJ. Mutations in collagen genes: causes of rare and some common diseases in humans. FASEB J 1991;5:2052–2060.
67. Byers PH. Brittle bones, fragile molecules: disorders of collagen gene structure and expression. Trends Genet 1990;6:293–300.
68. Ishimaru J, Handa Y, Kurita K, Goss AN. The effect of occlusal loss on normal and pathological temporomandibular joints: an animal study. J Craniomaxillofac Surg 1994;2:95–102.
69. Kawata T, Niida S, Kawasoko S et al. Morphology of the mandibular condyle in "toothless" osteopetrotic (op/op) mice. J Craniofac Genet Dev Biol 1997;17:198–203.
70. Stegenga B. Osteoarthritis of the temporomandibular joint organ and its relationship to disc displacement. J Orofac Pain 2001;15:193–205.
71. De Bont L, Dijkgraaf L, Stegenga B. Epidemiology and natural progression of articular temporomandibular disorders. Oral Surg Oral Med Oral Pathol Oral Radiol Endod 1997;83:72–76.
72. Lai YC, Shaftel S, Miller JH et al. Intraarticular induction of interleukin-1-beta expression in the adult mouse, with resultant temporomandibular joint pathologic changes, dysfunction, and pain. Arthritis Rheum 2006;54:1184–1197.
73. Sacapino RP. Histopathology associated with malposition of the human temporomandibular joint disc. Oral Surg Oral Med Oral Pathol 1983;55:382–397.
74. Wilkes CH. Internal derangement of the temporomandibular joint: pathologic variations. Arch Otolaryngol Head Neck Surg 1989;115:39–54.

75. Toller PA. Osteoarthrosis of the mandibular condyle. Br Dent J 1973;134:223–231.
76. Rasmussen OC. Description of population and progress of symptoms in a longitudinal study of temporomandibular arthropathy. Scand J Dent Res 1981;89:196–203.
77. De Leeuw R, Boering G, Stegenga B, de Bont LGM. Temporomandibular joint ostheoarthrosis: clinical and radiographic characteristics 30 years after nonsurgical treatment. A preliminary report. Cranio 1996;11:15–24.
78. Pereira FJ, Lundh H, Wetesson PL. Morphologic changes in the temporomandibular joint in different age groups. Oral Surg Oral Med Oral Pathol 1994;78:279–287.
79. Pullinger AG. Natural history and pathologic progression of internal derangement with persistent closed lock. In Sanders B, Murakami K-I, Clark GT (eds). Diagnostic and Surgical Arthroscopy of the Temporomandibular Joint. Philadelphia: WB Saunders, 1989:159–189.
80. Solovieva S, Kouhia S, Leino-Arjas P et al. Interleukin-1 polymorphisms and intervertebral disc degeneration. Epidemiology 2004;15:626–633.
81. Nishimura M, Segami N, Kaneyama K, Suzuki T, Miyamaru M. Relationships between pain-related mediators and both synovitis and joint pain in patients with internal derangements and osteoarthritis of the temporomandibular joint. Oral Surg Oral Med Oral Pathol Oral Radiol Endod 2002;94:328–332.
82. Goldring S, Goldring M. The role of cytokines in cartilage matrix degeneration in osteoarthritis. Clin Orthop Relat Res 2004;427:S27–36.
83. Milam S, Zardeneta G, Schmitz J. Oxidative stress and degenerative temporomandibular joint disease: a proposed hypothesis. J Oral Maxillofac Surg 1998;56:214–223.
84. Bonnet CS, Walsh DA. Osteoarthritis, angiogenesis and inflammation. Rheumatology 2005;44:7–16.
85. Lobbezoo F, Lavigne GJ. Do bruxism and temporomandibular disorders have a cause and effect relationship? J Orofac Pain 1997;11:15–23.
86. Roberts CA, Tallents RH, Katzberg RW et al. Comparison of internal derangements of the TMJ with occlusal findings. Oral Surg Oral Med Oral Pathol Oral Radiol Endod 1987;63:645–650.
87. Thorpy MJ. Parasomnias in International Classification of Sleep Disorders: Diagnostic and Coding Manual. Rochester, MN: American Sleep Disorders Association, 1990:142–185.
88. Lavigne GJ, Kato T, Kolta A, Sessle BJ. Neurobiological mechanisms involved in sleep bruxism. Crit Rev Oral Biol Med 2003;14:30–46.
89. Ohayon MM, Li KK, Guilleminault C. Risk factors for sleep bruxism in the general population. Chest 2001;119:53–61.
90. Lavigne GJ, Montplaisir J. Restless legs syndrome and sleep bruxism: prevalence and association among Canadians. Sleep 1994;17:739–743.
91. Laberge L, Tremblay RE, Vitaro F, Montplaisir J. Development of parasomnias from childhood to early adolescence. Pediatrics 2000;106:67–74.
92. Simonds JF, Parraga H. Prevalence of sleep disorders and sleep behaviors in children and adolescents. J Am Acad Child Adolesc Psychiatry 1982;21:383–388.
93. Fisher BE, Pauley C, McGuire K. Children's Sleep Behavior Scale: normative data on 870 children in grades 1 to 6. Percept Mot Skills 1989;68:227–236.
94. Lavigne GJ, Rompre PH, Monotplaisir JY. Sleep bruxism: validity of clinical research diagnostic criteria in a controlled polysomnographic study. J Dent Res 1996;75:546–552.
95. Kazuyoshi B, Tadasu H, Glenn C, Takashi O. Does tooth wear predict ongoing sleep bruxism in 30-year-old Japanese subjects? Int J Prosthodont 2004;17:39–44.
96. Ekfeldt A, Hugoson A, Bergendal T, Helkimo M. An industrial tooth wear index and an analysis of factors correlated to incisal and occlusal wear in an adult Swedish population. Acta Odontol Scand 1990;48:343.
97. Carlsson G, Johansson A, Lundqvist S. Occlusal wear: a follow-up study of 18 subjects with extensively worn dentitions. Acta Odontol Scand 1985;43:83–90.
98. Johansson A. A cross-cultural study of occlusal tooth wear. Swed Dent J Suppl; 1992;86:1–59.
99. Litonja L, Andreana S, Bush P, Cohen R. Tooth wear: attrition, erosion and abrasion. Quintessence Int 2003;34: 435–446.
100. Kelleher M, Bishop K. Tooth surface loss: an overview. Br Dent J 1999;186:61.
101. Dahl B, Øilo G. Wear of teeth and restorative materials. In: Öwall B, Käyser AF, Carlsson E (eds). Prosthodontics: Principles and Management Strategies. London: Mosby–Wolfe, 1996:187.
102. Kelleher M, Bishoo K. Tooth surface loss: an overview. Br Dent J 1999;186:61–66.
103. Hugoson A, Bergendal T, Ekfeldt A, Helkimo M. Prevalence and severity of incisal and occlusal tooth wear in an adult Swedish population. Acta Odontol Scand 1988;46: 255–265.
104. Seligman DA, Pullinger AG. The degree to which dental attrition in modern society is a function of age and canine contact. J Orofac Pain 1995;9:266–275.
105. Bernhardt O, Gesch D, Splieth C et al. Risk factors for high occlusal wear scores in a population-based sample: results of the study of health in Pomerania. Int J Prosthodont 2004;17:333–339.
106. Russell MD. The distinction between physiological and pathological attrition: a review. J Ir Dent Assoc 1987;33: 23–31.
107. Ramfjord SP, Ash MM . Occlusion, ed 3. Philadelphia: WB Saunders, 1983.
108. Solnit A, Curnutte DC. Occlusal Correlation: Principles and Practice. Chicago: Quintessence, 1988.
109. Greene CS, Laskin DM. Long-term evaluation of conservative treatment for myofascial pain-dysfunction syndrome. J Am Dent Assoc 1974;89:1365–1368.
110. Greene CS, Laskin DM. Long-term evaluation of treatment for myofascial pain-dysfunction syndrome: a comparative analysis. J Am Dent Assoc 1983;107:235–238.

111. Carraro JJ, Caffesse RG. Effect of occlusal splints on TMI symptomatology. J Prosthet Dent 1978;40:563–566.
112. Dohrmann RI, Laskin DM. An evaluation of electromyographic biofeedback in the treatment of myofascial pain-dysfunction syndrome. J Am Dent Assoc 1978;96:656–662.
113. Nel H. Myofascial pain-dysfunction syndrome. J Prosthet Dent 1978;40:438–441.
114. Heloe B, Heiberg AN. A follow-up study of a group of female patients with myofascial pain-dysfunction syndrome. Acta Odontol Scand 1980;38:129–134.
115. Paesani DA, Tallents RH, Murphy WC, Hatala MP, Proskin HM. Evaluation of the reproducibility of rest activity of the anterior temporal and masseter muscles in asymptomatic and symptomatic temporomandibular subjects. J Orofac Pain 1994;8:402–406.
116. Hough T. Ergographic studies in muscle soreness. Am J Physiol 1902;7:76–92.
117. Asmussen E. Observations on experimental muscle soreness. Acta Rheumatol Scand 1956;209:109–116.
118. Abraham WM. Factors in delayed muscle soreness. Med Sci Sports 1977;9:11–20.
119. Howell IN, Chila AG, Ford G, David D, Gates T. An electromyographic study of elbow motion during postexercise muscle soreness. J Appl Physiol 1985;58:1713–1718.
120. Travell JG, Rinzler S, Herman M. Pain and disability of the shoulder and arm: treatment by intramuscular infiltration with procaine hydrochloride. J Am Med Assoc 1942;120:417–422.
121. Lund JP. Pain and the control of muscles. In: Fricton JR, Dubner R (eds). Orofacial Pain and Temporomandibular Disorders. New York: Raven Press, 1995:103–115.
122. Lund JP, Donga R, Widmer CG, Stohler CS. The pain-adaptation model: a discussion of the relationship between chronic musculoskeletal pain and motor activity. Can J Physiol Pharmacol 1991;69:683–694.
123. Turp JC, Kowalski Cl, O'Leary TI, Stohler CS. Pain maps from facial pain patients indicate a broad pain geography. J Dent Res 1998;77:1465–1472.
124. Camparis CM, Siqueira JTT. Sleep bruxism: clinical aspects and characteristics in patients with and without chronic orofacial pain. Oral Surg Oral Med Oral Pathol Oral Radiol Endod 2006;101:188–193.
125. Lavigne GJ, Rompre PH, Montplaisir JY, Lobbezoo F. Motor activity in sleep bruxism with concomitant jaw muscle pain. Eur J Oral Sci 1997;105:92–95.
126. Kobs G, Bernhardt O, Kocher T, Meyer G. Oral parafunctions and positive clinical examination findings. Stomatologija 2005;7:81–83.
127. Kampe T, Tagdae T, Bader G, Edman G, Karlsson S. Reported symptoms and clinical findings in a group of subjects with longstanding bruxism behaviour. J Oral Rehabil 1997;24:581–587.
128. Van Selms M, Lobbezoo F, Wicks DJ, Hamburger HL, Naeije M. Craniomandibular pain, oral parafunctions, and psychological stress in a longitudinal case study. J Oral Rehabil 2004;31:738–745.
129. Ahlberg K, Ahlberg J, Könönen M et al. Perceived orofacial pain and its associations with reported bruxism and insomnia symptoms in media personnel with or without irregular shift work. Acta Odontol Scand 2005;63:213–217.
130. van der Meulen M, Lobbezoo F, Aartman I, Naeije M. Self-reported oral parafunctions and pain intensity in temporomandibular disorder patients. J Orofac Pain 2006;20:31–35.
131. Watanabe T, Ichikawa K, Clark G. Bruxism levels and daily behaviors: three weeks of measurement and correlation. J Orofac Pain 2003;17:65–73.
132. Baba K, Glenn C, Watanabe T, Ohyama T. Bruxism force detection by a piezoelectric film-based recording device in sleeping humans. J Orofac Pain 1993;7:378–385.
133. Ikeda T, Nishigawa K, Kondo K, Takeuchi H, Clark GT. Criteria for the detection of sleep-associated bruxism in humans. J Orofac Pain 1996;10:270.
134. Gallo LM, Salis Gross SS, Palla S. Nocturnal masseter EMG activity of healthy subjects in a natural environment. J Dent Res 1999;78:1436.
135. Lavigne GJ, Guitard F, Rompre PH, Montplaisir JY. Variability in sleep bruxism activity over time. J Sleep Res 2001;103:237.
136. Stegenga B, DeBont LGM, Boering G: Osteoarthrosis as the cause of craniomandibular pain and dysfunction. J Oral Maxillofac Surg 1989;47:249.
137. Stegenga B, DeBont LGM, Boering G et al. Tissue responses to degenerative changes in the temporomandibular joint: a review. J Oral Maxillofac Surg 1991;48:1079.
138. DeBont LGM, Stegenga B. Pathology of temporomandibular joint internal derangement and osteoarthrosis. Int J Oral Maxillofac Surg 1993;22:71–74.
139. Milam SB, Schmitz JP. Molecular biology of temporomandibular joint disorders: proposed mechanisms of disease. J Oral Maxillofac Surg 1995;53:1448.
140. Milam SB, Zardeneta G, Schmitz JP. Oxidative stress and degenerative temporomandibular joint disease: a proposed hypothesis. J Oral Maxillofac Surg 1998;56:214.
141. Christensen LV. Facial pain and internal pressure of masseter muscle in experimental bruxism in man. Arch Oral Biol 1971;16:1021–1031.
142. Christensen LW. Jaw muscle fatigue and pains induced by experimental tooth clenching: a review. J Oral Rehabil 1981;8:27–36.
143. Clark GT, Jow RW, Lee J. Jaw pain and stiffness levels after repeated maximum voluntary clenching. J Dent Res 1989;68:69–71.
144. Sessle BJ. The neural basis of temporomandibular joint and masticatory muscle pain. J Orofac Pain 1999;13:238–245.
145. Lavigne G, Woda A, Truelove E et al. Mechanisms associated with unusual orofacial pain. J Orofac Pain 2005;19:9–21.
146. Dao TT, Lund JP, Lavigne GJ. Comparison of pain and quality of life in bruxers and patients with myofascial pain of the masticatory muscles. J Orofac Pain 1994;8:350–356.

Chapter 17

# Pain and Bruxism

*Peter Svensson, Faramarz Jadidi, Taro Arima, and Lene Baad-Hansen*

## Introduction

Pain is commonly believed to be intimately linked to bruxism as a consequence of jaw muscle activity. However, recent insights into pain and bruxism have cautioned against establishing too simple a causal relationship. One of the problems we need to be aware of is that we often think in terms of linear relationships. For example, if a person has no or little activity in the jaw muscles this will cause no pain; if a person has moderate levels of activity this will lead to some pain; and if a person has very high levels of activity this will cause strong pain. Another problem is that the neurobiologic mechanism of pain related to bruxism is poorly understood. This chapter will review the current knowledge on pain mechanisms and critically discuss the potential relationships with bruxism.

## Overview of Pain Mechanisms

Pain has been defined as "an unpleasant and emotional experience associated with actual or potential tissue damage, or described in terms of such damage".[1] This definition captures the complexity of pain as being more than a simple sensation due to activation of specific pathways – which means that pain is not the same as nociception. This broad view on pain encompasses situations with overt tissue damage leading to activity in the nociceptive pathways but not necessarily reflected in comparable pain reports – if, for example, the subject is directing his or her attention to another event. Conversely, subjects without any visible signs of tissue damage or detectable activity in the nociceptive system may still report excruciating levels of pain. It is fair to state that there is no simple one-to-one relationship between potential "painful" stimuli and the reports of pain. During the last decades, significant progress has been made in our understanding of the neurobiologic mechanisms underlying pain and a classification system

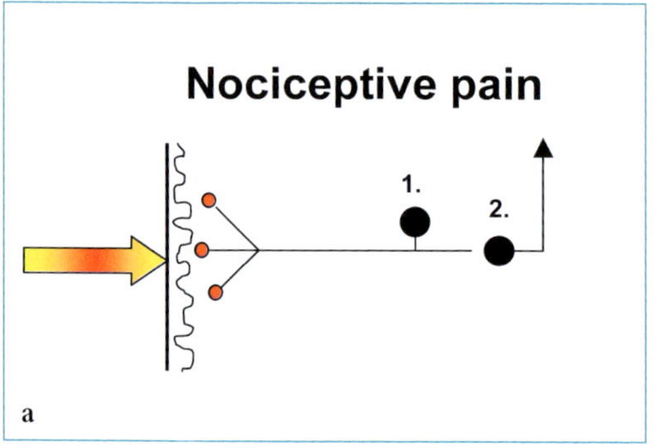


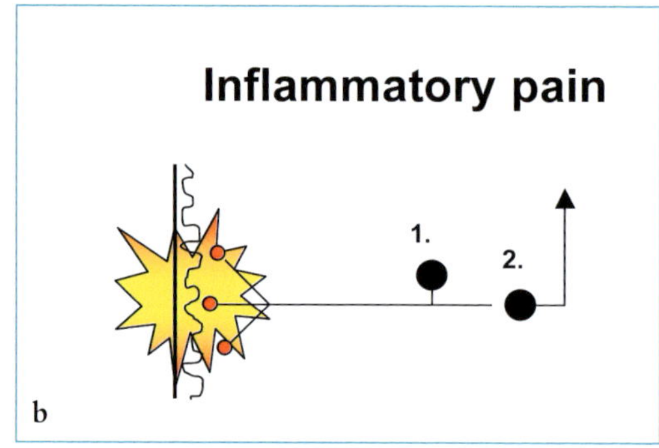


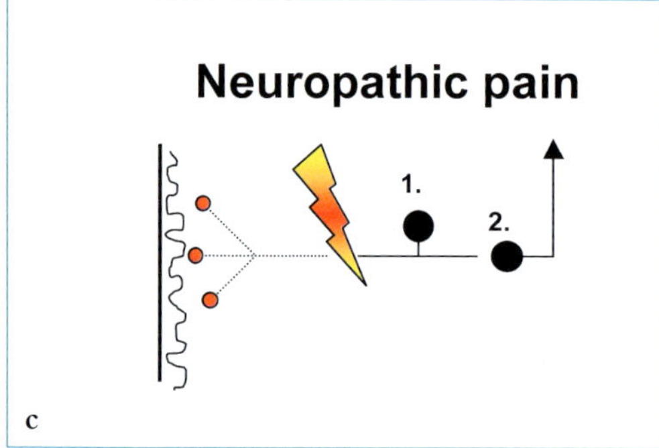


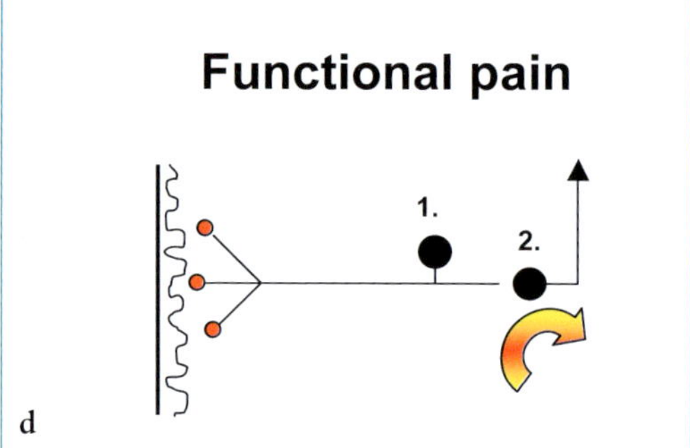


Fig 17-1 Schematic presentation of different types of pain. The first-order neuron (1) is located in the trigeminal ganglion and the primary afferent nerve fiber innervates, for example, the skin. **(a)** On the peripheral endings, many different ion channels and receptors are located (red circles) which can be activated by high-intensity and potentially tissue-damaging stimuli (arrow). **(b)** In conditions with inflammatory pain, the peripheral tissue is damaged and inflammatory cells (macrophages, mast cells, neutrophils, granulocytes) are accumulated and contribute to changes in the local environment. **(c)** Neuropathic pain is characterized by lesions or diseases affecting the somatosensory nerve system, for example cutting a peripheral nerve fiber (flash). **(d)** In functional pain conditions, the peripheral tissues look normal but apparently there is an increased amplification in the second-order neurons. (Modified from Woolf.[2])

based on mechanisms has been proposed.[2] The underlying mechanisms of pain are important to know not only for classification purposes but also for diagnostic and management reasons. The classification has four main categories (Fig 17-1) which will be described here with a particular reference to bruxism.

Transient or nociceptive pain may be the easiest type of pain to understand because we have all experienced this during daily life; for example, sharp or hot objects can produce a painful experience (see Fig 17-1a). Nevertheless, recent advances in molecular biology have shown the complex nature of even "simple" processing of pain.[3,4] The nociceptor is the basic receptor on primary afferent nerve fibers innervating the orofacial tissues. It is not an encapsulated ending like the mechanoreceptors (e.g., Pacinian corpuscules) but a free nerve ending with a multitude of transducing receptors and ion channels. The structure and function of many of these receptors and ion channels have been identified on the peripheral terminals – for example, acid-sensing ion channels (ASIC), a family of transient receptor potential receptors (TRPV1-8), P2X3 receptors, and many more.[5] These receptors are unique in the sense that they detect and respond to specific high-intensity stimuli (thermal heat, cold, mechanical, and chemical stimuli), which possibly could lead to tissue damage. Nociceptive pain can therefore be seen as a warning system and will contribute to survival by protecting the organism from injury.[2] In fact, patients with rare congenital diseases can be completely insensitive to pain but are at serious risk of suffering multiple life-threatening injuries and illnesses because the "warning system" is dysfunctional.

Nevertheless, in normal conditions, functional "awake" nociceptors are located in virtually all orofacial tissues including the teeth, periodontal ligament, skin, mucosa, muscle, joint, ligaments, etc.[6] From a pure neuroanatomic point of view, overloading of the jaw muscles or temporomandibular joints (TMJs) during bruxism could therefore lead to activation of nociceptors and pain. To what extent this may occur in experimental conditions mimicking bruxism will be discussed later in this chapter.

It is also common knowledge that overt tissue damage or injury (trauma, surgery) can be associated with pain[7] (see Fig 17-1b). In most cases this can be viewed as part of an inflammation process with (1) dolor (pain), (2) tumor (swelling), (3) rubor (redness), (4) calor (heat sensation), and (5) *functio laesae* (loss of function). Also for inflammatory pain, significant progress has been made in terms of understanding the neurobiologic changes in the nociceptive system in such conditions. A key point is that the local environment around the nociceptor is radically changed by a complex series of events involving breakdown of the tissue, migration of immune-competent cells, changes in vascular permeability, and activation of the autonomic system. Thus the "inflammatory soup" around the nociceptor will contain neurotrophins, neuroactive substances from the vessels, immune cell products, neuropeptides from the nerve fibers, and products of the tissue injury.[8] One important aspect is that this environmental change can trigger the nociceptor to become spontaneously active without being activated by a peripheral stimulus leading to spontaneous pain. Another important aspect is the phenomenon termed "sensitization", where the threshold for activation of the nociceptor is reduced and the responses are longer and stronger.[4] Furthermore, so-called "silent nociceptors" can be awakened and further contribute to pain. There is also good evidence that functional shifts occur in the number and activity of receptors and ion channels on the nociceptor. For example, receptors for nerve growth factor (NGF), bradykinin (BK), and prostaglandins (PGE) will be activated and lead to increased excitability of the cell membrane. It is also crucial to realize that second-order neurons in the trigeminal sensory nucleus complex react to the increased trafficking of action potentials from the nociceptor and, indeed, a sensitization of the neurons in the central nervous system can occur.[6] A cascade of biologic responses will take place in the second-order neuron involving phosphorylation of *N*-methyl-D-aspartate (NMDA) receptors and activation of neurokinin and neurotrophic receptors.[9] Our understanding of the intracellular pathways is fairly advanced and also includes alterations in gene expression of neurotransmitters and neuromodulators. Although the phenomenon of peripheral and central sensitization can develop within a time frame of minutes, these processes are, luckily, normally fully reversible in conditions with inflammatory types of pain. Inflammation can, of course, occur also in jaw muscles (myositis) and the TMJ (synovitis, capsulitis), and the question as to what extent clinical or biologic markers of inflammation have been identified in bruxism will be discussed later in this chapter.

Nervous system injury pain (neuropathic pain) can occur if the peripheral nerve fibers are damaged[2] (see Fig 17-1c), for example due to surgery (third molar surgery, orthognathic surgery on the maxilla and mandible, insertion of implants, etc.)

or due to diseases such as post-herpetic neuralgia or diabetic neuropathy. Neuropathic pain may also develop following injuries to the central somatosensory system, examples being stroke, multiple sclerosis, and spinal cord injuries. Neuropathic pain is defined as pain arising as a direct consequence of a lesion or disease affecting the somatosensory system.[10] The consequences of such lesions are spontaneous pain and hypersensitivity to painful stimuli. Thus, the primary afferent nerve fiber can start spontaneous discharges due to ectopic neural activity near the peripheral nerve lesion and there can be phenotypic changes and alterations in the expression and distribution of ion channels, which contribute to an increase in the excitability of the cell membrane.[9]

It is a major breakthrough to have discovered that expression of genes will change with up- or down-regulation of receptors, neurotransmitters, and neuromodulators involved in nociceptive processing. The term "neuroplasticity" is often used to describe these dynamic changes in the nociceptive system. Thus, it is easy to understand that sensitized nerve fibers play an important role in neuropathic pain. Unfortunately, the neurobiologic mechanisms underlying this dysfunctional neuroplasticity appear to be irreversible and resistant to current pharmacologic therapy. It should also be mentioned that the central nervous system, of course, has a significant role in neuropathic pain conditions. For example, one of the many responses at the second-order neuron is the loss of normal inhibitory mechanisms mediated by gamma-aminobutyric acid (GABA) and glycine.[9] Furthermore, there is, indeed, evidence that 1 week after nerve injury there are signs of apoptosis in dorsal horn neurons and there is therefore strong interest to develop therapies that prevent activation of apoptotic pathways to avoid disturbances in the delicate balance between inhibitory and excitatory pathways. The view that pain is not always just a "symptom" of a disease but may become a disease in its own right is evolving and it has been suggested that persistent types of pain are comparable to other neurodegenerative diseases such as Parkinson's or Alzheimer's disease.

A key message regarding neuropathic pain is that the underlying neurobiologic events cannot be detected by normal clinical inspection or radiology of the painful region; but even in the absence of visible signs of structural damage, the somatosensory system may have undergone pathologic changes that can explain many of the peculiar manifestations of neuropathic pain.[10] For example, gentle brushing or touching of the painful region can often elicit strong pain that lasts longer than the stimulus – a situation referred to as mechanical allodynia.[2] In relation to bruxism, it seems obvious that grinding or clenching the teeth cannot cause a complete injury (transsection) to nerves; but the intriguing question as to whether compression or stretching of the nerve fibers in the jaw muscles during bruxism can lead to demyelination or Wallerian degeneration (i.e., neurapraxia, axonotmesis, neurotmesis) will be discussed later in this chapter.

Finally, the concept of functional pain is evolving. From a clinical perspective there appears to be nothing wrong in the peripheral tissues, but the patients often complain about widespread pain in multiple parts and organs in the body (see Fig 17-1d). It is believed that for some unknown reasons there is an abnormal amplification and processing of peripheral stimuli in the central parts of the somatosensory system.[2] Examples of such disorders are fibromyalgia, irritable bowel syndrome, and probably also tension-type headaches and myofascial temporomandibular disorder (TMD) pain conditions. In contrast to inflammatory and neuropathic types of pain where there is a local hypersensitivity to painful stimuli, in the functional types of pain this hypersensitivity appears to be widespread and generalized. It is therefore believed that a comprehensive analysis of pain in addition to a careful elucidation of the many psychosocial aspects also needs to comprise a survey of the somatosensory function in the painful as well as pain-free parts of the body.[10] Simple tests of somatosensory function can, in fact, easily be done in the dental office whereas more elaborate tests such as quantitative sensory tests (QSTs) normally are available only at university clinics.[8] It is not well understood whether pain associated with bruxism could be considered a functional type of pain, although numerous studies discussed later in this chapter have reported associations between being stressed or tense and bruxism.

## Sex-related Differences in Pain Experience

Epidemiology has helped to identify a prominent feature of craniofacial pain – many more women than men complain about pain. This is true for TMD pain, tension-type headaches, migraine, burning mouth syndrome, and many other pain conditions. There can be many reasons for such differences in the way women and men experience and report pain, including pain from the craniofacial region. For example, some of these differences may be related to the multidimensional and complex nature of pain where gender expectations, societal influence on pain behavior, role models, and many other factors come into play. However, a series of recent studies have shown that there can be neurobiologic differences in the transmission and processing of nociceptive inputs.[11]

Neurophysiologic studies in laboratory animals have provided strong evidence that primary afferent nerve fibers in female rats are much more sensitive to nociceptive inputs from the jaw muscles and TMJ. Thus, a greater afferent barrage can be evoked by a painful stimulus applied to the masseter muscle or TMJ. The basis for this difference appears to be differences in the functional properties of the nerve fibers, for example by the expression of NMDA-receptor subtypes. Such studies in animals cannot, of course, be extrapolated directly to the clinical situation; but parallel studies in humans have, indeed, shown higher pain scores and greater pain areas in women than in men.[11]

Several studies have demonstrated also that the responsiveness of the second-order neurons in the trigeminal sensory nucleus complex following painful stimulation of the craniofacial region is significantly greater in females than in males. Also in terms of responsiveness to analgesics such as opioids, there is now good evidence for sex-related differences at both the peripheral and central levels in the nociceptive pathways.[11]

Finally, brain imaging techniques have been used to demonstrate that activation of endogenous pain inhibitory pathways following painful stimulation of jaw muscles differs between men and women, with women having much less inhibition.[12] It has also been shown that low-estradiol conditions are associated with increased pain sensitivity owing to a reduction in endogenous opioid receptor system function. This finding further substantiates the notion of sex-related differences in nociceptive processing of painful inputs from the jaw muscles. Several other studies are in accordance with this suggestion based on psychophysical examinations of the diffuse noxious inhibitory control phenomena.[13]

It is also noteworthy that there is a distinct age span where women of reproductive age are at higher risk of developing TMD pain, and sex hormones such as estradiol appear to be implicated in the pathophysiology of TMD.[14]

Overall, it seems that men and women are likely to have a number of significant functional differences in their nociceptive pathways, which therefore could contribute to the different expressions of pain often encountered in the dental office. One striking point, however, is that bruxism does not appear to follow the same epidemiologic trends; that is, women of reproductive age are not reported to have a higher prevalence of bruxism. In fact there appears to be no difference between men and women in terms of prevalence of bruxism,[15] and such discrepancies need to be considered when the relationship between pain and bruxism is examined.

## Pain Genetics

One of the most intriguing discoveries in the field of pain is the association between certain types of genes and the expression of pain.[16] It is common knowledge from the dental office that some patients are more susceptible to stimulation of the orofacial region; these patients may report very high levels of pain even in the absence of a strong nociceptive input via the primary afferent nerve fibers. And vice versa, there are patients who seem to be much more "pain resistant". Notwithstanding the significance of the many psychosocial aspects of pain, several genetic markers of "pain sensitive" and "pain resistant" patients have currently been identified. One of these markers is based on polymorphism of the catechol-O-methyl-transferase (COMT) gene. COMT is an enzyme that metabolizes catecholamines and is critically involved in pain perception, cognitive function, and affective mood with strong impacts on the efficacy of the endogenous pain modulatory systems.[17] Also, polymorphisms of the adrenergic-receptor-beta-2 gene have been linked with differences in pain sensitivity, and it is very likely that there are many more gene candidates that may contribute to individual differences in the expression of pain.[18] The significance of this new knowledge is that it provides a key to open up some of the "black boxes" in the understanding of individual pain experiences.

A genetic basis for bruxism is currently being investigated;[15] but bruxism, like pain, is not likely to be explained by a single gene expression and there can be multiple factors that may complicate a relationship, for example the influence of stress and anxiety. However, it is of interest to note that bruxism to some degree may also be linked to the release of catecholamines which appears important at least for the expression of pain. Further studies will be needed to address these questions and before the clinical relevance can be established.

In summary, there is an extensive body of knowledge about basic pain mechanisms and the challenge will be to link this information to bruxism.

## Experimental Bruxism and Craniofacial Pain

It is very straightforward to examine the relationship between bruxism and craniofacial pain by asking healthy subjects to perform "bruxism-like" activities in controlled laboratory settings.[19] The beauty of such experimental bruxism models is that a clear cause–effect relationship can be assumed under these specific conditions; but there are obviously also a number of limitations to extrapolating findings from an acute (minutes or hours) and highly controlled and standardized study to repeated (days, weeks, months, or even years) and more complex orofacial motor behaviors. Two different bruxism models have typically been used, one based on sustained concentric contraction, and the other based on repeated eccentric contractions.

### *Concentric Contraction Models*

Concentric dynamic and isometric contractions can, with sufficient loading and insufficient rest, lead to pain in leg and arm muscles.[20] This type of pain is thought to share the same pathophysiologic mechanisms as ischemic pain and can be viewed as a nociceptive or transient type of pain. Ischemia alone, however, is not sufficient to produce muscle pain, except when combined with contractions, strong pain can develop. Accumulation of metabolites, such as lactate, potassium, or the lack of oxidation of metabolic products, in addition to mechanical determinants such as the number of contractions, duration, and force have been shown to influence the development of muscle pain. Furthermore, hypoxia and the release of BK, PGE2, and CGRP, in association with a reduced pH, can cause sensitization of muscle nociceptors, leading to pain evoked by mechanical stimulation during contractions. This probably adds an inflammatory component to this kind of exercise-induced muscle pain.

In the craniofacial region, many studies have tried to establish an experimental model to induce jaw muscle pain. A combination of dynamic concentric contractions (chewing) and ischemic block of the superficial temporal artery in healthy subjects causes a continuously increasing, bilateral dull frontal headache with significantly more pain and significantly shorter onset of pain than chewing without an ischemic block. In this "headache" model, ischemia is achieved with the use of scalp sphygmomanometers wrapped around the head, which not only reduce blood circulation but may also cause activity in cutaneous and deep mechanoreceptors. The model has never been extensively used but may have some merits to further examine the question about headache, TMD pain, and repetitive masticatory muscle activity.

Sustained or repeated static tooth-clenching procedures have long been known and used to evoke a fairly intense pain with a rapid onset (for a review, see Svensson et al[19]). The pain nevertheless quickly disappears (transient pain), and most studies have failed to show any significant pain in the jaw muscles on the days following the exercise. Our own contributions to the literature have shown that even with 5 days of repeated submaximal tooth clenching, it is difficult to elicit longer-lasting muscle pain or soreness in healthy women.[21] Tooth clenching at 10% of the maximal voluntary bite force level for up to 60 minutes does not evoke much pain, but rather a pronounced fatigue sensation in the jaw muscles.Studies with sustained submaximal contraction of the frontalis muscles have failed to produce significant levels of headache.

Thus, it can be concluded that pain in the jaw muscles cannot be readily induced in healthy subjects using concentric contraction models. In fact, jaw muscles seem to be very resistant against development of fatigue and pain. In experimental studies, the contraction levels and duration have generally been in excess of what is found in clinical studies on bruxism, which seems to suggest that simple concentric contraction of muscles may be inadequate to explain the entire pathophysiology of myofascial TMD pain.

### *Eccentric Contraction Models*

In contrast to the immediate and rather short-lasting muscle pain evoked by concentric contractions, eccentric contractions which cause a lengthening of the muscle fibers despite an attempt to contract the muscle are more effective in inducing a delayed onset of muscle pain (DOMS) or soreness in healthy subjects.[22] One classical example is downhill walking where the contracting quadriceps muscle controls the rate of knee flexion against the force of gravity and in the process the muscle undergoes an eccentric contraction during each step. Under such circumstances there is usually no or only little pain immediately after the exercise, but significant levels of pain, soreness, and stiffness can develop in the leg or arm muscles on the following day and persist for up to 4–5 days after eccentric exercise. This condition is usually referred to as DOMS or post-exercise muscle soreness (PEMS), and it has been suggested that this type of pain is particularly related to bruxism.[23] The assumption is that unaccustomed eccentric exercise leads to localized areas of damage within the muscle which will be associated with inflammatory changes.[22] This inflammation can trigger some of the neurobiologic mechanisms as described above with peripheral sensitization of the primary afferent nerve fibers.

Some of the clinical characteristics of DOMS are quite different from other myofascial pain conditions. For example, there is no spontaneous pain but only pain on movement of the exercised limb or body part. Stretch and muscle contractions will increase the pain. An intriguing finding is that vibratory stimuli may increase the pain and soreness in DOMS rather than relieve it.[24]

The suggestion has been made that large-diameter muscle afferents could be involved in DOMS and that similar mechanisms such as secondary hyperalgesia and allodynia could be features in DOMS, a phenomenon coined "proprioceptive allodynia". The injuries to the muscle may include both contractile and cytoskeletal components of the myofibrils. Thus, the mechanisms underlying this kind of muscle pain are probably related to muscle injuries at the ultrastructural level or damage to the connective tissue. Histologic studies have, indeed, demonstrated disorganization of myofilaments and extensive disruption of muscle structures localized particularly in the regions of the Z-discs. Two possible initial events are discussed as being responsible for the subsequent damage.[22] One possibility is damage to the excitation–contraction coupling system, and the second is disruption at the level of the sarcomeres; most evidence favors the latter suggestion.

It is important to note that the magnitude of tissue damage induced by eccentric exercise does not correlate well with perceived intensity of DOMS, again substantiating the claim that there is no one-to-one relationship between tissue injury and pain.

Another typical feature of DOMS in limb muscles is the "training" effect: 1 week after the first eccentric exercise, a second exercise will cause much less damage and symptoms such as pain and soreness. It has been proposed that this adaptation process is based on an increase in sarcomere numbers in the muscle fibers that leads to a shift in the muscle's optimum length for active tension. A careful and controlled use of eccentric exercises has been suggested to be applied in the clinic as training or protection of muscles against major injuries. The concept of an exercise-induced pain followed by an exercise-mediated adaptation or training effect could possibly explain some of the characteristics observed in relation to bruxers and craniofacial pain: a single bout of bruxism would be able to trigger painful symptoms, but repeated "exercises" would tend to diminish the symptoms. The frequency and pattern of jaw muscle activity (temporal characteristics) could therefore be important determinants for the relationship between bruxism and craniofacial pain.

Several questions, however, need to be considered at this stage. For example, DOMS has in general been shown to be associated with lower pain scores in women than in men, which also has been shown for exercise-induced pain in jaw muscles. This is in contrast to the majority of both experimental and clinical studies demonstrating that women are more sensitive to painful stimulation of the muscles and outnumber men in the pain clinics.

Another concern is related to our current understanding of bruxism which includes both sleep bruxism and awake bruxism. It is not known at present whether the consequences of sleep bruxism are different from the consequences of awake bruxism. Probably there are differences in terms of type, duration, intensity, and frequency of jaw muscle contractions.

Although many experimental studies have attempted to apply different eccentric contractions of the jaw muscles, no studies so far have replicated all the features from DOMS in limb muscles. Forced lengthening of tetanic stimulated jaw muscles in mice has shown decreased contractile tension and elevated levels of plasma creatine kinase as indices of muscle injury. Experimental tooth grinding for 30 minutes, presumably also involving eccentric contractions, was originally reported to cause significant levels of jaw muscle pain lasting for several days in nine healthy subjects.[19] However, no exact information on pain intensity was provided for the days following tooth grinding. We have demonstrated that 45 minutes of strong tooth grinding activity at 50% maximum voluntary contraction (MVC) in 12 healthy subjects caused only low levels of pain and soreness on the following 3 days.[25] Thus, even with strong grinding activity, where part of the movement may involve eccentric contractions of the jaw muscles, there is little pain left the day after the exercise.[25]

These results from exercise-induced activation of human muscle nociceptors show that excessive and strong contractions of the jaw muscles can cause acute (transient) pain in the craniofacial region, but the pain is usually of rather short duration. There is no experimental evidence that a self-perpetuating, vicious cycle can be initiated by jaw muscle hyperactivity, leading to pain that again should lead to more jaw muscle hyperactivity.[26,27] So far the information from human experimental bruxism models does not indicate that prolonged symptoms with soreness, pain, and decrease in force can be triggered even by high-intensity contractions; but the critical caveat is the importance of repetition and frequency where experimental studies are short-lasting (minutes or hours) but where the clinical conditions may involve muscle contractions and work that are repeated over time (days, weeks months, or years). Therefore, it is necessary to consider clinical studies on bruxism and pain.

## Clinical Studies of Bruxism and Craniofacial Pain

There is a comprehensive clinical literature on the associations between craniofacial pain complaints and bruxism (for a review, see Svensson et al[19]). For example, one study has reported that self-reported bruxism is associated with an odds ratio of 4.8 for myofascial TMD pain and 1.2 for TMJ arthralgia. A remarkable 20-year follow-up study reported that bruxism was associated with TMD signs or symptoms assessed according to the Helkimo index.[28] Moreover, patients with long-standing sleep bruxism appear to be more likely to have craniofacial pain complaints than to have no pain problems. A study based on questionnaires demonstrated that craniofacial pain was significantly, and positively, associated with reports of frequent bruxism. In large-scale studies in 50- and 60-year-old subjects in Sweden, the strongest risk indicator for craniofacial pain and dysfunction was self-reported bruxism. Clenching habits during the day also appears to be associated with craniofacial pain. Recently, it has been shown that myofascial TMD pain patients report more frequent tooth contacts than control subjects and have higher levels of stress and tension.[29] From these studies, the case could seem clear: there is a strong relationship between bruxism and craniofacial pain.

However, many of the clinical studies have demonstrated significant associations and odds ratios, but these measures are not direct evidence of true cause–effect relationships between bruxism and craniofacial pain.[30] First, odds ratios indicate only associations and not necessarily the directions of the relationships. Thus, craniofacial pain could trigger bruxism although the experimental studies cited above do not seem to support this suggestion.[27] Bruxism and craniofacial pain could also be due to other pathologic mechanisms and simply co-vary. Second, most studies have used self-reported measures of bruxism which could be influenced by the patients' perception of their oral habits and being "tense" confounded by statements from clinicians. This point addresses our current abilities to accurately and reliably diagnose bruxism.

A study related to patients with fibromyalgia examined the relationships between physiologic muscle activity measured by electromyography (EMG) and the patients' own perception of being tense as well as muscle tension traits; surprisingly there were no correlations between these measures.[31] In contrast, the perception of being tense correlated with aspects of anxiety proneness, indicating that not all "tense" patients have increased EMG activity. We therefore have to be very careful because subject-based reports of grinding or clenching the teeth may not necessarily correspond to the physiologic measures in terms of EMG and tooth contacts.

A further word of caution needs to be said about a "common sense" relationship between muscle activity and pain. As clinicians we often think in linear terms: if patients grind or brux their teeth a little bit, this may not be associated with pain; if the patients have more muscle activity this may exceed a "threshold" and pain will emerge; and if the patients have a lot of muscle activity we expect a lot of pain (Fig 17-2). However, this assumption has never been thoroughly tested. There could be many other and maybe more complex relationships as illustrated in Figure 17-2. It also needs to be recognized that significant individual differences may influence the relationship between muscle activity and pain. Figure 17-3 shows data supporting the statement that muscle activity is not linearly related to pain.

The concept of a straightforward linear relationship between bruxism and craniofacial pain is furthermore challenged by several reports where patients with sleep bruxism, but without painful symptoms, have been found to have higher EMG activity than sleep bruxers with pain.[32,33] A very recent study showed that sleep bruxers with low frequencies of EMG activity were more at risk of reporting craniofacial pain.[34] It has also been reported that the amount of self-reported bruxism is not associated with more severe muscle pain, but remarkably is associated with less pain in the TMJ on palpation. Raphael and colleagues have pointed out that severity of bruxism may not be a good predictor of myofascial TMD pain, and they have recently strengthened this concern by the finding that tooth wear as a "cumulative" proxy of bruxism is negatively associated with measures of muscle sensitivity.[35,36] In fact all these studies support the general concept of the pain-adaptation model where pain inhibits muscle activity during voluntary movements as well as during sleep.[26,27]

In summary, the clinical literature has frequently linked bruxism and craniofacial pain and implied a linear cause–effect relationship with the possibility of establishing a threshold or cut-off point. However, several studies appear to challenge bruxism as a single, major risk factor for craniofacial pain. One important criticism is that none of the studies cited have attempted to further classify pain according to the underlying neurobiologic mechanisms. From the experimental bruxism studies in humans, it seems most likely that bruxism is associated with either transient or inflammatory types of pain. There is however, an intriguing possibility which will be discussed below.

Muscles, tendons, and bones will generally adapt to repetitive loading by appropriate remodeling. Highly repetitious low forces are, however, sufficient to trigger local responses in musculoskeletal tissues. The exact role of local changes in musculoskeletal tissues in generating pain in so-called repetitive strain injury (RSI) is far from being established,[37] but is of great interest and importance in, for example, occupational health and sports physiology. Local tissue level changes involving components of inflammation have typically not been considered the major source of continuing pain as seen in RSI because there are no visible clinical signs of inflammation. The exciting view has been developed that parallel changes may occur in peripheral nerves. For example, the median nerve has been shown to swell by 10% following only 5 minutes of hand activity. Reduced nerve movements due to low-grade and subclinical inflammation in the environment around the nerve could therefore be one possibility. Furthermore, full extension of the upper limbs causes the median nerve path to increase by 3 cm or more (corresponding to about 8–18%), which may be sufficient to reduce nerve blood flow and slow down nerve conduction. So far there is no direct evidence to support such mechanisms in relation to bruxism, although the thickness of the masseter muscle as assessed by ultrasonography is temporarily increased by 14% after static contractions at 15% of maximum effort until endurance in healthy subjects. Exercise-evoked swelling of the medial and lateral pterygoid

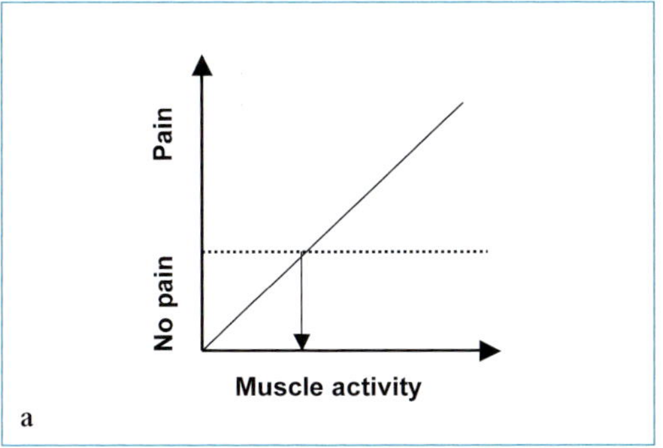


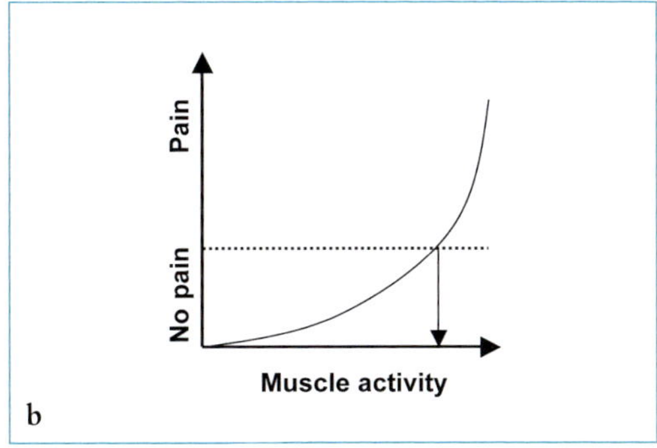


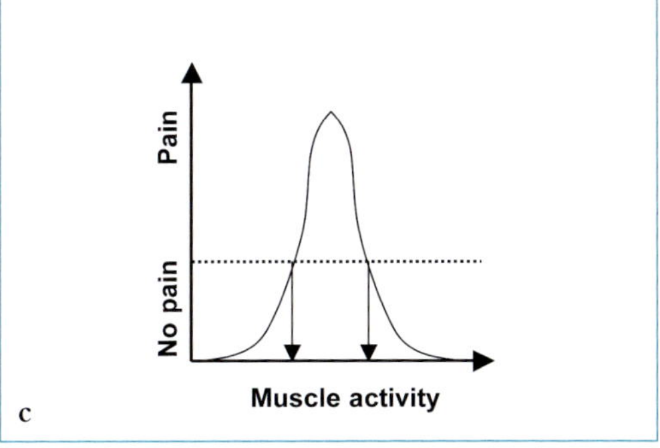


Fig 17-2 Examples of theoretical relationships between muscle activity and pain. **(a)** A common way to think about muscle activity and pain, where there is a linear relationship. Once the muscle activity exceeds a certain level (dashed line) symptoms will start to appear. **(b and c)** There can be other relationships, even some quite unexpected.

muscles could therefore theoretically lead to compression of the mandibular nerve. There is good evidence that the lateral pterygoid muscle is involved in force production during horizontal jaw movements, for example during protrusive or side-to-side movements in the presence of jaw-closing muscle activity. However, there is as yet no evidence to link the lateral pterygoid muscle specifically to bruxism-induced muscle pain, and there are significant concerns about the reliability of manual palpation of this muscle. Nevertheless, it remains a possibility that neuropathic pain mechanisms could contribute to bruxism-related craniofacial pain; but further studies will be needed to reject or substantiate this hypothesis.

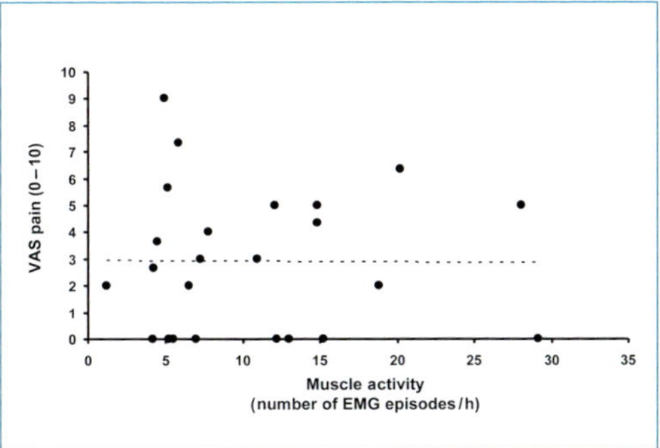


Fig 17-3 Illustration of relationship between muscle activity expressed as number of EMG episodes per hour of sleep in 24 subjects and their clinical pain level assessed on a 0–10 visual analog scale (VAS). No linear relationships can be established in this sample. Data are from Jadidi et al[47] and Baad-Hansen et al.[44]

In summary, experimental bruxism studies of tooth clenching or tooth grinding in healthy human subjects have consistently shown low grades of painful symptoms which quickly resolve, and no studies have so far been able to match the characteristics of DOMS in limb muscles. There may nevertheless still be merit in trying to understand the neurobiology and physiology of exercised jaw muscles; but it seems unlikely that transient or tissue injury-based pain alone can explain the clinical characteristics and manifestations of persistent craniofacial pain. Changes in central nociceptive mechanisms and endogenous pain control systems undoubtedly are also involved.

## Intervention Studies of Bruxism

Finally, we will examine the relationship between bruxism and craniofacial pain by looking at studies that have attempted to modify bruxism. So the question is whether reduction in loading and strain on the jaw muscles and TMJ will lead to changes in measures of craniofacial pain.

The literature shows a wide range of intervention or treatment methods that have been proposed over the last several decades to modify or decrease the level of bruxism.[38] These methods include physiotherapy, muscle relaxation exercises, acupuncture, biofeedback, hypnosis, occlusal adjustments, and occlusal splints. The most common treatment of bruxism involves protection of the teeth by occlusal splints.[39,40]

Although occlusal splints may be beneficial in protecting the dentition from attrition, the efficacy of intraoral appliances in reducing nocturnal jaw muscle activity and the report of craniofacial pain on awakening is unclear. When the efficacy of occlusal splints in the management of sleep bruxism is considered at the individual level, some authors have shown a decrease, no effect at all, or even an increase in muscle activity.[41,42] It is a common clinical observation that occlusal splints will be worn suggesting that a significant amount of jaw muscle activity will continue to be present. Polysomnographic (PSG) studies have documented that occlusal splints in patients with sleep bruxism are associated with great variability and found that approximately two-thirds of the subjects treated with appliances demonstrate either no change or an increase in masticatory muscle EMG activity. One PSG study showed that occlusal splints reduced the muscle activity associated with sleep bruxism in tooth grinding subjects 2 weeks after insertion.[43] However, this particular study evaluated the short-term effect of occlusal splints on sleep bruxism with a one-time measurement. Another recent study reported that occlusal splints reduced muscle activity associated with sleep bruxism but this effect was only temporary. Also, different variations of occlusal splints such as the "nociceptive trigeminal inhibitory" (NTI) splint have in a recent short-term study been shown to reduce the EMG activity during sleep but without significant effects on TMD pain complaints.[44] It has previously been emphasized that "mono-therapy" with occlusal appliances in order to reduce the muscle activity associated with bruxism may not result in predictable improvement of symptoms.

Comprehensive reviews have concluded that occlusal splints are useful adjuncts in the management of sleep bruxism, but are not definitive or "curative" treatment.[38,39] So far no definitive conclusions can be given in relation to the effects of occlusal splints on craniofacial pain because either the included patients in the above-cited studies were free of pain or there was no specific information on this important outcome parameter.

Another important point is illustrated in Figure 17-4. This figure shows the short-term effect (after 1 week) of an occlusal splint in 11 subjects. There is a significant decrease in the total number of EMG episodes per hour of sleep compared to baseline recordings – in accordance with the outcome described above. However, a further detailed analysis shows that there is a differential effect on the phasic EMG episodes, but no effect on the tonic or mixed EMG episodes according to the criteria proposed by Lavigne and co-workers.[45] This finding raises the fundamental question of whether it is the total amount of EMG activity, or a particular type of EMG activity (phasic, tonic, mixed), that is the most important for a treatment effect.

Biofeedback techniques appear to be promising treatment options for patients with sleep bruxism. For example, EMG-activated alarms have been tested. Although the EMG suppression induced by auditory stimulation is interesting, a consistent return to pre-treatment bruxism levels has been reported in all studies that have monitored bruxism after stopping the feedback. Aversive gustatory stimuli have also been attempted to modify bruxism. However, the disadvantage of auditory (and gustatory) feedback is that they may interfere with sleep stage and quality because of arousal reactions.

Case reports have shown that contingent vibratory stimulation delivered to the maxillary teeth via an occlusal splint can lead to a significant decrease in the number of EMG events per hour (25% reduction) and the duration of each event (44% reduction). One potentially stronger form of afferent biofeedback is low-level electrical stimulation of the trigeminal nerve innervation area. It is well known and well researched that perioral electrical stimulation causes inhibitory responses in the contracting jaw muscles, the so-called exteroceptive suppression periods.[46] Recently, a study reported the use of contingent electrical stimulation of the perioral region in seven subjects and showed a decrease in the EMG activity by 37% over five nights. We have shown that the effect of conditioning electrical stimulation during sleep is a significant decrease (53%) in the EMG events per hour of sleep, and the study raised the question whether learning or conditioning effects could take place over time.[47] However, further studies will be required to determine the long-term effects on jaw muscle activity.

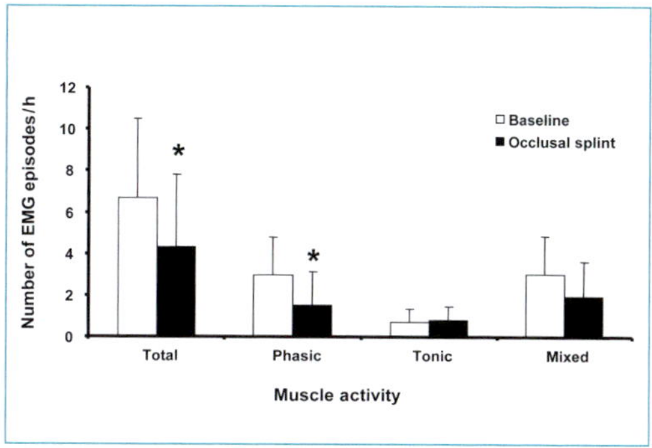


Fig 17-4 Short-term effects of an occlusal splint on muscle activity expressed as total number of EMG episodes per hour of sleep in 11 subjects (mean values + standard deviations). There is a significant decrease after 1 week's use of the splint, mainly due to a decrease in the phasic type of EMG episodes (* paired $t$-test: $P < 0.05$). Unpublished data from Drs Toyota and Arima.

It also needs to be pointed out that there were no significant effects of biofeedback on craniofacial pain parameters. This could be due to the low levels of painful problems at the time of inclusion, lack of statistical power, or dissociation between levels of jaw muscle activity and craniofacial pain.

In summary, the reviewed studies have shown that different therapeutic interventions have at least a temporary effect on muscle activity. However, these changes are not directly translated into changes in craniofacial symptoms – pain and unpleasantness.

## Conclusion

This chapter has focused on some of the problems related to the understanding of the relationship between bruxism and craniofacial pain. While it is clear that there are associations, one has to be cautious about inferring direct and simplistic causal relationships. One reason is the problem with operationalized definitions of bruxism.

In research settings and advanced university-based clinics it may be possible to use PSG recordings that will be the "gold standard" because EMG activity, jaw movements, and noises can be recorded and detected. However, this is also a limitation because the majority of clinical research will be unable to apply such sophisticated and resource-demanding techniques. Furthermore, there may be reasons to differentiate between sleep bruxism and awake bruxism, and these potentially different entities may have different associations with TMD pain.

We also need to know whether the most relevant parameters are the total amount of EMG activity or specific fractions of the EMG signal – for example, the phasic, tonic, or mixed bursts. Related to this issue is whether the intensity and frequency of bruxism is mainly dependent on patient-based measures (self-report of perceived tension, awareness of tooth grinding or clenching habits, bed-partner reports of noises, etc.) or objective measures of jaw movements and jaw-muscle EMG activity. A better characteristic of the temporal aspects, for example infrequent (<1 day/month), intermittent (1–15 days/month), or frequent (>15 days/month) types of bruxers could also be valuable. Furthermore, a grading system of the diagnostic probability (definite, probable, possible, and unlikely bruxers) might be useful to further advance the field. A diagnosis of definite sleep bruxism could be suggested to comprise a PSG recording, a series of ambulatory EMG recordings, reports from bed-partners about clenching or grinding activity during sleep, and self-reported awareness of grinding or clenching the teeth. Similarly, there would have to be operationalized criteria for a definitive awake bruxism diagnosis. Further research will allow improvement on the current classification of bruxism.

It is a surprise that jaw muscle pain associated with bruxism has not been better characterized. It seems worthwhile to examine neurobiologic and physiologic features of jaw muscles. Animal as well as human experimental models to examine these features will be needed. For example, one way to investigate the underlying mechanisms of pain related to bruxism could be to use the recent observations on "proprioceptive allodynia"; that is, to test for changes in vibratory sensation as well as other somatosensory modalities (QST). Another approach would be to use microdialysis and get an insight into potential inflammatory mediators in muscles of bruxers. Simple provocation tests like "clenching on a tooth" should also be more systematically examined in patient populations and may be able to provide important diagnostic information. Careful analyses of the phenotypes of bruxers may, together with advances in genotyping, also hold promise for a better understanding of the relationships between bruxism and craniofacial pain.

The take-home message for clinicians is that it is important to understand the concept of "non-linear" relationships between bruxism and craniofacial pain to avoid oversimplification of diagnosis and management. Craniofacial pain and bruxism should be managed as separate problems in individual patients.

## References

1. Merskey H, Bogduk N (eds). Classification of Chronic Pain: Descriptions of Chronic Pain Syndromes and Definitions of Pain Terms. Seattle: IASP Press, 1994.
2. Woolf CJ. Pain: moving from symptom control toward mechanism-specific pharmacologic management. Ann Intern Med 2004;140:441–451.
3. Julius D, Basbaum AI. Molecular mechanisms of nociception. Nature 2001;413:203–210.
4. Hucho T, Levine JD. Signaling pathways in sensitization: toward a nociceptor cell biology. Neuron 2007;55: 365–376.
5. Marchand F, Perretti M, McMahon SB. Role of the immune system in chronic pain. Nat Rev Neurosci 2005;6:521–532.
6. Sessle BJ. Acute and chronic craniofacial pain: brainstem mechanisms of nociceptive transmission and neuroplasticity, and their clinical correlates. Crit Rev Oral Biol Med 2000;11:57–91.
7. McMahon SB, Bennett DLH, Bevan S. Inflammatory mediators and modulators of pain. In: McMahon SB, Koltzenburg M (eds). Wall and Melzack's Textbook of

Pain, ed 5. Edinburgh: Elsevier Churchill Livingstone, 2006: 49–72.

8. Svensson P, Sessle BJ. Orofacial pain. In: Miles TS, Nauntofte B, Svensson P (eds). Clinical Oral Physiology. Copenhagen: Quintessence, 2004:93–139.
9. Woolf CJ, Salter MW. Plasticity and pain: role of the dorsal horn. In: McMahon SB, Koltzenburg M (eds). Wall and Melzack's Textbook of Pain, ed 5. Edinburgh: Elsevier Churchill Livingstone, 2006:91–106.
10. Treede RD, Jensen TS, Campbell JN et al. Neuropathic pain: redefinition and a grading system for clinical and research purposes. Neurology 2008;70:1630–1635.
11. Cairns BE. The influence of gender and sex steroids on craniofacial nociception. Headache 2007;74:319–324.
12. Zubieta JK, Smith YR, Bueller JA et al. mu-opioid receptor-mediated antinociceptive responses differ in men and women. J Neurosci 2002;22:5100–5107.
13. Greenspan JD, Craft RM, Le Resche L et al. Studying sex and gender differences in pain and analgesia: a consensus report. Pain 2007(Suppl 1):S26–45.
14. Le Resche L, Drangsholt M. Epidemiology of orofacial pain: prevalence, incidence and risk factors. In: Sessle BJ, Lavigne GL, Lund JP, Dubner R (eds). Orofacial Pain and Related Conditions, ed 2. Chicago: Quintessence, 2008.
15. Lavigne G, Khoury S, Abe S, Yamaguchi T, Raphael K. Bruxism physiology and pathology: an overview for clinicians. J Oral Rehabil 2008;35:476–494.
16. Couzin J. Genetics. Unraveling pain's DNA. Science 2006;314:585–586.
17. Zubieta JK, Heitzeg MM, Smith YR et al. COMT val158met genotype affects mu-opioid neurotransmitter responses to a pain stressor. Science 2003;299:1240–1243.
18. Diatchenko L, Nackley AG, Tchivileva IE, Shabalina SA, Maixner W. Genetic architecture of human pain perception. Trends Genet 2007;23:605–613.
19. Svensson P, Jadidi F, Arima T, Baad-Hansen L, Sessle BJ. Relationships between craniofacial pain and bruxism. J Oral Rehabil 2008;35:524–547.
20. Newham DJ, Edwards RHT, Mills KR. Skeletal muscle pain. In: Wall PD, Melzack R (eds). Textbook of Pain. Edinburgh: Churchill Livingstone, 1994:423–440.
21. Svensson P, Arendt-Nielsen L. Effects of 5 days of repeated submaximal clenching on masticatory muscle pain and tenderness: an experimental study. J Orofac Pain 1996;10:330–338.
22. Proske U, Morgan DL. Muscle damage from eccentric exercise: mechanism, mechanical signs, adaptation and clinical applications. J Physiol 2001;537:333–345.
23. Lund JP, Stohler CS. Effects of pain on muscular activity in temporomandibular disorders and related conditions In: Stohler CS, Carlson DS (eds). Biological and Psychological Aspects of Orofacial Pain [Craniofacial Growth Series 29]. Ann Arbor: Center for Human Growth and Development, University of Michigan, 1994:75–91.
24. Weerakkody NS, Percival P, Hickey MW et al. Effects of local pressure and vibration on muscle pain from eccentric exercise and hypertonic saline. Pain 2003;105: 425–435.
25. Arima T, Svensson P, Arendt-Nielsen L. Experimental grinding in healthy subjects: a model for postexercise jaw muscle soreness. J Orofac Pain 1999;13:104–114.
26. Lund JP, Donga R, Widmer CG, Stohler CS. The pain-adaptation model: a discussion of the relationship between chronic musculoskeletal pain and motor activity. Can J Physiol Pharmacol 1991;69:683–694.
27. Svensson P, Graven-Nielsen T. Craniofacial muscle pain: review of mechanisms and clinical manifestations. J Orofac Pain 2001;15:117–145.
28. Carlsson GE, Egermark I, Magnusson T. Predictors of signs and symptoms of temporomandibular disorders: a 20-year follow-up study from childhood to adulthood. Acta Odontol Scand 2002;60:180–185.
29. Chen CY, Palla S, Erni S, Sieber M, Gallo LM. Nonfunctional tooth contact in healthy controls and patients with myogenous facial pain. J Orofac Pain 2007;21: 185–193.
30. Lobbezoo F, Lavigne GJ. Do bruxism and temporomandibular disorders have a cause-and-effect relationship? J Orofac Pain 1997;11:15–23.
31. Kendall SA, Elert J, Ekselius L, Gerdle B. Are perceived muscle tension, electromyographic hyperactivity and personality traits correlated in the fibromyalgia syndrome? J Rehabil Med 2002;34:73–79.
32. Arima T, Arendt-Nielsen L, Svensson P. Effect of jaw muscle pain and soreness evoked by capsaicin before sleep on orofacial motor activity during sleep. J Orofac Pain 2001;15:245–256.
33. Lavigne GJ, Rompré PH, Montplaisir JY, Lobbezoo F. Motor activity in sleep bruxism with concomitant jaw muscle pain. A retrospective pilot study. Eur J Oral Sci 1997;105:92–95.
34. Rompré PH, Daigle-Landry D, Guitard F, Montplaisir JY, Lavigne GJ. Identification of a sleep bruxism subgroup with a higher risk of pain. J Dent Res 2007;86: 837–842.
35. Raphael KG, Marbach JJ, Klausner JJ, Teaford MF, Fischoff DK. Is bruxism severity a predictor of oral splint efficacy in patients with myofascial face pain? J Oral Rehabil 2003;30:17–29.
36. Janal MN, Raphael KG, Klausner J, Teaford M. The role of tooth-grinding in the maintenance of myofascial face pain: a test of alternate models. Pain Med 2007;8: 486–496.
37. Lynn B. Repetitive strain injury. In: McMahon SB, Koltzenburg M (eds). Wall and Melzack's Textbook of Pain, ed 5. Edinburgh: Elsevier Chuchill Livingstone, 2006:709–720.
38. Lobbezoo F, van der Zaag J, Selms MKA, Hamburger HL, Naeije M. Principles for the managment of bruxism. J Oral Rehabil 2008;35:509–523.

39. Dao TT, Lavigne GJ. Oral splints: the crutches for temporomandibular disorders and bruxism. Crit Rev Oral Biol Med 1998;9:345–361.
40. Macedo CR, Silva AB, Machado MA, Saconato H, Prado GF. Occlusal splints for treating sleep bruxism (tooth grinding). Cochrane Database Syst Rev 2007;4:CD005514.
41. Harada T, Ichiki R, Tsukiyama Y, Koyano K. The effect of oral splint devices on sleep bruxism: a 6-week observation with an ambulatory electromyographic recording device. J Oral Rehabil 2006;33:482–488.
42. van der Zaag J, Lobbezoo F, Wicks DJ et al. Controlled assessment of the efficacy of occlusal stabilization splints on sleep bruxism. J Orofac Pain 2005;19:151–158.
43. Dubé C, Rompré PH, Manzini C et al. Quantitative polygraphic controlled study on efficacy and safety of oral splint devices in tooth-grinding subjects. J Dent Res 2004;83:398–403.
44. Baad-Hansen L, Jadidi F, Castrillon E, Thomsen PB, Svensson P. Effect of a nociceptive trigeminal inhibitory splint on electromyographic activity in jaw closing muscles during sleep. J Oral Rehabil 2007;34:105–111.
45. Lavigne GJ, Rompré PH, Montplaisir JY. Sleep bruxism: validity of clinical research diagnostic criteria in a controlled polysomnographic study. J Dent Res 1996;75:546–552.
46. Lund JP, Murray GM, Svensson P. Pain and motor reflexes. In: Sessle BJ, Lavigne GL, Lund JP, Dubner R (eds). Orofacial Pain and Related Conditions, ed 2. Chicago: Quintessence, 2008.
47. Jadidi F, Castrillon E, Svensson P. Effect of conditioning electrical stimuli on temporalis electromyographic activity during sleep. J Oral Rehabil 2008;35:171–183.

# Part 3

# Clinical Approaches

Chapter 18

# Pharmacologic Considerations in Bruxism

*Marcelo Kreiner*

## Introduction

The effects of various medicines and social drugs on orofacial motor disorders and bruxism has been a major clinical concern in recent years. However, the possibility of effective pharmacologic treatment has been hindered by the lack of appropriate evidence. Often, pharmacologic treatment is implemented without sound scientific support. It is also relevant to understand that various drugs may worsen parafunctional orofacial activity. When a person has bruxism as an adverse effect of a drug treatment, the cause of the condition needs to be ascertained. If the clinician does not take this into consideration, any treatment instituted will result in failure.

Although there is still no thorough understanding of the pharmacologic and neurophysiologic central mechanisms related to bruxism, scientific data suggest that several neurotransmitters and centers are involved in the effect of various drugs on bruxism. Participation of the dopaminergic systems in the striated body (striatum) and frontal lobe of the brain is of special importance, since their hyperactivity generates bruxism-like mandibular movement with tooth grinding.[1,2] Research has suggested the participation of dopaminergic receptors D2 of the striated body in the bruxism mechanism.[3] The adrenergic system may be involved together with the dopaminergic ones, even in children.[4]

Serotonergic mechanisms also play an important role not only in the physiologic regulation of the orofacial motor activity, but also in the effect of some drugs on bruxism,[5] either improving or worsening the parafunctional activity. Although independent analysis of the dopaminergic and of the serotonergic systems is useful, we should also consider the complex functional relations among them and other systems within the central nervous system. The influence of the serotonergic neurons of the raphe nucleus on dopaminergic neurons that later project themselves over the prefrontal cortex[6] gives us an idea of the complexity of the physiologic processes that regulate the extrapyramidal system and influence the mechanisms of some drugs on bruxism.

The aim of this chapter is to review the effects of various medicines and addictive drugs on bruxism, based on the scientific data available.

## Anxiolytic Drugs

### *Benzodiazepines*

Benzodiazepines comprise a group of drugs that have hypnotic, anxiolytic, anticonvulsive and myorelaxing effects. Their effect in the central nervous system (CNS) is focused on inhibitory neurotransmitters, mainly the GABA (gamma-aminobutyric acid). Such effect is mediated by the interaction of these drugs with specific membrane receptors, the so-called "benzodiazepinic receptors". There are at least two membrane receptors involved in the mechanisms of these drugs: the BZ1 and BZ2 receptors. The BZ1 receptor is related to sleeping mechanisms while the BZ2 receptor is related to motor, sensory, and memory functions.

The action of these drugs occurs at various CNS levels. The effects on the spine are mainly related to their muscle relaxing effect, while their action in the limbic system and cortical areas is connected with their effect on behavior and emotions. The anticonvulsive properties are mainly related to their action on structures of the encephalic trunk. One distinctive feature of these drugs is their wide safety margin with regard to therapeutic doses and drug toxicity, and they also have a long half life, which may reach 100 hours for some of the drugs of this group. The most frequently used benzodiazepines are alprazolam, bromazepam, clonazepam, diazepam, flunitrazepam, and lorazepam.

Owing to the possible relationships between stress, anxiety, and parafunctional activity of the stomatognathic system,[7,8] it has been proposed that anxiolytic drugs may have a beneficial effect in the treatment of bruxism. Clinicians often prescribe this type of drug for this purpose. However, evidence for this is scarce and sometimes contradictory. There are few controlled studies of the effect of benzodiazepines on bruxism, so most of the information currently available is anecdotical or based on reports of uncontrolled clinical cases. Nevertheless, a placebo-controlled study on the effect of clonazepam on bruxism was published.[9] It studied the effect of 1 mg of clonazepam administered to patients half an hour before going to bed. Positive results were obtained in relation to the bruxism rate. To date, clonazepam is featured as one of the drugs of this pharmacologic group with the most promising results. Although diazepam has been historically used in the treatment of bruxism, there is not enough evidence of its positive effect.

### *Buspirone*

Buspirone is an anxiolytic drug whose chemical structure relates neither to the benzodiazepines nor to the barbiturate. Unlike the benzodiazepines, it has no anticonvulsive or myorelaxing effects. Its mechanism of action is based on its agonism for serotonergic receptors, interacting mainly with the 5-HT1A receptor,[10] at both the presynaptic and postsynaptic levels. Its affinity with the D2 dopaminergic receptors has also been proved.[10] Its possible use in the treatment of bruxism has been considered owing to its anxiolytic action and its interaction with the serotonergic and the dopaminergic systems.

Although no randomized or placebo-controlled studies of the effect of buspirone on bruxism have been conducted, it has been reported that it has a beneficial effect on patients who suffer from bruxism induced by antidepressive drugs of the selective serotonin-reuptake inhibitor (SSRI) class.[5,11] Considering that buspirone does not present the side-effects of other anxiolytic drugs (e.g., addiction or sedation), its use seems promising in the treatment of bruxism. Further research with an appropriate experimental design will be necessary.

*Table 18-1*

Pharmacologic profiles of common antidepressant drugs.

| Name | Adverse effects | | | Effect on neurotransmitter reuptake mechanisms | | Half-life (h) | Dose (mg/day) |
|---|---|---|---|---|---|---|---|
| | Anticolinergic | Sedation | Orthostatic hypotension | Norepinephrine | Serotonin | | |
| Amitriptyline | High | High | Moderate | Moderate | High | 31–46 | 10–300 |
| Imipramine | Moderate | Moderate | High | Moderate | High | 11–25 | 30–300 |
| Nortriptyline | Moderate | Moderate | Low | Moderate | High | 18–44 | 30–100 |
| Trazodone | No | High | Moderate | No | High | 4–9 | 150–600 |
| Bupropion | Moderate | Moderate | Low | No | Low | 8–24 | 200–450 |
| Venlafaxine | No | No | No | High | High | 5–11 | 75–375 |
| Fluoxetine | Low | Low | Low | Low | High | 1–16 days | 20–80 |
| Paroxetine | No | Low | No | Low | High | 10–24 | 10–50 |
| Sertraline | No | Low | No | Low | High | 1–4 days | 50–200 |

## Antidepressant Drugs

Antidepressants are common drugs. Many of them are used to treat chronic pain, including neuropathic and myofascial pain, whether or not the patient has depression. While some of these drugs relieve the symptoms of patients who suffer different types of craniofacial pain, others worsen the symptoms because they can trigger or aggravate bruxism. Clinicians who prescribe antidepressants are not always aware that some drugs from this group may have a negative effect on bruxism.

Antidepressants include mainly the following drugs or groups of drugs: tricyclic antidepressants, tetracyclic antidepressants, bupropion, venlafaxine, trazodone, selective serotonin-reuptake inhibitors (SSRIs), and monoamino oxidase inhibitors (MAOIs). Table 18-1 illustrates some of the characteristics of the most frequently used antidepressants. We next discuss those antidepressants that have been considered to be related to bruxism.

### *Tricyclic Antidepressants*

Tricyclic antidepressants are so-called because of their molecular structure, which is composed of three rings of atoms. For a long time they were the preferred drugs to treat depression, but in the last few years they have been substituted by other drugs, mainly belonging to the SSRI group (see below). Their mechanism of action is centered on their inhibitory effect on the reuptake mechanisms of the adrenergic and serotonergic neurons of the CNS. These drugs have been widely used in general medicine and dentistry owing to their positive effect in the management of chronic pain,[12] in the treatment of some neuropathies and myofascial pain syndromes.

Amitriptyline is the most commonly used tricyclic antidepressant for the clinical treatment of craniofacial pain of muscular origin. This fact, together with its effect on the sleeping architecture (mainly during the rapid-eye-movement period) and on depression, led scientists to think about its positive effect on bruxism. Raigrodski and co-workers[13] conducted a double-blind, randomized, crossover study to evaluate its effect. Ten patients were given 25 mg amitriptyline per night for 28 nights, and they also received 25 mg of a placebo for the same number of nights in a crossover design. No significant statistical differences between amitriptyline and placebo were found regarding bruxism levels. However, it is important to point out that amitriptyline dose used was extremely low, as was the number of participating patients (n = 10). The authors concluded that 105 patients would be the ideal sample to prove a significant effect of amitriptyline on EMG activity. In another paper, this same group of researchers evaluated the effectiveness of amitriptyline on facial pain related to bruxism, though they could not prove a positive effect.[14] Although these studies have not been able to confirm a positive effect for amitriptyline, the experimental design problems means that the results should be viewed very cautiously.

### *Selective Serotonin-reuptake Inhibitors*

SSRIs are antidepressant drugs that are used mainly to deal with depression, anxiety, panic attacks, obsessions, and some eating disorders. The mechanisms of these drugs are related to their action on the serotonin carriers at the neuronal membrane level. Such carriers are proteins that allow neurons and other cells of the body, such as platelets, to accumulate serotonin at the intracellular level. These carriers play an important role at the synaptic button since they allow the reuptake of serotonin by the neuron, thus regulating the concentration of this neurotransmitter in the synaptic cleft. As a result, it affects the postsynaptic neuron. The main mechanism of action of SSRI drugs consists of inhibiting the serotonin reuptake by the synaptic button, allowing the neurotransmitter to remain in the synaptic cleft for longer and, as a result, the postsynaptic neuron is more stimulated.

The scientific dental community is highly concerned about the possible connection between SSRIs and bruxism. Day after day, more data are found to suggest that some drugs from this group may trigger and even worsen bruxism in some patients (Table 18-2). Ellison and Stanziani[15] reported four clinical cases in which the use of fluoxetine and sertraline was associated with a worsening of bruxism, which decreased when the dose of SSRI was reduced. Paroxetine has also been associated with the manifestation and worsening of bruxism in patients who had not had a previous history of parafunction.[16,17] Fitzgerald and Healy[18] reported six cases of SSRI medication-induced bruxism; five also had symptoms during the day. Data obtained in an experiment conducted in the Netherlands, in collaboration with general physicians' offices, suggest a strong connection between SSRIs and bruxism, mainly fluoxetine and paroxetine.[17] To a lesser extent, severe cases of citalopram-induced bruxism have been reported.[19] In one of the cases, bruxism caused teeth loss.

### *Venlafaxine*

Venlafaxine is an antidepressant that is not chemically related to the tricyclics or SSRIs. Nevertheless, its mechanism of action is based on the inhibition of neurotransmitter reuptake. This drug potentially inhibits the neuronal reuptake of serotonin and norepinephrine, but the dopamine reuptake inhibition is weak. Its possible connection with the manifestation of bruxism was reported by Brown and Hong[20] and later by Jafee and Bostwick.[11] In the latter report, it is interesting to note that one of the patients had also developed bruxism 2 years before that, in relation to the use of paroxetine. This may mean that some patients are prone to developing bruxism when consuming different types of antidepressant, though the biological mechanisms of that are still unknown.

*Table 18-2*

**Effect of some drugs on bruxism.**

| Drug | Effect on bruxism | Author | Study design |
|---|---|---|---|
| Clonazepam | Improvement | Saletu et al[9] | Placebo-controlled |
| Diazepam | Improvement | Rosales et al[56] | Experimental (animals) |
| Buspirone | Improvement | Bostwick and Jafee[5] | Case report |
| Buspirone | Improvement | Jafee and Bostwick[11] | Case report |
| Amitriptyline | No effect | Raigrodski et al[13] | Double-blind, crossover |
| Amitriptyline | No effect | Mohamed et al[14] | Double-blind, crossover |
| Fluoxetine | Worsening | Ellison and Stanziani[15] | Case report |
| Fluoxetine | Worsening | Lobbezoo et al[17] | Case report |
| Sertraline | Worsening | Fitzgerald and Healy[18] | Case report |
| Paroxetine | Worsening | Romanelli et al[16] | Case report |
| Citalopram | Worsening | Wise[19] | Case report |
| Venlafaxine | Worsening | Jafee and Bostwick[11] | Case report |
| Chlorpromazine | Worsening | Amir et al[30] | Case report |
| Amphetamines | Worsening | Baylen and Rosenberg[33] | Meta-analysis |
| Cocaine | Worsening | Fazzi et al[39] | Descriptive |
| Propranolol | Improvement | Amir et al[30] | Case report |
| Propranolol | No effect | Huynh et al[50] | Placebo-controlled |
| Clonidine | Improvement | Huynh et al[50] | Placebo-controlled |

## Neuroleptics

Neuroleptics are used to treat psychiatric disorders such as schizophrenia, depression, delirious states, and hallucinations. They have also been used to treat some chronic pain syndromes. Their mechanism of action is centered on their antagonism with the dopaminergic receptors at the CNS.

Since their therapeutic introduction over 50 years ago, it has been observed that some patients have developed motor disorders of the craniofacial muscles and other areas of the body, associated with the use of this type of drug. These motor disorders include distonia, dyskinesia, and bruxism. The disorders most commonly described in relation to the use of neuroleptics are tardive dyskinesia and dystonia,[21] which consist of involuntary and repetitive muscular contractions of the affected muscles. Chlorpromazine is one of the drugs in this pharmacologic group used by clinicians and is also the most commonly reported as the cause of motor disorders. These disorders can be caused by either the abrupt interruption of the use of the drug or during their period of use. It has been observed that cervical and craniofacial muscles are the most commonly affected ones, and the disorder is frequently accompanied by facial pain.[22]

The pathophysiological mechanisms of these disorders are related to the neurotoxic effects of these substances, mainly at the membrane level of some neurons. These membrane alterations include synaptic alterations at the extrapyramidal system in the area of the striated body,[23] as well as severe neuronal and glial alterations at different levels of the basal ganglia.[24] The structural alterations in the basal ganglia have been observed through functional magnetic resonance imaging,[25] and the neuronal metabolic changes have been studied with tomographic techniques with positron emission.[26] The considerable increase in the production of free radicals after the prolonged use of neuroleptic drugs seems to play an important role in their adverse effects on motor systems.[27,28]

The high therapeutic efficiency of these drugs to treat various psychiatric disorders makes their use common in many countries, in spite of the motor disorders they provoke.[29] Taking into account that these disorders tend to be irreversible if not treated in time, and that many times they manifest first as bruxism or worsening of already present bruxism,[30] it is essential that the dental practitioner is aware of the patient's drug history so as to make an appropriate diagnosis and provide early treatment. The development of bruxism due to the intake of neuroleptic drugs tends to be acute and responds positively to treatment with propranolol[30] if diagnosed in time. It is likely that the beneficial effect of propranolol on bruxism symptoms is not based on its beta-blocking effect, but on the fact that it has a cross affinity with various serotonergic receptors.[29] An early diagnosis of this problem is vital in order to avoid the irreversibility of the process.

## Addictive Social Drugs

Addiction to drugs is a chronic disease characterized by compulsive behavior with a tendency to look for and consume drugs, and by important neurochemical changes in the brain. The use of social drugs has significant harmful effects at different levels of the organism, and the effects on craniofacial structures and functions, mainly on bruxism, are of great interest to clinicians.

### *Amphetamines*

Amphetamines are addictive drugs with a strong stimulant effect on the central nervous system. The group includes various substances with similar structure and effects: amphetamine, dextroamphetamine, and metamphetamine. The strongest of the group is metamphetamine. The term "amphetamine" is used also to refer to stimulants that chemically derive from this group, such as metilendioximetamphetamine (MDMA), commonly known as "Ecstasy".

The amphetamines originally derive from ephedrine, and since this is a sympathomimetic drug, its mechanism of action is mediated by its effect on the catecholaminergic neurons, thus stimulating the liberation of neurotransmitters. Since this drug easily crosses the blood–brain barrier, its mechanism of action has an important stimulant effect on the CNS. The elevation of central levels of norepinephrine (noradrenaline) and dopamine by the amphetamine is strengthened by the blocking effect of this drug on the presynaptic transporters which are involved in the of reuptake of these neurotransmitters into the intracellular space. This generates a significant increase in the concentration of these neurotransmitters in the synaptic space, strengthening their stimulant action.

MDMA is used with the intention of increasing energy level, improving mood, and inhibiting appetite. The metamphetamines were originally used as components of nasal decongesting medicines and bronchodilating inhalers. The molecular structure is similar to that of the amphetamines, but its effect on the CNS is more powerful. Its effect usually lasts for 6–8 hours and it may generate significant behavioral changes, including agitation, euphoria, and even violence. The adverse effects of these drugs are varied, including cardiovascular and behavioral disorders, insomnia, hallucinations, and motor alterations of varying degrees. Most of these disorders are caused by the harmful effect of this substance on the membrane function of various groups of neurons of the CNS, mainly on the dopaminergic and serotonergic ones.[31]

Among the motor disorders generated by these drugs we should highlight bruxism, which was first reported in the 1970s,[32] but later more widely considered and described.[33] The drug from the group that has generated most concern in relation to bruxism is MDMA, which is associated with severe day and night parafunctional activity. Ecstasy-generated bruxism can be associated with lingual and other facial muscle dystonias.[34] These motor disorders induced by MDMA have their pathophysiologic basis in the damage this drug causes at some neurons in the CNS, mainly on the dopaminergic and serotonergic neural circuits.[35] It has been estimated that bruxism is a side-effect of MDMA intake in at least one-third of the people addicted to this drug.[36] Considering that the treatment should be primarily etiologic, dental practitioners must know about this side-effect of the amphetamine group, and the amphetamine-derived drugs, so as to make a correct diagnosis and follow the appropriate interdisciplinary approach to treatment.

### *Cocaine*

Cocaine is a CNS stimulant that derives from the cocoa plant. Chlorhydrate is its most common presentation, and for over a century it has been used for various purposes. At the beginning of the 20th century, this substance was frequently used as the component of various medicines, mainly tonics. Once consumed, the effects are rapidly observed and they include the feeling of confidence, excitation, and irritability. When its effects end, after 20–50 minutes, it produces a high level of anxiety. It is highly addictive and its side-effects are so severe that it may cause death. Owing to its anesthetic-like effect, its use was widespread until its highly adverse effects were detected. Like other stimulant drugs, its mechanism of action is based on its effect on certain neuronal transmitters in the brain. Although the affected neurotransmitters include dopamine as well as glutamate,[37] it has been observed that the dopaminergic systems are the most involved.[38]

It is essential for dental practitioners to be familiar with the adverse effects that cocaine has on the stomatognathic system. This drug can provoke ischemic necrosis at the palatal level, gingival ulcers, and severe bruxism.[39] Experiments in rats have demonstrated that cocaine causes bruxism and severe attrition. This adverse effect can be irreversible, since it does not decrease with the administration of haloperidol, a dopaminergic receptor inhibitor.[8] The clinical dental treatment of cocaine-addicted patients is complex and must be based on an interdisciplinary approach that considers the biologic and the psychosocial aspects of the patient.[40] Managing bruxism in this type of patient is a key factor in the dental treatment, with the aim of lessening the consequences provoked by muscle hyperactivity.

### *Alcohol*

Evidence indicates that excessive consumption of alcohol constitutes a risk factor for bruxism.[41] The mechanisms of action of alcohol in the CNS include alterations of levels of glutamate, dopamine, and serotonin, even in the extrapyramidal regions such as substantia nigra.[42] This explains the occurrence of motor disorders when a person consumes alcohol. This effect decreases the modulating role that the glutamate neurons play on the dopaminergic system in the CNS, thus generating important alterations in behavior and motor activity.

Reports of clinical cases had suggested a possible relation between alcohol intake and bruxism.[43]

However, it was not until recently that a research study reported that the quantity of alcohol consumed was related to the electromyographic activity of the masseter muscle during sleep in young women.[44] In this study, the EMG night recordings were carried out by a portable device and the threshold of the EMG activity was pre-established as 20% of the maximum level of voluntary contraction. The duration of the bruxism episodes showed positive correlation with alcohol intake. An increase of 10 mg in the intake of ethanol led to an increase of 5.1 seconds in the EMG activity.

## Adrenergic Antagonists and Agonists

The antagonist drugs of beta-adrenergic receptors are commonly used to treat hypertension, ischemic cardiopathies, and some arrhythmias. In the last few years, this drug group has received considerable attention owing to its potentially beneficial effect on the treatment of bruxism. The hypothesis stating that adrenergic antagonist drugs may be useful in the clinical management of bruxism emerged from the fact that the cardiac rhythm increases during episodes of bruxism during sleep,[45,46] suggesting a possible relation between the activation of the sympathetic system and bruxism. It has been observed that, at the start of the bruxism episodes, periods of tachycardia occur, lasting at least 10 seconds each, generally preceded by changes in the electroencephalographic activity.[47] These data strongly suggest a possible relation between the activity of the autonomous nervous system and the mechanisms of bruxism. In line with these data, propranolol, a beta-blocking agent, showed positive effects on bruxism in reports of clinical cases.[30,48]

Beta-blocking drugs have important effects on the cardiovascular system, affecting both beta-1 and beta-2 receptors.[49] These effects become evident in the cardiac rhythm and automatism, reducing the sinus rhythm and slowing down the conduction of impulses in the cardiac muscle. Another drug group that has important antihypertensive cardiovascular effects is the selective alpha-2 adrenergic agonists. One of the most commonly used drugs from this group is clonidine, and its main pharmacologic effects consist of generating changes in arterial pressure and heart rate.[49]

Considering the effects of these drugs on the autonomous nervous system, scientists have developed a hypothesis regarding their possible effect on the central mechanisms of bruxism. Based on this, a research study analyzed the effect of propranolol and clonidine on night bruxism, using a placebo-controlled, randomized, crossover design.[50] Patients who had at least four episodes of bruxism per hour confirmed through polysomnography were included in the study. No significant statistical differences between the propranolol and the placebo groups were found. However, clonidine was superior to the placebo since it decreased bruxism by 62% ($P < 0.02$). An interesting result from this research study was that, although both propranolol and clonidine decreased the global sympathetic activity during sleep, only clonidine decreased sympathetic tone during the minutes preceding the onset of sleep bruxism.

The differences found between these two drugs are due to differences between their pharmacokinetic and pharmacodynamic characteristics. Apparently, clonidine has a more potent inhibiting action on the sympathetic system than propranolol. Also, it may have a direct effect on the regulating mechanisms of bruxism as well. Further research with a bigger sample size will be needed in order to verify the effect of these drugs on bruxism.

## Agonists of Dopaminergic Receptors

A functional study of the central nervous system in patients who suffer from bruxism, using single-photon emission computed tomography (SPECT), specific radiomarkers, and a controlled design has revealed the existence of a significant asymmetry of the density of dopaminergic receptors type D2 at the nigrostriatal level.[51] This finding has led into the possible relation of these receptors to bruxism mechanisms.

With the aim of evaluating the clinical use of these neurophysiologic findings, a placebo-controlled, double-blind research study of the effect of bromocriptine in patients with bruxism was carried out.[3] Bromocriptine is a dopaminergic D2 agonist that works at both central and peripheral levels. Based on the previous findings which state the possible relation between D2 receptors and bruxism, the hypothesis of this research study stated that small doses of bromocriptine should reduce bruxism. Polysomnographic evaluation and a specific radiomarker (I-123 iodobenzamide) were used to estimate and compare the relative concentration of sites of union of D2 receptors after the administration of bromocriptine or placebo. Although several patients who participated in the research study abandoned it because of the side-effects of bromocriptine, analysis of the data of those patients who were able to finish the 2-week treatment revealed a significant decrease of EMG levels compared with those of the placebo. Likewise, analysis of the distribution of D2 receptors at the striatum region and the nigrostriatal level showed a significant improvement after the use of bromocriptine.

In line with these findings, a dopaminergic (pergolide) D1/D2 agonist was recently used in the treatment of a patient with severe bruxism.[52] The history of this patient revealed that the severity of bruxism provoked the fracture of an extensive implant-supported rehabilitation. With the purpose of reducing the frequency and intensity of the bruxism episodes prior to a new implant, the patient was prescribed pergolide, starting with a 0.05 mg dose which gradually reached a 0.5 mg dose. Polysomnographic studies revealed a significant improvement in bruxism episodes. It is also interesting to note that this improvement was seen even a year after the administration of the medication was interrupted, which suggests that pergolide would have been able to interrupt, in some way, the mechanism that tends to keep bruxism relatively constant in a patient.

The results of these studies support the theory implicating of dopaminergic pathways in the mechanisms of bruxism, and show the necessity for further investigations in this pharmacologic field.

## Antiepileptics

Antiepileptic drugs are commonly used in the clinical management of orofacial pain, mainly in neuropathic cases such as idiopathic trigeminal neuralgia and postherpetic neuralgia. This clinical indication, together with their beneficial effects on neuromotor diseases such as epilepsy, has led clinicians to test their use in the treatment of bruxism.

The possible beneficial effect of gabapentin in cases of bruxism induced by antidepressant SSRI drugs has been reported. Brown and Hong[20] described a 50-year-old man with a clinical history of bipolar disorder who started psychiatric treatment with venlafaxine at an initial dose of 37.5 mg twice a day, which was doubled after a week. A few days after the beginning of the treatment, the patient was diagnosed with severe bruxism, with both daytime and night-time tooth grinding. He responded well to gabapentin 300 mg per day given for a 3-month period.

Another antiepileptic drug was successfully used by Kast[53] in a series of clinical cases. He used tiagabine, an antiepileptic that inhibits the reuptake of the neurotransmitter GABA, at the synaptic terminals. Specifically, tiagabine inhibits the reuptake system GAT-1.[54] Besides its anticonvulsive action, it has been observed that – unlike other antiepileptics – it increases the sleep stages III and IV in humans,[55] which has encouraged its use in the treatment of bruxism. Four out of the five patients presented by Kast were women. The ages of these patients ranged between 24 and 48. Four of the patients suffered from night bruxism with severe morning symptoms, while one female patient (age 48) suffered parafunction mainly during the day. The oral administration of tiagabine in doses ranging from 4 mg to 16 mg per day caused a total reduction of symptoms in four of the patients who suffered from night bruxism, while the female patient with day parafunction did not show significant improvement.

These case studies suggest the possibility of using some antiepileptic drugs in the clinic management of sleep bruxism.

## References

1. Tan EK, Chan LL. Severe bruxism following basal ganglia infarcts. J Neurol Sci 2004;217:229–232.
2. Chen WH, Lu YC, Lui CC, Liu JS. A proposed mechanism for diurnal/nocturnal bruxism: hypersensitivity of presynaptic dopamine receptors in the frontal lobe. J Clin Neurosci 2005;12:161–163.
3. Lobbezoo F, Soucy JP, Hartman NG, Montplaisir JY, Lavigne GJ. Effects of the D2 receptor agonist bromocriptine on sleep bruxism: report of two single-patient clinical trials. J Dent Res 1997;76:1610–1614.
4. Vanderas AP, Manetas C, Papagiannoulis L. Urinary catecholamine levels and bruxism in children. J Oral Rehabil 1999;26:103–110.
5. Bostwick JM, Jafee MS. Buspirone as an antidote to venlafaxine-induced bruxism. J Clin Psychiatry 1999;60: 857–860.
6. Kapur S, Remington G. Serotonin–dopamine interaction and its relevance to schizophrenia. Am J Psychiatry 1996; 153:466–476.
7. Pingitore R, Chrobak B, Petrie J. The social and psychologic factors of bruxism. J Prosthet Dent 1991;65: 443–446.
8. Gomez FM, Areso MP, Giralt MT, Sainz B, García-Vallejo P. Effects of dopaminergic drugs, occlusal disharmonies, and chronic stress on non-functional masticatory activity in the rat, assessed by incisal attrition. J Dent Res 1998;77:1454–1464.
9. Saletu A, Parapatics S, Saletu B et al. On the pharmacotherapy of sleep bruxism: placebo-controlled polysomnographic and psychometric studies with clonazepam. Neuropsychobiology 2005;51:214–225.
10. Tunnicliff G. Molecular basis of buspirone's anxiolytic action. Pharmacol Toxicol 1991;69:149–156.
11. Jafee MS, Bostwick JM. Buspirone as an antidote to venlafaxine-induced bruxism. Psychosomatics 2000;41: 535–536.
12. Cayley WE. Antidepressants for the treatment of neuropathic pain. Am Fam Physician 2006;73:1933–1934.
13. Raigrodski AJ, Christensen LV, Mohamed SE. The effect of four-week administration of amitriptyline on sleep bruxism: a double-blind crossover clinical study. Cranio 2001;19:21–25.
14. Mohamed SE, Christensen LV, Penchas J. A randomized double-blind clinical trial of the effect of amitriptyline on nocturnal masseteric motor activity (sleep bruxism). J Craniomandibular Pract 1997;15:326–332.
15. Ellison JM, Stanziani P. SSRI-associated nocturnal bruxism in four patients. J Clin Psychiatry 1993;54:432–434.
16. Romanelli F, Adler DA, Bungay KM. Possible paroxetine-induced bruxism. Ann Pharmacother 1996;30: 1246–1248.
17. Lobbezoo F, van Denderen RJA, Verheij JGC, Naeije M. Reports of SSRI-associated bruxims in the family physician's office. J Orofac Pain 2001;15:340–346.
18. Fitzgerald K, Healy D. Dystonias and dyskinesias of the jaw associated with the use of SSRIs. Hum Psychopharmacol 1995;10:215–220.
19. Wise M. Citalopram-induced bruxism. Br J Psychiatry 2001;178:182.
20. Brown ES, Hong SC. Antidepressant-induced bruxism: successfully treated with gabapentin. J Am Dent Assoc 1999;130:1467–1469.
21. Burke RE, Fahn S, Jankovic J et al. Tardive dystonia: late-onset and persistent dystonia caused by antipsychotic drugs. Neurology 1982;32:1335–1346.
22. Kiriakakis V, Bhatia KP, Quinn NP, Marsden CD. The natural history of tardive dystonia: a long-term follow-up study of 107 cases. Brain 1998;121:2053–2066.
23. Benes FM, Paskevich PA, Davidson J, Domesick VB. The effects of haloperidol on synaptic patterns in the rat striatum. Brain Res 1985;329:265–273.
24. Jellinger K. Neuropathologic findings after neuroleptic long-term therapy. In: Roizin L, Shiraki H, Greevic N (eds). Neurotoxicology. New York: Raven Press, 1977: 25–41.
25. Mion CC, Andreasen NC, Arndt S, Swayze VW, Cohen GA. MRI abnormalities in tardive dyskinesia. Psychiatry Res 1991;40:157–166.
26. Pahl JJ, Mazziotta JC, Bartzokis G et al. Positron-emission tomography in tardive dyskinesia. J Neuropsychiatry Clin Neurosci 1995;7:457–465.
27. Cadet JL, Lohr JB. Possible involvement of free radicals in neuroleptic induced movement disorders: evidence from treatment of tardive dyskinesia with vitamin E. Ann N Y Acad Sci 1989;570:176–185.
28. Lohr JB. Oxygen radicals and neuropsychiatric illness-some speculations. Arch Gen Psychiatry 1991;48: 1097–1106.
29. Wirshing W. Movement disorders associated with neuroleptic treatment. J Clin Psychiatry 2001;62(Suppl 21): 15–18.
30. Amir I, Hermesh H, Gavish A. Bruxism secondary to antipsychotic drug exposure: a positive response to propanolol. Clin Neuropharmacol 1997;20:86–89.

31. Peterson JD, Wolf ME, White FJ. Repeated amphetamine administration decreases D1 dopamine receptor-mediated inhibition of voltage-gated sodium currents in the prefrontal cortex. J Neurosci 2006;26:3164–3168.
32. Ashcroft GW, Eccleston D, Waddell JL. Recognition of amphetamine addicts. Br Med J 1965;1:57.
33. Baylen CA, Rosenberg H. A review of the acute subjective effects of MDMA/ecstasy. Addiction 2006;101:933–947.
34. See SJ, Tan EK. Severe amphetamine-induced bruxism: treatment with botulinum toxin. Acta Neurol Scand 2003; 107:161–163.
35. Goñi-Allo B, Ramos M, Hervas I, Lasheras B, Aguirre N. Studies on striatal neurotoxicity caused by the 3,4-methylenedioxymethamphetamine/malonate combination: implications for serotonin/dopamine interactions. J Psychopharmacol 2006;20:245–256.
36. Liester MB, Grob ChS, Bravo GL, Walsh RG. Phenomenology and sequelae of 3,4-methylenedioxymethamphetamine use. J Nerv Ment Dis 1992;180: 345–352.
37. Fernández-Espejo E. The neurobiology of psychostimulant addiction. Rev Neurol 2006;43:147–154.
38. Nader MA, Morgan D, Gage HD et al. PET imaging of dopamine D2 receptors during chronic cocaine self-administration in monkeys. Nat Neurosci 2006;9: 1050–1056.
39. Fazzi M, Vescovi P, Savi A, Manfredi M, Peracchia M. The effects of drugs on the oral cavity (review). Minerva Stomatol 1999;48:485–492.
40. Friedlander AH, Gorelick A. Dental management of the cocaine addict. Oral Surg Oral Med Oral Pathol 1988;65: 45–48.
41. Ohayon MM, Li KK, Guilleminault C. Risk factors for sleep bruxism in the general population. Chest 2001;119: 53–61.
42. Brancucci A, Berretta N, Mercuri NB, Fransesconi W. Gamma-hydroxybutyrate and ethanol depress spontaneous excitatory postsynaptic currents in dopaminergic neurons of the substantia nigra. Brain Res 2004;997: 62–66.
43. Hartman E. Alcohol and bruxism. N Engl J Med 1979;301:333–334.
44. Hojo A, Haketa T, Baba K, Igarashi Y. Association between the amount of alcohol intake and masseter muscle activity levels recorded during sleep in healthy young women. Int J Prosthodont 2007;20:251–255.
45. Macaluso GM, Guerra P, Di Giovanni G et al. Sleep bruxism is a disorder related to periodic arousals during sleep. J Dent Res 1998;77:565–573.
46. Huynh N, Kato T, Rompre PH et al. Sleep bruxism is associated to micro-arousals and an increase in cardiac sympathetic activity. J Sleep Res 2006;15:339–346.
47. Bader GG, Kampe T, Tagdae T, Karlsson S, Blomqvist M. Descriptive physiological data on a sleep bruxism population. Sleep 1997;20:982–990.
48. Sjoholm TT, Lehtinen I, Piha SJ. The effect of propranolol on sleep bruxism: hypothetical considerations based on a case study. Clin Auton Res 1996;6(1):37–40.
49. Goodman y Gilman. Las bases farmacológicas de la terapéutica, ed 10. México DF: McGraw-Hill Interamericana Editores, 2003.
50. Huynh N, Lavigne GJ, Lanfranchi PA. The effect of two sympatholytic medications – propranolol and clonidine – on sleep bruxism: experimental randomized controlled studies. Sleep 2006;29:307–316.
51. Lobbezoo F, Soucy JP, Montplaisir JY, Lavigne GJ. Striatal D2 receptor binding in sleep bruxism: a controlled study with iodine-123-iodobenzamide and single-photon-emission computed tomography. J Dent Res 1996;75:1804–1810.
52. Van Der Zaag F, Lobbezzoo F, Van Der Avoort PGGL et al. Effects of pergolide in severe sleep bruxism in a patient experiencing oral implant failure: case report. J Oral Rehabil 2007;34:317–322.
53. Kast RE. Tiagabine may reduce bruxism and associated temporomandibular joint pain, Anesth Prog 2005;52: 102–104.
54. Soudijin W, van Wijngaarden I. The GABA transporter and its inhibitors. Curr Med Chem 2000;7:1063–1079.
55. Mathias S, Wetter TC, Steiger A et al. The GABA uptake inhibitor tiagabine promotes slow wave sleep in normal elderly subject. Neurobiol Aging 2001;22:247–253.
56. Rosales VP, Ikeda K, Hizaki K, Naruo T, Nozoe S, Ito G. Emotional stress and brux-like activity of the masseter muscle in rats. Eur J Orthod 2002;24:107–117.

# Chapter 19

# Dental Materials for the Bruxing Patient

*Marta M. Barreiro and Ricardo L. Macchi*

## Introduction

The clinical use of dental materials requires their careful selection. Each restoration aims to obtain a final result with esthetic harmony, correct anatomic form, avoidance of recurrent lesions, and the re-establishment of biomechanical behavior. Biocompatible materials are needed with adequate mechanical properties to withstand applied forces.

Initial biocompatibility can be affected by degradation processes that take place during clinical use. Materials degrade as a consequence of their interaction with the environment in which they are placed. Any material can experience chemical or physical degradation, or both, under specific conditions. Common metals can corrode if not protected by covering them with ceramics or polymers than can better withstand the action of some environmental conditions. However, several chemical reactions can modify the mechanical behavior of these materials. For example, ceramics such as silicates can fail by fatigue in the presence of water.[1] This situation can be observed when a feldespar-based dental porcelain (an aluminum and potassium silicate) is placed in an aqueous environment such as saliva. The mechanical properties of the polymers can be altered in the presence of humidity or if they come into contact with organic solvents, as polymers can react with them – this phenomenon has been observed in dentures made of acrylic resins.

So, conditions in the oral environment affect the behavior of materials. Some materials are affected by the wide range of forces applied on them, the reciprocating movements of opposing dentitions, sudden thermal changes that can be considered as thermal shocks, and acid attacks.[2] Vale Antunes and Ramalho[3] have provided data on this (Table 19-1). These conditions could be worsened by the presence of parafunctional habits, pathologies such as xerostomia, and other changes in the environment.

The regular use of composite resins as restorative material in molar teeth has provided crucial

*Table 19-1*

**Conditions found within the oral cavity (Vale Antunes and Ramalho[3]).**

| | |
|---|---|
| Temperature | −10–50°C |
| Lubricant (saliva) | Saline solution – complex proteins |
| pH values | 1–9 |
| Loads during contact | 1–700 N |
| Loads during mastication | 6–130 N |
| Load rate | Up to 1500 cycles/day |
| Sliding distance | 0.6 km/year |

knowledge on the wear behavior of materials. Pathologies that accelerate physiologic tooth wear – such as bruxism, bulimia, and gastroesophageal reflux – are additional factors, as is the consumption of beverages with acidic pH and sugar content, which leads to dental erosion. All of these factors can have an impact on the surface of teeth and dental restorative material.

Normal tooth wear in non-bruxing people is considered to be ~29 μm per year in molars and ~15 μm in premolars.[4] Dental enamel loss of 10–40 μm per year occurs as a consequence of friction while biting or chewing.[2] The forces generated during mastication are between 20 and 120 N (newtons). With bruxism the load can be increased to values as high as 1000 N,[5] thus changing normal physiologic wear to severe wear and finally leading to fatigue failure. Wear and fractures that are found in bruxism are mainly due to the increase in load and movement. Fracture is seen when the increase in stress (force applied per unit of surface area) reaches the maximum material strength.[6] Metals exhibit better behavior under bruxing conditions since they can dissipate stresses by plastic deformation before fracturing. The many factors that are present in the clinical condition complicate the correct selection of materials under bruxism and severe wear conditions.

When significant dental tissue is lost due to wear, rehabilitation of affected teeth is indicated. Traditional approaches use crowns, bridges, and dentures, but the development of composite resins and adhesive techniques now allows for more conservative or minimally invasive procedures – while in cases of severe destruction, ceramic veneers, inlays, or crowns are also used.[7] According to Mount and Ngo,[8] amalgam should be considered as an option owing to its high resistance and good behavior in large restorations. Minimal intervention principles, designed to limit the loss of natural tooth structure, should be applied to all restorative dentistry even when none of the available restorative materials is entirely satisfactory in the long term.[7,8] The results depend on the possibility of eliminating or controlling etiologic factors.

This chapter will describe criteria for selection of materials, and will analyze wear mechanisms and other degradation mechanisms that can affect restorative materials. Emphasis will be placed on the bruxing patient.

## Criteria for Material Selection

When the moment comes, the clinician has to consider the material that he or she will want to use, the environment in which it will be used, and the patient conditions that can modify both material and environmental behavior[9] (Fig 19-1).

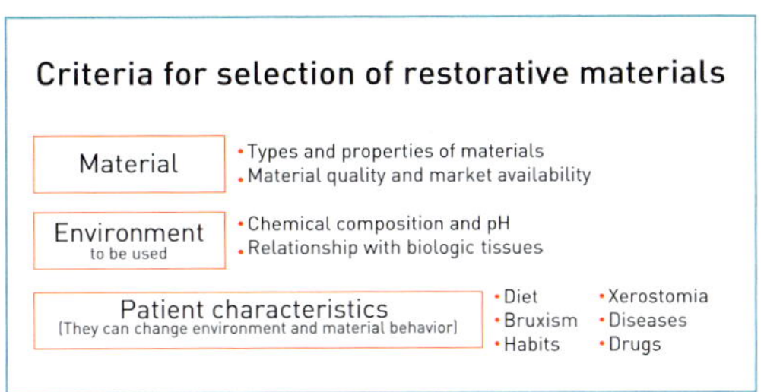


**Fig 19-1** Considerations in selection of the most appropriate material.

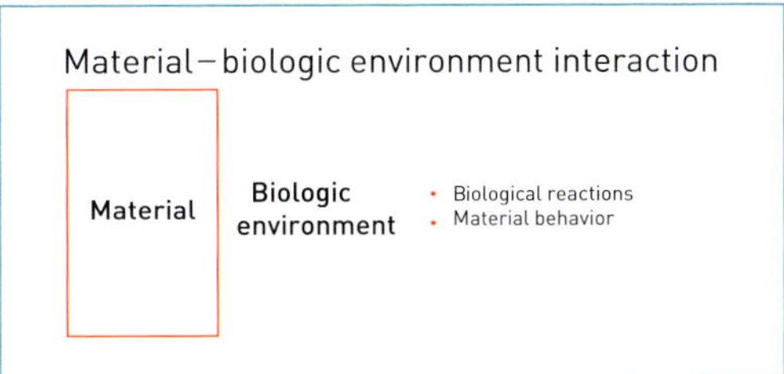


**Fig 19-2** Interaction between a restorative material and the oral environment.

## *Material Types*

We can consider materials to belong to four groups: metallic, ceramic, organic, and composites.

### *Metallic materials*

Metals are not esthetic in the mouth, and they can corrode. On the other hand, it is not difficult to obtain good mechanical properties with them. Most of them are ductile, and that means they are capable of permanent strain before fracture. Alloys that are indicated in prosthodontics and orthodontics, as well as dental amalgam and implant materials, are included in this group. The wear characteristics of many alloys are similar to those seen in dental structures.

### *Ceramic materials*

Ceramics are stable in the oral environment, and visually they have characteristics that make them esthetic over long periods. Their brittleness and rigidity are sometimes a disadvantage. They may need reinforcement or need to be supported by a rigid understructure to avoid flaw propagation and fracture. They can produce wear on other structures (enamel, composite resins, metals).

### *Organic materials*

Organic materials used in dentistry are synthetic polymers obtained at low temperatures using chemical or physical activation. They can be easily worked and can wear when occluding against dental enamel. They shrink as a consequence of polymerization. Their properties are significantly improved when combined with ceramic materials.

### *Composite materials*

These are the result of combinations of two or three of the material types already described. They are combined to improve on the individual properties of the components. They usually have a binding matrix and a reinforcement or filler. When a ceramic reinforcement is added to an organic matrix, mechanical properties and dimensional stability are improved. Handling is easier than in the case of ceramic products. Lack of adhesion between the two constituent phases can become a problem with loss of reinforcing particles after matrix wear.

## *Interaction with the Environment*

Restorative materials can behave differently when interacting with a biologic environment. They can generate a favorable response, stay inert, or start some type of dissolution process. In all cases they have to be biocompatible and produce no adverse effect. A material that is ideally biocompatible is the one that produces an appropriate response that is of benefit to the living organism. Materials that produce no response, those known as inert, can be used but with not so favorable results. Unfavorable responses due to the presence of the material within the biologic environment – such as allergic reactions and toxic effects – are not considered to be acceptable (Fig 19-2).

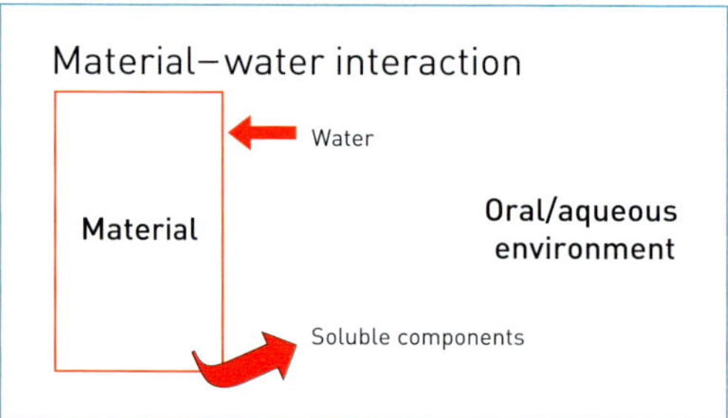


Fig 19-3 Interaction between a restorative material and an aqueous environment such as saliva.

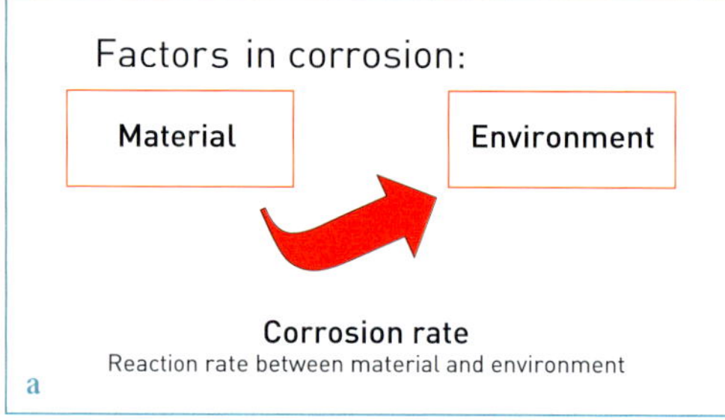


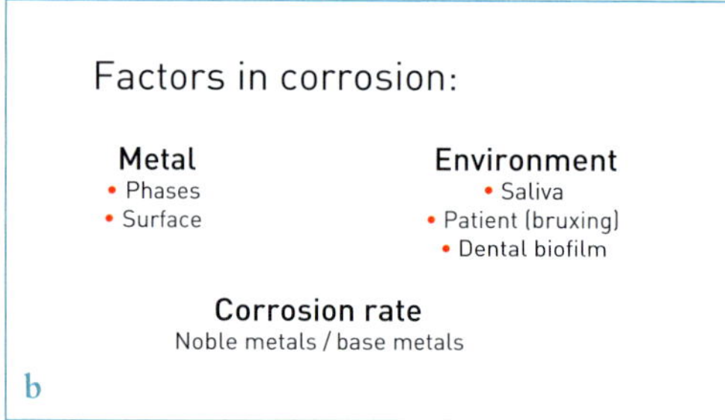


Fig 19-4 **(a and b)** Factors that determine corrosion rate according to material characteristics and patient condition.

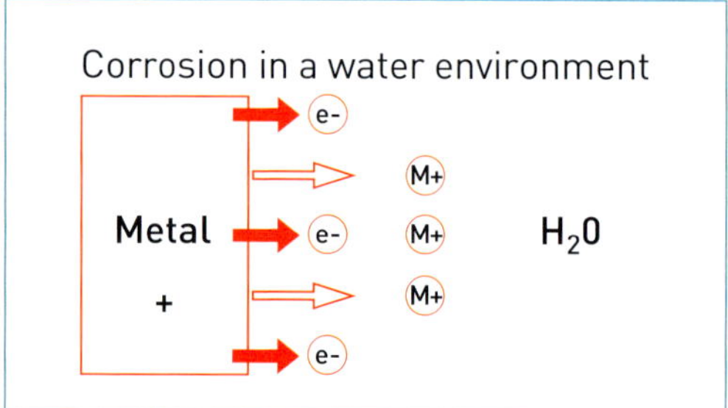


Fig 19-5 Oxidizing and reducing reaction with electron or metallic ion liberation.

As a product of the interaction between materials and the biologic environment, the following consequences can be observed.

- *Corrosion.* This can be defined as the degradation of a material and its properties due to a chemical or electrochemical reaction between the material and its environment.[10,11]
- *Fatigue.* This is failure that is produced when stresses are repeatedly applied for some time. It can generate fracture, loss of elasticity, or wear. It is greatly influenced by the environment. It can be either static or dynamic depending on how the load is applied.[12]
- *Wear.* This is characterized by loss of material in contact surfaces. It will be further defined later.
- *Allergic reactions and hypersensitivity.* These are reactions of the immunologic system owing to the presence of the material.
- *Toxicity.* More severe adverse effects are produced when particles are drawn into the internal environment and are deposited in different organs, affecting their function.

Corrosion, fatigue, and wear are the most frequent forms of degradation within the oral cavity. The consequences of fatigue in dental restorations can be seen as marginal fractures, loss of layers of material, wear, and fractures.

Soluble products can leak out of a material towards an aqueous environment; the degree of solubility of cements determines the time during which they can be useful within the oral cavity. A material can also incorporate water from the environment, a phenomenon described as "water sorption" that can take place in organic materials such as acrylic resins and in composite resins (Fig 19-3).

Certain materials can react with the biologic environment, and corrosion products leak from them and generate reactions in neighboring tissues or systemic reactions. Patients who are especially sensitive can show an allergic reaction to minute amounts of a material. A good example is nickel allergy, but reactions to cobalt or mercury can also occur. This situation arises not only due to the leakage of corrosion products but also due to the presence of particles (debris) produced by friction wear.

The factors determining corrosion rate are material and patient characteristics (Fig 19-4). During the corrosion process, oxidation–reduction reactions take place and electrons and metallic ions are liberated[9] (Fig 19-5). Corrosion products are chemical compounds generated by interaction with the environment.

### *Patient Factors*

Factors related to diet – mainly sugar-containing food and beverages, and low pH, increase degradation. The consumption of these types of beverage has increased in recent years. A "cola" type beverage that is drunk slowly produces a sugar-containing oral environment for more than 1 hour. Bacteria degrade the sugar into acids, and the more frequently this takes place, the more difficult it is for saliva to neutralize the acidity with buffering reactions. Enamel demineralization and erosion is the result. The corrosive potential of acidic beverages is not only pH-dependent; saliva buffering properties, the chelating of acids, and the frequency and duration of consumption are also factors that influence the development of the process.[13]

Several studies carried out in rats showed a change in dietary habit in animals that were fed with sugar-containing "cola" beverages. A significant increase in liquid ingestion was seen in these animals with a simultaneous 50% reduction in the consumption of solid food when compared to animals that drank plain water.[14] It can be speculated that enamel wear could also increase due to addiction to beverages.

The increase in occlusal loading and the frequent action on teeth that is seen in bruxism can also increase not only wear but the possibility of fatigue fracture. Some habits such as biting on hard objects (pencils, pipes, etc.) can also generate wear and fatigue.

Some diseases that produce chronic inflammation can be accompanied by a pH decrease to a value around 5.2. Metallic materials are more prone to corrode in this situation.

Xerostomia that is associated with rheumatic diseases, the use of certain drugs, and some other factors increases wear both in teeth and in restorative materials. This phenomenon is due not only to the decrease in salivary flow but also to changes in its composition. Medicines such as acetyl salicylic acid (aspirin) or vitamin C can also degrade materials.

## General Wear Processes

Following their eruption, teeth are subjected to a wear process that can be considered physiologic. Although wear resistance is considered the "gold standard" when evaluating dental materials, the ideal material to replace a tooth structure is the one that can follow normal tooth wear without affecting opposing teeth.

A few problems arise with terminology when talking about wear. Some terms used regularly in clinical dentistry for years conflict with those used by experts in the study of materials wear. What is the importance of a correct definition of each term? The idea is that this might help in establishing the etiology of every lesion found in tooth structures. An understanding of the mechanisms that take place and their interactions could help in differential diagnosis and planning effective prevention and treatment.[15]

Traditional terminology used in dentistry to describe wear phenomena within the oral cavity will be described (see also Chapter 9). Wear of materials according to the terminology regularly used in materials science will then be discussed, and differences will be analyzed.

### *Definitions*

In a simple way, wear can be considered as the loss of material from the surface of a solid. Actually, though, it is a complex phenomenon that is controlled by both mechanical and chemical variables. Here are some definitions:

- Wear is a process of degradation in which material is moved within, or removed from, the surface of a material as a result of the action of loads generated by movement.
- Wear is a phenomenon that is characterized by a loss of the original anatomic form of teeth and can be produced by physiologic or pathologic causes.[16]
- During wear, material is moved or removed by interfacial forces generated when two surfaces slide against each other.

When two bodies in contact slide against each other, several wear mechanisms start. A great loss of mass is not always needed before damage can affect function.

Another factor that has to be taken into consideration is friction (or resistance) that is found with sliding. If we invert these concepts, we can say that if there is neither movement nor force or friction, no wear will be registered.

Wear cannot be avoided under the conditions that are found within the oral cavity (see Table 19-1). The factors that interact simultaneously are contact surfaces, the applied force, movement, and friction; the factors that influence the process are movement speed, force intensity between the surfaces, the load that is present in the system, and specific characteristics of each of the surfaces (roughness, texture, smoothness, hardness, chemical composition, etc.).

Fragile materials such as dental porcelain show wear mechanisms that are different from those observed in ductile materials such as metals. The latter are capable of permanent mechanical deformation before rupture is produced. Temperature or load increases can also be expected to modify the wear mechanism as wear progresses.

### Types of Dental Wear

Traditional dental terminology divides wear into attrition, abrasion, erosion, and abfraction. Grippo and co-workers[15,17] suggest replacement of the term "erosion" by "corrosion" and describe a series of combined mechanisms:

- *Attrition.* This results from oclussal contact between opposing teeth (Fig 19-6).
- *Abrasion.* This incorporates an exogenous abrasive agent between surfaces (see Fig 19-6).
- *Erosion.* This describes loss of dental structure produced as a result of a non-bacterial chemical process.[18] It is also considered as the gradual destruction of dental hard tissue as a consequence of acid attack or chelation that is not the consequence of intraoral microflora.

This classification tries to differentiate the phenomena and identify their etiologies so as to decide on the most appropriate treatment. Some cases

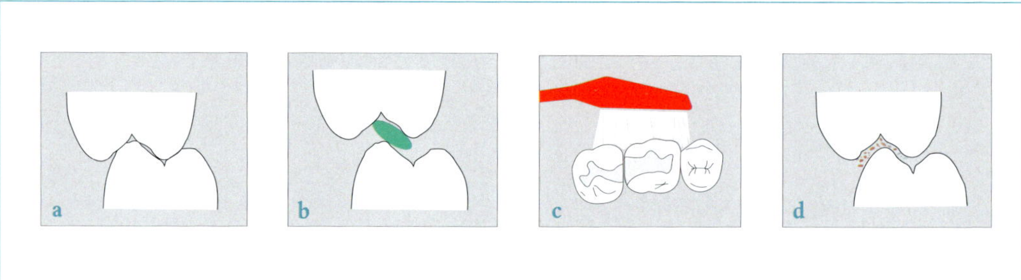


Fig 19-6 **(a)** Two-body wear or attrition. **(b)** Three-body wear by food or mastication. **(c)** Three-body wear by abrasion (tooth brushing). **(d)** Abrasive particles in between surfaces. (Modified from Söderholm.[28])

*Table 19-2*

**Wear type classification used to describe material wear.**

| | | |
|---|---|---|
| Abrasive | Hard and rough surface sliding on a softer one | |
| | Two-body | Particles detached during sliding that adhere to the softer surface |
| | Three-body | Particles that roll between the two surfaces with similar hardness |
| Adhesive | | Two surfaces slide, particles detached from one of them adhere to the other |
| Corrosive | | Sliding of surfaces in a corrosive environment |
| Due to surface fatigue | | Cyclic forces parallel to the surface generate cracks that progress and generate loss of mass |

might require restorative materials as the solution, while others might not.

Grippo[15,19] explains that the process that is identified as erosion in dentistry is best described as corrosion since it is the physical deterioration of a material by a chemical or electrochemical attack. This thinking takes into consideration the definitions included in the glossary of metallurgical terms and tables of the American Society for Metals, which also defines erosion as the abrasive destruction of a material by the movement of a liquid or a gas with or without solid particles.[17] We consider that both terms can be used as synonyms in practice since both are understood in dentistry to describe the same phenomenon even when they are not the same in materials science.

### *Wear Mechanisms in Materials*

Different types of wear can be found in materials used within the oral cavity.[20,21] The mechanism that produces loss of material, and the amount of wear, is dependent mainly on mechanical behavior and the characteristics of the surfaces that come into contact. Different types of wear, the conditions under which they take place, and similarities and differences with dental terminology are described in Table 19-2.

*Abrasive wear*

This is seen when a hard and rough surface slides on a softer one. Depending on the surfaces that interact, two- or three-body wear or abrasion can be differentiated.

- *Two-body abrasion.* Particles are drawn from one of the surfaces in contact during sliding. They adhere themselves to the other surface – usually the softer one – with generation of a groove (see Fig 19-6).
- *Three-body abrasion.* Particles move between two surfaces with similar hardness with a different body between them (see Fig 19-6). When this type of wear is produced by food it is also known as "demastication".

Three-body abrasion is the most important wear mechanism in mastication. The forces are generated by muscles, and when teeth are in contact they are concentrated on the occlusal area. When food is present, forces are distributed and their intensity will depend on the food's hardness. When the food bolus is compressed, the contact surface increases and so the load per unit area decreases.[22]

So, when there is direct contact between tooth surfaces a two-body abrasion is generated. Many

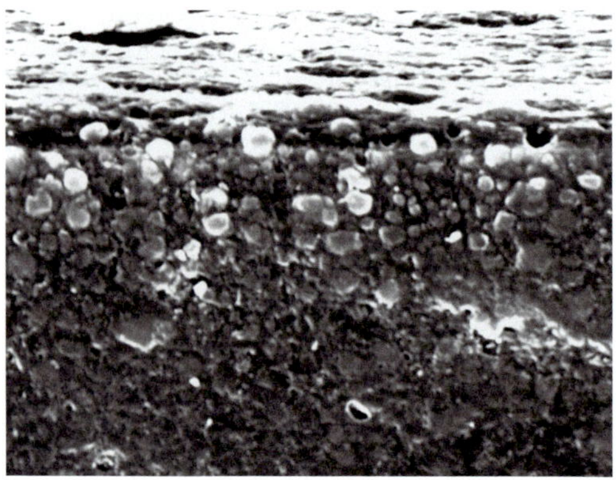

Fig 19-7 Secondary electron microscopy (SEM) image of wear area (top) during roll-on-disk test. Detached filler (bottom, debonding) in a composite with irregular shaped particles.

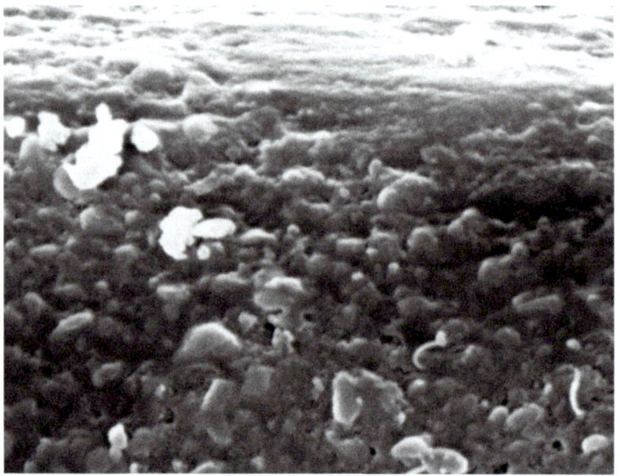

Fig 19-8 Wear area (top) after a test similar to the one in Figure 19-7. Round filler particles (bottom) with no detached particles observed under scanning electron microscopy.

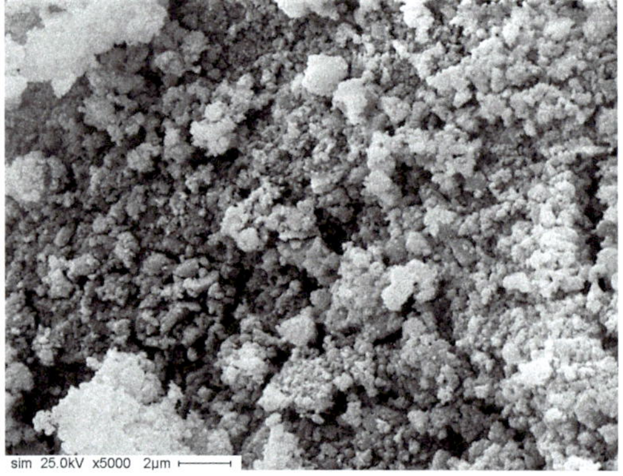


Fig 19-9 Filler particles seen after organic matrix elimination by heat.

dental practitioners call this process "attrition", and they describe "abrasion" as a three-body mechanism that takes place in mastication by the interposition of food and during tooth brushing with abrasive dentifrices. It is important to remember that for a third body to be considered as such it has to behave as an abrasive; so saliva cannot be considered a third body, but it can be thought to behave as a lubricant diminishing friction.

It is also possible for the phenomenon to begin as a two-body wear and then become a three-body one. This situation can be observed in composite resins by the popping out of reinforcing particles (debonding) that become a third body in abrasion. Figure 19-7 shows reinforcing particles that came out of the resin during wear testing. Irregular particles were present in this case, while rounded ones are demonstrated in Figure 19-8; the appearance of the abraded surface is different with evidence of no particles by scanning electron microcopy. Figure 19-9 shows a composite resin after elimination of the polymeric matrix by heat.

*Adhesive wear*

This is produced when two smooth surfaces slide on each other. Fragments of one surface are loosened and adhere to the other one.

*Fatigue wear*

This type of wear is produced by surface sliding of one material on another one. Fissures are generated by the action of cyclic loading and their progression is then facilitated.

Fissures can be present immediately under the surface and parallel to each other, or they can join together. An incubation period can be identified in which the fissures connect between themselves and generate a damage area that eventually can fail to maintain the surface attached (delamination). A rough surface is generated after large plastic deformation.[12]

Tooth geometry determines the stress concentration immediately under the surface, generating a net of fissures. This type of wear can be seen when an important compression load is applied to a solid element by an opposing tooth on hard bodies during mastication.

*Corrosive wear*
This takes place in a corrosive environment and under sliding. Chemical attack on surfaces in contact is associated with mechanical wear. Both the action of forces and surface chemical reactions with the environment are responsible for deterioration.[23,24] Corrosion is a degradation phenomenon of materials within the environment in which they are employed. Metals are the most corrosion-prone materials.

Saliva is an aqueous solution that contains electrolytes that are potentially aggressive. Foods, drinks, and microorganisms can also produce chemical attack. The process of corrosive wear in the oral cavity is still only partially understood and only a few clinical data are available. This phenomenon is considered to play an important role in intraoral wear and is associated with other wear mechanisms. As already mentioned, it is equivalent to what is referred to as "erosion" in traditional dental terminology.

### *Wear Mechanisms in the Oral Cavity*

As soon as teeth contact their antagonists a physiologic wear process is started. According to the area that is involved, it can be occlusal or proximal.

*Physiologic wear*
Once teeth are erupted and in contact with opposing teeth, occlusal and proximal wear is compensated by slow post-eruptive movements. At the same time, structural changes take place with deposition of secondary or cellular cement mainly in the apical area. The apposition of cement is enough to compensate for the physiologic wear and ensure maintenance of occlusal equilibrium.

*Occlusal wear*
The wear mechanisms that predominate are two-body wear or attrition in areas with occlusal contact, and three-body wear or abrasion in areas without occlusal contact.

The opposing cusp introduces stress in regions on which food is triturated when primary cusps come into contact. Wear in occlusal contact areas is approximately 2.5 times greater than in non-occlusal contact areas.[25] Forces around 10–12 N are estimated to be present on surfaces without contact.[26,27] Those values are increased to 50–150 N when tooth surfaces contact directly against each other and two-body wear or attrition is generated.[25]

*Proximal wear*
This is found in proximal surfaces as a consequence of sliding and compressive loads that appear during function. The mechanism is two-body wear or attrition. The presence of associated periodontal problems with great tooth mobility can intensify wear. Composite resin restorations that include proximal surfaces show greater proximal wear than unrestored surfaces.

Contact between different materials can be seen in Figure 19-10. This type of wear produces a shortening of the dental arch[28] (Fig 19-11) and not an opening of the interproximal space such as can be found after restoring a lesion.[29,30] When proximal contact has been lost, abrasion or three-body wear is found.

*Comment*
All of the mechanisms that have been mentioned can be found within the oral cavity, both when tooth tissues or restorative materials are considered, but attrition and abrasion predominate. Generally speaking they are the consequence of occlusal interactions. The most frequent wear is produced by physiologic or pathologic factors or by dental hygiene. The different types of wear along with their causes, terminology equivalence, and the

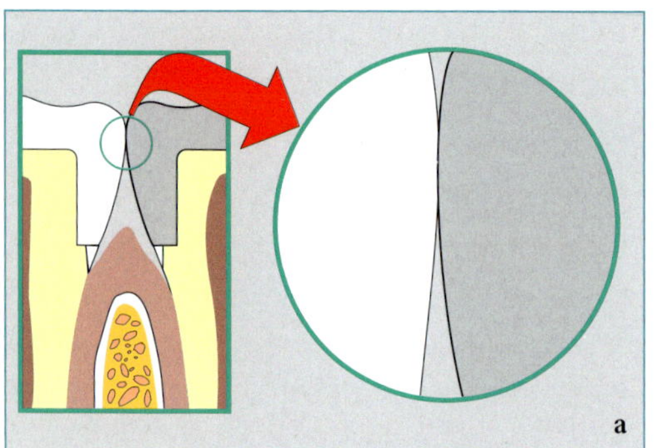


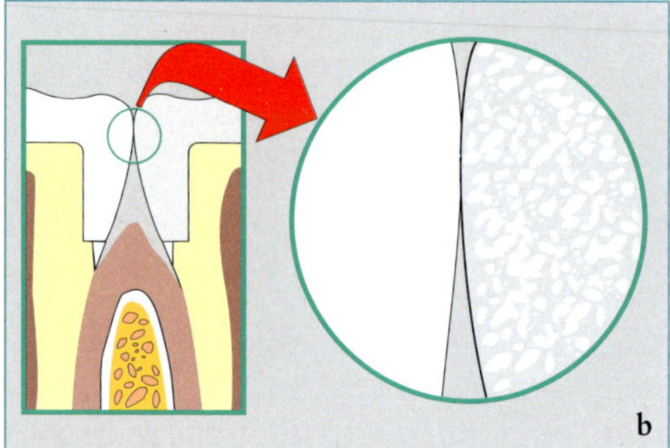


Fig 19-10 Proximal contact between restorations with different hardnesses: **(a)** porcelain–metal, and **(b)** porcelain–composite. Several mechanisms are present – two-body, three-body, and corrosive wear.

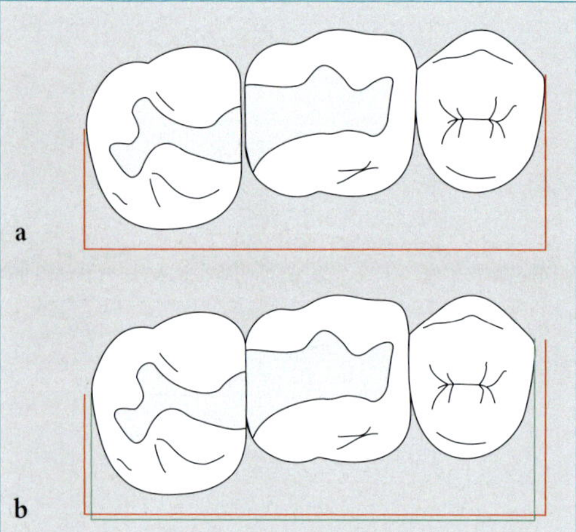


Fig 19-11 **(a and b)** Proximal wear in teeth with proximal composite resin restorations. This type of wear is also seen on enamel and is increased in the presence of periodontal mobility. (Modified from Söderholm.[28])

lubricant that acts in each case can be seen in Table 19-3. The contacts can be tooth against tooth, tooth against restoration, restoration against restoration, as well as a tooth brush or other foreign body – which includes foods.

Corrosive wear or erosion can take place when a chemical process is added, as happens by the effect of acid in bulimic patients. Wear by superficial fatigue can be the consequence of a habit such as biting on a solid object (e.g., a pen), which involves the application of high compressive loads.

In the case of bruxism, two-body wear or attrition is found. Tooth surfaces come into direct contact, the frequency of sliding is incremented as well as the loads that are applied, and all these factors lead to significantly greater wear and increased possibility of fatigue failure.[15]

## Evaluation of Wear Behavior

Laboratory simulator and clinical studies can be used to evaluate intraoral wear.

### *In-vitro Laboratory Studies*

The use of in-vitro studies provides an approximation of the evaluation of wear of new materials before their clinical application.[31,32]

Is the prediction of wear behavior of dental materials possible? One important point to keep in mind when evaluating lab studies is the difficulties that appear when attempting to simulate conditions present in the oral cavity. The very many variables that participate in wear make its measurement with a single parameter difficult, even when variations seen from patient to patient are not considered.[31]

The weak correlation that is seen between mechanical properties and wear is remarkable. Some physical properties such as water sorption can give just a hint of potential wear, particularly when corrosive wear is considered.

*Table 19-3*

**Most frequent wear types within the oral cavity: comparison between dental and materials science terminology (modified from Vale Antunes and Ramalho[3]).**

| Causes of wear | Dental term | Material terminology | Lubricant/abrasive |
|---|---|---|---|
| *Physiologic* | | | |
| Without occlusal contact | Abrasion | Three-body | Saliva/food |
| Direct contact | Attrition | Two-body | Saliva |
| Contact and sliding | Attrition | Two-body | Saliva |
| *Pathologic* | | | |
| Bruxism | Attrition | Two-body | Saliva |
| Xerostomia | Attrition | Two-body | – |
| Chemical attack | Erosion | Corrosion | Saliva |
| Negative habits | Attrition/abrasion | Two- or three-body | – |
| *Hygiene* | | | |
| Tooth brushing | Abrasion | Three-body | Water/dentifrice |

### *Clinical Studies*

Understanding clinical wear requires studies in which the different factors that interact are taken into account. Clinical studies are the best option in the actual evaluation of wear, but they are expensive and need to be long term.[33–35]

Clinical wear can be expressed by the amount (in micrometers) of material loss per year, using normal tooth wear for comparison. For example, the American Dental Association considers that a loss no greater than 50 μm per year has to be established by means of systematic clinical studies if a material is to be used in posterior restorations.

Both direct and indirect methods are used in these studies. Most of the direct studies follow criteria that have been established by Ryge:[36] color matching, marginal integrity, secondary caries, anatomic form, and surface roughness. Some changes in categorization are introduced according to each study's specific needs. Inter-examiner variability is the main limitation to obtaining adequate discrimination in the use of scales.

Indirect methods use impressions and models, which are evaluated, or epoxy resin replicas that can reproduce worn surfaces, and scanning electron microscopy observation.

Loss of vertical dimension is commonly measured in clinical studies. Visual examination is fast and no additional cost is required, but it is prone to subjective variation; often just changes in anatomic force are registered without any quantification. Special optical or scanning electron microscopes and profilometers allow for greater precision in the evaluation of material loss. Surface changes in exposed cavity walls can be evaluated so as to establish the types of wear that are present.

Many discrepancies are seen between results from in-vitro lab studies and observation in long-term clinical studies. The evaluation of actual behavior with reliable measurements is still a problem to be solved. Present efforts are focused on the use of wear simulators for wear studies, and these results have be corroborated later by clinical studies.[31]

## Degradation of Restorative Materials

The degradation that restorative materials suffer has to be considered when selecting a specific product. Not very much is known about the clinical effects, local or systemic, that can appear when corrosion products or particles of a worn material are inhaled or ingested. Consequences within the stomatognathic system are seen as tissue alteration due to loading, and changes in the distance between jaws and in arch dimensions[31] (see Fig 19-11).

Since restoration longevity is affected, one of the factors to consider is the cost in terms of sound remaining structure and in function that replacement represents. Health risks that can arise through corrosion and wear have been mentioned. The loss of vertical dimension and loss of reinforcing particles when composite resin restorations are used are of special interest.[23]

Restorative materials ideally should match the wear characteristics in the dental structure they replace. Surprisingly, the evidence suggests that the behavior of dental enamel has not been reproduced yet, even when very good esthetic appearance is obtained. A sound knowledge of the enamel wear mechanism could lead to optimization of materials used. However, the principle to be followed today is that the best material is sound tooth structure, which makes a minimally invasive technique the best choice. Since composite resin is the material that best fulfills what is needed,[37] most wear studies concentrate on these products.

It is to be expected that materials with different surface characteristics and mechanical behavior will wear differently. For example, a very hard material such as dental porcelain can lead to wear in the opposing tooth. However, this material is a silicate and its surface is modified in the presence of water, with a reduction in hardness mainly in an acidic environment.[16] A decrease in salivary flow produces an effect that is opposite to what is expected and wear possibilities are reduced.

Since wear is a multifactorial process, hardness is just one variable to be considered. Failure due to fatigue can be seen in prosthodontic devices and dental restorations as wear, marginal fracture, delamination, and fracture. The mechanisms that can induce fracture by fatigue depend on material ductility.[12] Plastic deformation before fracture allows for stress dissipation, so avoiding crack propagation. This effect is seen in metallic restorations, while brittle materials are susceptible to catastrophic fractures owing to the propagation of cracks since no stress dissipation can occur. Toughness in fracture measures the resistance to crack propagation, and it is an important property when estimating the possible longevity of restorations.

### *Composite resins*

Composite resins have a polymeric matrix and a ceramic filler. They can be considered as a three-dimensional combination of two chemically different materials with a bond between them. Dental composites differ in shape, size, and the amount of filler particles, as well as in the polymeric matrix.[6] A great variety of commercial products can be found in the dental market.

These materials can be used in plastic restorations since their polymeric matrix allows for their direct insertion in a dental preparation and followed by a polymerization reaction and hardening within the oral cavity. They are mainly indicated for less than extensive restorations without a high occlusal involvement, and where esthetics is important.[3] Disadvantages include polymerization shrinkage and wear, but improvement in both aspects has been made by manufacturers in recent years. The selection of a specific product is not easy owing to the large choice.

Its success as an amalgam replacement is limited by the extent of the restoration. Amalgam or inlays – metallic or composite – have to be considered as alternatives in these situations. It is convenient to have a high ceramic filler content, small distance between reinforcing particles, a smooth surface,

*Table 19-4*

**Clinical wear values: in-vivo measurements (modified from Heintze[31]).**

| Type of restoration material | Wear localization | Wear (μm) |
|---|---|---|
| Class I/II composite | Occlusal contact<br>Without contact<br>Occlusal surface(overall)<br>Proximal contact | 72–172<br>20–101<br>64–208<br>114–243 |
| Class V composite | | 20 |
| Composite crown | Occlusal contact<br>Occlusal surface(overall) | 238 (8 months)<br>60–170 |
| Amalgam | Occlusal contact<br>Occlusal surface(overall) | 120<br>28 |
| Enamel | Occlusal contact<br>Occlusal surface(overall)<br>Proximal contact | 54–91<br>41<br>17 |

good mechanical behavior, and good wear resistance in composites that are designed for posterior restorations.

One of the first clinical studies on the use of posterior composite restorations was published in 1973. Phillips and co-workers[38] observed that only 15% of the restorations that were analyzed maintained adequate anatomic form after 3 years, owing to excessive wear. They concluded that composite resins were contraindicated for Class II restorations in those days. In 1984, Lutz and co-workers[25] evaluated the influence of cavity size and curing mode in MOD (mesio-occlusal–distal) restorations with products that were available then. They concluded that wear resistance increased as cavity size decreased and when light-curing was used. Their opinion was that wear in composite resins was not acceptable and could not be considered as an amalgam alternative in large restorations.

A review published in 2006 by Heintze[31] compared enamel, composite, and amalgam wear after 2 years in the oral cavity (Table 19-4). Amalgam had less wear than composite mainly in occlusal surfaces. Approximate values were 28 μm for amalgam, 64–208 μm for composite, and 41 μm for enamel. These data take into consideration the whole occlusal surface and they change when proximal areas are analyzed. It has to be recognized that this review includes studies in different types of subjects, with different selection criteria and different methods to evaluate wear. Even then it is interesting on a comparative basis.

Clinical wear in posterior composite restorations has improved considerably thanks to changes in formulation, and some authors consider that today it is a problem solved.[39] However, only a small part of the dental literature gives evidence to support this statement in the case of large restorations – chiefly when they include main functional cusps. The evidence shows minimal wear in small- and medium-sized restorations, but higher failure rates and significant wear in large posterior restorations in patients with bruxism and sliding habits.[32]

These considerations were looked at in 2006 by Ferracane[32] after many publications on the subject[40] and a symposium on intraoral wear of restorative materials that was organized by the International Association for Dental Research (IADR) with the participation of members from around the world. The question of whether composite wear was still a clinical problem to consider was raised, and whether in-vitro wear simulating devices were needed in research. It has to be stated that Ferracane designed and optimized his research with these devices. The different types of wear mechanism found in materials and the need for in-vitro evaluation before clinical use has been covered already in this chapter.

Wear in composite resins is considered to be a complex and multifactorial phenomenon that is difficult to reproduce in the laboratory. It includes adhesion, abrasion, attrition, chemical degradation, and fatigue.[40,41] The detaching of filler particles, water sorption, and the viscoelastic behavior of the matrix are other factors to be considered. The effect of dental plaque-generated acids, foods, and enzymes produce softening and roughness on the surfaces. As a consequence corrosive wear can be present under loading. The literature is in agreement on recognizing the process as complex with simultaneous or sequential effects of different mechanisms that influence each other, so prediction of the progression of the process becomes a very difficult task.[23,24,41] Abrasive or three-body wear is considered the main reason for loss of composite mass in occlusal surfaces. This can happen during tooth brushing or by the action of abrasive food.[23] Proximal wear can also be seen depending on the contacting element; Figure 19-10b shows how it can be increased in the composite if a ceramic structure is involucrated.

*Comment*

If present criteria on minimal invasion and tooth structure conservation are considered, composite resin is the first choice. Unfortunately, degradation of the composite within the oral cavity limits the longevity of restoration. There is good clinical evidence of good results in small- and medium-sized posterior restorations. Composite seems to be contraindicated in large restorations that include functional cusps and in bruxing patients. Whenever possible, composite restoration repair is preferred to replacement to avoid unnecessary tooth structure sacrifice.

### *Dental Porcelains*

Dental porcelains are ceramic materials that show excellent chemical and optical properties; a good initial and long-lasting appearance can be obtained. They are indicated in various types of restoration. If processing technique is considered, products can be classified as sintered, injected, and machined (by CAD-CAM). With regard to the type of mechanical reinforcement, classification includes feldspar-based porcelains with a metallic understructure, porcelains with an alumina core, alumina and zirconia porcelains, and porcelains with high leucite or lithium disilicate content. Many of these systems can be processed with different techniques; lithium disilicate, for instance, can be injected or machined.

Porcelains are used as an alternative to cast metal alloy restorations mainly owing to their esthetics. If wear behavior is considered, gold alloys produce minimum enamel wear while traditional porcelains could be very abrasive.[42,43] The situation is then complicated by occlusal disorders. Feldspar-based porcelains that are used in ceramometallic crowns generate wear of the opposing tooth, and this is more evident if the opposing surface is composite resin.

The presence of defects within the porcelain structure compromises its strength. Defects can be generated during processing or during occlusal adjustment by grinding. Microscopic cracks can be present within the microstructure of the material.[16,44,45] Micro-cracks can be seen in feldspar-based porcelain surrounded by leucite crystals that are included in a vitreous matrix; they are generated by thermal changes during cooling owing to martensitic transformations.[45] Another factor is the presence of porosity that is present even after vacuum processing. Porosity decreases as sintering temperatures are increased. The relationship between phases can be modified by thermal treatments; if they are prolonged a different crystalline phase can appear and leucite content could diminish. This process depends on processing temperature and time.[46,47] Structural changes are followed by changes in optical and mechanical properties.

During load application and in a water environment, stress concentration is generated around pores and cracks. This stress concentration in the end-zone of cracks leads to the catastrophic failure that is characteristic of ceramics.[1] It has to be remembered that these are brittle materials and no plastic strain takes place before rupture.

Porcelain is practically insoluble in neutral pH water under 250°C. However, chemical dissolution can take place in an acidic environment; hydroxyl ions are produced and they then react with alkaline ions such as potassium or sodium to maintain neutrality. As a consequence, what is known as "chemical progression of cracks" is observed.[16,48]

Low-fusion porcelains have been developed in an attempt to decrease wear through lower hardness, lower concentration of crystalline phase, and a significant reduction in crystal size. These factors were discussed in a review published by Oh and co-workers,[16] and some of their conclusions – later corroborated by other authors – will be analyzed.

Hardness in dental porcelain has been considered the most important factor in the acceleration of loss of mass. However, research does not show a high correlation between hardness and enamel wear. It seems to be related to the ceramic microstructure, the roughness of the surfaces in contact, and environmental influence. Porosity as well as other defects are stress concentration determinants and increase wear. A glazed or polished surface only has influence initially since it is lost when occlusal contact appears.[16,49] External use should be limited to areas with no occlusal contact in esthetic restorations. Ceramic surfaces can degrade in an acidic or alkaline environment. Dietary habits and some diseases can modify a neutral pH, and wear can accelerate in bruxing patients (the overnight use of muscle relaxing devices is recommended as a solution). Finally, Oh and co-workers conclude that occlusion plays an important role in wear mechanisms. To keep it low, equilibrium in load distribution is needed with multiple contact areas. Sliding contacts in centric and eccentric positions have to be avoided or eliminated when installing a ceramic restoration.

Modern ceramic materials offer excellent esthetics and improvement in mechanical properties that have widened the scope of their use. Lithium disilicate-based porcelains have double the strength of conventional feldspar-based products, even if they are not better if esthetics is the main consideration. Alumina- or zirconia-reinforced porcelains can be chosen when higher mechanical requirements have to be met. Zirconia-based porcelains are considered to be tough ceramics since they can absorb stress without fracture. They are used when superior mechanical properties are a must, even when metal feldspar-based products are preferred for posterior work in bruxing patients. This preference is based on clinical experience, but long-term clinical studies are needed to evaluate the actual behavior of these new materials.

### *Dental Amalgam*

Dental amalgam has been used for over 150 years as a plastic restoration in premolars and molars.[50] It is a metallic alloy with silver, tin, and copper as main constituents. The alloy powder is mixed with mercury at room temperature and condensed into a cavity preparation. Hardening takes place at 37°C owing to the precipitation of solid phases that are generated when the alloy components interact with liquid mercury. As in any other solidification, the process ends when no more liquid is available.

Amalgams are characterized by their good mechanical behavior and wear resistance. This allows for easy and low-cost rehabilitation of occlusal function.[3] On the other hand they are not esthetic materials since the color is different from dental tissues, so they are limited to posterior restorations. Cavity preparations with specific morphology are needed so that amalgams can be mechanically retained. This, unfortunately, creates the need for removal of extra sound dental structure.

It is necessary to take precautions in the handling of mercury owing to its toxicity. Inhalation of mercury vapor or skin contact should be avoided. Manufacturers provide pre-measured mercury to make handling safer.

If the restoration is in direct contact with a noble metal, galvanic corrosion can result. Amalgam dissolution rate is increased, and the leaking of electrons can generate electric currents that a patient can feel in vital pulps; "a metallic taste" is another symptom that can be present. When these problems arise the choice of replacing the restoration with a ceramic or composite resin should be considered.

Metallic particles detached from amalgam can produce changes in neighboring tissues with time. Postoperative thermal sensitivity can be experienced owing to the metallic condition of amalgam. Some soft tissue reactions are occasionally seen, as well as hypersensitivity.

When all the foregoing aspects of amalgam are considered, it is not difficult to understand the urge to seek other materials that might ensure a better combination of mechanical, chemical, and physical properties.[51] However, at present amalgam cannot be completely discounted as a material in restorations that demand high mechanical strength and wear resistance.

### *Other Alloys*

Gold has been the first-choice material in dentistry for many years owing to its biocompatibility, longevity, and wear behaviors, which are similar to those of dental structures.[43,52] Gold alloys are used that include silver, copper, and other minor elements. Noble-metal content is over 75% by weight in most alloys. The alloys that are used in restorative dentistry and prosthodontics include both noble and base metals. They are usually worked by casting molten metal into a mold. Adequate precision is obtained using this procedure.[53]

The original alloys that were used in dentistry with high noble-metal content had good corrosion resistance, adequate mechanical properties, and the best wear behavior available within restorative materials. Metals allow for plastic strain under load without generation of internal cracks. Gold, palladium, and platinum can be found as the main components in noble-metal based alloys; other metallic elements are used to adjust properties to the intended use. The weight percentage of noble metal varies, and silver is not considered within this group since it oxidizes in the oral cavity and has to be used in combination with palladium.

An alloy to be used for a totally metallic inlay is designed with lower stiffness and hardness than one that is to be used as a metallic understructure in a ceramo-metallic prosthesis. Such an inlay avoids wear in the opposing tooth, and a metallic understructure will be rigid enough to avoid porcelain flexure. A high fusion temperature is required for porcelain firing, as well as the possibility of producing an oxide layer to favor a chemical bond between metal and porcelain.

Base-metal alloys that are used are cobalt, nickel, copper, and titanium based. An oxide layer covers these alloys, protecting them from corrosion. The phenomenon known as passivation is also found in the stainless steel that is used in orthodontic appliances. The contact of aggressive ions (e.g., chloride) is to be avoided since they can disrupt the oxide layer and eliminate protection

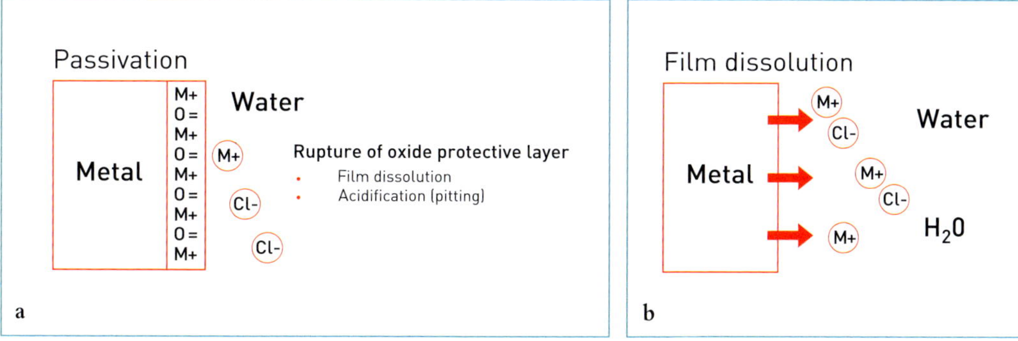


**Fig 19-12** **(a and b)** Protective oxide layer (passivation), possible rupture, and dissolution due to changes in the environment with localized acidification and pitting.

(Fig 19-12). With regard to wear behavior, it is advisable to avoid the use of the most rigid alloys on occlusal surfaces.

The best wear behavior is seen when alloys with high gold content are chosen, and they can be considered the best choice if esthetics is not taken into account.

## Conclusion

Success in posterior composite resin restorations depends mainly on their size. Minimun wear is seen in medium- and small-sized restorations. Composites are contraindicated for large restorations in bruxing patients. The use of inlays or amalgam, if possible, is to be considered in those cases.

The longevity of porcelain restorations can be affected by the presence of micro-cracks. Under some conditions, such as a very acidic environment or high loads, they could progress and lead to restoration fracture.

The newest ceramics show significant improvement in mechanical properties but clinical studies are needed to evaluate their long-term behavior. The use of porcelain with a metallic understructure is preferred in the posterior region of the mouth in bruxing patients. Some cases could be treated with zirconia-based ceramic, considering the unfavorable conditions present in this area.

A ceramic system has to be selected after considering both esthetic and mechanical requirements in the case to be treated, and this means differentiation between anterior and posterior restorative needs. The possibility of wear in the opposing teeth has to be considered in some cases.

Both amalgam and dental alloys can be chosen for posterior work if esthetics is not the prime consideration. They have good wear behavior and wear values of gold alloys and are the closest to dental enamel. The creation of galvanic couples by direct contact between metals with different electrode potential, as well as the use of very rigid alloys on occlusal surfaces, must be avoided.

As a final remark it can be stated that all the materials that have been used up to now, as well as tooth structures, will show increased wear in bruxing patients and have to be appropriately protected.

## References

1. Shackelford JF, Güemes A. Degradación y fallo de materiales. In: Introducción a la Ciencia de Materiales para Ingenieros. Madrid: Prentice-Hall, 1998:525–566.
2. Sajewicz E. On evaluation of wear resistance of tooth enamel and dental materials. Wear 2006;260:1256–1261.
3. Vale Antunes P, Ramalho A. Study of abrasive resistance of composites for dental restoration by ball-catering. Wear 2003;255:990–998.

4. Lambrechts P, Braem M, Vuylsteke-Wauters M, Vanherle G. Quantitative in-vitro wear of human enamel. J Dent Res 1989;68:1752–1754.
5. Heinze SD. Wear in ceramic materials. In: Ivoclar Vivadent Reports (eds). Metal Free Ceramics. Lichtenstein, 2006: 27–30.
6. Macchi RL. Materiales Dentales. Buenos Aires: Panamericana, 2007.
7. Jaeggi T, Grüninger A, Lussi A. Restorative therapy of erosion. In: Lussi A (ed). Dental Erosion. Monogr Oral Sci 2006;20:200–214.
8. Mount GJ, Ngo H. Minimal intervention: advanced lesions. Quintessence Int 2000;31:621–629.
9. Van Noort R. Basic science for dental materials. In: Introduction to Dental Materials. London: Mosby, 1994:2–4.
10. Fontana M. Corrosion Engineering. New York: McGraw-Hill, 1986.
11. Duffó GS, Galvele JR. Procesos de Corrosión. San Martín, Buenos Aires: Instituto de Tecnología Prof. Jorge Sábato, Universidad Nacional de Gral, 2002.
12. Baran G, Boberick K, McCool J. Fatigue of restorative materials. Crit Rev Oral Biol Med 2001;12:350–360.
13. Lussi A. Detal erosion: clinical diagnosis and case history taking. Eur J Oral Sci 1996;104:191–198.
14. Grana DR, Barreiro MM, Botana A et al. Efecto de bebida cola sobre el desarrollo y la mineralizaciòn en ratas inmaduras. La Prensa Médica Argentina 2004;91:68–73.
15. Grippo JO, Simring M, Schreiner S. Attrition, abrasion, corrosion and abfraction revisited: a new perspective on tooth surface lesions. J Am Dent Assoc 2004;135: 1109–1118.
16. Oh W, De Long R, Anusavice KJ. Factors affecting enamel and ceramic wear: a literature review. J Prosthet Dent 2002; 87:451–459.
17. Grippo JO, Simring M. Dental erosion revisited. J Am Dent Assoc 1995;126:619–630.
18. Imfeld T. Dental erosion: definition, classification and links (review). Eur J Oral Sci 1996;104:151–155.
19. Grippo JO. Erosion vs. corrosion. J Am Dent Assoc 2007; 138:1535.
20. Barlett DW, Shah P. A critical review of non-carious cervical (wear) lesions and the role of abfraction, erosion, and abrasion. J Dent Res 2006;85:306–312.
21. Mair LH. Understanding wear in Dentistry. Compendium 1999;20:19–30.
22. De Long R. Intra-oral restorative materials wear: rethinking the current approaches. How to measure wear. Dent Mater 2006;22:702–711.
23. Lambrechts P, Goovaerts K, Bharadwaj D et al. Degradation of tooth structure and restorative materials: a review. Wear 2006;255:980–986.
24. Pedroso Turssi C, De Moraes Purqueiro B, Campos Serra M. Wear of dental resine composites: insights into underlying processes and assesment methods, a review. J Biomed Mater Res Appl Biomater 2003;65B:280–285.
25. Lutz F, Phillips RW, Roulet JF, Setcos JC. In-vivo and in-vitro wear of potential posterior composites. J Dent Res 1984;63:914–920.
26. De Gee AJ, Pallav P. Occlusal wear simulation with the ACTA wear machine (review). J Dent 1994;22(Suppl 1): S21–7.
27. Pallav P, de Gee AJ, Werner A, Davidson CL.Influence of shearing action of food on contact stress and subsequent wear of stress-bearing composites. J Dent Res 1993;72: 56–61.
28. Söderholm KJ. Degradation mechanisms of dental resin composites. In: Eliades G, Theodore E, Brantley WA, Watts DC (eds). Dental Materials In Vivo: Aging and Related Phenomena. Hong Kong: Quintessence, 2003:99–122.
29. Hickel R, Manhart J. Longevity of restorations in posterior teeth and reasons for failure. J Adhes Dent 2001;3: 45–64.
30. Brunthaler A, Konig F, Lucas T, Sperr W, Schedle A. Longevity of direct resin composite restorations in posterior teeth. Clin Oral Investig 2003;7:63–70.
31. Heintze SD. How to qualify and validate wear simulation devices and methods. Dent Mater 2006;22:712–734.
32. Ferracane JL. Is the wear of dental composites still a clinical concern? Is there still a need for in-vitro wear simulating devices? Dent Mater 2006;22:689–692.
33. Pallesen U, Qvist V. Composite resin fillings and inlays: an 11-year evaluation. Clin Oral Investig 2003;7:71–79.
34. Van Dijken JW. Direct resin composite inlays/onlays: an 11 year follow-up. J Dent 2000;28:299–306.
35. Van Nieuwenhuysen JP, D'Hoore W, Carvalho J, Qvist V. Long-term evaluation of extensive restorations in permanent teeth. J Dent 2003;31:395–405.
36. Ryge G. Clinical criteria. Int Dent J 1980;30:347–358.
37. Degrange M, Roulet JF. Minimally invasive restorations with bonding. Chicago: Quintessence, 1997.
38. Phillips RW, Avery DR, Mehra R, Swartz ML, McCune RJ. Observations on a composite resin for Class II restorations: three-year report. J Prosthet Dent 1973;30:891–897.
39. Söderholm KJ, Richards ND. Wear resistance of composites: a solved problem? Gen Dent 1998;46:256–263.
40. Ferracane JL. Current trends in dental composites. Crit Rev Oral Biol Med 1995;6:302–318.
41. Lim BS, Ferracane JL, Condon JR, Adey JD. Effect of filler fraction and filler surface treatment on wear of microfilled composites. Dent Mater 2002;18:1–11.
42. Hudson JD, Goldstein GR, Georgescu M. Enamel wear caused by three restorative materials. J Prosthet Dent 1995;74:647–654.
43. Monasky GF, Taylor DF. Studies on the wear of porcelain, enamel, and gold. J Prosthet Dent 1971;25:299–306.
44. Drummond JL. Ceramic behavior under different environmental and loading conditions. In: Eliades G, Theodore E, Brantley WA, Watts DC (eds). Dental Materials In Vivo: Aging and Related Phenomena. Hong Kong: Quintessence, 2003:35–45.

45. Barreiro MM, Riesgo O, Vicente EE. Phase identification in dental porcelains for ceramo-metalic restorations. Dent Mater 1989;5:51–57.
46. Barreiro MM, Vicente EE. Kinetics of isothermal phase transformations in a dental porcelain. J Mater Sci Mater Med 1993;4:431–436.
47. Catell MJ, ChadwickTC, Knowies JC, Clarke RL. The crystallization of an aluminosilicate glass in the KO–AlO–SiO system. Dent Mater 2005;21:811–822.
48. Taskonak B, Griggs JA, Mecholsky JJ, Yan JH. Analysis of subcritical crack growth in dental ceramics using fracture mechanics and fractography. Dent Mater 2008;24:700–707.
49. Heintze SD, Cavalleri A, Forjanic M, Zellweger G, Rousson V. Wear of ceramic and antagonist: a systematic evaluation of influencing factors in vitro. Dent Mater 2008;24: 433–449.
50. Bergman M. Side-effects of amalgam and its alternatives: local, systemic and environmental. Int Dent J 1990;40: 4–10.
51. Anusavice KJ. Phillip's Science of Dental Materials. St Louis: Elsevier, 2003:666–670.
52. Jacobi R, Shillingburg HT, Duncanson MG. A comparison of the abrasiveness of six ceramic surfaces and gold. J Prosthet Dent 1991;66:303–309.
53. Brantley WA. Aging of casting alloys used in prosthodontics and restorative dentistry. In: Eliades G, Theodore E, Brantley WA, Watts DC (eds). Dental Materials In Vivo: Aging and Related Phenomena. Hong Kong: Quintessence, 2003:23–34.

Chapter 20

# Evidence Related to the Treatment of Bruxism

*Daniel A. Paesani*

## Introduction

"Treatment" can be defined as any attempt to solve a health problem, generally preceded by a diagnosis. If we follow this definition, the first step is to confirm that bruxism is really the cause of the patient's problem. As mentioned in Chapter 2, diagnosing bruxism is not easy, and this is closely linked to paradigms deeply rooted in the dental profession: practitioners' historical tendency to link bruxism with tooth wear and masticatory system dysfunctions. Although earlier chapters have dealt with these fallacies, their ongoing influence cannot be over-emphasized.

As in any medical specialty, thorough knowledge of the patient's history is key, since it will provide extremely important data regarding the subject's general health status. A detailed list of any medications taken by the patient will allow identifying or excluding potential secondary bruxism (pharmacologic bruxism). By means of accurate diagnosis, the need for treating bruxism specifically or for managing other etiologies which may be related to bruxism will be determined. In the latter case, treatment protocols may also need to involve other healthcare specialists.

Before discussing the treatment of bruxism, we must distinguish between sleep bruxism and awake bruxism, since they are different entities, each having its own etiology, diagnosis, effects, and treatment. Distinguishing between these two types of activity is important, because interchanging their respective protocols will usually prevent the therapeutic goal from being attained.

## Treatments for Sleep Bruxism

Sleep bruxism consists of a stereotyped movement which results in tooth grinding and/or tooth clenching; the American Academy of Sleep Medicine has classified it as a sleep-related disorder.[1] Although its etiology remains unclear, there is evidence suggesting the existence of a regulating mechanism dependent on the central nervous system (CNS).[2] The latest research studies have shown bruxism to be related to very brief cortical activation episodes (3–15 seconds) known as "micro-arousals", which are associated with increased sympathetic nervous system activity.[3]

As discussed in Chapter 18, several pharmacologic trials aimed at intercepting bruxism have been conducted; and, although up to the present they have not been fully successful, this proved to be the right track. Several teams of researchers are carrying out trials, so perhaps in the near future a "pill" that fully inhibits sleep bruxism may be available.

### Risk Factor Control

Alcohol, tobacco, and caffeine consumption has been shown to exacerbate the development of sleep bruxism. Nicotine stimulates the dopaminergic system; this would account for bruxism being twice as prevalent in cigarette smokers as it is in non-smokers, and for bruxism episodes per night being five times as frequent.[4] Also, the number of bruxism-related symptoms is three times as high in smokers as it is in non-smokers.[5]

Bruxism development has also been related to the consumption of one glass (or more) of alcoholic drink per day,[6] although some claim that, in order for alcohol to become a risk factor, at least four glasses of alcoholic drink per day need to be consumed.[7] People who drink a lot of coffee (six cups a day) are exposed to a higher risk of tooth grinding during sleep.[6]

Based on this evidence, Morin[8] suggests keeping adequate sleep hygiene, avoiding consumption of the above-mentioned stimulants at least a couple of hours before going to bed. He recommends sticking to an orderly, regular sleep schedule in order to attain and maintain a deep, refreshing sleep-stage regime.

Thus, when assisting patients with a history of sleep bruxism, the first step will be to recommend limiting the consumption of these risk factors. This will not really stop bruxism, but it will help to prevent it becoming worse.

### Occlusal Splints

Since no specific, definitive treatment capable of canceling bruxism is yet available, all efforts are directed towards the prevention of bruxism's destructive effects. Occlusal splints (also known as "bruxism splints", "splints", "night guards", "dental orthoses", "occlusal devices", etc.) are, undoubtedly, the means more commonly used to preserve dental structures.

A survey conducted among dental practitioners in the USA found that around three million splints are fabricated each year, most of them in managing bruxism cases.[9] Another survey recently conducted in Sweden showed that acrylic rigid splints would be indicated, first, for counteracting tooth wear, and, second, for treating muscle pain.[10]

Before going into this subject in detail, it is important to make it clear that we will deal with splints used as treatment for bruxism exclusively. We will not deal with splints used in the management of patients with temporomandibular disorders (TMD), 78% of whom have dysfunction and pain as a result of internal disorders and temporomandibular joint (TMJ) osteoarthritis[11] (of course, these patients can also suffer from bruxism). While splints are used in bruxers just to protect their teeth, in the case of patients with TMD the therapeutic approach aims at restoring the function and eliminating pain.

However, due to very deep-rooted traditional paradigms, many clinicians still consider bruxism and TMD to be synonymous in cause and effect. In fact, not all bruxers have TMD, and not all patients suffering from TMD are bruxers. The relationship between bruxism and TMD is far from being clear; in a significant number of patients, it is very possible that both entities can simply coexist.[12] Any treatment plan for patients with TMD which considers bruxism as an intermediate variable should be considered to be mere speculation.[13]

*Objectives of splint use*

The use of splints in bruxers is aimed mainly at protecting their teeth. Evidence suggests that wearing a splint during sleep does not guarantee that the parafunctional activity will be interrupted.[14] Studies of patients with TMD treated with occlusal splints confirmed that 54% of the participants showed bruxism scars as early as 1 week after they started wearing the splint, and after 10 weeks bruxism marks were present on the occlusal surfaces of the devices of 88% of the participants. Most of the splints (52%) reflected a bilateral grinding bruxism pattern.[15] In a study of 31 subjects who were aware of their sleep bruxism habit, who had morning symptoms and wore full-occlusal-coverage splints during sleep time, all of the splints showed signs of bruxism on their surface. In the control visits every 2 weeks, the splints of most of the subjects (61%) were found to be worn out; facets were observed in the rest of the splints (31%) over longer periods of time. This confirms that bruxism varies over time. The study of wear patterns showed that most subjects (71%) grinded their teeth laterally in both directions; 13% of the subjects showed a unilateral pattern, 3% showed a protrusive, straight-line pattern, and another 13% presented static tooth clenching.[16] A very similar study was conducted in which a scanner was used to measure wear volume and depth; a lateral tooth grinding pattern was found to prevail. Owing to the objectivity of such measurements, wear was shown to be asymmetric in volume and depth despite being bilateral. The canine and molar areas were the ones most affected by wear; there was an intermediate area – the premolar area – where less substance loss occurred. These results may be ascribed to several factors, among them increased muscle force in the posterior segment plus the fact that molars have a larger number of cusps. Wear in the canine area can be ascribed to the sharp shape of canine cusp tips.[17]

Sleep bruxism is characterized by tooth grinding being more frequent than clenching, which was proved through polysomnography (PSG).[18] These two different types of sleep bruxism have been confirmed through electromyography (EMG). During tooth clenching, tonic, simultaneous contraction of both masseters is seen on the EMG; in contrast, during tooth grinding such contractions occur unilaterally and alternately, at intervals of approximately 1 second.[19] Figure 20-1 shows different impressions left on splints by SB tooth grinding and clenching activities.

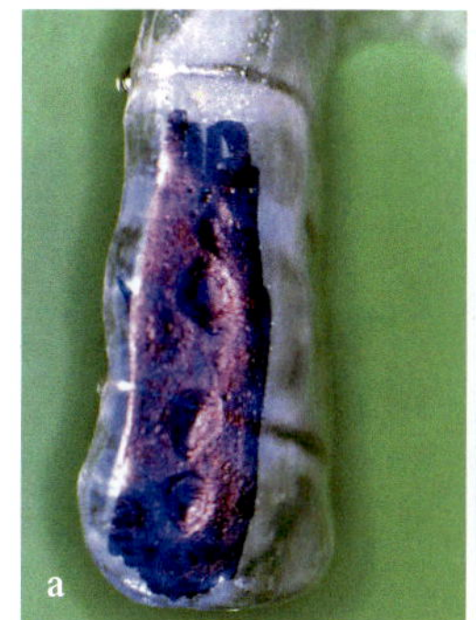

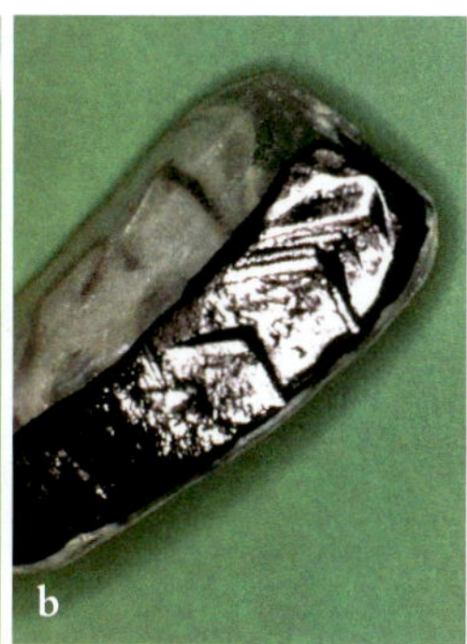


Fig 20-1 Splints: **(a)** tooth clenching impressions left during sleep; **(b)** tooth grinding scars. These splints have been stained for better appreciation of wear.

Splints can be said to be to bruxism what umbrellas are to rain. Both splints and umbrellas can offer protection, but the process cannot be prevented by them. Thus, the major advantage of splints is their ability to protect teeth – both natural teeth and prosthetic restorations, including implants. Splints not only prevent wear, they also prevent potential fractures in teeth, restorations, prostheses, and implants. They also provide temporary splinting of teeth, thus preventing undesirable mobility caused by the strong forces generated during bruxism activities. Splints are also beneficial for the pulp and the periodontium, since they distribute the forces evenly and prevent them from affecting the teeth individually. They also eliminate the pain that patients commonly complain of on waking. Splints also help alleviate fatigue and morning muscle pain.

The relationship between bruxism and pain is very complex (see Chapter 17). Bruxers will not usually feel pain, but whenever they do, they suffer from morning pain on waking.[20] Although the evidence on the mechanism causing such pain is very controversial, patients who wear night guards will not feel pain or muscle fatigue on waking. Last, but not least, splints will reduce the unpleasant grinding noise that is so annoying to room or bed partners.

*Evidence on the effects of splints worn during sleep*
As far as bruxism treatment is concerned, it is important to be aware of the effect of splints on the masticatory muscles, which are the ones producing bruxism. In the past, splints were thought to inhibit bruxism because they would reduce jaw bone pain, which was deemed to result from muscle hyperactivity. One of the names for splints, "muscle relaxant splint", probably originated from this. Some studies of patients wearing bruxism splints during sleep are now available which deal with the effects of splints on EMG activity. The two variables measured are masseter muscle activity and sleep factors. However, a review of the literature shows that not many research studies have been conducted on this subject: only 16 studies were published in 30 years (Table 20-1).

The effects of splints on bruxism was first studied through ambulatory surface EMG, and more recently through PSG. The first study in which masseter activity was objectively measured through EMG was published in 1975 by Solberg and coworkers,[21] who used first-generation EMG – a system that had the ability only to take amplitude cumulative measurements expressed in microvolts (μV). Eight bruxers wearing rigid full-occlusal-coverage splints were studied in their sleep. While wearing the device, all of them showed decreased masseter activity. The EMGs done after the subjects stopped wearing the splints showed increased masseter activity in seven of the eight participants.

This trial was reproduced by other researchers who trebled the number of study subjects. Different results were obtained, since only 52% of the participants showed decreased EMG activity, 28% showed no changes, and the remainder (20%) showed increased EMG activity.[22]

Another trial using similar equipment compared the effects of hard and soft splints. While the former decreased bruxism in eight of the 10 participants, soft splints increased bruxism in five subjects.[23]

Various splint designs have been studied. Canine-disclusion splints and molar-disclusion splints have been compared. Similar results were obtained for both splints increased activity in one-third of the subjects and decreased activity in another third; in the rest of the participants no differences were found.[24]

Technologic developments have allowed for improved ambulatory EMG. Kydd and Daly[19] studied 10 female bruxers and compared them to 10 female non-bruxers. For this purpose, they used ambulatory equipment with several channels and the ability to record multiple events (EMG, electrocardiogram, body movements) and measure the duration of bruxism episodes. Bruxism episodes were detected in all the participants, both bruxers and non-bruxers; however, while average masseter activity in bruxers was 11.4 minutes per night, in non-bruxers it was just 3.1 minutes per night. The use of splints made no difference to the duration of bruxism episodes, although the participants felt more comfortable while wearing the splints. The authors detected a sudden and significant increase in pulse rate at the end of each episode; then, the pulse rate quickly returned to normal. They were also able to distinguish clearly between tooth clenching episodes (bilateral masseter contraction) and grinding episodes (unilateral, alternate contractions).

A group of scientists – led by the deeply rooted paradigm that considers occlusion to be the origin of bruxism – compared the effects of full-occlusal-coverage splints and "placebo splints". (The latter are more correctly called "palatal splints", since

*Table 20-1*

**Evidence of the effects of different splint designs on bruxism during sleep.**

| Study | Method | Splint | Effect on EMG activity during splint wear (%) | Number of study subjects | Effect on EMG activity after splint wear (%) |
|---|---|---|---|---|---|
| Solberg et al[21] | EMG | Occlusal | ↓100 | 8 | ↑87.5 |
| Clark et al[22] | EMG | Occlusal | ↓52 = 28 ↑20 | 25 | ↑100 |
| Kydd and Daly[19] | EMG | Occlusal | = 100 | 20 | ND |
| Okeson[23] | EMG | Rigid | ↓80 = 20 | 10 | ND |
| | | Resilient | ↑50 = 40 ↓10 | | |
| Rugh et al[24] | EMG | Canine disclusion | ↓37.5 = 12.5 ↑50 | 8 | ↑92 |
| | | Molar disclusion | ↓37.5 = 25 ↑37.5 | | |
| Cassisi et al[25] | EMG | Occlusal | ↓100 | 1 | ↑100 |
| | | Palatal | | | |
| Pierce and Gale[26] | EMG | Occlusal | ↓100 | 20 | ↑100 |
| Hiyama et al[27] | EMG | Occlusal | ↓100 | 6 | ↑100 |
| Harada et al[28] | EMG | Occlusal | ↓100 | 16 | ↑100 |
| | | Palatal | | | |
| Okkerse et al[31] | PSG | Jeanmonod's | ↓100 | 10 | ND |
| Sjöholm et al[34] | PSG | Occlusal | ↓36 = 21 ↑43 | 14 | ND |
| Dube et al[35] | PSG | Occlusal | ↓51 | 9 | ND |
| | | Palatal | ↓55 | | |
| Van der Zaag et al[36] | PSG | Occlusal | ↓19–29 = 50 ↑33–48 | 11 | ND |
| | | Palatal | | 10 | |
| Landry et al[38] | PSG | Anterior repositioning | ↓77–83 | 13 | ND |
| | | Occlusal | ↓42 | | |
| Baad-Hansen et al[32] | EMG | Occlusal | Non-significant decrease | 10 | ND |
| | | NTI | Very significant decrease | | |
| Hasegawa et al[29] | EMG | 4 types of palatal splints | Significant decrease obtained with the thick palatal splint | 8 | ND |

PSG = polysomnography; ND = no data

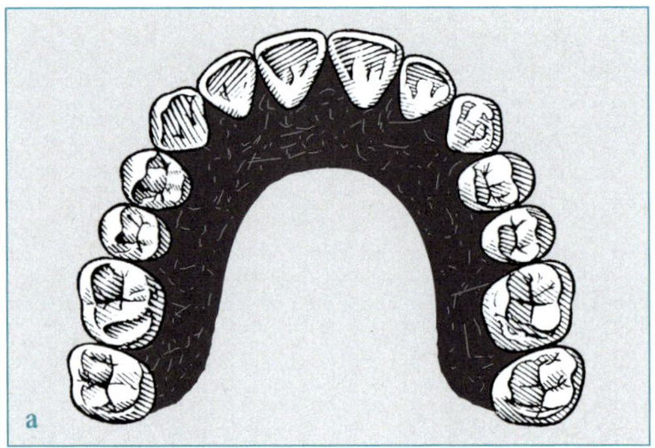
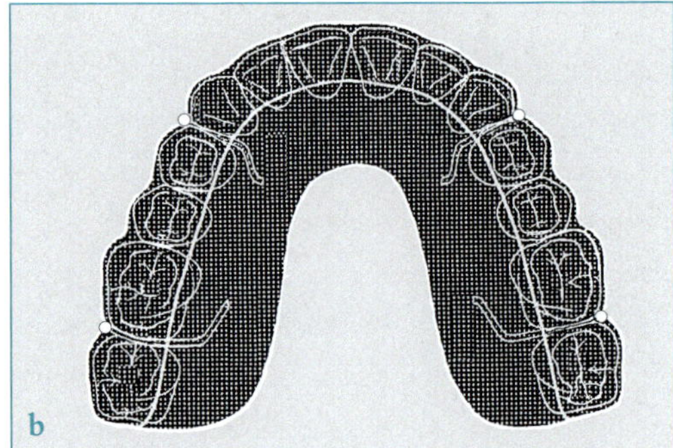

Fig 20-2 **(a)** Palatal-coverage splint that does not affect occlusion. **(b)** Full-occlusal-coverage splint.

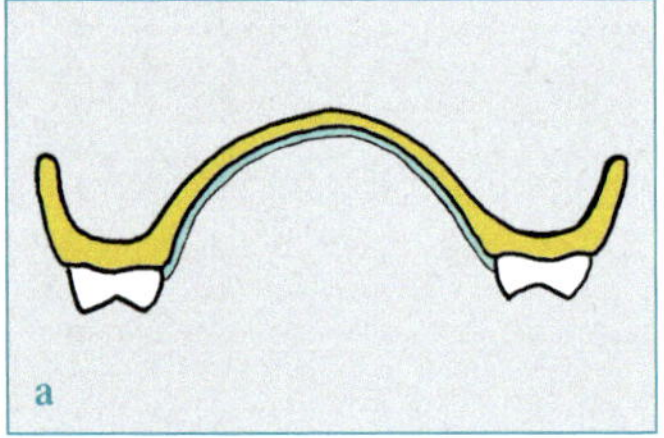
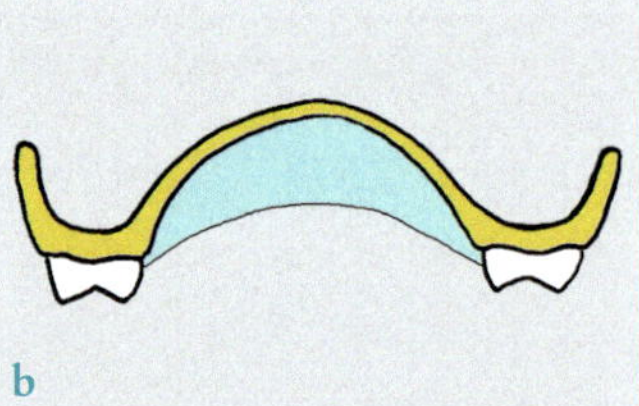
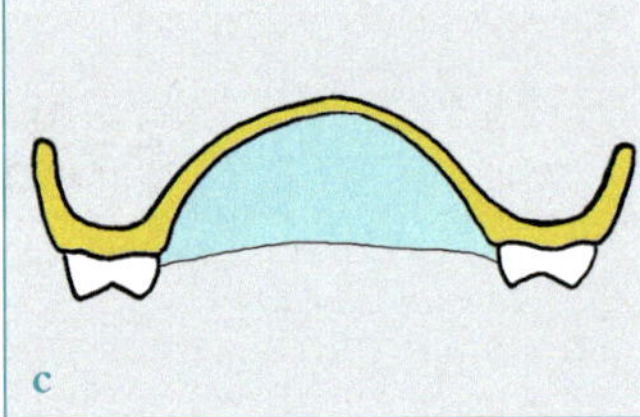

Fig 20-3 Palatal-coverage splint thickness variations: **(a)** thin, **(b)** medium, and **(c)** thick.

they cover only the hard palate without modifying dental occlusion.) Use of either type resulted in decreased EMG activity; when the use of either type was interrupted, EMG activity returned to its initial values. This study was conducted on just one bruxer, so its results have limited scientific relevance. However, it showed so much creativity that it set a precedent for future, more controlled studies.[25]

Within a period of 2 weeks, Pierce and Gale[26] were able to reduce the frequency and duration of bruxism episodes in 20 bruxers by means of occlusal splints. However, the activity returned to its initial values when the patients interrupted the use of the splints.

Trials have recently been carried out with four-channel equipment that allows evaluation of both masseter and temporalis muscles. Researchers who use this new equipment stress the fact that it has the capability of filtering the noise from body movements, allowing one to record muscle activity without interference and to overcome the drawbacks of older equipment. By means of this technology, reduced masseter and temporalis muscle activity during sleep when rigid splints were worn was demonstrated.[27]

Another group of researchers used similar equipment in a controlled study.[28] Once again, the effects of full-occlusal-coverage splints and of partial-palatal-coverage splints (not affecting occlusion) proved to be similar. Figure 20-2 exemplifies the use of these splints. Both types of devices proved to reduce sleep bruxism in the study subjects. The splints were fast-acting, but after 2 weeks bruxism levels returned to their initial values. The authors ascribed this to an adaptation of the stomatognathic system to the splint.

Perhaps motivated by the results of studies on splints that do not interfere with occlusion, researchers carried out studies on the relationship between sleep bruxism and palatal-coverage splint thickness variations (Fig 20-3). The thickest

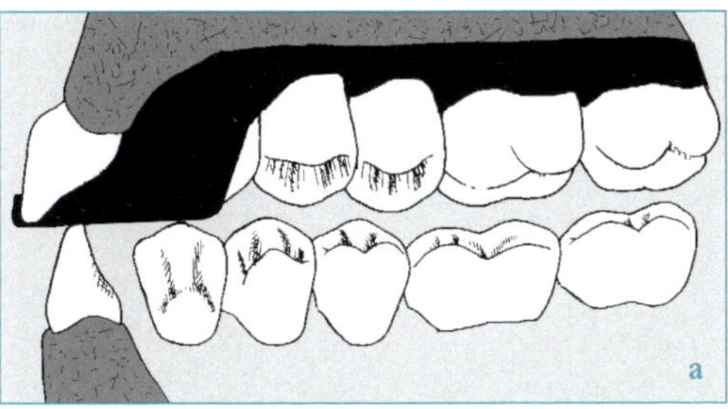


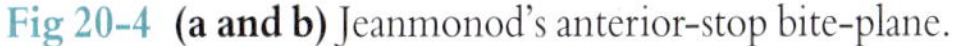

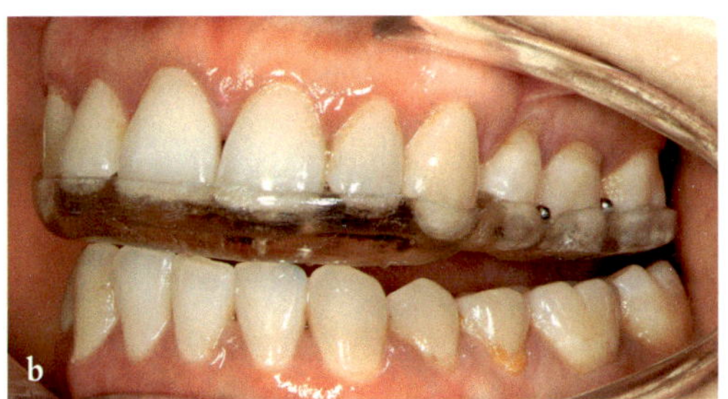


Fig 20-4 **(a and b)** Jeanmonod's anterior-stop bite-plane.

palatal-coverage splints produced a significant decrease in EMG activity with respect to basal records without splint use.[29]

Undoubtedly, the most accurate studies are those conducted in a sleep laboratory. Trials carried out in sleep labs are constantly monitored by specialized staff and they allow recording of multiple aspects of body physiology (sleep, breathing, deglutition, pulse rate, etc.). These studies are routinely supplemented by audio and video recordings that can distinguish between bruxism episodes and other episodes not consistent with bruxism. The disadvantages of these trials include cost, a strange environment for participants, and the difficulties related to the requirement for patients to report to the lab. These drawbacks make it difficult to carry out studies on a great number of subjects and over long periods. Despite this, some studies on the effects of splints have been conducted which contributed valuable scientific information.

A group of 10 bruxers was evaluated in a sleep lab over two nights. The recordings were taken before and after the use of an "anterior-stop" bite-plane made according to Jeanmonod's principles[30] and which can be appreciated in detail in Figure 20-4. This splint allows contact of the six anterior teeth only, premolars and molars being in complete disclusion. The participants wore splints 24 hours a day for 3–4 weeks. At the end of this period, another sleep recording was taken. All the patients showed decreased bruxism while wearing Jeanmonod's bite-plane. On comparing the recordings taken while the patients were wearing Jeanmonod's splint with the recordings taken when the patients were not wearing the splint, no differences in the distribution of sleep stages were found. Jeanmonod's splint is the only splint whose use resulted in decreased individual bruxism activity in all the research participants. However, due to its peculiar design, it is not advisable to wear it for more than 3–4 weeks, since prolonged use may result in the eruption of the posterior antagonist teeth.

In the USA, the use of a type of splint that is said to be effective in the treatment of headaches has lately become widespread. The name "nociceptive trigeminal inhibition (NTI) splint" has been suggested for it. In fact, it is just a variation of Jeanmonod's splint, the only difference being that nociceptive trigeminal inhibition splints do not extend beyond the incisors (Fig 20-5). EMG sleep evaluation showed significant muscle activity inhibition in patients who wore NTIs, in contrast with those patients who wore conventional splints – though it needs to be pointed out that these effects were evaluated over a short period.[32] Others have reported occlusal changes in a patient who wore this device for a long period.[33]

An abstract published by Sjöholm and coworkers[34] reports the EMG effects of occlusal stabilization splints. Recordings were taken before participants started wearing such devices and after

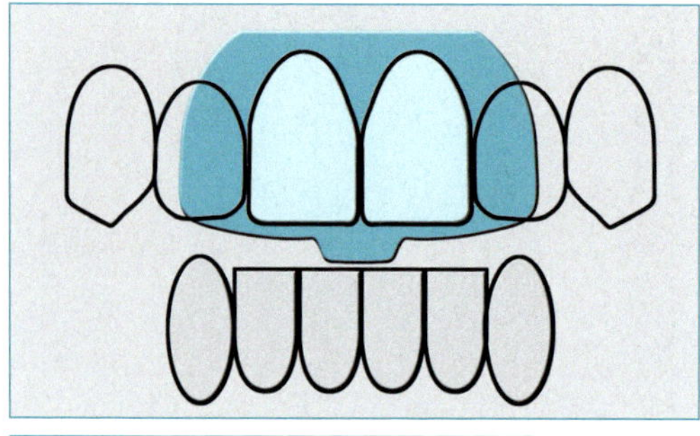

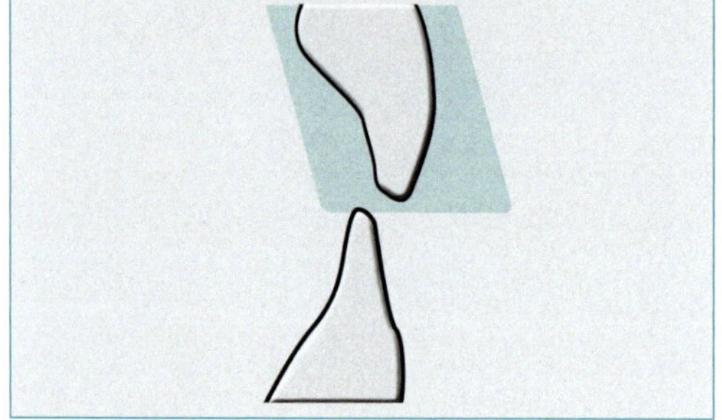

Fig 20-5 The NTI splint.

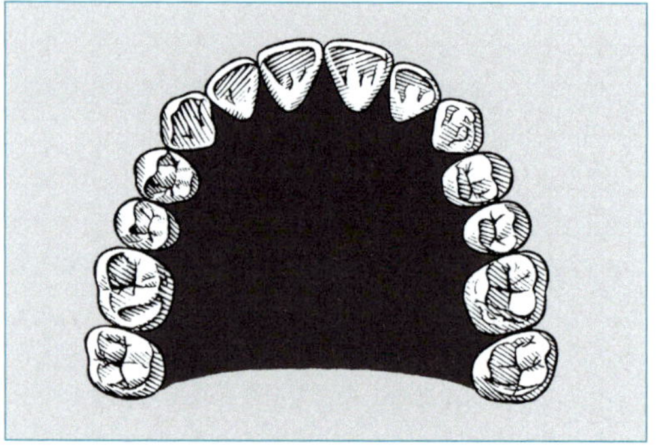

Fig 20-6 Splint fully covering the palate but not affecting occlusion.

2 months of wearing them. Bruxism levels decreased in only 36% of participants; 43% of participants showed increased activity, and no changes were observed in the remainder (21%). The use of these splints significantly altered sleep-stage proportions: a decrease in the duration of rapid-eye-movement sleep was observed, while slow-wave sleep lasted longer.

The effects of occlusal-coverage splints and palatal-coverage splints (Fig 20-6) were also compared through PSG. Both types of splint produced a decrease in tooth grinding frequency during sleep (with the exception of one patient who showed increased activity). Recordings were taken before the participants started wearing the splints and after two weeks of alternating one type of splint and the other. Again, the results of this research proved the lack of correlation between bruxism and dental occlusion. With regard to sleep, splint wear did not affect the number of arousals, although they caused restorative sleep (i.e., slow-wave sleep; non-REM stages 3 and 4) to decrease by one-third.

Another controlled, randomized double-blind study using PSG was also unable to find significant differences between two groups of subjects confirmed to be tooth grinders by their bed partners.[36] Subjects in one group wore occlusal-coverage splints, as in Figure 20-2b; the other group wore splints covering only the palate, similar to the one shown in Figure 20-2a. However, when the results were analyzed individually, the activity increased by 50% in some subjects, while in other subjects it decreased by 50%. Again, these results clearly show the differences between a significant statistical relationship at group level and clinical significance at individual level. Neither of the two types of splint altered sleep parameters, nor did they cause breathing variables, apnea, or hypoapnea to increase – their levels remained low during the whole duration of the study.

Patients suffering from sleep apnea will commonly be prescribed intraoral mandibular or lingual advancement devices which increase airway space. Mandibular advancement splints have proved to be very popular, and they have been useful in preventing sleep apnea.[37] A group of scientists conducted research on the effect of these devices on bruxism, and they compared them to traditional occlusal splints.[38] In their controlled, randomized, crossover study of 13 heavy bruxers,

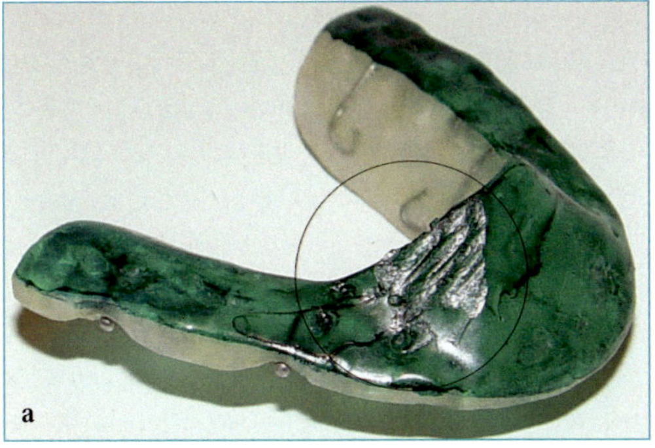

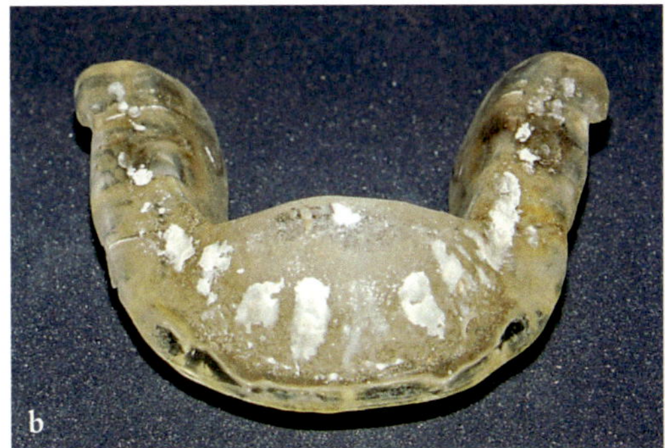

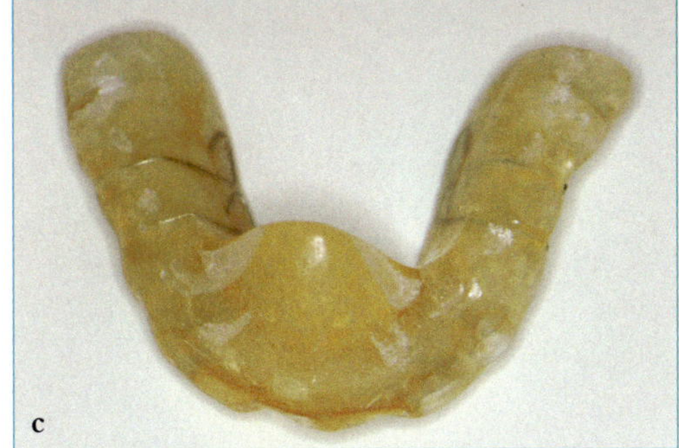

Fig 20-7 **(a–c)** Anterior repositioning appliances showing signs of wear from bruxism.

PSG recordings were taken before and during the alternate use of both types of splint; also recordings were obtained for different degrees of mandibular protrusion. Both splints were found to decrease bruxism levels significantly. Traditional occlusal splints caused the number of bruxism episodes per hour to decrease by 42%. Mandibular advancement splints performed much better; at minimum advancement, bruxism decreased by 77%, while at maximum protrusion it decreased by 83%. At individual level, one of the study subjects showed bruxism exacerbation, with tooth grinding episodes while wearing the splints. Sleep parameters remained stable; no variations were observed with any of the devices used. Interestingly, when requested to choose between the occlusal splint and the mandibular advancement device, none of the patients showed a preference for the latter.

This trial – the first and only one at the time of writing – proved that this type of device performs much better in terms of bruxism inhibition than traditional occlusal splints. According to the results of this study, such a device seems to be the most appropriate for the treatment of subjects suffering from sleep apnea who are also bruxers. However, owing to the above-mentioned drawbacks related to the type of technology used, this research study monitored the effects for only a very short period; thus, there are doubts regarding potential long-term effects. Such uncertainty originates in the evidence from clinics where patients with internal TMJ disorders are assisted. In these clinics, mandibular anterior repositioning appliances are commonly used in the treatment of intermittent joint locking occurring on waking. After some weeks, the effects of bruxism will usually be clearly visible on these appliances; this clearly proves that such devices have failed to inhibit bruxism (Fig 20-7).

Reaching a final conclusion from the results of all these research studies is not an easy task because they are very different. Such differences include:

- different splint designs
- different evaluation and recording methods
- lack of homogeneity between the different study populations
- different monitoring durations and different intervals between measurements
- different "bruxism episode" definitions.

So, the mechanism of action of splints remains unclear. Furthermore, such action may not even be directly related to a specific splint design. The fact that coverage and non-coverage splints seemed to produce similar effects suggests, once again, that there is scarce or no relationship at all between dental occlusion and sleep bruxism etiology. Further evidence of this is found in the results of recent sleep research studies, which corroborate that tooth contact (bruxism) does not set parafunction cycles in motion; quite the contrary: tooth grinding is the last link of a chain of physiologic events which start with a temporary microarousal.[3,39,40] Those studies in which decreased bruxism levels while a splint was being used were reported seem to agree that such effect stops taking place when the splint is no longer worn.

Finally, there is total consensus that bruxism splints play a positive role in protecting dental hard tissues.

*EMG studies of splints with canine guidance*

The addition of canine guidance to bruxism splints was first suggested in 1966 by Ramfjord and Ash[41] with the aim of preventing dental interference on the non-working side during the lateral movements of the jaw. This proposal gave rise to much debate over the validity of the use of canine guidance in bruxism splints.

Williamson and Lundquist,[42] who compared the EMG effects of splints with canine guidance and splints with group function, were the first to advocate canine guidance. Canine guidance significantly reduced temporalis muscle and masseter muscle EMG activity. The authors emphasize that this result should not be ascribed to stimulation due to canine contact, but to the effect produced by the canine eliminating interferences at the level of posterior teeth. Shupe and co-workers[43] obtained similar results in a controlled trial comparing splints with canine guidance and splints with group function; the use of canine guidance caused muscle activity to decrease during the lateral tooth grinding episodes. Some years later, another group of researchers also compared the effects of splints with group function with those of splints with canine guidance; the latter were found to reduce levator muscle activity during lateral movements.[44]

Such muscle activity decrease was initially ascribed to increased vertical dimension (VD). Upon analysis of the three last studies, VD should be excluded as a factor in EMG-activity decrease, since both types of splint compared in these trials were found to equally increase VD. In short, the success of canine disclusion splints seems to be attributable to the contact of this tooth with the splint during lateral movements. Subsequent investigations reported a significant reduction in the muscle activity developed through tooth clenching during the maximum dental intercuspation when such activity was performed laterally over canine guidance.[45–47]

In an attempt to elucidate the true cause of muscle-activity reduction, Graham and Rugh[48] carried out an interesting laboratory experiment. They compared splints in disclusion with canines with splints in disclusion with first molars. Both types of splint were found to reduce muscle activity in a similar way during lateral movements under tooth clenching in the lateral jaw position. The final conclusion drawn by the authors was that the reduced EMG activity resulted from the contact with one tooth only (canine or first molar), thus no longer ascribing the results exclusively to canines.

However, in a study of asymptomatic subjects during wakefulness, Borromeo and co-workers[49] reported similar decreased EMG activity both when splints with canine guidance and splints with group function were used.

Is it important to emphasize that study subjects were awake while these trials were being carried out. This is not ideal, since it does not reproduce real conditions. Splints are usually worn during sleep; rarely are they used in the treatment of awake bruxism. For this reason, Rugh and co-workers corroborated the results they had obtained in the lab, but this time they studied participants during sleep.[24] Both types of splint (canine disocclusion and molar disocclusion) produced similar effects while worn during sleep. However – as was the case with other studies already mentioned – results showed significant variations at the individual level. Reduced EMG activity was reported in three of the eight study subjects; another three subjects showed increased EMG activity; and no changes were observed in another subject. These results were similar for both types of splints. The remaining subject showed increased EMG activity while wearing the splint with canine guidance and no variation while wearing the molar disclusion splint.

Other studies conducted on awake subjects showed that the maximum voluntary bite force in intercuspal position recorded in the masseter muscle increased by 13% when patients bit over a smooth bruxism splint.[45] These results are consistent with the results reported by Manns and co-workers.[44] Undoubtedly, the occlusal stability achieved through the use of splints allows for muscles to exert all their power; in tune with this, Bakke and co-workers[50] found a correlation between intercuspal-position stability and masseter-muscle EMG activity level.

In agreement with the latter, another research study conducted on a group of asymptomatic subjects compared the daytime effects of anterior-stop bite planes and mandibular stabilization splints. In the mandibular resting position, neither of the splints caused EMG variations. However, during maximum voluntary contraction, when compared with mandibular stabilization splints, the anterior-stop bite planes significantly reduced EMG activity. This effect has also been ascribed to the scarce number of teeth in contact with the splint, and especially due to their being located in the anterior sector.[51]

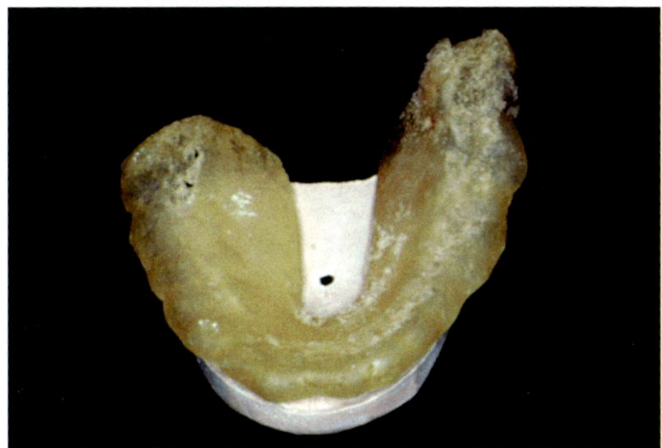

Fig 20-8 Soft vinyl splint that has been significantly deformed by bruxism. When compared to the cast of the patient's maxilla, it looks stretched.

*Soft splints*

Made of thermoplastic vinyl, soft splints were originally developed as tooth protectors to be used in the practice of some contact sports. However, since they are inexpensive and they can be easily and rapidly manufactured, today they are fabricated in many dental offices as protection against bruxism. In Sweden, general practitioners will usually make soft splints for patients suffering from tooth wear ascribed to bruxism.[10]

However, this type of device may produce unwanted occlusal changes.[52] Shore also warns that soft splints may become perforated due to the action of sleep bruxism, thus turning them into orthodontic-action devices.[53] There is evidence that occlusal changes in the form of dental intrusion occurred after use of these splints.[54] One publication reported mild premolar and molar intrusions in 67% of the participants in a trial who wore

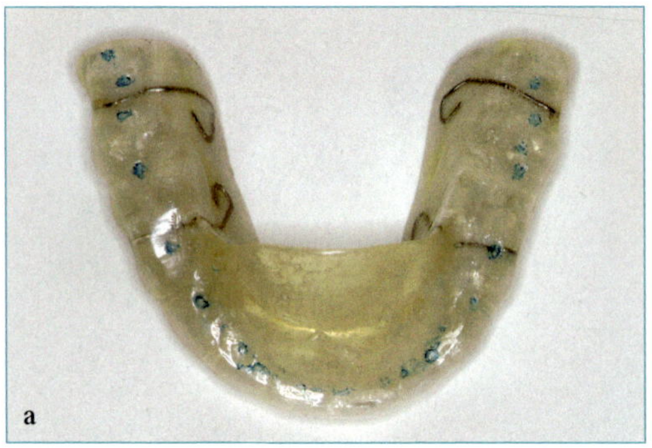

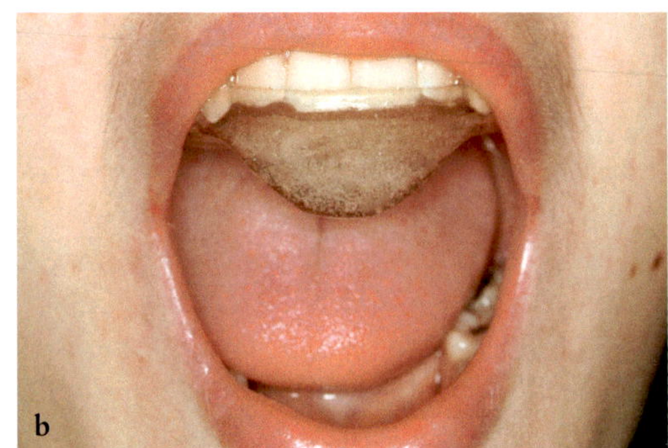

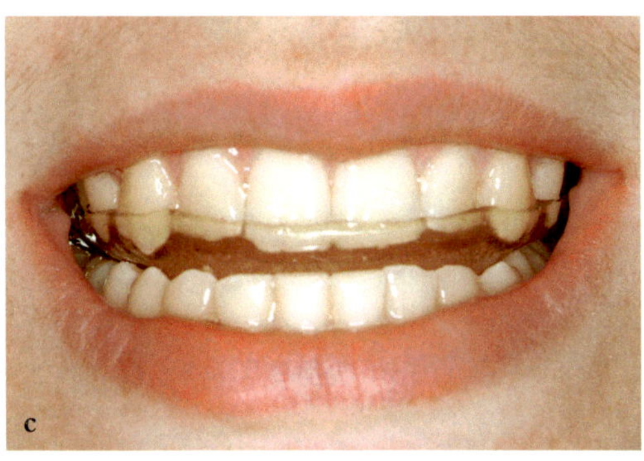

Fig 20-9 **(a)** Mandibular repositioning splint used in patients with morning intermittent locking. **(b and c)** Patient who wears a repositioning appliance during sleep. Previously, she wore a conventional bruxism splint and would systematically find her temporomandibular joint was locked on waking.

soft splints.[55] Others have reported opposite results and failed to prove the occurrence of such occlusal changes.[56,57] Ramfjord and Ash[58] suggested that these splints are unlikely to inhibit bruxism, since clenching on a resilient surface is stimulating for patients; this, however, was not scientifically proved. Okeson would later confirm this hypothesis.[23] Through ambulatory EMG, he reported that this type of splint increased sleep bruxism by 50% in his study population.

Figure 20-8 shows a vinyl splint worn by a bruxer for a year. Note the difference in size when the splint is compared with the patient's actual cast; this is due to the splint having stretched considerably. With regard to acceptance by patients, some authors report that some people will complain that these splints are too bulky and make the oral cavity stick out.[55,56] Others report that vinyl splints and acrylic splints have the same level of acceptance.[57]

Many research studies have been conducted on the effects of soft splints in patients with temporomandibular disorders (TMD). However, some of the variables evaluated in these studies (e.g., mouth opening, muscle pain on palpation, pain grading) are not specific bruxism signs, which is why they have not been included in this review.

It is very difficult to take a solid stand based on the outcomes of the published literature. However, no valid reason seems to exist for prescribing soft splints as bruxism treatment, since, far from reducing bruxism, they seem to exacerbate it. Besides, despite soft splints being easily and rapidly fabricated (which quite simplifies daily tasks for clinicians), the reported potential occlusal changes they may produce may be another problem associated with their use.

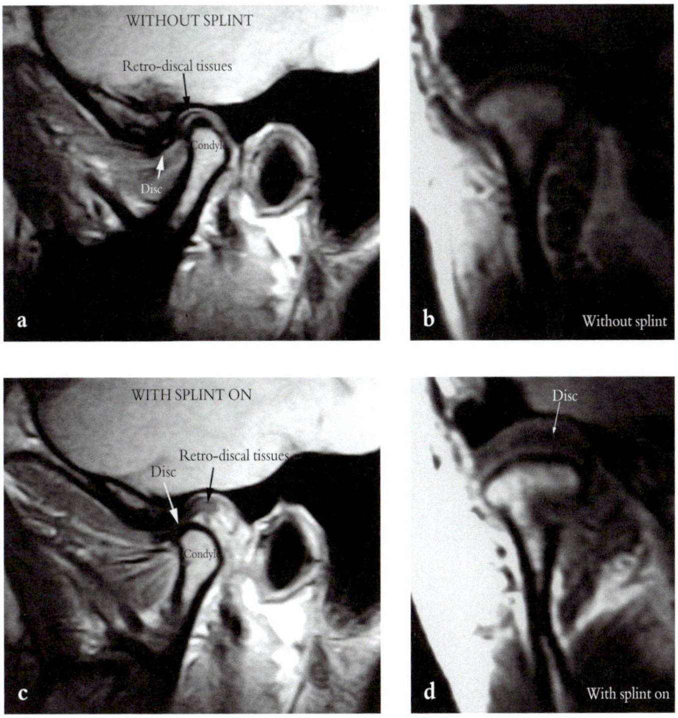

Fig 20-10 **(a and b)** Magnetic resonance imaging of a temporomandibular joint in the intercuspal position: **(a)** sagittal plane – anterior disc displacement and the condyle resting on the retro-discal tissues; **(b)** coronal plane – the disc is displaced in a more anterior plane and thus is not visible. **(c and d)** Sequences obtained during use of the mandibular repositioning appliance: **(c)** sagittal plane – the disc has been relocated perfectly, and the retro-discal tissues can be seen behind the condyle, free from compression; **(d)** coronal plane – the disk has been relocated into a normal position between the fossa and the condyle.

*Mandibular anterior repositioning appliances*

Usually, patients will first present to clinics specializing in craniomandibular dysfunction (CMD) complaining of jaw locking. Sometimes these patients will refer to the difficulties they face every morning in opening their mouth for the first time after waking from restorative sleep, since their jaw is usually locked on waking. After making some lateral movements or by remaining still and relaxed for a while, they usually manage to unlock their jaw. This impairment is known as "intermittent locking", and it is considered to be a precursor to permanent joint locking or "closed lock".[59]

Intermittent joint locking consists of transient condyle failure to reduce the articular disc displaced from its normal upper position. Although this problem is usually related to TMJ pathologies, sleep bruxism may be involved too. At night, when increased muscle activity occurs, the condyle is resting on the retro-discal tissues, which are very easily compressed. The two aggravating factors which may complicate this would be bruxism and an unfavorable mandibular or decubitus position during sleep. Though no research has been conducted on this specific subject, the cases seen in specialized clinics reflect a reality that demands therapeutic address. Since they do not modify the condyle–disc relationship, traditional bruxism splints will not help solve this problem.[60] Wearing a mandibular advancement device (Fig 20-9) will reorganize the relationship between articular structures, thus preventing jaw lock on waking.

Figure 20-10 shows disc displacement in the intercuspal position and the disc subsequently going back to normal while the splint was being worn. However, it has been shown also that the prolonged use of mandibular advancement devices may produce slight orthodontic-type changes in patients with sleep apnea.[61] The case presented in Fig 20-11 exemplifies and proves the occurrence

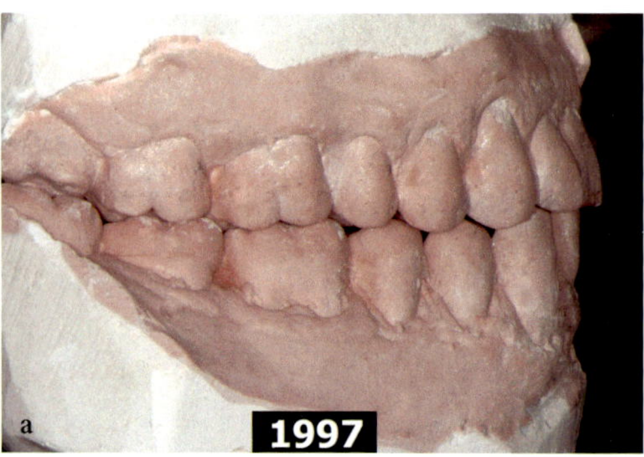


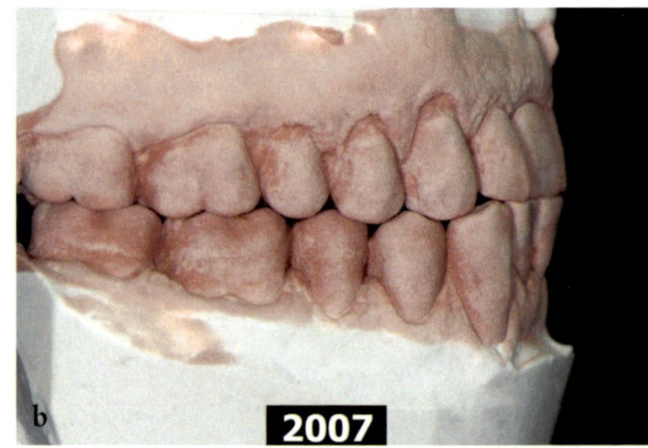


Fig 20-11 **(a and b)** Casts of a patient with sleep apnea who used a mandibular advancement device for 10 years. Polysomnography tests showed complete absence of apnea while the device was being worn. Comparison between the initial casts and the current ones allows the clinician to appreciate how a new intercuspal position has been established in which anterior teeth are in an end-to-end relationship. As a consequence of the loss of the overjet and the overbite, the patient will keep biting his soft tissues accidentally during mastication.

of such complications. For this reason, it is advisable to take some precautions. For example, these splints should not be used for more than a year; all the teeth should be covered by the splints so as to prevent extrusion; and, of course, contact should exist between the occlusal table and all antagonist pieces. Once the 1-year period has elapsed, the repositioning appliance should be replaced by a conventional bruxism splint and the results should be evaluated.

### *Can Splints Cause Bruxism?*

According to the results of some of the research studies discussed here, the effects splints may have on bruxism are unpredictable. They may cause EMG activity levels to decrease, increase, or simply remain unchanged. The reasons for such enigmatic variations remain unclear. At the time of writing, the only research study to have reported decreased bruxism levels in the 10 study subjects used an anterior-stop bite plane.[31] The outcomes of such a trial should be treated with caution, since the reported effects concerned just a short period of 3–4 weeks. On the other hand, if the splints had been worn for a longer time, extrusion of the teeth which were not in contact with the appliance would possibly have occurred. However, when on some occasions we have prescribed these splints – though for short periods – we noticed tooth grinding impressions on the anterior platform. Although clinical case reports should never replace research, at least they provide a direction for future research.

The reported increase in bruxism from the use of splints[22,24,34,36] explains some of the comments we hear from patients with TMDs. Some subjects suffering from TMDs and treated with splints will commonly complain of finding themselves clenching their teeth on waking. Our explanation for this used to be that wearing a splint caused these subjects to become aware of their bruxing habit, which they were not aware of before. However, the evidence recently reported may force us to admit that these patients are right. As a case example, a splint made for a 15-year-old can be seen showing signs of sleep tooth grinding in Figure 20-12. Before he started wearing the splint his teeth had shown no signs of tooth grinding at all. His brother, who was his roommate, reported never having heard any tooth grinding sounds.

A similar situation is depicted in Figure 20-13. This was a 20-year-old man treated for osteo-

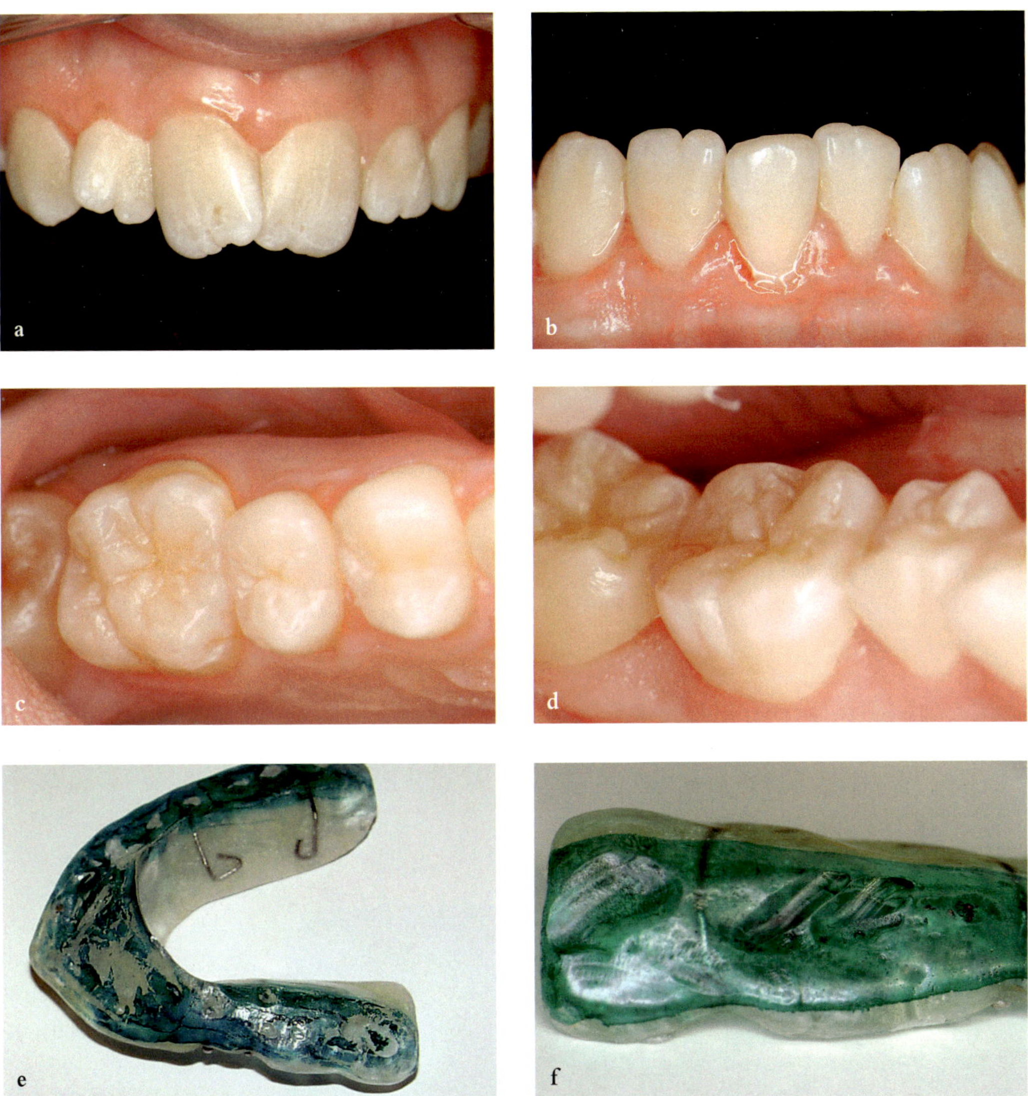

Fig 20-12 **(a–d)** Teeth belonging to a teenager who, as inferred by the total lack of attrition in his teeth and by his never having been heard to grind his teeth during sleep, was not a bruxer. **(e and f)** Tooth grinding impressions left on his mandibular repositioning appliance during sleep.

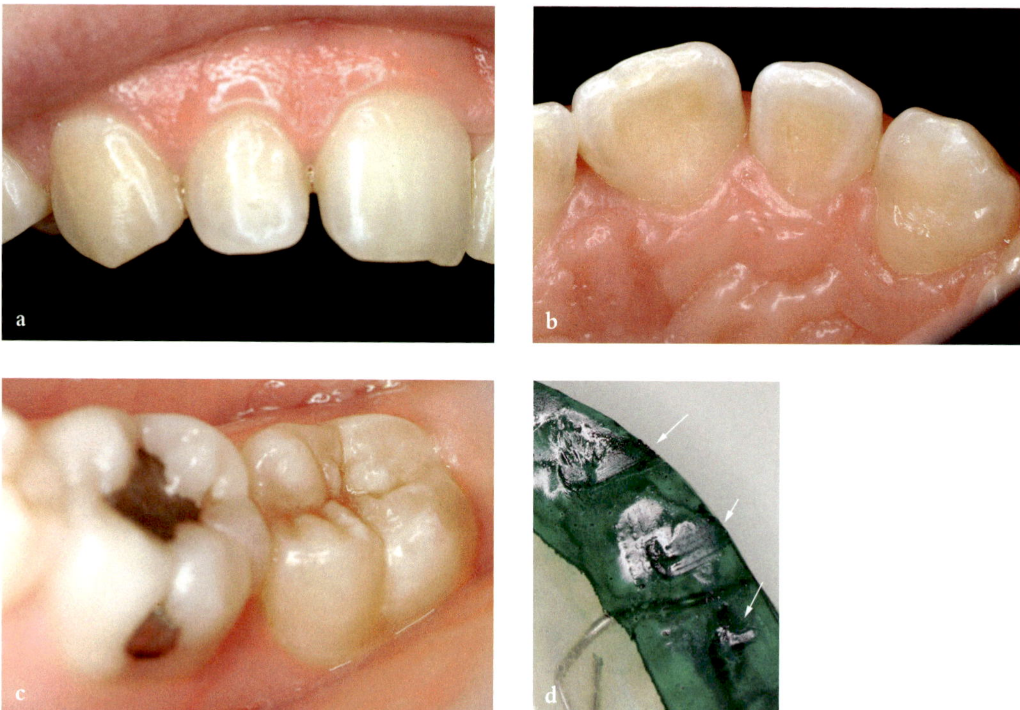

Fig 20-13 **(a–c)** Dentition of a 20-year-old man without a bruxism history and no signs of attrition. **(d)** This splint, which was prescribed to the patient as treatment for symptomatic osteoarthritis, shows the impressions (arrows) left by tooth grinding bruxism during sleep.

arthritis. Though he had no history of bruxism, his splint shows marked signs of it. One possibility is that these patients' enamel is so hard that no traces of potential bruxism are left on the teeth when the patients are unaware of their habit. However, neither of the two above-mentioned patients had been heard grinding their teeth during sleep.

The outcomes of the trial carried out by Okkerse and co-workers[31] suggest that the decrease in bruxism is ascribable to the uncoupling of the posterior teeth. However, other authors, who used palatal-coverage splints that did not alter tooth contacts, have reported similar results – although not in all the patients studied.

## Awake Bruxism

People can suffer from awake bruxism only, or from both awake and sleep bruxism.[62] Awake bruxism consists mainly of sustained tooth clenching episodes. Although the subject is awake, they are unaware that they are grinding or clenching their teeth, or at least they admit to noticing their bruxing activity but fail to determine when it starts. There are scarce scientific data on awake bruxism. Undoubtedly this can be attributable to the difficulties involved in the study of this kind of bruxism – which is not to imply that sleep bruxism research is easy to carry out.

The etiology of awake bruxism is currently considered to be related to emotional factors (see Chapter 6). It was Olkinuora[63] who suggested this hypothesis 30 years ago, and it was confirmed some years later by Rao and Glaros,[64] who proved that awake bruxers will respond differently from non-bruxers to stressful stimuli. In contrast with sleep bruxism, which has been shown to be associated with pulse rate acceleration, no significant correlation was found between masseter activation and pulse rate in this research study.

Since there is consensus about the role of emotional factors in awake bruxism, this section will now review the literature on treatments based on behavior modification.

### Treatments Based on Behaviour Modification

*First steps*

Bruxism being a "habit" (awake bruxism specially, since sleep bruxism is considered to be a sleep disorder, a parasomnia), many techniques have been proposed to eliminate such behaviour. Among them are massed therapy, biofeedback, habit-reversal training, hypnosis, progressive relaxation, and lifestyle changes. All these treatments have the same goal: addressing emotional factors and reducing stress. Such emotional factors are more closely related to awake bruxism than to sleep bruxism (see Chapter 6).

The first step is to make patients aware of their unconscious behavior. Although many patients identify and admit their tooth clenching habit, others are completely unaware of it. When we see these patients and while we explain to them the fascinating, uncontrollable mechanism they show, we will usually be surprised to see the masseter-muscle fibrillation movements showing in their cheeks; that is, they clench their teeth while they are being told that they should not do it. This gives an idea of how difficult it is for awake bruxers to control their habit. Close relatives should be asked to help by watching these patients' cheeks and making them aware that they are clenching their teeth. This is not likely to eradicate the problem, but at least it will help the person to recognize the reality and possibly reduce the amount of time they spend bruxing. Once these patients become aware of their automated reaction, they will be able to start controlling it.

*Psychoanalysis and autosuggestion*

Olkinuora[65] was the first to propose using these techniques from the psychiatric field in order to control bruxism. Unfortunately, no research has been conducted on the use of these techniques.

*Habit awareness*

A suggestion was made for patients to be trained so that they can control daytime tooth clenching. This type of treatment was suggested by Rosen[66] as a way to monitor daytime bruxism. The author recommends that, whenever a bruxer notices that they are bruxing, they should note it down and keep count. This will allow them to become aware of the frequency with which they involuntarily clench their teeth. Although this proposal is very interesting, no data are provided to assess its efficacy.

*Habit-reversal therapy*

This therapy was developed in the 1970s by psychologists Aznin and Nunn as treatment for some automated habits, like nervous tics. It was then adapted for odontologic purposes; the aim is to exercise the opening of the mouth, thus producing an effect opposite to bruxism.[67,68] A variant consists of avoiding tooth clenching and keeping a free space between the teeth.[69] No evidence has been offered to confirm the effectiveness of this therapy – as seems to be the norm with these types of proposal.

*Relaxation techniques*

In the early 1980s, Pear[70] was the first to suggest the use of meditation and relaxation as a way to control the body. Later, these techniques were mentioned by Cannistraci and Friedrich,[71] though no published evidence on their effectiveness exists.

Positive results have been recently reported by a group of researchers who were able to reduce bruxism levels in 3- to-6-year-old children with primary teeth. With the help of a psychologist, the authors used two relaxation techniques: guided muscle relaxation and competency reaction. However, the results reported by the authors regarding the decrease in bruxism were indirectly inferred from the lower number of objective signs and subjective symptoms associated to TMD.[72]

Muscle-awareness relaxation training (MART) is a technique aimed at becoming aware of the stress signals affecting the whole body. This philosophy pays much attention to posture, to the identification of muscle groups, and to breathing control. This technique was applied and assessed in a group of bruxers with TMD for 4 months.[73] Its success in reducing bruxism was inferred, though, from the increase in mouth opening and the decrease in masseter EMG activity in the resting state shown by the patients; no direct measuring of the bruxism episodes was performed. Interestingly, the author also reports decreased breathing rate per minute, as he emphasizes that breathing is behind sleep arousal episodes.

*Biofeedback*

Research on the use of biofeedback as treatment for bruxism was first carried out by Solberg and Rugh.[74] Biofeedback is based on the paradigm which considers that bruxers can control their bruxing behavior by means of a stimulus that causes them to become aware of the negative activity they are engaged in. This method uses EMG technology; a threshold is set, and whenever the patient exceeds the set value, they will hear an unpleasant sound alarm through an earphone. In order to determine the proper threshold, the subject is requested to move their face and masticatory muscles.

Lund and Widmer[75] warn about the great inter- and intra-variability of cumulative EMG, which makes it difficult to determine which values should be considered normal. Another of the problems with the use of ambulatory EMG is that it is difficult to distinguish between bruxism and non-bruxing muscle activity, since there is no supervision.

The first trials conducted to evaluate the use of biofeedback (all over short periods) have been considered to be successful, since they reduced average night-time EMG activity duration without increasing the number of events.[76,77] After biofeedback is discontinued, the activity returns to its original levels.[78,79] Trials conducted over longer periods have been reported by others to have had successful results.[80] Pierce and Gale[26] were successful in reducing the number and duration of events; however, as was the case with the other studies noted above, the values returned to their original levels when use of the equipment was discontinued. Pierce and Gale also researched the use of biofeedback during the day and its subsequent effect on sleep bruxism; negative results were obtained. The authors admit that, perhaps, they should have evaluated its effect purely on awake bruxism since the patients, having been trained to achieve deep muscle relaxation while awake (conscious state), became considerably different when asleep (unconscious state). Results were therefore not completely reliable or consistent.

Resting EMG activity of a group of bruxers treated with biofeedback and transcutaneous electrical neuromuscular stimulation (TENS) has lately been studied.[81] Although the study did not involve direct bruxism measurements, no resting EMG muscle activity decrease was observed during the application of these two treatments. Nissani[82] devised another type of biofeedback technique. A capsule containing a nasty flavored product is placed inside the splint (the patient can choose between garlic, mustard, ginger, etc.); the product is then released into the mouth whenever the subject clenches their teeth, which helps them become aware of their activity. After testing the method in only one patient, the author deemed it to be infallible. The only controlled clinical trial which assessed the use of biofeedback during sleep showed good results when compared to control subjects who were not treated.[83]

On critical analysis, the use of biofeedback during sleep is tinged with contradictions which are difficult to understand. Some will use a sound alarm to alert the patient about the need to stop bruxing; others have resorted to the same principle to produce sounds and vibratile stimuli – only to prove later, through polysomnography, that such sounds and stimuli had been able to provoke bruxism episodes during sleep.[84,85] Perhaps the strongest criticism one can make about biofeedback is that it constantly interrupts sleep, which causes the subject to be exhausted and sleepy the rest of the day.[86] Aware of this problem, a group of researchers conducted a pilot study with a female bruxer as participant.[87] What was new about this trial was that the sound alarm was replaced by a vibratile stimulation system. The patient used two splints, an upper and a lower. Inside them a thin sensor was placed which, on activation by either clenching or grinding, would emit a vibratile discharge. By means of a radio frequency (no wires involved), a signal was simultaneously transmitted to a receptor, where all the information was stored. The authors reported a significant decrease in the number (25%) and duration (44%) of events per hour. Unfortunately, since the researchers did not assess the situation after the use of the vibratile device was discontinued, it is not known whether bruxism returns or not to its initial values. Interestingly, the patient did not report any subjective disturbance in sleep quality.

A study of seven subjects, based on a similar principle, used (non-harmful) electrical stimuli applied to the upper lip simultaneously with the beginning of each bruxism episode.[88] The aim was to inhibit bruxism without waking the subjects. The results of this trial were similar to the results obtained by the previous one. The number and duration of the bruxism episodes was reduced without altering sleep – this latter piece of information, though, was subjectively reported by the participants.

The two research studies we have just analyzed, though still in the experimental stage, have showed very promising results. However, it should be noted that both included a factor which, as we have already discussed in this chapter, leads to confusion – the unpredictable effects of splint wear.

This short review of the literature on the use and effectiveness of biofeedback does not provide enough evidence that this technique really helps to reduce bruxism. In some of these studies, the populations consisted of patients with TMDs, and the fact that they got relief from their symptoms was inferred to represent a decrease in bruxism. Once the sound stimulation is discontinued, bruxism will return to the values it showed before the treatment.

Future controlled trials monitored through PSG may finally determine whether the technique meets the desired goals while not interfering with normal sleep architecture. Provided that researchers are successful in demonstrating through PSG that no sleep interference exists, they will have solved the most important difficulty shared by all previous studies on biofeedback.

*Massed therapy*

This method consists of an aware tooth-clenching exercise program. Each clenching action lasts approximately 5 seconds and is repeated 10 times, with a 5-second relaxation period between each clenching. The whole routine is repeated six times a day.

This technique is based on "learning theory". The approach was advocated in the 1950s by Yates,[89] who developed the concept of "reactive inhibition". The basic idea is that the unconscious mind perceives tooth clenching as disagreeable, while the relaxation periods are perceived as comfortable. It has been speculated that this therapy is successful in reducing bruxism levels during sleep. Ayer and Levin,[90] its developers, reported bruxism eradication in 11 of the 14 patients who participated in a trial, and they established a 10-day training period as the minimum needed in order to get a successful outcome. This has limited scientific value, since the authors requested the patients to evaluate the results of the treatment themselves.

A partial reproduction of this trial by Heller and Forgione[91] measured results in a more objective way by means of a Bruxcore plate (described in Chapter 2). These researchers compared the effects of the massed negative practice with the effects of a technique called "automated relaxation training"; neither of them, however, was successful in modifying bruxism levels. This type of treatment was subsequently tested in a group of patients monitored through ambulatory EMG, and it too failed to render positive results in the patients who were treated with it.

Although it is obvious that this massed therapy is not harmful for patients, no objective evidence exists to prove it is helpful in the treatment of bruxism.

*Hypnosis*

The use of hypnosis as bruxism treatment was first mentioned in the literature in 1973 by Goldberg.[92] Far from demonstrating the therapeutic effectiveness of hypnosis, this author just provided three case reports as examples. Another study was successful in proving a decrease in bruxism levels through EMG done before and immediately after hypnosis therapy; however, the long-term results were subjectively established by means of a questionnaire.[93] From that moment onwards, literature reviews include just two reports which merely praise hypnosis as treatment and describe only one clinical case.[94,95] The existing material is scarce and its scientific validity is questionable, which makes it unsuitable for drawing valid conclusions on the effects of hypnosis on bruxism.

## References


1. American Academy of Sleep Medicine. International Classification of Sleep Disorders, ed 2. Diagnostic and Coding Manual. Westchester: AASM, 2005:297.
2. Lobbezoo F, Naeije M. Bruxism is mainly regulated centrally, not peripherally. J Oral Rehabil 2001;28:1085–1091.
3. Kato T, Rompre P, Montplaisir JY, Sessle BJ, Lavigne GJ. Sleep bruxism: an oromotor activity secondary to microarousal. J Dent Res 2001;80:1940–1944.
4. Lavigne GL, Lobbezoo F, Rompre PH, Nielsen TA, Montplaisir J. Cigarette smoking as a risk factor or an exacerbating factor for restless legs syndrome and sleep bruxism. Sleep 1997;20:290–293.
5. Madrid G, Vranesh JG, Hicks RA. Cigarette smoking and bruxism. Percept Mot Skills 1998;87:898.
6. Ohayon MM, Li KK, Guilleminault C. Risk factors for sleep bruxism in the general population. Chest 2001;119:53–61.
7. Hartmann E. Bruxism. In: Kryger MH, Roth T, Dement WC (eds). Principles and Practice of Sleep Medicine, ed 2. Philadelphia: Elsevier Saunders, 1994:598–602.
8. Morin CM. Psychological and behavioral treatments for primary insomnia. In: Kryger MH, Roth T, Dement WC (eds). Principles and Practice of Sleep Medicine, ed 4. Philadelphia: Elsevier Saunders, 2005:726–733.
9. Pierce CJ, Weyant RJ, Block HM, Nemir DC. Dental splint prescription patterns: a survey. J Am Dent Assoc 1995;126:248–254.
10. Lindfors E, Magnusson T, Tegelberg A. Interocclusal appliances: indications and clinical routines in general dental practice in Sweden. Swed Dent J 2006;30: 123–134.
11. Paesani D, Westesson PL, Hatala M, Tallents RH, Kurita K. Prevalence of temporomandibular joint internal derangement in patients with craniomandibular disorders. Am J Orthod Dentofacial Orthop 1992;101:41–47.
12. Lobbezoo F, Lavigne GJ. Do bruxism and temporomandibular disorders have a cause-and-effect relationship? J Orofac Pain 1997;11:15–23.
13. Marbach JJ. The "temporomandibular pain dysfunction syndrome" personality: fact or fiction? J Oral Rehabil 1992;19:545–560.
14. Yap AUJ. Effects of stabilization appliances on nocturnal parafunctional activities in patients with and without signs of temporomandibular disorders. J Oral Rehabil 1998;25: 64–68.
15. Chung SC, Kim YK, Kim HS. Prevalence and patterns of nocturnal bruxofacets on stabilization splints in temporomandibular disorder patients. Cranio 2000;18:92–97.
16. Holmgren K, Sheikholeslam A, RiiseC. Effect of a full-arch maxillary occlusal splint on parafunctional activity during sleep in patients with nocturnal bruxism and signs and symptoms of craniomandibular disorders. J Prosthet Dent 1993;69:293–297.

17. Korioth TWP, Bohlig KC, Anderson GC. Digital assessment of occlusal wear patterns on occlusal stabilization splints: a pilot study. J Prosthet Dent 1998;80:209–213.
18. Lavigne GJ, Rompre PH, Montplaisir JY. Sleep bruxism: validity of clinical research diagnosis criteria in a controlled polysomnographic study. J Dent Res 1996;75: 546–552.
19. Kydd WL, Daly C. Duration of nocturnal tooth contact during bruxing. J Prosthet Dent 1985;53:717–721.
20. Lavigne GJ, Rompre PH, Montplaisir JY, Lobbezoo F. Motor activity in sleep bruxism with concomitant jaw muscle pain: a retrospective pilot study. Eur J Oral Sci 1997;105:92–95.
21. Solberg WK, Clark GT, Rugh JD. Nocturnal electromyographic evaluation of bruxism patients undergoing short term splint therapy. J Oral Rehabil 1975;2: 215–223.
22. Clark GT, Beemsterboer PL, Solberg WK, Rugh JD. Nocturnal electromyographic evaluation of myofascial pain dysfunction in patients undergoing occlusal splint therapy. J Am Dent Assoc 1979;99:607–611.
23. Okeson JP. The effects of hard and soft occlusal splints on nocturnal bruxism. J Am Dent Assoc 1987;114:788–791.
24. Rugh JD, Graham GS, Smith JC, Ohrbach RK. Effects of canine versus molar occlusal splint guidance on nocturnal bruxism and craniomandibular symptomatology. J Craniomandib Disord 1989;3:203–210.
25. Cassisi JE, McGlynn FD, Mahan PE. Occlusal splint effects on nocturnal bruxing: an emerging paradigm and some early results. Cranio 1987;5:64–68.
26. Pierce CJ, Gale EN. A comparison of different treatments for nocturnal bruxism. J Dent Res 1988;67:597–601.
27. Hiyama S, Ono T, Ishiwata Y, Kato Y, Kuroda T. First night effect of an interocclusal appliance on nocturnal masticatory muscle activity. J Oral Rehabil 2003;30: 139–145.
28. Harada T, Ichiki R, Tsukiyama Y, Koyano K. The effect of oral splint devices on sleep bruxism: a 6-week observation with an ambulatory electromyographic recording device. J Oral Rehabil 2006;33:482–488.
29. Hasegawa K, Okamoto M, Nishigawa G, Oki K, Minagi S. The design of non-occlusal intraoral appliances on hard palate and their effect on masseter muscle activity during sleep. Cranio 2007;25:8–15.
30. Jeanmonod A. Occlusodontie, applications, cliniques. Paris: Editions CdP, 1988.
31. Okkerse W, Brebels A, De Deyn PP et al. Influence of a bite-plane according to Jeanmonod, on bruxism activity during sleep. J Oral Rehabil 2002;29:980–985.
32. Baad-Hansen L, Jadidi F, Castrillon E, Thomsen PB. Effect of a nociceptive trigeminal inhibitory splint on electromyographic activity in jaw closing muscles during sleep. J Oral Rehabil 2007;34:105–111.
33. Magnusson T, Adiels AM, Nilsson HL, Helkimo M. Treatment effect on signs and symptoms of temporomandibular disorders: comparison between stabilization splint and a new type of splint (NTI). A pilot study. Swed Dent J 2004;28:11–20.
34. Sjöholm T, Lehtinen I, Polo O. The effect of mouth guard on masseter muscle activity during sleep. J Sleep Res 2002;11(Suppl 1):209–210.
35. Dube C, Rompre PH, Manzini C et al. Quantitative polygraphic controlled study on efficacy and safety of oral splint devices in tooth-grinding subjects. J Dent Res 2004;83:398–403.
36. van der Zaag J, Lobbezoo F, Wicks DJ et al. Controlled assessment of the efficacy of occlusal stabilization splints on sleep bruxism. J Orofac Pain 2005;19:151–158.
37. Mehta A, Oian J, Petocz P, Darendeliler MA, Cistulli PA. A randomized, controlled study of a mandibular advancement splint for obstructive sleep apnea. Am J Respir Crit Care Med 2001;163:1457–1461.
38. Landry ML, Rompre PH, Manzini C et al. Reduction of sleep bruxism using a mandibular advancement device: an experimental controlled study. Int J Prosthodont 2006; 19:549–556.
39. Lavigne GJ, Rompre PH, Poirier G et al. Rhythmic masticatory muscle activity during sleep in humans. J Dent Res 2001;80:443–448.
40. Huynh N, Kato T, Rompre PH et al. Sleep bruxism is associated to micro arousals and an increase in cardiac sympathetic activity. J Sleep Res 2006;15:339–346.
41. Ramfjord SP, Ash MM. Occlusion. Philadelphia: WB Saunders, 1966.
42. Williamson EH, Lundquist DO. Anterior guidance: its effect on electromyographic activity of the temporal and masseter muscles. J Prosthet Dent 1983;49:816–823.
43. Shupe RJ, Mohamed SE, Christensen LV, Finger IM, Weinberg R. Effects of occlusal guidance on jaw muscle activity. J Prosthet Dent 1984;51:811–818.
44. Manns A, Miralles R, Valdivia J. Influence of variation in anteroposterior occlusal contacts on electromyographic activity. J Prosthet Dent 1989;61:617–623.
45. Fitins D, Sheikholeslam A. Effect of canine guidance of maxillary occlusal splint on level of activation of masticatory muscles. Swed Dent J 1993;17:235–241.
46. MacDonald JWC, Hannam AG. Relationship between occlusal contacts and jaw-closing muscle activity during tooth clenching: Pt I. J Prosthet Dent 1984;52:718–728.
47. Manns A, Chan C, Miralles R. Influence of group function and canine guidance on electromyographic activity of elevator muscles. J Prosthet Dent 1987;57:494–501.
48. Graham GS, Rugh JD. Maxillary splint occlusal guidance patterns and electromyographic activity of the jaw-closing muscles. J Prosthet Dent 1988;59:73–77.

49. Borromeo GL, Suvinen TI, Reade PC. A comparison of the effects of group function and canine guidance interocclusal device on masseter muscle electromyographic activity in normal subjects. J Prosthet Dent 1995;74: 174–180.
50. Bakke M, Michler M, Møller E. Occlusal control of mandibular elevator muscles. Scand J Dent Res 1992;100: 284–291.
51. Dalström L, Haraldson T. Immediate electromyographic response in masseter and temporal muscles to bite plates and stabilization splints. Scand J Dent Res 1989;97: 533–538.
52. Nevarro E, Barghi N, Rey R. Clinical evaluation of maxillary hard and resilient occlusal splints. J Dent Res 1985; 64:318 (abstract 1246).
53. Shore N. Temporomandibular Joint Dysfunction and Occlusal Equilibration, ed 2. Philadelphia: Lippincott, 1976:238–249.
54. Singh BP, Berry DC. Occlusal changes following use of soft occlusal splints. J Prosthet Dent 1985;54:711–715.
55. Harkins S, Marteney JL, Cueva O, Cueva L. Application of soft occlusal splints in patients suffering from clicking temporomandibular joints. Cranio 1988;6:71–76.
56. Wright E, Anderson G, Schulte J. A randomized clinical trial of intraoral soft splints and palliative treatment for masticatory muscle pain. J Orofac Pain 1995;9:192–199.
57. Truelove E, Huggins KH, Manci L, Dworkin SF. The efficacy of traditional, low-cost and nonsplint therapies for temporomandibular disorder: a randomized controlled trial. J Am Dent Assoc 2006;137:1099–1107.
58. Ramfjord SP, Ash MM. Occlusion, ed 3. Philadelphia: Lippincott, 1983:359–383.
59. Tallents RH, Katzberg RW, Macher DJ, Roberts CA. Use of protrusive splint therapy in anterior disk displacement of the temporomandibular joint: a 1- to 3-year follow-up. J Prosthet Dent 1990;63:336–341.
60. Anderson GC, Schulte JK, Goodkind RJ. Comparative study of two treatment methods for internal derangement of the temporomandibular joint. J Prosthet Dent 1985;53:392–397.
61. Marklund M, Franklin KA, Persson M. Orthodontic side-effects of mandibular advancement devices during treatment of snoring and sleep apnea. Eur J Orthod 2001; 23:135–144.
62. Glaros AG. Incidence of diurnal and nocturnal bruxism. J Prosthet Dent 1981;45:545–549.
63. Olkinuora M. Psychosocial aspects in a series of bruxists compared with a group of non-bruxists. Proc Finn Dent Soc 1972;68:200–208.
64. Rao SM, Glaros AG. Electromyographic correlates of experimentally induced stress in diurnal bruxist and normals. J Dent Res 1979;58:1872–1878.
65. Olkinuora M. A review of the literature on, and a discussion of, studies of bruxism and its psychogenesis and some new psychological hypotheses. Suom Hammaslaak Toim 1969;65:312–324.
66. Rosen JC. Self-monitoring in the treatment of diurnal bruxism. J Behav Ther Exp Psychiatry 1981;12:347–350.
67. Rosenbaum MS, Ayllon T. Treating bruxism with the habit-reversal technique. Behav Res Ther 1981;19:87–96.
68. Blore D. Grinding down. Nurs Times 1995;91:46–47.
69. Zeldow LL. Treating clenching and bruxing by habit change. J Am Dent Assoc 1976;93:31–33.
70. Pear JH. Holistic care concepts, bruxism and necrotizing ulcerative gingivitis. Dent Hyg (Chic) 1982;56:24–29.
71. Cannistraci AJ, Friedrich JA. A multidimensional approach to bruxism and TMD. N Y State Dent J 1987; 53:31–34.
72. Restrepo CC, Alvarez E, Jaramillo C, Velez C, Valencia I. Effects of psychological techniques on bruxism in children with primary teeth. J Oral Rehabil 2001;28: 354–360.
73. Treacy K. Awareness/relaxation training and transcutaneous electrical neural stimulation in the treatment of bruxism. J Oral Rehabil 1999;26:280–287.
74. Solberg WK, Rugh JD. The use of bio-feedback devices in the treatment of bruxism. J South Calif Dent Assoc 1972;40:852–853.
75. Lund JP, Widmer CG. Evaluation of the use of surface electromyography in the diagnosis, documentation, and treatment of dental patients. J Craniomandib Disord 1989;3:125–137.
76. Kardachi BJ, Clarke NG. The use of biofeedback to control bruxism. J Periodontol 1977;48:639–642.
77. Rugh JD, Johnson RW. Temporal analysis of nocturnal bruxism during EMG feedback. J Periodontol 1981;52: 263–265.
78. Rugh JD, Solberg WK. Electromyographic studies of bruxist behavior before and during treatment. J Calif Dent Assoc 1975;3:56–59.
79. Kardachi BJ, Bailey JO, Ash MM. A comparison of biofeedback and occlusal adjustment on bruxism. J Periodontol 1978;49:367–372.
80. Hudzinski LG, Walters PJ. Use of a portable electromyogram integrator and biofeedback unit in the treatment of chronic nocturnal bruxism. J Prosthet Dent 1987;58: 698–701.
81. Wieselmann-Penkner A, Janda M, Lorenzoni M, Polansky A. A comparison of the muscular relaxation effects of TENS and EMG-biofeedback in patients with bruxism. J Oral Rehabil 2001;28:849–853.
82. Nissani M. Can taste aversion prevent bruxism? Appl Psychophysiol Biofeedback 2000;25:43–54.
83. Casas JM, Beemsterboer P, Clark GT. A comparison of stress-reduction behavioral counseling and contingent nocturnal EMG feedback for the treatment of bruxism. Behav Res Ther 1982;20:9–15.
84. Satoh T, Harada Y. Tooth-grinding during sleep as an arousal reaction. Experientia 1971;27:785–786.
85. Kato T, Thie NM, Huynh N, Miyawaki S, Lavigne GJ. Topical review: sleep bruxism and the role of peripheral sensory influences. J Orofac Pain 2003;17:191–213.

86. Roehrs T, Carskadon MA, Dement WC, Roth T. Daytime sleepiness and alertness. In: Kryger MH, Roth T, Dement WC (eds). Principles and Practice of Sleep Medicine, ed 4. Philadelphia: Elsevier Saunders, 2005:39–50.
87. Watanabe T, Baba K, Yamagata K, Ohyama T, Clark GT. A vibratory stimulation-based inhibition system for nocturnal bruxism: a clinical report. J Prosthet Dent 2001;85:233–235.
88. Nishigawa K, Kondo K, Takeuchi H, Clark GT. Contingent electrical lip stimulation for sleep bruxism: a pilot study. J Prosthet Dent 2003;89:412–417.
89. Yates AJ. The application of learning theory to the treatment of tics. J Abnorm Psychol 1958;56:175–182.
90. Ayer WA, Levin MP. Elimination of tooth grinding habits by massed practice therapy. J Periodontol 1973;44:569–571.
91. Heller RF, Forgione AG. An evaluation of bruxism control: massed negative practice and automated relaxation training. J Dent Res 1975;54:1120–1123.
92. Goldberg G. The psychological, physiological and hypnotic approach to bruxism in the treatment of periodontal disease. J Am Soc Psychosom Dent Med 1973;20:75–91.
93. Clarke JH, Reynolds PJ. Suggestive hypnotherapy for nocturnal bruxism: a pilot study. Am J Clin Hypn 1991;33:248–253.
94. Somer E. Hypnotherapy in the treatment of the chronic nocturnal use of a dental splint prescribed for bruxism. Int J Clin Exp Hypn 1991;39:145–154.
95. LaCrosse MB. Understanding change: five-year follow-up of brief hypnotic treatment of chronic bruxism. Am J Clin Hypn 1994;36:276–281.

Chapter 21

# Introduction to Complex Oral Restoration

*Daniel A. Paesani and Fernando Cifuentes*

## Introduction

Bruxism is a habit that directly affects human dentition. Its effects range from simple facets to total destruction. For this reason, this chapter will deal with the questionable and controversial subject of "occlusion" because dental practitioners frequently need not only to protect occlusion but also to reconstruct it. The aim of this chapter is to discuss the different points of view, which are subject of infinite controversies generated by a permanent disagreement between mechanisist concepts and biologic reasoning. In order to progress this discussion, we must be willing to highlight evidence resulting from scientific methods rather than concepts based on dogma, mysticism, or the experts' clinical experiences. Finally, we will formulate a clear, "simple" proposal to be applied in clinicians' offices every day.

## Centric Relation

This may be one of the most controversial issues regarding occlusion and oral restoration. It is sarcastically said among dental practitioners that there are three topics people will never agree on – religion, politics, and centric relation. Different aspects of this last topic will be analyzed as sensibly as possible, trying to encourage readers to tackle it in a clear, simple and tangible manner to avoid generating a contradiction between what is being said and what is actually being done.

### *A Question of Context*

The need for a reference occlusal position arose a long time ago when well-known pioneers such as Gysi, Hannau, and Bennet faced the necessity of establishing parameters to be used in prosthetic treatments. If we could go back in time, let us say to 1900, we would find a great number of young edentulous individuals owing to the lack of technology and current preventive concepts. Caries and periodontal diseases developed fast and they prematurely destroyed the dentition. We must bear in mind that, at that time, there were no X-ray facilities, antibiotics, periodontal probes, etc. Once the teeth were lost, it was difficult for clinicians to select a mandibular position to make a denture prosthesis. From then onwards, the most retruded mandibular position (RP) was used as an anatomic parameter leading to the first concept of centric relation (CR) – defined as "the most retruded position of the condyles from where all the mandibular movements start".

Early pioneers in dentistry rapidly designed different methods to put this theory into practice. In view of this, in 1905 Christensen[1] published the first bite registration in this position by means of using a wax piece placed between the edentulous alveolar ridges of a patient. Later on, in 1910, Gysi[2] designed an extraoral anterior bite plane in order to locate this position; and, in 1927, Phillips[3] provided an intraoral version of it. The original aim of the localization of the mandibular centric relation was to obtain a reference border position which, owing to its closeness to the intercuspal position (IP), allows the prosthetist to establish a relationship between the maxilla and the mandible and start with the lining up of the teeth. Throughout history, an innumerable amount of complete prostheses were fabricated following this method. This acceptance of the CR as a starting point in obtaining a therapeutic position (TP) slightly more forward than the CR is called the "classic school of occlusion".

### *Philosophical Conflicts Among Schools of Occlusion*

As new schools of occlusion appeared, new proposals came up and diverging points of view emerged, which have still not been sorted out.

In 1938, McCollum[4] founded the "California Gnathologic Society" that proposed the use of CR not only as a reference point but also as the ideal position for dental occlusion reconstruction, the so-called "occlusion in centric relation".

Another occlusal philosophy was introduced by Schuyler[5] in 1935, when he set up the "long centric" school and proposed "freedom in centric". This school, as well as the gnathologic one, suggests the coincidence between the maximal occlusion and the CR but with the addition of a carved groove or occlusal anterior bite plane so that the mandible can perform horizontally, avoiding occlusal surface interferences. Time has gone by, the school of "long centric" has started to lose relevance, while the gnathologic school has an important number of enthusiastic followers and practitioners.

### *Anatomic and Orthopedic Principles*

Accepting CR as a final treatment position implies putting the temporomandibular joint (TMJ) under tension. The maneuver of retruding the mandible is limited by the TMJ ligaments such as the capsular and lateral ligaments and the horizontal part of the TM ligaments.[6–9] This is supported by research carried out on corpses. According to basic orthopedic principles, articulations cannot function in a constant strained position as they are limited by ligaments. The main function of these tissues is to restrain articulation movements and to avoid luxations and preserve anatomic structures. With regard to the TMJ, its capsule and temporomandibular ligament force the condyle to a minimal retrusion in order to preserve the retro-discal tissues, which are very fragile since they are made of a fundamental vascular plexus and numerous elements of the nervous system.

An experimental study carried out on monkeys showed that if the mandible is kept in the final position, significant structural modifications take place in the TMJ.[10] In another similar study performed on rabbits, the mandible remained retruded for 33 days and some damage was seen in the articular tissues.[11] Cholasueksa and co-workers[12] obtained the same results using lab rats.

Needless to say, beyond research, if we retrude our mandible, we will have an unpleasant sensation which cannot be sustained over time. In their publications, McMillan and co-workers define retrusion not only as "non-functional" but also as a forced mandibular position. In a study carried out on people who were asked to maintain a retruded mandibular position voluntarily, McMillan and co-workers[13] reported that the individuals were only able to keep it for a short period of time and their efforts resulted in a tremor followed by jerky movements toward a more forward position where the tremor continued but with less intensity.

The mandible is a bone capable of moving in multiple ways. It is articulated to the skull by means of both temporomandibular articulations and dental occlusion. The masticatory muscles are in charge of producing the mandible movements and of maintaining the relation between the skull and the mandible. This last function is carried out by means of the development of muscular engrams, a kind of muscular program that contributes to the achievement of a certain function. In the specific case of the mandible, these engrams develop in the masticatory muscles so that all the masticatory system functions are efficiently and safely achieved. Despite the numerous three-dimensional mandibular movements (opening, closing, protrusion, retrusion, lateral, and their combinations) the mandible always reaches the intercuspal position thanks to the engrams. None of us wonders "how to bite". However, on many occasions during our lifetime, the masticatory cycle ends in maximal intercuspation (MI) without causing contact or undesirable interferences between the antagonist teeth even though most of the time there is no ideal occlusion. This wonderful system of engrams makes all this possible by means of a synchronized relaxation and contraction of the different muscle groups with the purpose of effectively and accurately carrying out the masticatory cycle, speech, and swallowing. All the masticatory muscles have force vectors acting upward and forward. Two important conclusions can be drawn from this simple anatomo-physiologic truth.

- Anatomically, the mandible is not able to maintain a retruded position for a period of time.
- Before any clinical maneuver aimed at retruding the mandible, the masticatory muscles must be at rest.

The retruded mandibular position must be used as a reference point that will enable us to compare its location with respect to the therapeutic position. This last position must be placed within a small area, not larger than 1 mm. If MI cannot be found, or if a new intercuspal relation must be built up in another vertical dimension (VD), RP localization will be essential. In all situations, to achieve a retrusive movement of the mandible, the patient must be requested to cooperate and relax their masticatory muscles. If these minute but powerful muscles are not at rest, it will be useless to try to fight against them.

### *Discrepancy*

"Discrepancy" is defined as the spatial difference between the MI and the mandible RP (or CR for others), measured in millimeters. According to many epidemiologic studies, 1 mm discrepancy between the IP and the RP is common in most individuals with complete natural dentition. This means that when the mandible moves backwards from the MI, a small retrusion takes place[14–17] (Fig 21-1).

The above discrepancy value applies to 90% of the general population. This high number may suggest that discrepancy, far from being an exception, is common among humans. Moreover, one might wonder whether the 10% of people with matching mandibular positions were able to relax their masticatory muscles, or perhaps these potent muscles offered resistance to the mandibular retrusion and remained active throughout the maneuver. Frequently, patients have difficulty in reaching a retrusive position because, regardless of their wish to cooperate, they find it hard to achieve

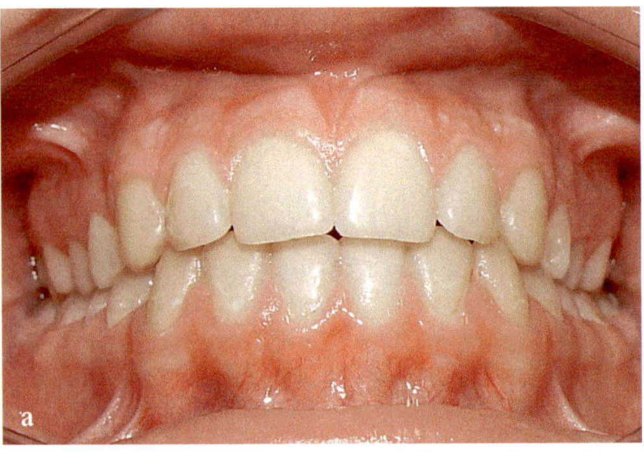

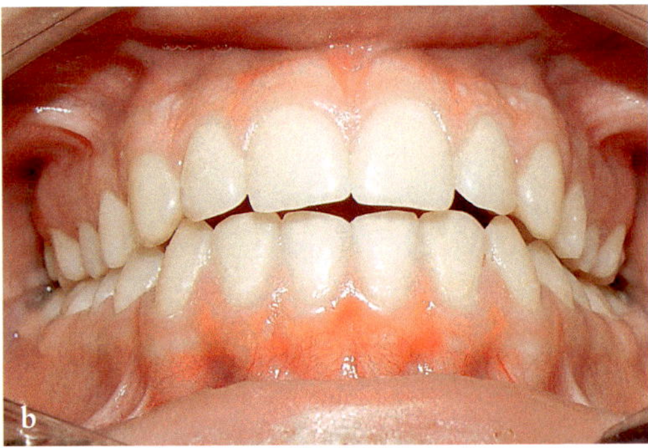

Fig 21-1 **(a)** Intercuspal position, and **(b)** retrusive position. Note the minimal discrepancy between the two positions.

muscle relaxation and they cannot accomplish the desirable mandibular retrusion. In these situations, the practitioner should take enough time to persuade the patient to relax his or her muscles.

Mandibular retrusion always results in a slight mandibular distalization and in a modification in the cusp–fossa relationship, characteristic of MI. This new maxillo-mandibular relation will be extremely unstable since only two teeth will make contact, one superior and one inferior (Fig 21-2).

The above-mentioned contacts have been thought of as dental occlusal "interferences" by some authors, especially by the gnathologic school. They propose to eliminate them by means of a procedure called "selective grinding" or "occlusal adjustment". Nevertheless, others do not favor this preventive elimination of the contacts because they do not take place during functional mandible movements.[18] MI is the only fixed occlusal relation since the close meshing of the cusp and the fossa dynamically keeps control over dental stability. Any tooth adjustment carried out outside this position will not prevail. So, when the mandible returns to the MI functional position, the eliminated contact (interference in CR) will possibly reappear after a short period. This statement is supported by the results of a longitudinal clinical study carried out on 53 children and teenagers. Only one of them did not have interference while the remaining 52, who did have interference, had them preventively eliminated. When the whole group was examined a year later, all of them had interference in CR again, which was eliminated for a second time. After a year, on examination of the group, only six of the subjects had no interferences. The rest went through another round of selective grinding once again. The following year, only nine individuals did not show interferences.[19] From this we can infer that it is impossible to think that when the mandible is retruded, no "interference" will appear. It seems more appropriate to call these interferences "dental contacts in the retrusive position" because they are far from interfering with the mandible physiology.

It is possible that a great discrepancy results from a retrusive excursion, that is, the space between both arches in the axial plane is greater than 1 mm. When this happens, an analysis must be made to find the origin of the discrepancy. Below, two large discrepancy types are explained, one real and one relative.

- *Large real discrepancies.* Discrepancies bigger than the ones illustrated by the epidemiologic studies mentioned above have been found in patients with TMJ diseases, with a specific diagnosis of osteoarthritis[20,21] (Fig 21-3). These results show that the discrepancy increase may be the consequence of the degenerative state of the TMJ in these patients. For this reason, we suggest that TMJ clinical examinations should be carefully car-

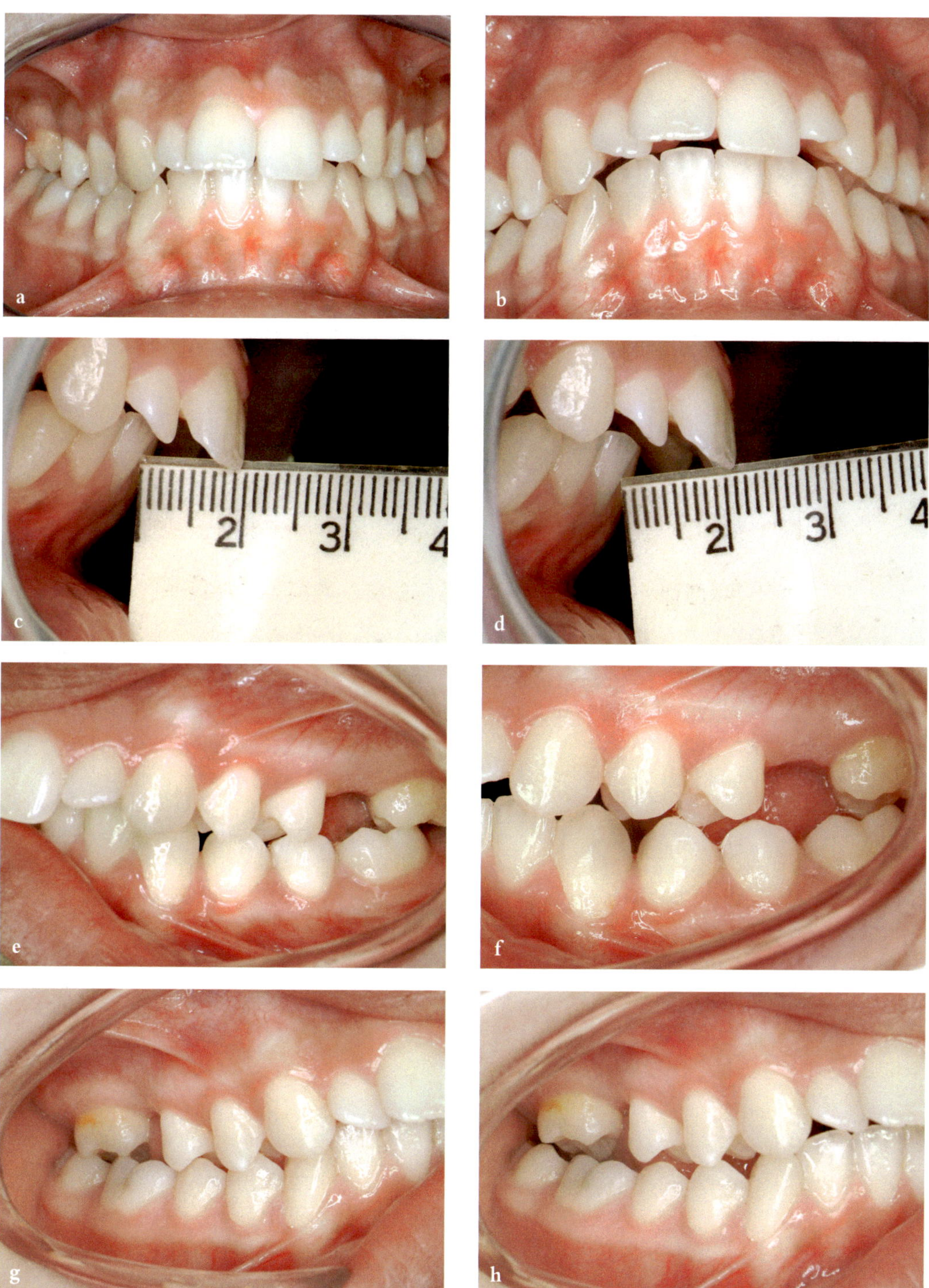


Fig 21-2 **(a and b)** Intercuspal and retrusive positions. **(c and d)** Intercuspal position and retrusive position – discrepancy does not exceed 1 mm. **(e and f)** Intercuspal position, left lateral view, and retrusive position, right lateral view – only the second molar comes into contact. **(g and h)** Intercuspal position and retrusive position – there is no tooth contact.

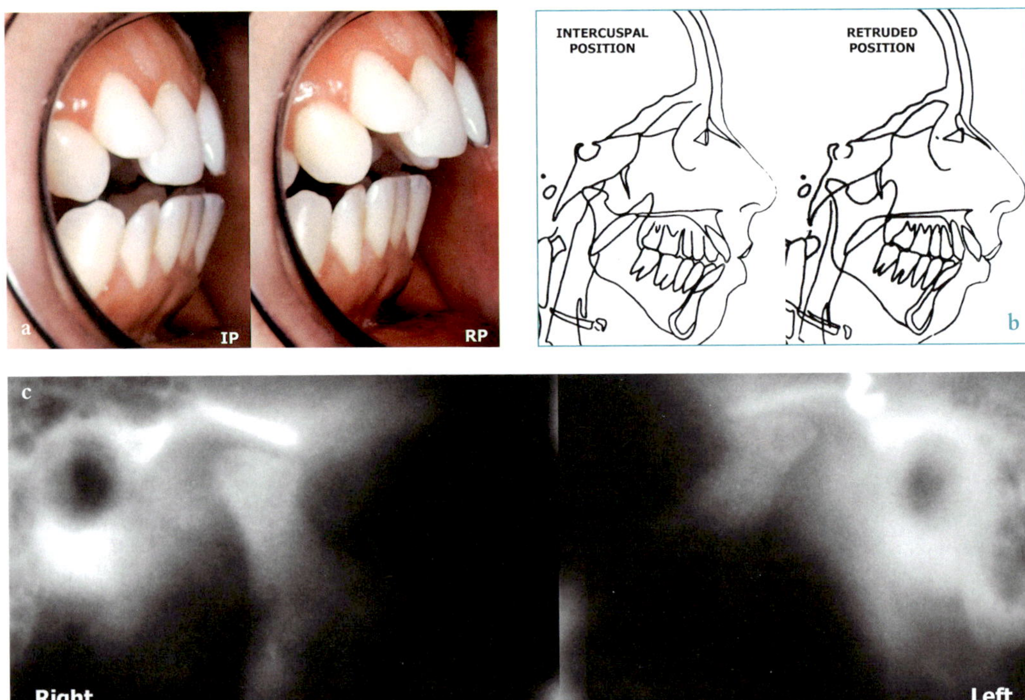


Fig 21-3 **(a)** Sixteen-year-old patient with juvenile rheumatoid arthritis. There is significant discrepancy (10 mm) between the intercuspal position and the retrusive position, as a consequence of degenerative arthritis. **(b)** Lateral cephalograms done in intercuspal and retrusive positions. **(c)** Linear tomography of both TMJs; condyle remodeling and significant glenoid cavity flattening can be observed.

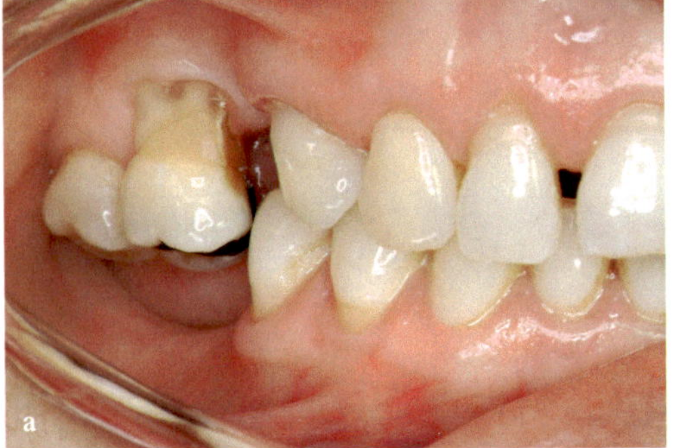

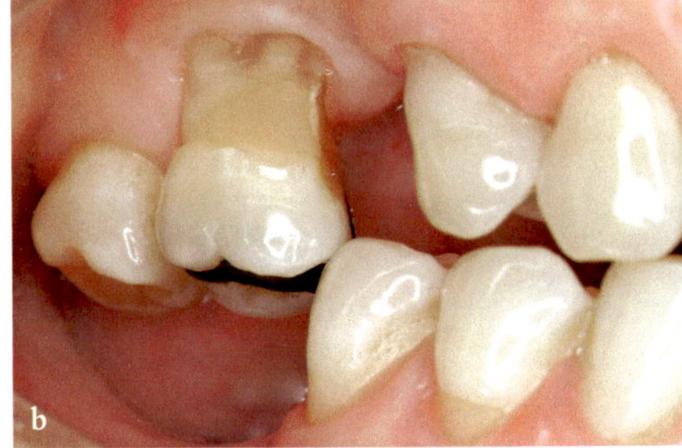

Fig 21-4 **(a)** Maximum dental intercuspation in a subject who lost his mandibular molars; this caused extrusion of the maxillary molars. **(b)** In order to retrude the jaw, the dental locking should first be unlocked. This results in a significantly increased vertical dimension, which produces the impression of greater discrepancy. This greater discrepancy is "relative".

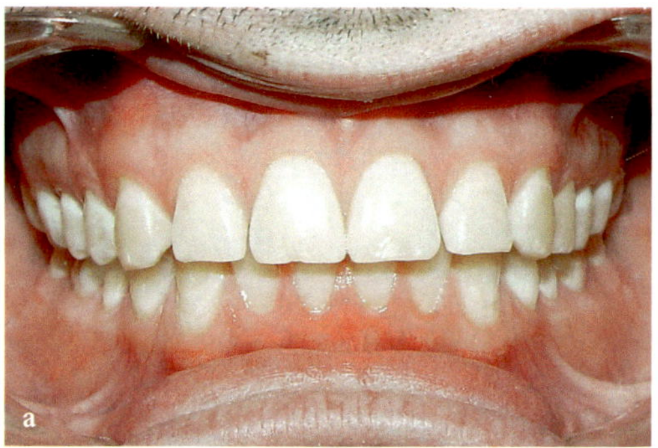

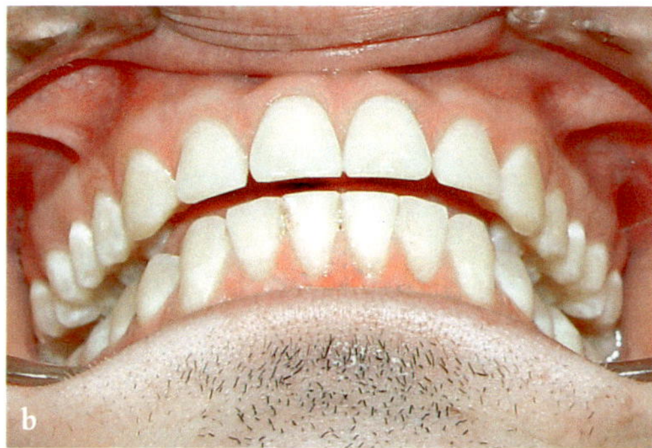

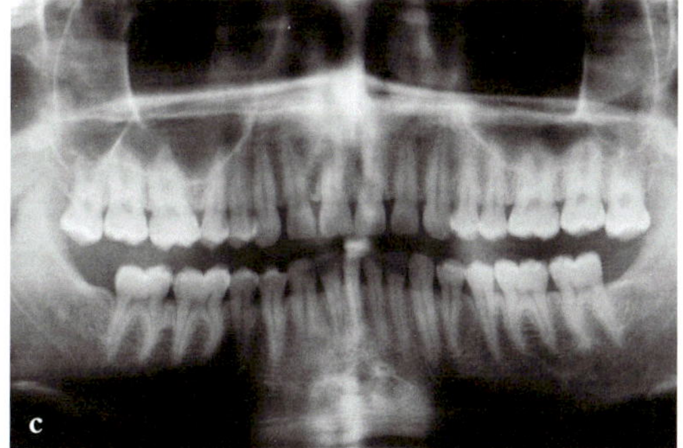

Fig 21-5 **(a)** Intercuspal position, and **(b)** retrusive position showing a large (relative) discrepancy. **(c)** On this panoramic radiograph, note how both third molars are extruded owing to the absence of antagonists. During jaw retrusion, the mandibular second molars come into contact with the third molars, and this results in a significantly increased vertical dimension, which gives the impression of a large (relative) discrepancy.

ried out on patients who are diagnosed with a discrepancy larger than 1 mm, to rule out the presence of a degenerative articular pathology that could be asymptomatic.

- *Large relative discrepancies.* Although the IP–RP discrepancy is determined by the retrusion allowed by the TMJ ligaments (large real discrepancy), it could be inherently influenced by some dental occlusion characteristics resulting in a misleading large mandible retrusion.

Whenever we try to guide a patient with complete or incomplete dentition into a retrusive excursion, first we need to break the connections between the teeth and their IP and consequently the maxillomandibular VD will increase (Fig 21-4). This VD increase will be proportional to the dental height to be dealt with so as to set the mandible free and allow the required retrusion. Undoubtedly, the dental occlusion condition can cause variations on this measure.

A typical example is a patient with a third unerupted mandibular molar, or a patient who had this third molar extracted a long time ago. Because of the molar's absence, the antagonist maxillary molar erupts without limitation, possibly supra-erupting by quite a few millimeters. In order to perform the maneuver of retrusion, first we have to get round this third molar causing an increase in the VD (Fig 21-5). While the patient opens their mouth, it gradually forms a posterior concave arch (Fig 21-6), and the bigger the mouth opening is, the more retruded are the mandibular incisors. This gives the impression that there is a big discrepancy between the two positions because, when we compare the overjet in IP with that in RP, the resulted measure is considerably bigger

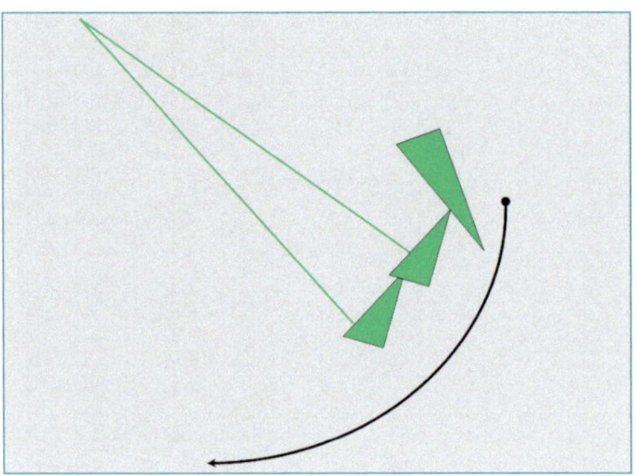

Fig 21-6 Diagram showing how, as vertical dimension increases, the distance between mandibular and maxillary incisors increases as well.

than 1 mm. This is called a large false (or relative) discrepancy that is not related to the mandibular retrusion but to the increase in VD.

Something similar could happen to patients who have had a tooth extracted which has not been replaced. This situation helps the distally located tooth to bend over, and so the antagonist tooth is left with no occlusal control. Therefore it can extrude freely. In an attempt to achieve retrusion in these cases, an increase in the VD must be previously reached, which undoubtedly causes inferior teeth distalization. This can also be seen in cases of tooth rotations and in direct relation to the malocclusion situation in general. Every time we compare the MI with the RP this effect should be borne in mind to avoid judgment errors such as the one mentioned above.

This kind of error can be made in a patient with prognathism in whom the mesial position of the mandible prevents the second superior molar from making occlusal contact with its inferior antagonist allowing it to extrude passively. In these cases, mandible retrusion must be performed along with a significant increase in VD (to get round the superior second molar), causing the visual impression that there is a big discrepancy but this picture is the result of a combination of the performed retrusion (which is generally within the normal statistical parameters) and the large VD increase (Fig 21-7).

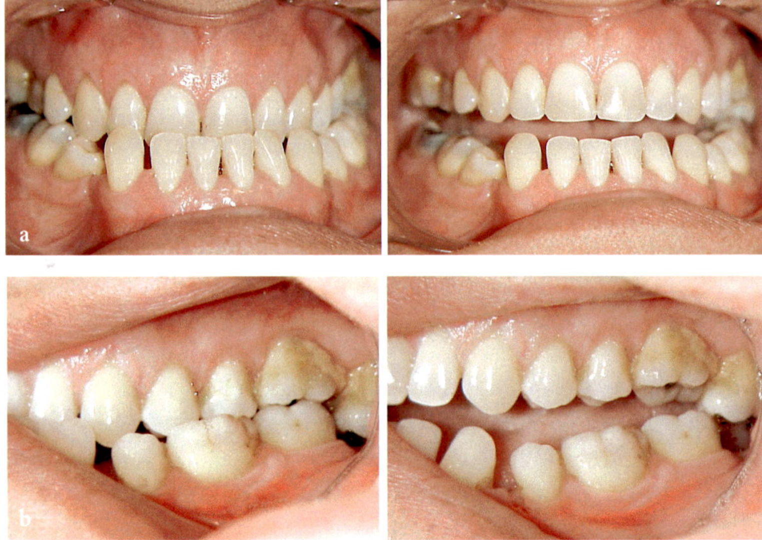


Fig 21-7 **(a)** Patient with intercuspal position prognathism, and the retrusive position showing a great (false) discrepancy. **(b)** Mandibular prognathism results in the absence of an antagonist for the maxillary second molar, which can extrude freely. In the retrusive position, the contact between second molars significantly increases vertical dimension. The combined effect of a normal retrusion and a significantly increased vertical dimension produces the impression of a large discrepancy.

### *Chronology of Centric Relation Definition*

Time has passed and the CR definition has been continuously modified. In order to appreciate its progressive mutation one just has to look at the Glossary of Terms of the American Academy of Prosthodontics, which is published every 6 years in the *Journal of Prosthetic Dentistry*.

In its first edition in 1956, CR was defined as "the most posterior relation between the mandible and the maxilla, from which every lateral movement in a specific VD can be performed". In 1987, in the fifth version, the definition changed into "the most retruded physiologic position of the mandible with respect to the maxilla from which lateral movements can be executed. It's the condition that emerges when there are several grades of intercuspal separation. This appears around the terminal hinge axis". In 1994, in the sixth version, the CR was defined as:

> *maxillo-mandibular relationship in which the condyles articulate with the thinnest avascular portion of their respective disks with the complex in the anterior–superior position against the slopes of the articular eminences. This position is independent of tooth contact and it is clinically discernable when the mandible is directed superiorly and anteriorly and restricted to a purely rotary movement about a transverse horizontal axis.*

This last definition has not changed in the following versions in 1999 and 2005, thus it is still in use.[56]

On analyzing the different definitions, we can see the changes from the most posterior condyle position to the most anterior and superior one. Peculiarly, despite radical changes in the definition, the same clinical maneuvers are still used in order to obtain CR. But, in all cases, it does not matter what maneuver is being used to guide the mandible into a centric position, the final noticeable result is that the inferior incisors are always in a more posterior position than the one they were in MI. That is why we think it is wiser to define it as a retruded mandible position because, in this way, there will be a logical correspondence between what we have defined, what we do, and the results we will see.

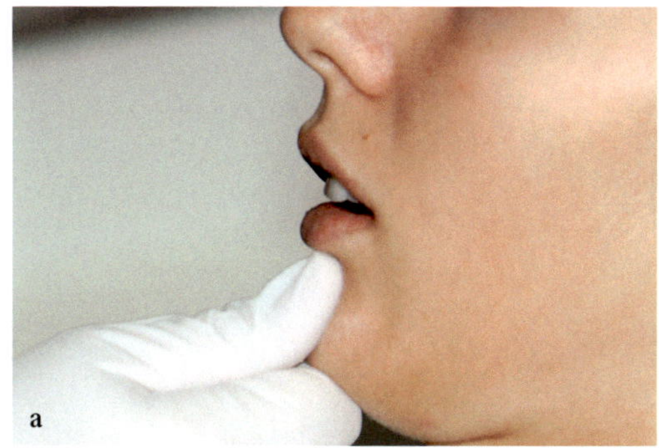

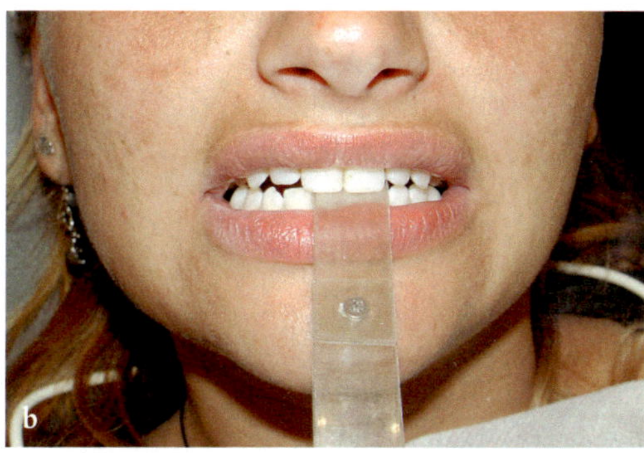

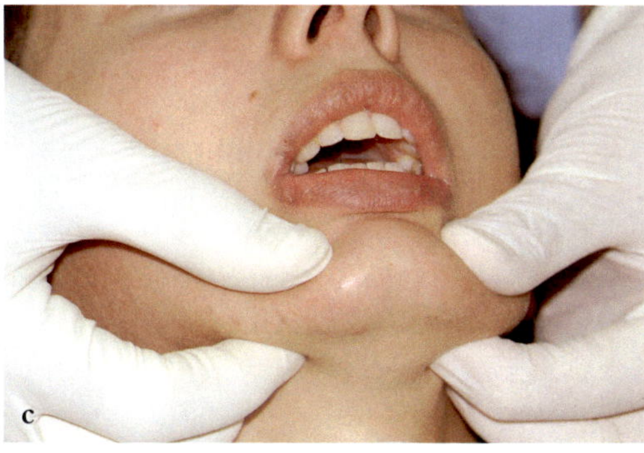

Fig 21-8 Clinical maneuvers used to retrude the jaw: **(a)** chin point method; **(b)** Long's leaf gauge; **(c)** Dawson's manipulation technique.

### *Reaching a Retruded Position*

Many methods have been proposed to guide the mandible into a centric relation position (retruded). Some of the best known methods are: pushing the

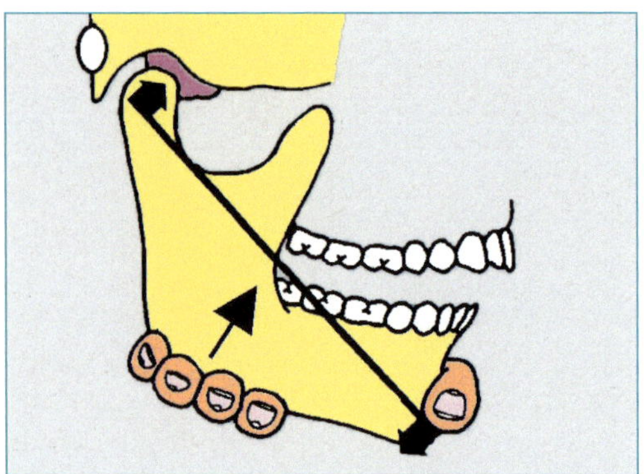

Fig 21-9 Manipulation technique suggested by Dawson.[55]

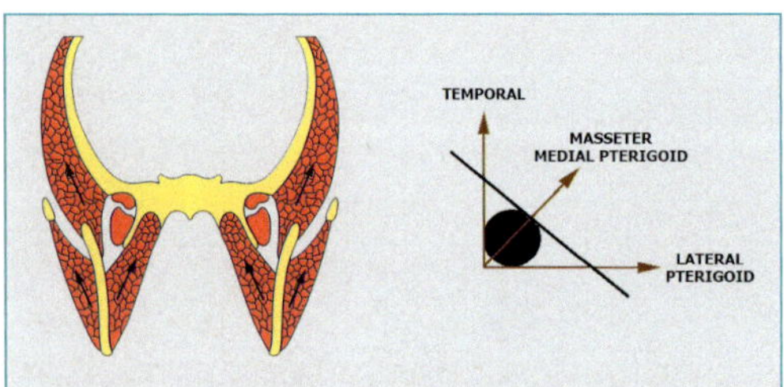


Fig 21-10 Force vectors of the levator muscles. Their tone keeps articular structures always in contact.

chin backwards with the thumbs, biting a cotton roll, biting a tongue depressor, using a Long leaf gauge, making use of a Lucia jig, swallowing saliva, closing the mouth while the tongue and palate keep in contact, asking the patient to voluntarily close their mouth in retrusion, or applying Dawson bimanual manipulation (Fig 21-8). To a greater or lesser degree, all these methods invariably result in mandible retrusion since all of them have been presented to satisfy the CR definitions which describe CR as the most posterior position of the condyles. Later on, bearing in mind the new definition of CR which states that it is the most superior and anterior position, all these methods seem to be out of context.

Without offering proof, Dawson proposes a bimanual manipulation technique which aims to fit the new CR definition – the antero-superior position of both condyles[22] (Fig 21-9). If we analyze this technique, it is difficult to understand how condyles can move upwards and forwards as the elevator muscle tones are permanently doing this themselves, at least during wakefulness.

According to basic physiologic principles of the synovial joint, there must be permanent and close contact between the articular bone ends in order to avoid disarticulation. There is no empty anatomic space between the condyle, the disc, and the articular ends, so they must always be in contact. As mentioned before, this function is carried out by the masticatory muscles that keep the corporal posture when their muscle tone is unstrained (Fig 21-10). When disc displacement occurs, other tissues – such as the retro-discal ones, the capsule, or a collateral ligament – fill the empty space.

This can be clearly understood if we consider patients who suffer from osteoarthritis and whose condylar anatomy undergoes permanent deformations and reductions. The muscle tone permanently raises the affected condyle to be able to maintain contact with the upper structures. Day after day, we meet patients who suffer from this degenerative articular disease, which causes progressive mandibular asymmetries and permanent occlusal overload on the affected side (Fig 21-11). The same happens to patients whose condyle must rest on tissues histologically different from the tissues of the disc because of a chronic disc displacement without reduction. In these cases, an occlusal overload is also seen on the affected section because the muscle raises the condyle in order to ensure permanent contact, causing early tooth contacts on that side (Fig 21-12).

Once this has been understood, then we can realize that there is no chance to guide the condyle upwards and forwards without introducing it into the cranium. The roof of the glenoid fossa inclines up from the back of the joint and down at the front. Thus, if the condyle achieves the most superior position, retrusion is also attained infallibly. Likewise, if the condyle is

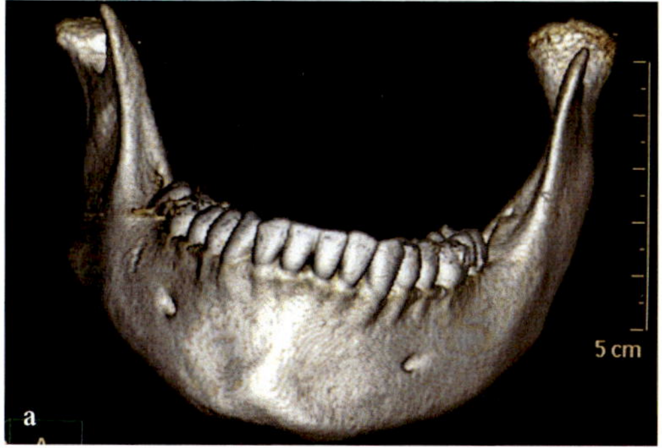


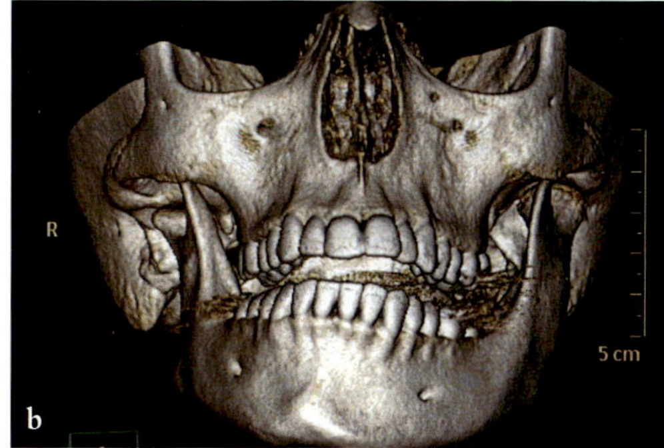


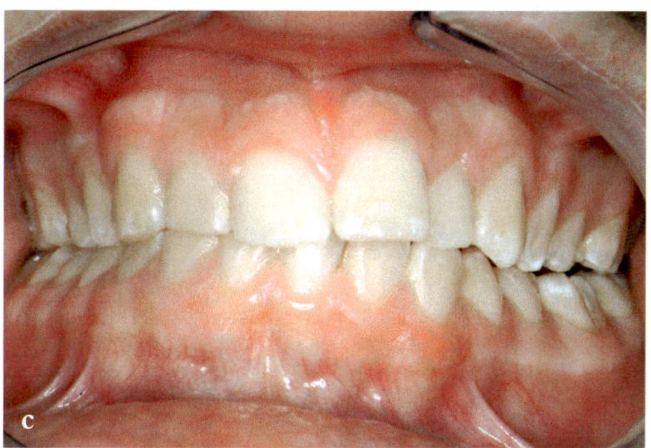


Fig 21-11 **(a)** Three-dimensional CT of a patient with osteoarthritis in the right TMJ. **(b)** In the resting position, the tone of the levator muscles raises both condyles. Note the difference of spacing between the mandibular right and left molars when compared to their respective maxillary antagonists. **(c)** Intercuspal position: note the occlusal overload on the affected side, as a result of the constant deterioration of the right joint by the disease.

guided forward, a condyle protrusion systematically takes place (see Fig 21-12).

The muscle tone is responsible for this constant state of contact that is common in every articulation of economy. Something different happens during sleep when the musculature is at rest, and thus we cannot sleep standing up or simply keep our head up.

Returning to the maneuver proposed by Dawson, it was proved that it caused condyle retrusion in all the observed patients in a study carried out by Muraoka and Iwata.[23] They obtained similar results when they analyzed the technique of the thumb on the chin. These conclusions have been supported by similar studies.[24,25] The possibility of guiding the condyle a bit upwards and forwards does exist when the bite at IP is strong. This last state should not be considered as a condyle repositioning, but rather

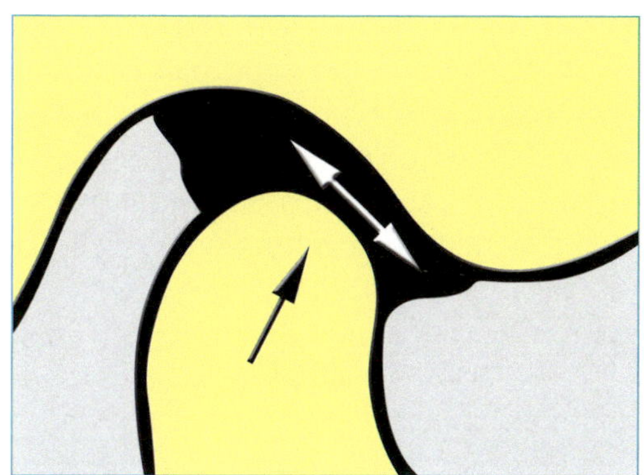

Fig 21-12 The tone of the masticatory muscles keeps articular structures in close contact. When there is condyle elevation, the condyle will also retrude.

the result of narrowing of the disc or other tissue that has been in the disc place owing to the strong muscle force performed.[26]

Moreover, the terminal condyle position after biting the Long leaf gauge has been analyzed and all the studied subjects showed condyle retrusion directly proportional to the biting force.[27] The positioning of this leaf gauge leads to a directly inclined posterior plane. When the patient bites it, the mandible moves in a caudal direction, causing mandibular distalization towards retrusion.

## Axis of Rotation of the Mandible

The idea that the mandible rotates around a transversal hinge axis dates back to before 1900. As early as 1860, based on cadaveric dissections, Langer[28] stated that, during small mouth openings, condyles apparently remain motionless – suggesting the existence of an axis of rotation. This theory has gained a lot of support.[29–32] The most acknowledged work may be that presented in 1952 by Ulf Posselt.[33] In his publication he showed mandibular movements illustrated at the inferior incisor level in three dimensions. Posselt suggested that the mandible can achieve pure rotation around a hinge axis for the first 20 mm of the opening of the mouth. He also stated that, in order to achieve rotation, the mandible must perform the act of opening and closing in its most retruded position. For this reason, Posselt presented this view to the prosthodontic community not as an axis to use during functional mandibular movements, but as a reference point to be later transferred to the articulating device.

Sicher,[34] the celebrated anatomist, concluded that the hinge axis position is achieved from the most retrusive position of the condyles obtained by means of the patients' own muscles. These concepts are refuted by Shanahan and Leff's work; these authors assert that an artificial mandibular axis can be obtained with opening and closing of the mouth and the chin directly upwards. However, they state that this is not helpful because the discovered axis is part of a non-physiologic mandibular position.[35–38]

The existence of a unique transverse axis for mandibular rotation common for both condyles has been strongly defended by gnathologists who put this idea into action and laid the foundations for this school of thought – to the point of justifying the execution of permanent facial tattoos. The first actual kinematic location of the hinge axis was carried out by the California Gnathologic Society under the leadership of Dr B. B. McCollum who used a Snow facebow to achieve his goal – and it took him 8 hours to do so.[29] Modified reproductions of the instrument used at that time are used by gnathologists today.

Nevertheless, others have disagreed with this notion and have proposed an "instantaneous centers of mandibular rotation" hypothesis.[39–41] According to this, when the mouth opens, the mandible always performs combined rotation and translation movements around a unique axis; therefore there may exist an axis for each VD.

Disagreement goes beyond the discussion about whether or not a mandibular axis of rotation exists. Another source of disagreement is where this questionable axis could be located. In 1919, Gysi[42] was the first to state that it is impossible that the center of rotation is located at the levels of condyles. Brewka's work[43] along with that of Nattestad and Vedtofte[44] supports this idea; their investigations revealed that the center of rotation is located *behind* the condyles. Nevekari[45] maintains that the center of rotation is *outside* the condyles and that it could be located at the level of the mastoid process. Koski[46] agrees with that, and he also proposes that the axis is located somewhere in the mastoid apophysis.

Whereas mechanical methods were used in the first studies carried out as corroboration, contemporary researchers have been using new technology for measurement and verification, and the new results deny the existence of a hinge axis. A

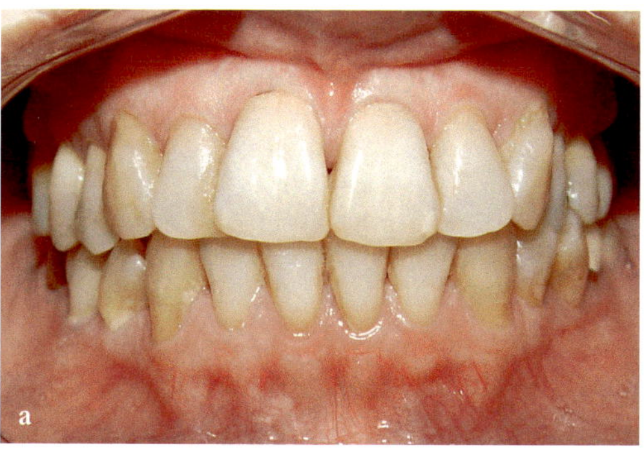

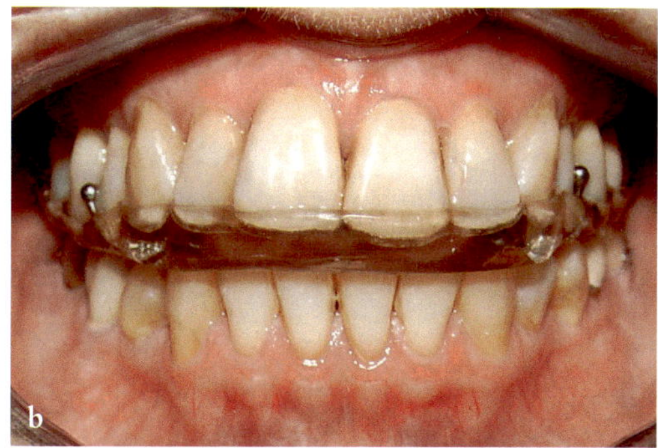

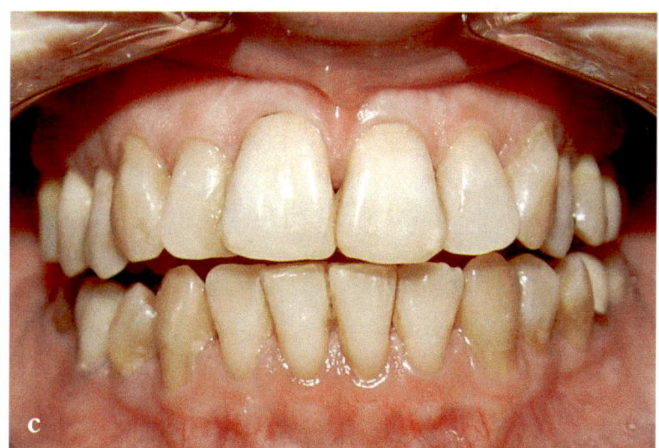

Fig 21-13 Female bruxer who wears a night guard. **(a)** Maximum dental intercuspation. **(b)** Maximum dental intercuspation on the splint. **(c)** On waking after 8 hours of sleep and removing the splint, the maximum intercuspation is different from the original one.

subtraction radiographic technique was used in a study in which the position of the condyles was recorded starting from a retruded mandibular position, and eventually the VD of the occlusion was gradually increased.[47] The researchers concluded that the opening movements of the mandible from a retruded position have mainly rotational characteristics, although none of the eight subjects studied showed a pure rotational movement and the direction and axis translation amount varied from one subject to another.

In addition, condyle position has been studied in eight subjects with common characteristics by means of a sophisticated three-dimensional system of digitalization.[48] In this research the starting point was the dental MI, and then mouth opening increased from a distance of 3 mm to 25 mm at the molar level. The eight subjects (16 condyles) showed simultaneous rotation and translation, mainly in an anteroinferior direction. These authors support the concept of an instantaneous axis of rotation and they suggest mounting the cast on articulators to use the constructive bites obtained during treatment.

By means of magnetic resonance imaging, McDevitt and co-workers have noted the translation of the center of rotation while small mouth openings increase progressively.[49]

Ferrario and co-workers' studies have shown that, along its physiologic cycles (normal) of opening and closing, the mandible never performs a pure rotation movement round an intercondylar axis – confirming in this way the truth of the theory of instantaneous centers of rotation.[50] Similar conclusions have been reached by others who used kinesiography as a method of verification.[51]

In an interesting study using computerized tomography, Kuboki and co-workers[26] observed condyle translation when they compared the condyle position during MI with the result obtained from biting a 2 mm flat splint. This experience acquires great significance because it answers a question that often arises in dental offices. Patients who use bruxism splints every night while sleeping frequently inform us that, when they wake up and remove the device, they find it impossible to achieve dental intercuspation until some minutes later (Fig 21-13). Why does this happen?

The commonly given answer is that mandibular deprogramming takes place, but this is not correct. For a better understanding, we make use of the valuable information from the above-mentioned research which rejects the existence of a pure axis of mandibular rotation. The existence of such an axis would imply that, when the bruxism splint is removed after being used for some hours, teeth will reach intercuspation without problems. But evidence shows a different reality. When the splint is placed, an increase in the VD takes place and consequently both condyles rotate (mainly) but they also move to another position (slightly). So, condyles are in a position during dental intercuspation (at occlusal VD) but they are in a different position while the splint is being used (at a larger VD). This means that the patient's system of muscle engrams to perform in MI has been replaced by another one (reprogramming) as occlusion and VD have changed. This does not mean that the use of the splint has brought about a mandibular deprogramming and it moves to another position, but the VD increase implies roto-translation of both condyles. Then, if the person has the splint in their mouth for several hours, new muscle engrams develop to keep condyles in this last position. When the patient takes out the splint after using it all night, the condyles are still governed by those engrams and thus dental intercuspation cannot be achieved. A few minutes later, these engrams fade, IP is possible again, and it is governed by a new engram system.

If the patient wears the splint for only a few minutes and then takes it out, the effect mentioned above is not present. Wearing the splint for a short period does not lead to new engram development, and the patient can normally reach intercuspation. In contrast, if the device is used all night or for 24 hours, as in the case of patients with TMJ disorders, the neuromuscular system will require a period of time to adapt the condyles to a new position in the glenoid fossa. Consequently, the term "deprogramming" must not be used for the reason that this "engram reprogramming" is the result of VD increase and not of a splint "magical" effect.

To confirm this, a bruxism splint must be made and occlusal contact points must be indicated in a permanent way (with an acrylic of different color) before giving it to the patient (Fig 21-14). In a subsequent appointment, after the patient has used the splint for a significant amount of time, the occlusion in the splint is checked by using articulating paper. It can then be observed that the maxillomandibular relation has not changed; that is, the marks on the articulating paper match the color marks on the splint even though the patient cannot achieve tooth contact after taking out the device.

When starting significant occlusal reconstructions of the masticatory system, it is very important to decide whether or not to accept the existence of an intercondylar center of rotation. If there *is* a center of rotation, the VD can be modified directly in the articulator. Otherwise, it will be necessary to have clinical records of the bite at the exact VD at which place the reconstruction is going to take place. The same happens when making a bruxism splint; at the moment of recording the maxillomandibular relation to mount the lower cast on the articulator, it is necessary to leave a separation between both dental arches that represents the thickness that the splint will be.

A very simple and effective method for making a bruxism splint is presented below. This method can also be used when prosthetically restoring the masticatory system in a larger VD.

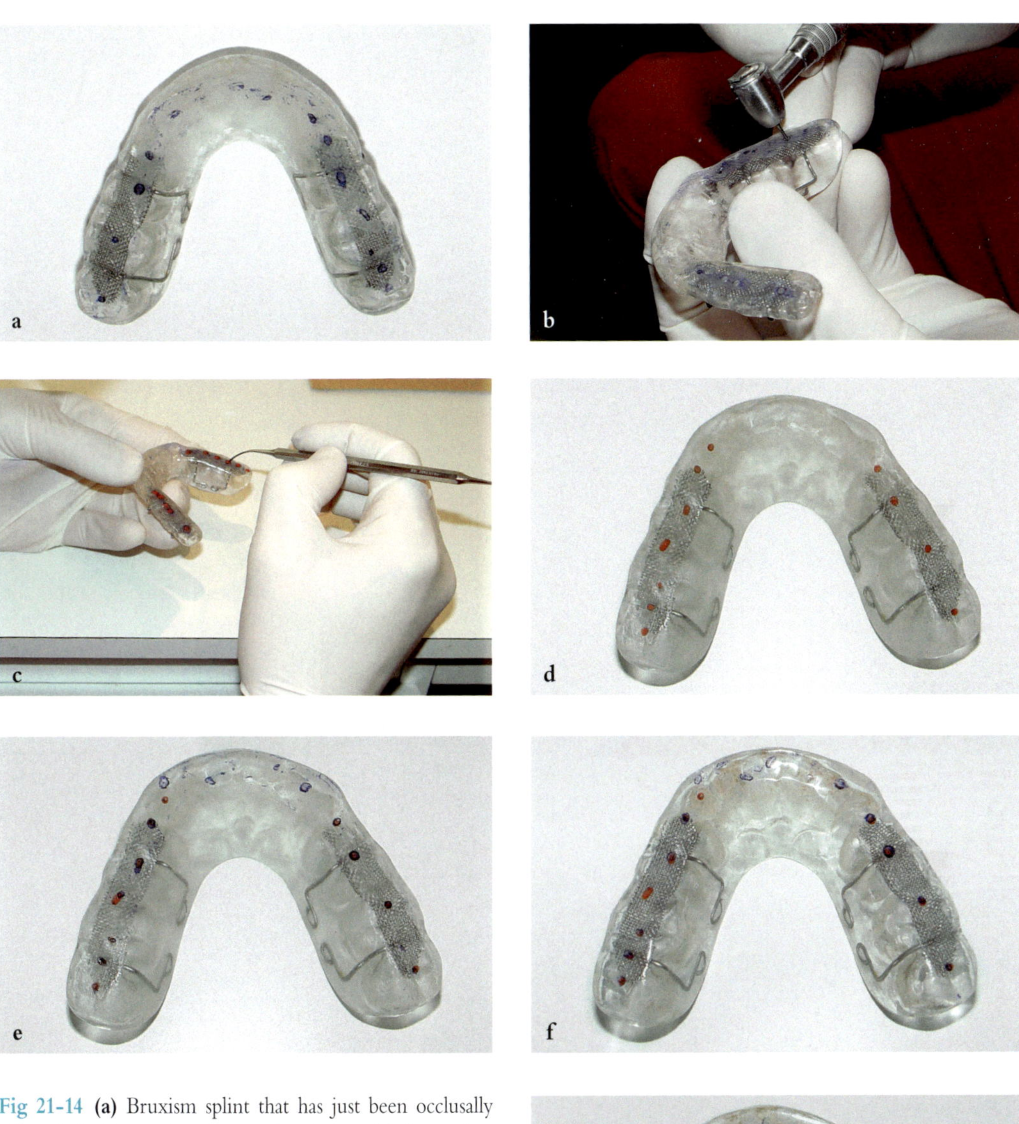

Fig 21-14 **(a)** Bruxism splint that has just been occlusally adjusted; the blue marks correspond to the mandibular vestibular cusps. **(b)** With a round bur, a cavity (1 mm deep) is carved in the center of the blue marks. **(c)** The cavities are filled with red fluid acrylic (Duralay). **(d)** Once polymerized, they are polished to the level of the surface of the splint. **(e)** The splint is placed in the mouth and articulating paper is used to verify that there is coincidence with the red acrylic dots. **(f)** Six months later, the occlusion is checked by using articulating paper, and no changes in the position of the jaw are observed, since there is still coincidence with the red dots. **(g)** The splint after 2 years of use. It shows wear, but coincidence with the dots still remains. Note: This patient mentioned that, upon removal of the splint after wearing it the whole night, intercuspation did not immediately occur; but 30 minutes later, occlusion has returned to normal.

## The Anterior bite Plane Method

The anterior bite plane method is highly efficient and so simple that it can be carried out by anyone ranging from the most experienced clinician to an undergraduate student. It is helpful when determining the new VD and when controlling and recording mandibular position in the axial plane. It is essential also in the following clinical situations:

- oral rehabilitation – when performing a complete prosthetic restoration of the patient's occlusion
- bruxism – when making a splint.

*Making the anterior bite plane*
It can be made by means of a direct technique (in the patient's mouth) or indirectly (on the maxilla model).

*Direct technique*
This technique is quite simple and consequently quicker than the indirect one. However, it requires a higher degree of skill. As the job is done directly in the patient's mouth using plastic acrylic, when the patient has a crown or a facial surface made of acrylic, it should be previously lubricated using solid Vaseline. Then, self-curing acrylic is prepared and, when it has reached a plastic state, it is manually placed on the patient's maxillary incisors (Fig 21-15). Before the acrylic polymerization takes place, it is convenient to take it out and put it back again twice or three times to prevent this from sticking under the pontics in patients with a fixed bridge or between dental pieces, since the presence of empty interdental spaces is very common. When the acrylic has polymerized, it is removed from the mouth and its edges are shaped by means of burs for acrylic. It is always convenient to remove all the imperfections on the entire interior walls to prevent any fractures on the plaster cast, but this has to be done very carefully to avoid going too far and eliminating the minimal retention needed for the next clinical maneuvers.

*Indirect technique*
A maxillary model is needed. Aluminum foil is placed on the model, where the teeth are located, preferably between the first premolars (Fig 21-16). This step has two aims: to prevent the acrylic from sticking, and to leave a small space between the cast and the acrylic, which is useful to ensure the model's integrity. As in the direct technique, after polymerization, it is convenient to take the acrylic out and put it in again several times so that the anterior bite plane is not attached to empty spaces that the model could have. Once the acrylic polymerizes, the anterior bite plane is removed, the aluminum foil is removed and the undercuts created by the interdental spaces are eliminated. The next step consists in testing the anterior bite plane on the model. This must be done carefully to avoid breaking the teeth, and if there is too much friction, it is recommended grinding the areas of the anterior bite plane which show abrasion as many times as necessary until the splint can be placed and taken out with certain ease. Finally it is smoothened using an acrylic bur for the initial check in the mouth.

*Clinical procedure*
*Anterior bite plane requirements*

- The anterior bite plane must remain closely attached to the teeth while the patient performs opening and closing mouth movements.
- It must not change the upper lip position significantly. So the wall of the anterior bite plane must be extremely thin (almost transparent) (Fig 21-17).
- Its surface must be completely flat and it must diverge from the upper occlusal plane at 14 degrees (Fig 21-18) so that the dental tapping of the mandibular incisors take place in a smaller area.[52]

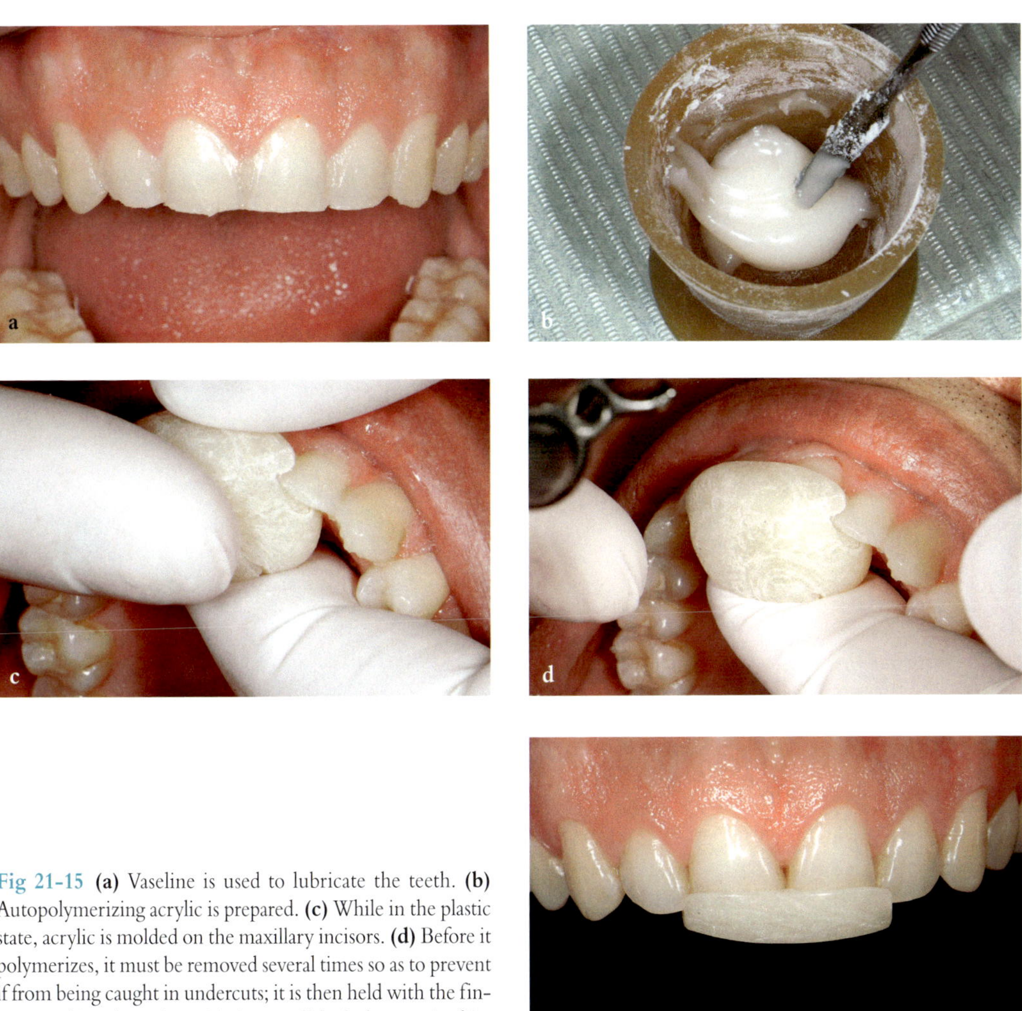

Fig 21-15 **(a)** Vaseline is used to lubricate the teeth. **(b)** Autopolymerizing acrylic is prepared. **(c)** While in the plastic state, acrylic is molded on the maxillary incisors. **(d)** Before it polymerizes, it must be removed several times so as to prevent if from being caught in undercuts; it is then held with the fingers until it polymerizes. **(e)** Once polished, the anterior bite plane is fitted over the incisors.

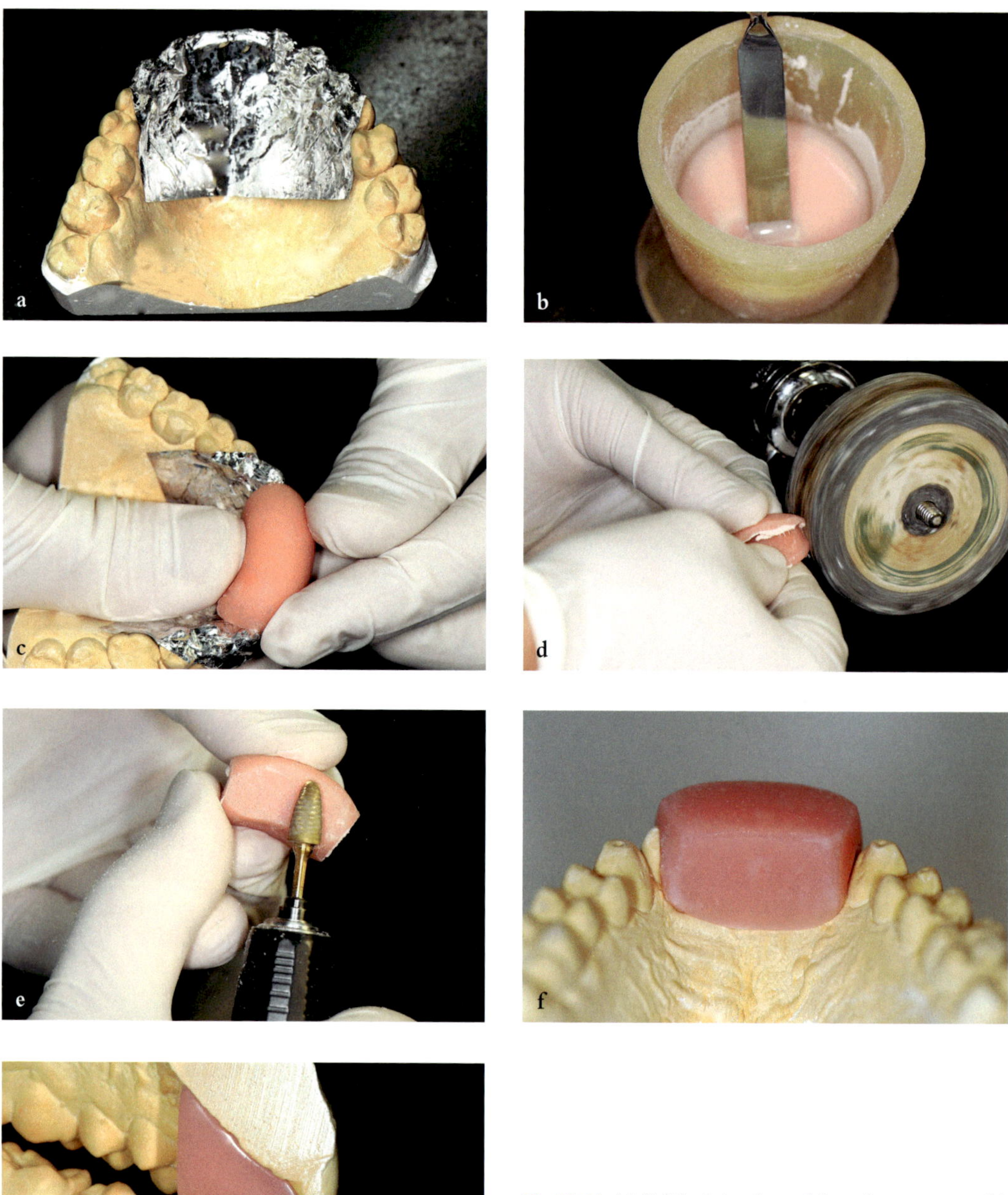


Fig 21-16 **(a)** Polished aluminum foil on the upper cast. **(b)** Self-cure acrylic is prepared. **(c)** An acrylic mass in the plastic state is molded on the cast. **(d)** It is shaped with a lathe. **(e)** An acrylic bur is used to polish the piece to a smooth finish. **(f)** The anterior bite plane finished and ready to be used. **(g)** Articulated-cast section which allows anterior bite plane features to be observed.

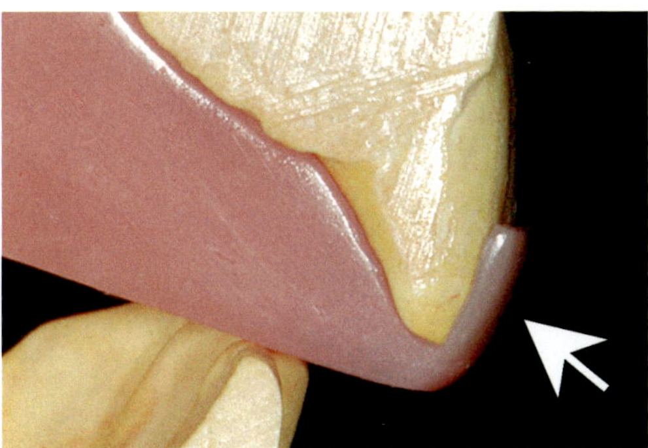

Fig 21-17 The vestibular wall of the anterior bite plane should be extremely thin (arrow), so as not to cause the upper lip to stick out.

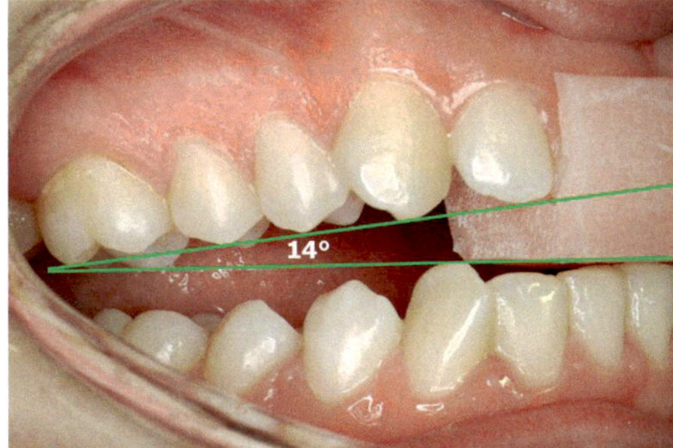


Fig 21-18 The flat surface of the anterior bite plane should diverge approximately 14 degrees from the occlusal plane.

- When occluding, it must make contact in only one spot (or two), the place that is closest to the middle line.

*Aims*

- In oral rehabilitation, the aim is to make it easier for clinicians to determine a new VD based on facial esthetics and lip competence; and to allow establishment of a relationship between both arches after the teeth have been shaped and the IP eliminated.
- In bruxism splint fabrication, the aim is to facilitate the correct separation between the arches in order to determine splint thickness.
- Another aim is to corroborate mandibular closing movement repetition in the TP (equivalent to the MI but with a larger VD).
- A further aim is to measure the distance between the TP (voluntary) and the reference RP (guided).

*Technique*

*Position of the patient*

The mandible is a movable bone that has its own specific gravity and so it is subjected to the physical laws of gravity. Thus, the patient's position depends on the treatment. If a bruxism splint to be worn while sleeping (supine position) is to be fabricated, the patient must be lying down at the moment of obtaining the record. If the purpose is oral rehabilitation and the restoration is going to be used during mastication, the patient must be seated.

*Vertical dimension selection*

At the beginning, an arbitrary VD determined by the acrylic anterior bite plane thickness is used. For the development of a bruxism splint, the thickness at the level of the second molars is 2 mm. So, it must be confirmed that when the patient is asked to close their mouth, there is a 2 mm separation between the cusps of the already mentioned teeth (Fig 21-19). This ensures enough acrylic thickness

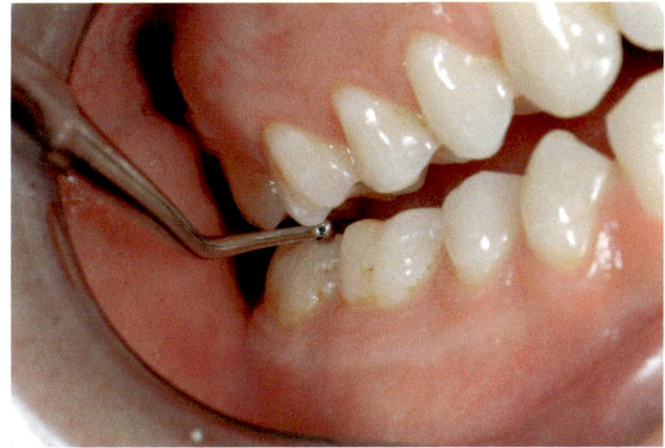

Fig 21-19 While the patient occludes over the anterior bite plane, the existence of a suitable space required at the level of the molars is verified with the end of a tool whose size matches the thickness desired for the splint.

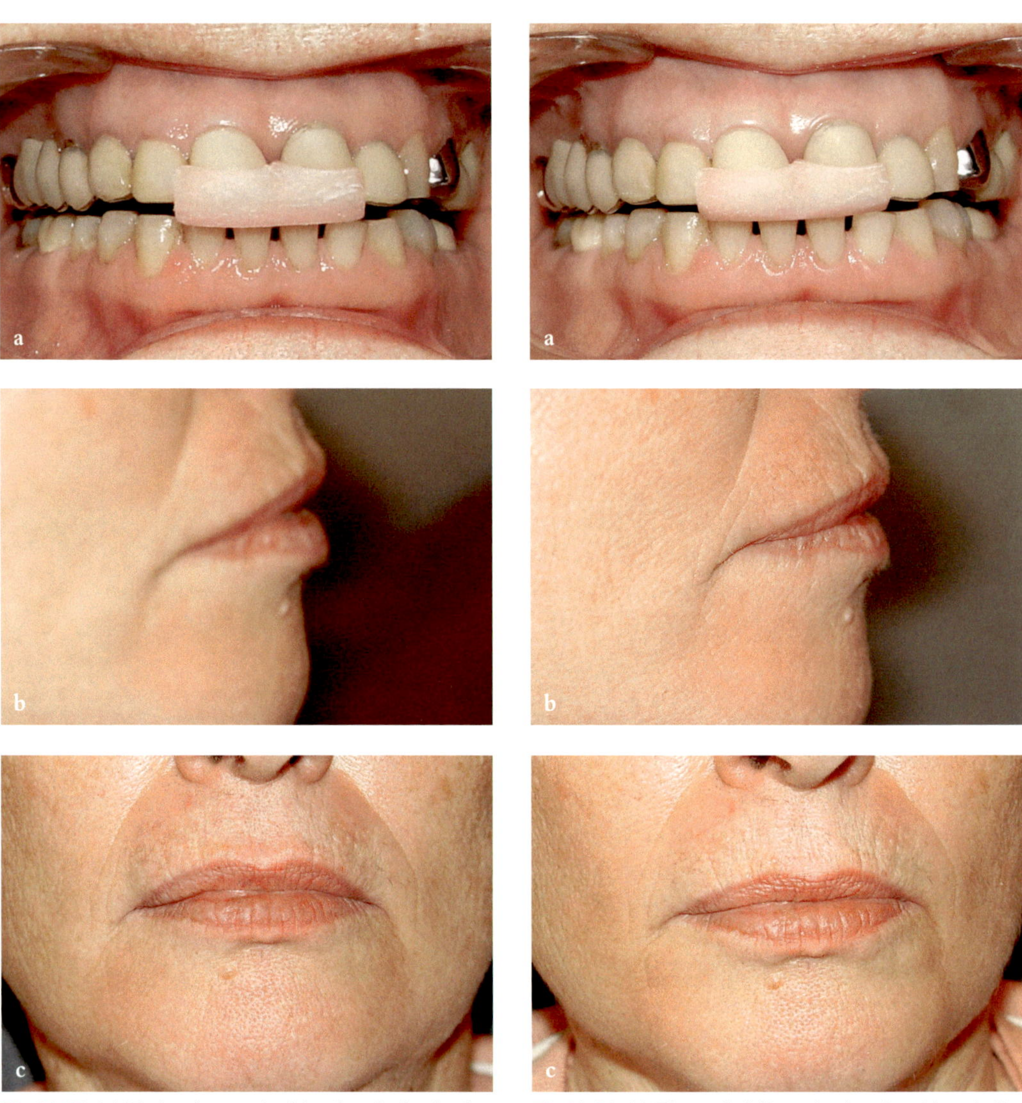

**Fig 21-20** **(a)** Trying the anterior bite plane in for the first time. **(b and c)** The vertical dimension is excessively high, and the patient must make an effort to maintain her lips in contact.

**Fig 21-21** **(a)** The vertical dimension is reduced by grinding away the anterior bite plane. **(b and c)** Now the patient can comfortably maintain her lips in contact.

so that the future splint will be resistant to the possible clenching and grinding of teeth at night.

If the aim is oral rehabilitation, the anterior bite plane thickness is determined by the characteristics of each case. VD restitution is an empirical process. Unfortunately, and despite technologic advances, there is no precise method that enables us to determine VD, but the use of two subjective clinical principles has led to accurate results (Figs 21-20 to 21-22).

- First, the patient must be comfortable when closing their lips without forcing their muscles while the mandible is at the rest position and the mandibular incisors are occluding with the anterior bite plane. For this reason, it is convenient to make a thicker anterior-bite plane than the one needed, and then gradually reduce its thickness until reaching the desired lip competence.
- Second, the patient is asked to look at themself in a mirror and make an esthetic evaluation. It is recommended that the patient comes with somebody they trust so that they can express their opinions. It is hugely important that the upper lip position does not change owing to the thickness of the walls of the anterior bite plane, because this leads to an unattractive look that is not related to a VD increase.

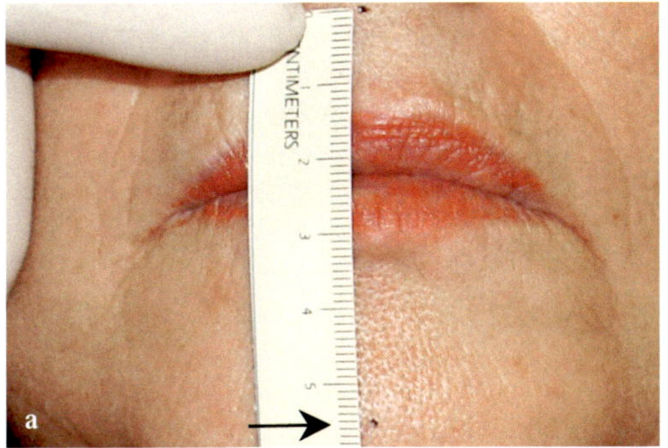


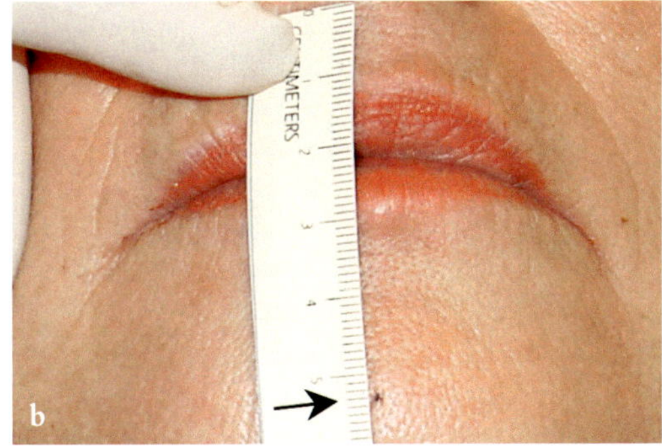


Fig 21-22 **(a)** Before anterior bite plane height is reduced, two dots are marked on the skin for reference. **(b)** A 2 mm reduction at the level of the anterior bite plane resulted in reduced VD, and the patient achieved comfortable lip competence.

*Therapeutic position attainment and repetitiveness*

As stated before, the TP is determined by the patient's own musculature without the clinician's guidance. The TP must be repeatable and, as it is an intraborder position, it must be slightly anterior to the RP at a distance not larger than 1 mm (Fig 21-23). The patient will be required to perform closing movements repeatedly (like tapping on the anterior bite plane) while the clinician places an articulating paper (Fig 21-24).

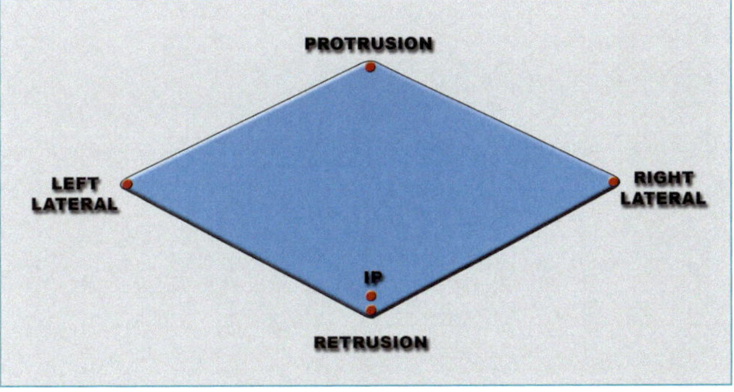


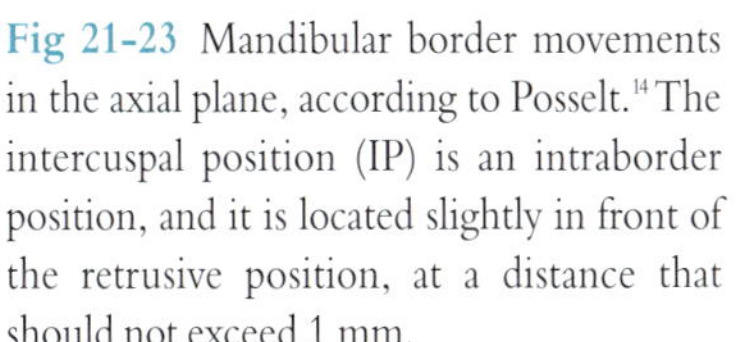

Fig 21-23 Mandibular border movements in the axial plane, according to Posselt.[14] The intercuspal position (IP) is an intraborder position, and it is located slightly in front of the retrusive position, at a distance that should not exceed 1 mm.

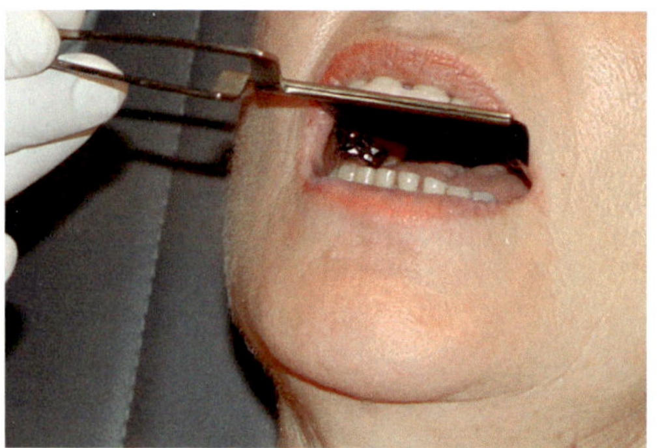

**Fig 21-24** The patient is requested to tap (3 or 4 per second) with her teeth on the surface of the anterior bite plane, as the operator places articulating paper in between the arches.

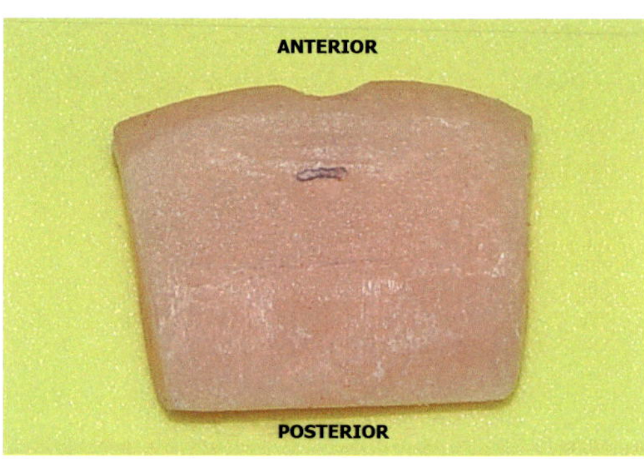


**Fig 21-25** Impressions from the taps are left on the anterior bite plane. Note how closures repeat and converge into only one impression.

These taps should be performed quickly, at least three or four per second. Studies have proved that opening and closing movements are more accurate and systematic when they are performed quickly than when they are carried out rather slowly.[53,54] In order to increase the number of taps, the mouth opening must be small; an opening of approximately 20 mm is recommended. It is advisable that the patient carries out these movements first as a test, so that they get used to them and perform them naturally. To summarize, the aim is to get a unique mark that will represent the places where the three or four mandible closings coincide (Fig 21-25). If this is not achieved in the first attempt, the procedure must be repeated as many times as necessary. It is recommended that the patient is observed while carrying out this test so that the clinician will be able to corroborate reproducibility of the final position and consequently confirm that the muscles allow reaching that position naturally and that the patient will be able to reach it again.

*Determination of the reference retruded position*

To achieve this purpose, the mandible must be guided to its most retruded position that will be the reference point. First, the patient will be asked to relax their mandible muscles and then their chin is gently pushed backwards by the clinician's thumb (Fig 21-26). This is not simple because it is not about forcing the mandible; on the contrary, the patient must let the dentist guide their mandible. The desired mandible retrusion cannot be achieved without proper relaxation of the masticatory muscles, and it is naive to think that the force of the hand will be stronger than the power of the masticatory muscles.

When the retrusion is accomplished, the clinician then manually induces two or three closings similar to the teeth tapping after previously placing articulating paper of a different color from the one used for the registration of the therapeutic position. In that way, a distinction can be made between the two positions (Fig 21-27).

*Verification of the distance between positions*

This step is executed to dismiss the possibility that the patient has carried out the voluntary closings in a protrusive position. The TP (voluntary) must be no more than 1 mm away from the reference RP (guided).

From a statistical standpoint, it is known that 90% of individuals have their IP slightly forward from the reference RP (at a distance smaller than 1 mm),[14–17] and both positions coincide for the

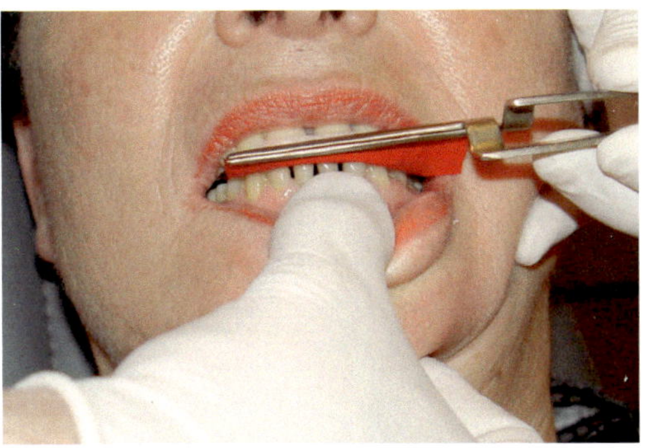

Fig 21-26 With one hand, the operator gently manipulates the jaw into a more retrusive position, from which several taps are given on the anterior bite plane. At the same time, the operator places articulating paper of another color in between the teeth with the other hand.

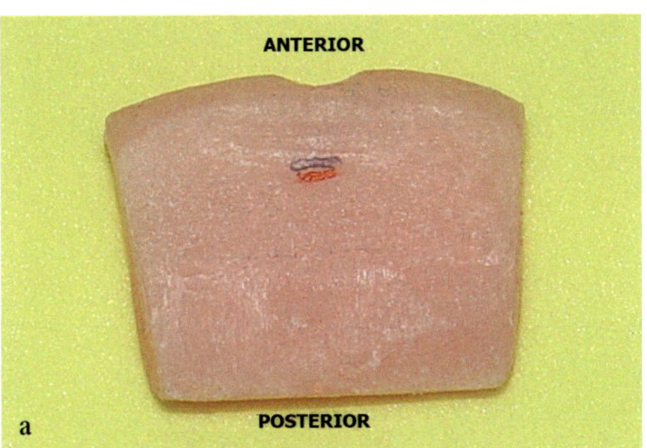


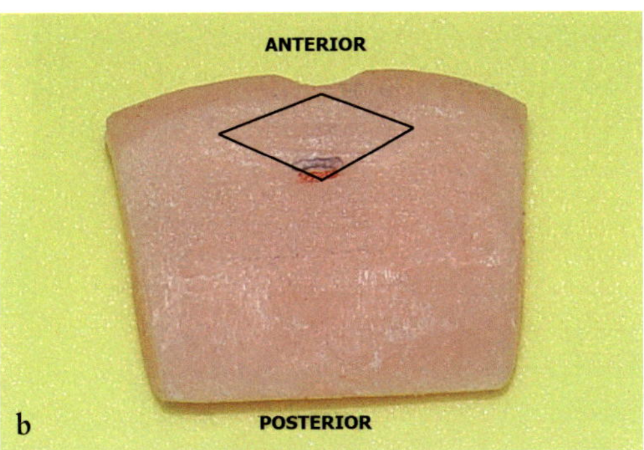


Fig 21-27 **(a)** The blue mark corresponds to the series of taps made freely by the patient (intercuspal position); the red mark corresponds to the retruded position. The distance between these marks is within the normal parameters. **(b)** For illustrative purposes, Posselt's rhomboid has been drawn in the axial plane on the anterior bite plane. The red mark corresponds to the retruded position (border), the blue mark to the maximum intercuspation (intraborder).

remaining 10%. If the result is within these parameters, the clinician can go to the next step, which is to obtain the maxillomandibular registeration. If the distance between the positions is larger than 1 mm, the registeration of the TP must be repeated because the patient has surely occluded in a protrusive position. In this case, it is best for the clinician to ask the patient to let him or her gently guide the mandible into the reference RP, and after that ask the patient to relax and try to let the mandible go down a few millimeters under its own weight (to the physiologic rest position) so that they can start again with the tapping. As this procedure is cheap, it can be done as many times as necessary until the patient gets used to it.

Another clinical step that is worth doing can be carried out to control the accuracy of the register, since placing wax between the posterior dental pieces may pose the risk of stimulating the sensory receptors of the periodontal ligament and the patient could move the mandible to an undesired position. This can be prevented by adding a closing acrylic key on the anterior bite plane. While the patient's incisors are in contact in TP, a small amount of self-curing acrylic is placed in the angle formed by the vestibular surfaces of the mandibular central incisors and the anterior bite plane by means of a Peter K. Thomas (PKT) dropper for wax (Fig 21-28). The patient must not move until the acrylic polymerizes. In this way, a key that makes the patient occlude in the exact position during the registration of the maxillomandibular record will be made. At this point, the most important steps are achieved; a new VD and a treatment position given by the patient's musculature itself are obtained. Besides, it will be corroborated that muscles are able to reach the same position repeatedly and that the distance between RP and TP is within the admissible parameters.

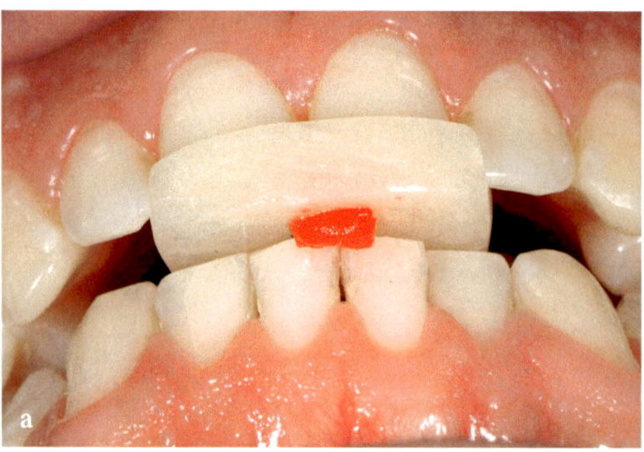

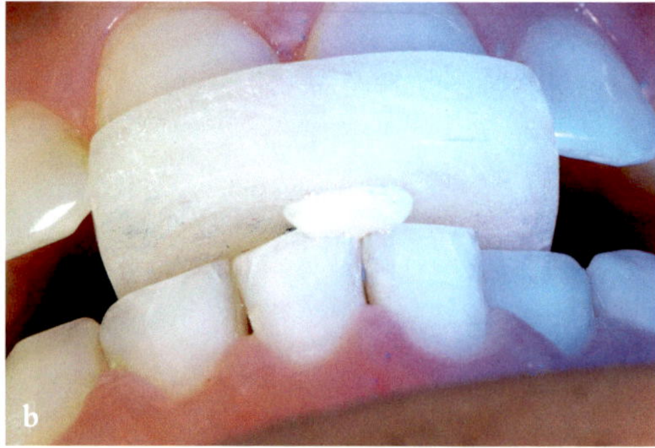

Fig 21-28 **(a)** Using a self-cure acrylic key is a good resource that guarantees an accurate procedure whenever wax is used for registrations. **(b)** The key can also be made of light-cured composite.

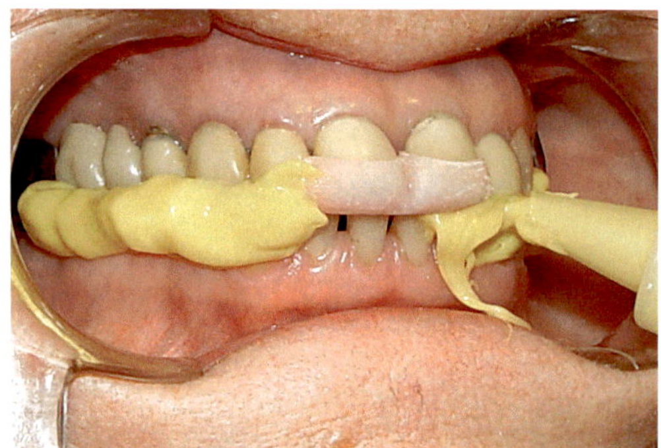

Fig 21-29 "Closed-mouth" interjaw registration. While the patient bites in the therapeutic position, silicon registration material is injected with a syringe.

*Obtaining the maxillomandibular record*

The maxillomandibular record can be obtained by using a silicone or polyether material placed with a syringe (Fig 21-29) or by using the traditional wax that guarantees greater stability during mounting in the articulator (Fig 21-30). Registrations recorded by means of elastic material can lead to a loss of accuracy to a greater or lesser degree as a consequence of the material's own elasticity. Thus, wax is recommended for an occlusal restoration treatment with fixed prosthesis. When making a bruxism splint, which does not require absolute accuracy, the record can be obtained by injecting silicone or recording polyether using a syringe.

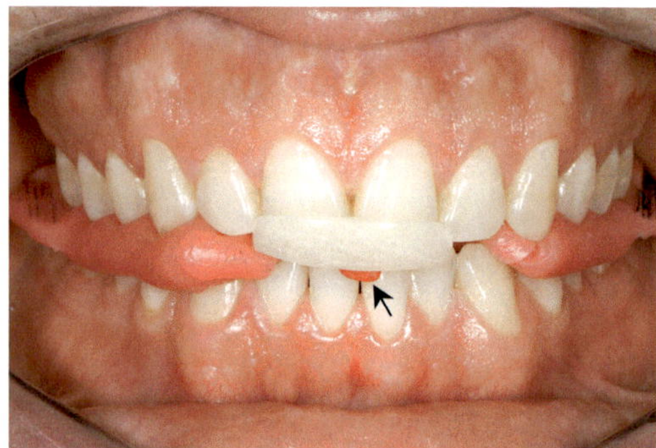

Fig 21-30 Interjaw wax registration. The use of a bite key (arrow) is advisable in order to improve control of the procedure.

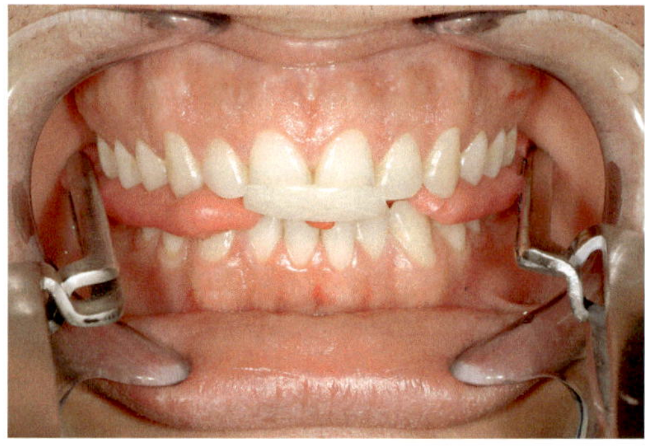

Fig 21-31 With the aid of Miller pliers, wax is placed deeply over the posterior segments.

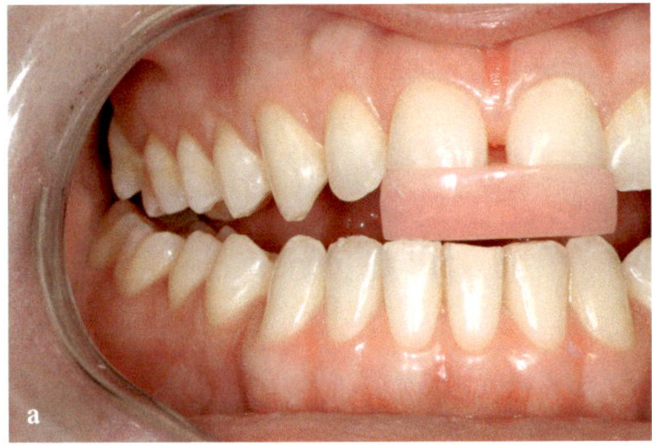

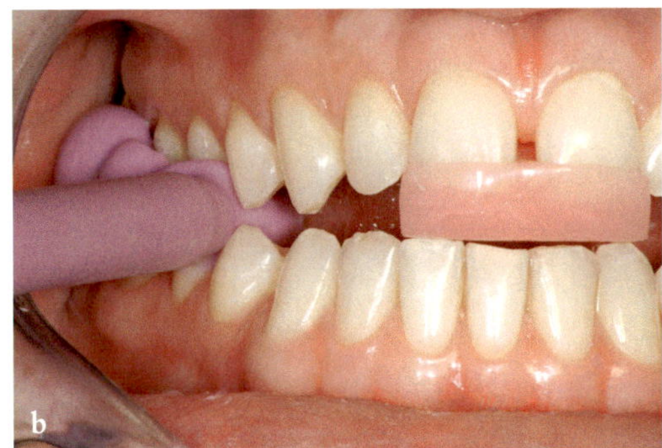

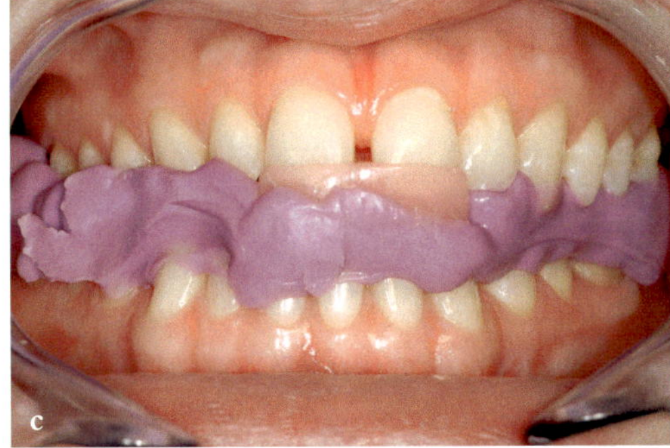

Fig 21-32 Lateral movement registration. **(a)** The patient is requested to make a lateral movement until the cusps of both canines are opposite each other. **(b)** Silicone registration material is injected to obtain an impression of the position. **(c)** When registration has been completed, a similar procedure is performed to obtain an impression of the lateral movement towards the other side.

So as to work with better visibility, it is convenient to retract the soft tissues using a lip retractor (Spandex). It is also advisable to use Miller articulating paper forceps to manipulate the wax and place it deep into the oral cavity. In this way, a record will be obtained of every tooth, even the most posterior ones (Fig 21-31). As the maxillo-mandibular registeration is a highly important clinical step for occlusal treatment, it is worth using a kind of wax capable of stability even at ambient temperature.

Subsequently, the records of the lateral movements are obtained. These can be done by using wax, polyether, or silicone (Fig 21-32). The position of the maxilla can be recorded with the facebow of a semi-adjustable articulator (Fig 21-33). This must be performed by following the common procedures for this kind of mounting.

*Mounting of dental models on the articulator*

First, the upper model is mounted using the record taken previously with the facebow. Then the same procedure is done with the lower model. As stated earlier, the VD cannot be changed on the articulator, so the incisal pin must be arranged in such a way that the articulator arms are parallel to each other. It is advisable to place a bit of adhesive tape on the superior part of the pin as an indicator and to avoid a VD

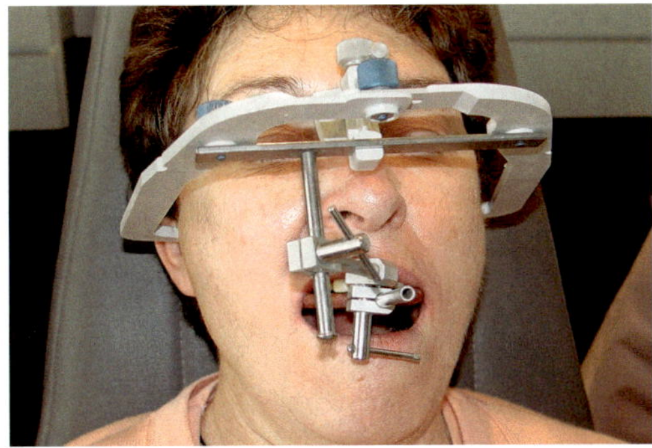

Fig 21-33 Registration of the position of the maxilla by means of a facebow.

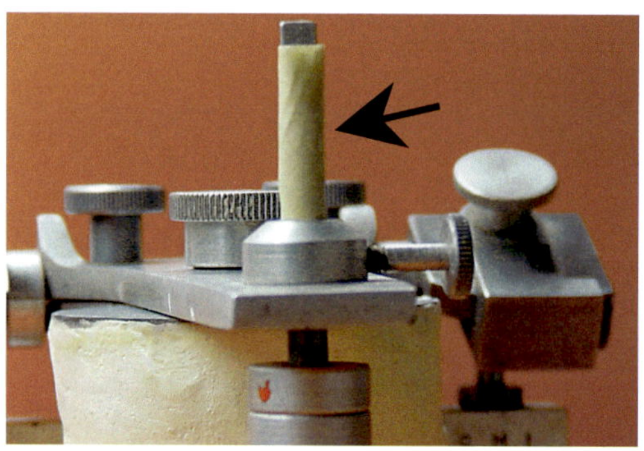

Fige 21-34 Before mounting the lower cast, and keeping the two arms of the articulator parallel to each other, the upper end of the incisal pin is "sealed" with adhesive tape (arrow). This allows easy relocation of the incisal pin without modifying VD in case the screw which attaches the pin is loosened by accident.

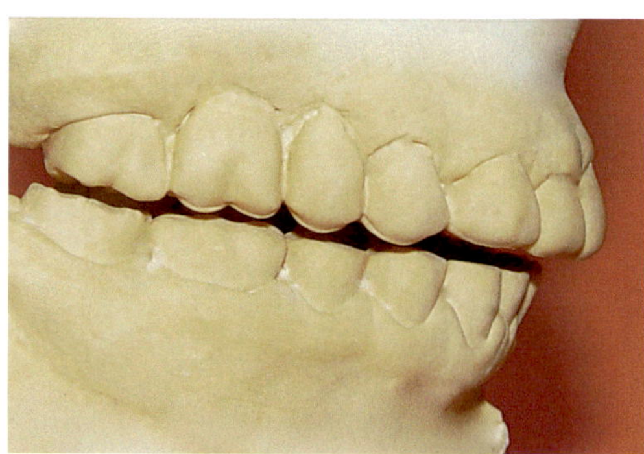

Fig 21-36 The mounted casts are ready for laboratory work using the VD established by means of the anterior bite plane.

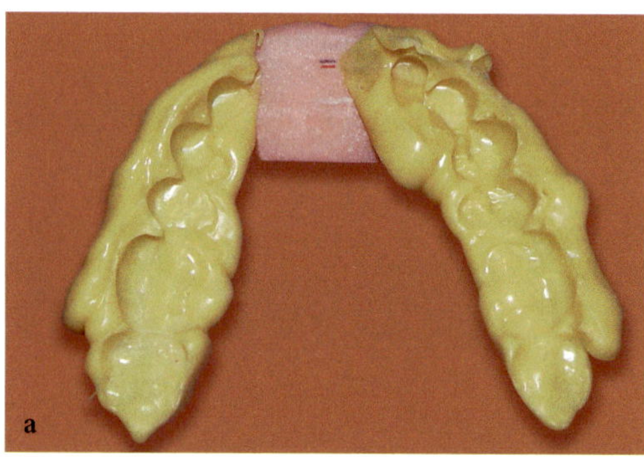

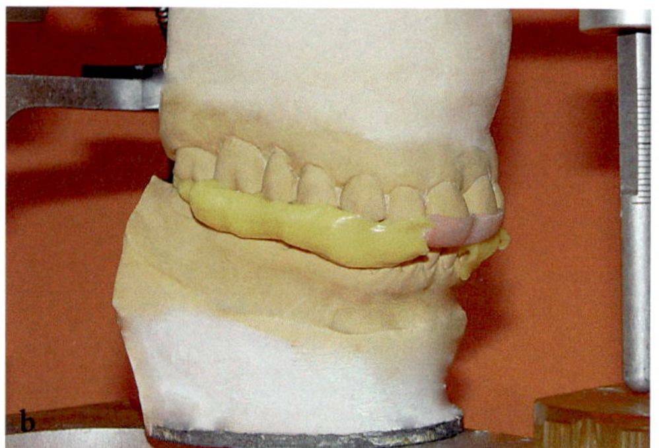

Fig 21-35 **(a and b)** For better lower cast stability during the mounting process, it is advisable to use the interjaw registration (wax or silicone) along with the anterior bite plane.

change in case the screw that fastens the pin becomes loose (Fig 21-34).

To ensure stability, it is always convenient to place the maxillomandibular record on the models with the anterior bite plane all together at once (Fig 21-35). The models, the register, and the anterior bite plane are stuck together by means of wax to avoid movements that can happen when manipulating the mounting plaster. When the plaster has hardened, the whole set is washed with hot water to eliminate the wax, and subsequently the maxillomandibular record and the anterior bite plane can be removed (Figs 21-36 to 21-39). At this point, the articulator already has the models at the working position, and the desired space between the maxilla and the mandible to accomplish the intended task.

Figures 21-40 and 21-41 show other complex uses of the anterior bite plane in cases where the IP and VD has been lost.

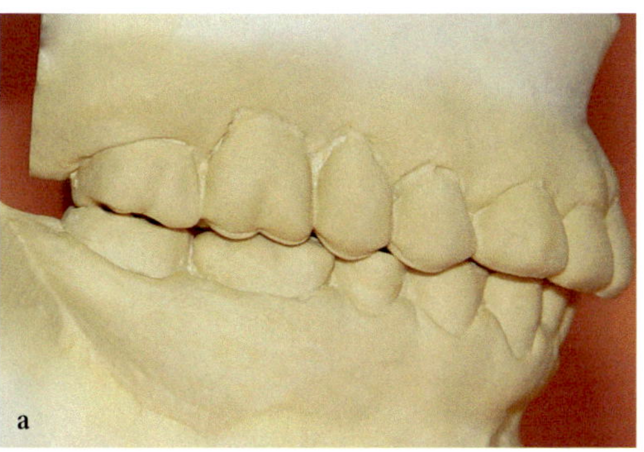
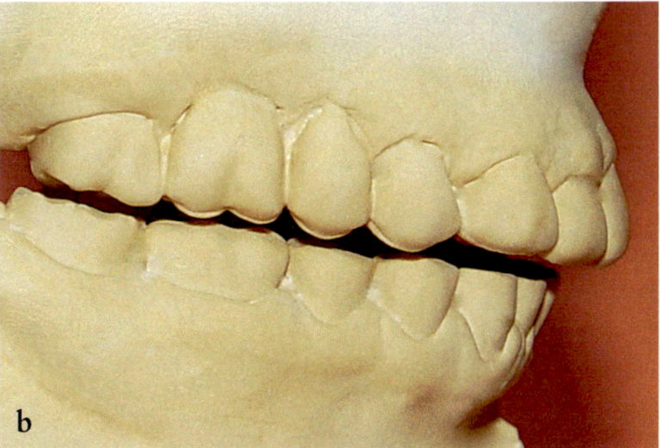

Fig 21-37 Cast comparison: **(a)** original (reduced) VD study models in the intercuspal position; **(b)** mounted models, with VD already increased.

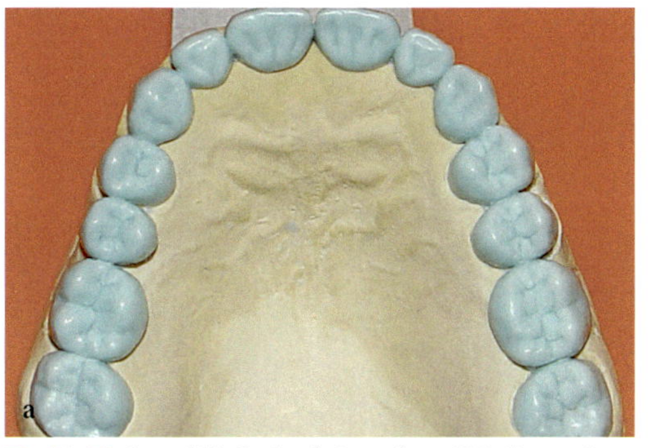
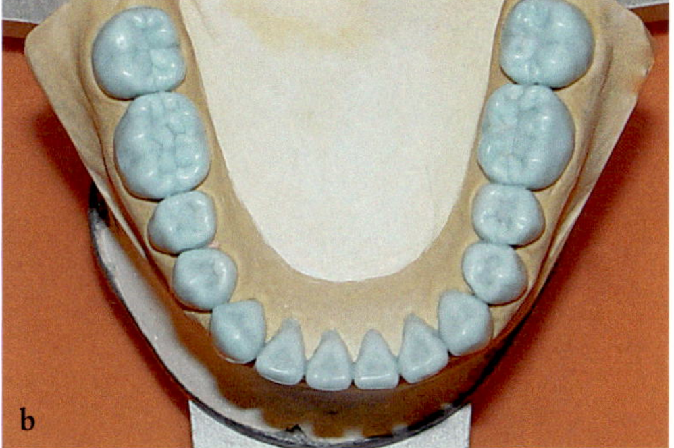

Fig 21-38 **(a and b)** Occlusal view of new VD diagnostic waxing.

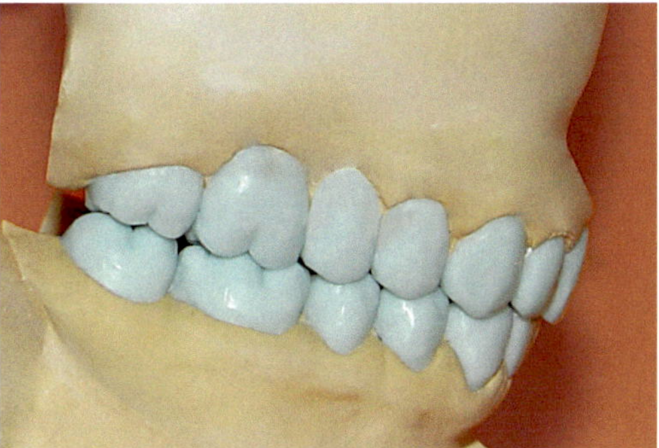

Fig 21-39 Sagittal view: waxing has been done in order to plan occlusal rehabilitation.

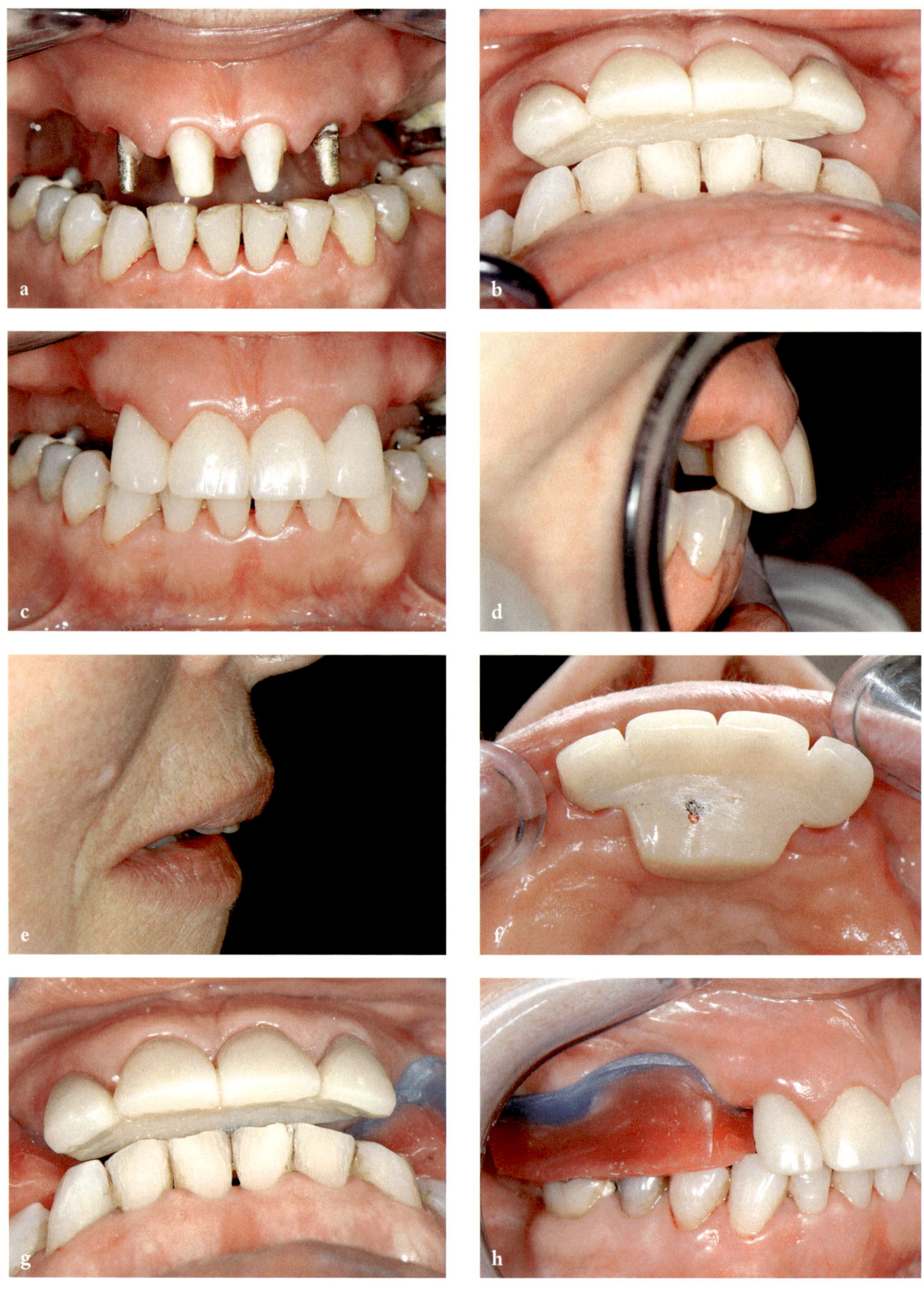
a
b
c
d
e
f
g
h

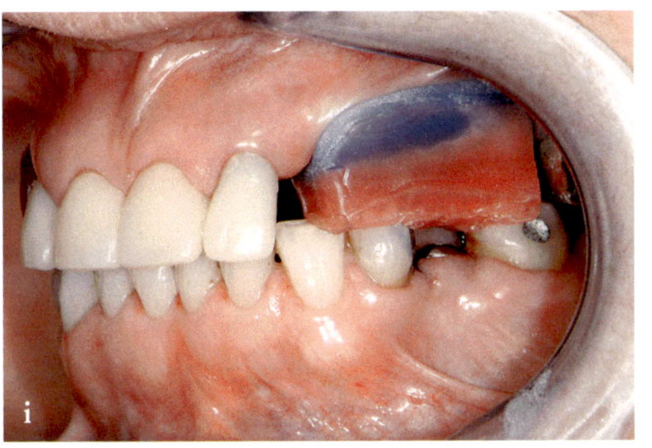

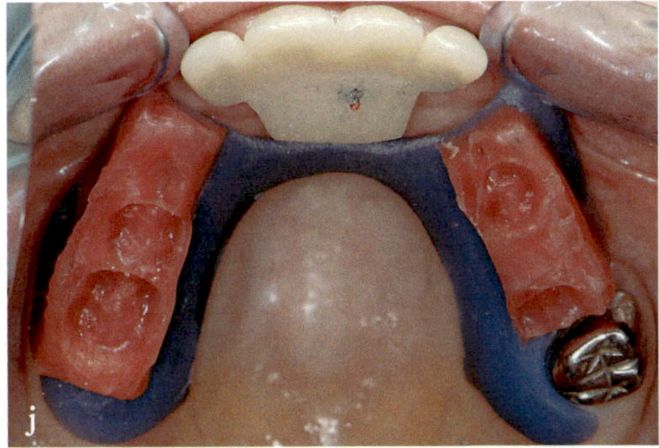

Fig 21-40 **(a)** Female patient who lost maximum intercuspation completely. Rehabilitation will consist of a combination of fixed and removable prostheses. **(b)** The provisional crowns and the anterior bite plane are made from just one block. **(c)** Front view of the provisional crowns. **(d)** Lateral view of the crowns and the anterior bite plane. **(e)** Esthetic try-in of the provisional crowns. **(f)** The blue mark corresponds to the intercuspal position, the red mark to the retrusive position used as reference. **(g)** Bite registration in the intercuspal position. **(h)** Right lateral view with bite plate. **(i)** Left lateral view. **(j)** Bite registration view. **(k)** Registration placed in the upper cast, which is ready to be mounted on the articulator.

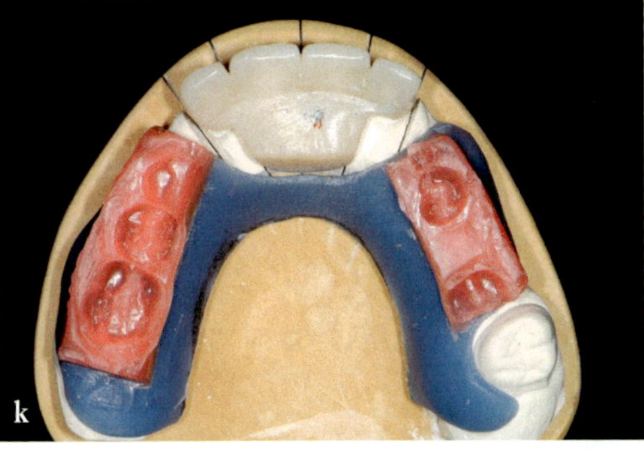

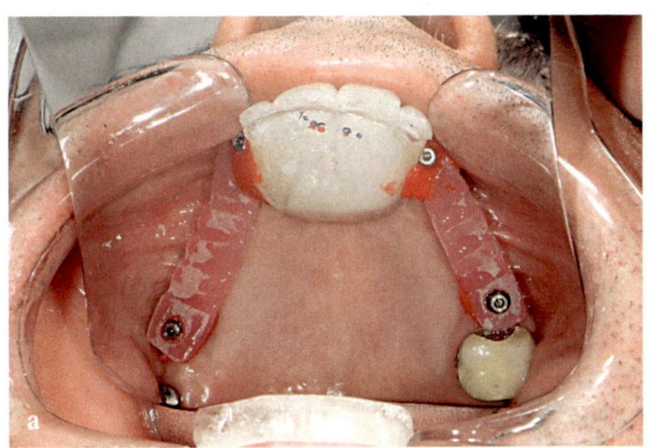

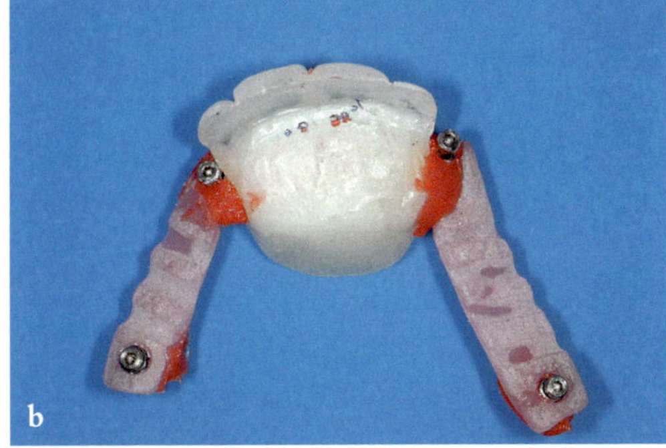

Fig 21-41 **(a)** Bite registration of a patient who will undergo implant-supported fixed-prosthesis rehabilitation. A mono-block appliance was made which includes the anterior bite plane, four transparent acrylic incisors, and the registration plate. The group will be attached to the implants by means of screws. **(b)** Mono-block appliance view; note the marks corresponding to the intercuspal position (blue) and the retrusive position used as reference (red). **(c)** Making a registration with bite wax.

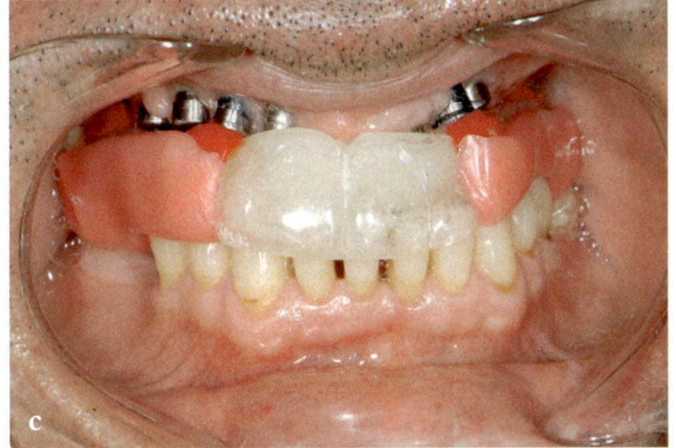

## References


1. Christensen C. The problem of the bite. Dental Cosmos 1905;47:1184.
2. Gysi A. The problem of articulation. Dental Cosmos 1910;52:1.
3. Phillips GB. Fundamentals in the mandibular movements in edentulous mouth. J Am Dent Assoc 1927;14:409.
4. McCollum BB. Considering the mouth as a functioning unit as the basis of a dental diagnosis. J Calif Dent Assoc 1938;5:268–276.
5. Schuyler CH. Fundamental principles in the correction of oclusal disharmony, natural and artificial. J Am Dent Assoc 1935;22:1193–1202.
6. Aprile H, Saizar P. Gothic arch tracing and temporomandibular anatomy. J Am Dent Assoc 1947;35:256–261.
7. Arstad T. The Capsular Ligaments of the Temporomandibular Joint and Retrusion Facets of the Dentition in Relationship to Mandibular Movements. Oslo: Akademisk Forlag, 1954.
8. Page HL. Temporomandibular joint physiology and jaw synergy. D Digest 1954;60:54–59.
9. Steinhardt G. Anatomy and physiology of the temporomandibular joint: effect on function. Int Dent J 1958;8: 155–156.
10. Isberg A, Isacsson G. Tissue reactions of the temporomandibular joint following retrusive guidance of the mandible. J Craniomandibular Pract 1986;4:143–148.
11. Desai S, Johnson DL, Howes RI, Rohrer MD. Changes in the rabbit temporomandibular joint associated with posterior displacement of the mandible. Int J Prosthodont 1996;9:46–57.
12. Cholasueksa P, Warita H, Soma K. Alterations of the rat temporomandibular joint in functional posterior displacement of the mandible. Angle Orthod 2004;74: 677–683.
13. McMillan DR, McMillan AS. A comparison of habitual jaw movements and articulator function. Acta Odontol Scand 1986;44:291–299.
14. Posselt U. Studies in the mobility of the human mandible. Acta Odontol Scand 1952;10(Suppl 10):1–160.
15. Ingervall B. Retruded contact position of the mandible: a comparison between children and adults. Odontol Revy 1964;15:130–149.
16. Hodge L, Mahan PE. A study of mandibular movement from centric occlusion to maximum intercuspation. J Prosthet Dent 1967;18:19.
17. Rieder CE. The prevalence and magnitude of mandibular displacement in a survey population. J Prosthet Dent 1978;39:324.
18. De Boever JA, Carlsson GE, Klineberg IJ. Need for occlusal therapy and prosthodontic treatment in the management of temporomandibular disorders. I: Occlusal interferences and occlusal adjustment. J Oral Rehabil 2000;27:367–379.
19. Kirveskari P, Alanen P, Jämsä T. Association between craniomandibular disorders and oclusal interferences. J Prosthet Dent 1989;62:66–69.
20. Tsuruta A, Yamada K, Hanada K et al. Comparisons of condylar position at intercuspal and reference positions in patients with condylar bony changes. J Oral Rehabil 2004;31:640–646.
21. Selligman DA, Pullinger AG. Association of occlusal variables among refined TM patient diagnostic groups. J Craniomandib Disord 1989;3:227–236.
22. Dawson PE. Centric relation: its effect on occluso-muscle harmony. Dent Clin North Am 1979;23:169–180.
23. Muraoka H, Iwata TA. Comparative study on manipulation for centric relation. J Gnathol 1982;1:47–57.
24. Simon RL, Nicholls JI. Variability of passively recorded centric relation. J Prosthet Dent 1980;44:21–26.
25. Kantor ME, Silverman SI, Garfinkel L. Centric-relation recording techniques: a comparative investigation. J Prosthet Dent 1972;28:593–600.
26. Kuboki T, Azuma Y, Orsini MG et al. The effect of oclusal appliances and clenching on the temporomandibular joint space. J Oral Rehabil 1977;11:67–77.
27. Fenlon MR, Woelfel JB. Condylar position recorded using leaf gauges and specific closure forces. Int J Prosthodont 1993;6:402–408.
28. Langer C. Kiefergelenk des Menschen. Sitzungsber Heidelb Akad Wiss Math Naturwiss Kl 1860;39:457–71.
29. McCollum BB. Fundamentals involved in prescribing restorative dental remedies. Pt 1. Dent Items Interest 1939;61:522–535.
30. Lucia VO. The fundamentals of oral physiology and their practical application in the securing and reproducing of records to be used in restorative dentistry. J Prosthet Dent 1953;3:213.
31. Kornfield M. The problem of function in restorative dentistry. J Prosthet Dent 1955;5:670.
32. Granger ER. Centric relation. J Prosthet Dent 1952;2:160.
33. Posselt U. Range of movement of the mandible. J Am Dent Assoc 1958;56:10.
34. Sicher H. Positions and movements of the mandible. J Am Dent Assoc 1954;48:620.
35. Shanahan TEJ, Leff A. Mandibular and articulator movements. Pt 1. J Prosthet Dent 1959;9:941–945.
36. Shanahan TEJ, Leff A. Mandibular and articulator movements. Pt 2: Illusion of mandibular tracings. J Prosthet Dent 1962;12:82–85.
37. Shanahan TEJ, Leff A. Mandibular and articulator movements. Pt 3: The mandibular axis dilemma. J Prosthet Dent 1962;12:292–297.
38. Shanahan TEJ, Leff A. Mandibular and articulator movements. Pt 4: Mandibular three-dimensional movements. J Prosthet Dent 1962;12:678–684.
39. Luce CE. The movements of the lower jaw. Boston Med Surg J 1889;121:8–11.

40. Bennett NG. A contribution to the study of the movements of the mandible. Proc R Soc Med 1908;1:79–95.
41. Trapozzano VR, Lazzari JB. A study of hinge axis determination. J Prosthet Dent 1961;11:858.
42. Gysi A. The problem of articulation. Dental Cosmos 1910;52:1.
43. Brewka RE. Pantographic evaluation of cephalometric hinge axis. Am J Orthod 1981;79:1–19.
44. Nattestad A, Vedtofte P. Mandibular autorotation in orthognatic surgery: a new method of locating the centre of mandibular rotation and determining its consequence in orthognatic surgery. J Craniomaxillofac Surg 1992;20: 163–170.
45. Nevekari K. An analysis of the mandibular movement from rest to occlusal position: a Roentgenographic–cephalometric investigation. Acta Odontol Scand 1956; 14(Suppl 19):9–129.
46. Koski K. Axis of the opening movement of the mandible. J Prosthet Dent 1962;12:888–894.
47. Hellsing G, Hellsing E, Eliasson S. The hinge axis concept: a radiographic study of its relevance. J Prosthet Dent 1995;73:60–64.
48. Lindauer SJ, Sabol G, Isaacson RJ, Davidovitch M. Condylar movement and mandibular rotation during jaw opening. Am J Orthod 1995;107:573–577.
49. McDevitt WE, Brady AP, Stack JP. A magnetic resonance imaging study of centric maxillomandibular relation. Int J Prosthodont 1995;8:337–391.
50. Ferrario VF, Sforza C, Miani A, Serrao G, Tartaglia G. Open–close movements in the human temporomandibular joint: does a pure rotation around the intercondylar hinge axis exist? J Oral Rehabil 1996;23:401–408.
51. McMillan AS, McMillan DR, Darvell BW. Centers of rotation during jaw movements. Acta Odontol Scand 1989;47:323–328.
52. Rahman MD, Kohno S, Kobayashi H, Sawada K. Influence of the inclination of the plate of an intra-oral tracing device on the condilar position registered by tapping movement. J Oral Rehabil 2004;31:546–553.
53. Widmalm SE, Hedegård B. Kinematics of the tooth tapping movement. J Oral Rehabil 1977;4:237–246.
54. Naeije M, Honée GL. The reproducibility of movement parameters of the empty open–close–clench cycle in man and their dependency on the frequency of movements. J Oral Rehabil 1979;6:405–415.
55. Dawson PE. New definition for relating occlusion to varying conditions of the temporomandibular joint. J Prosthet Dent 1995;74:619–627.
56. Glossary of prosthodontic terms. J Prosthet Dent 2005; 94:10–92.

Chapter 22

# Restoration of the Worn Dentition

*Anders Johansson, Ann-Katrin Johansson, Ridwaan Omar, and Gunnar E. Carlsson*

## Introduction

This chapter discusses approaches to the rehabilitation of teeth with wear based on an appraisal of the available literature, and goes on to describe various methods of reconstructing worn teeth. As background information, and in order to contextualize the topic, some brief historic, epidemiologic, and etiologic perspectives of tooth wear are provided, although these are more comprehensively dealt with in Chapter 9.

## Historical Aspects

Extensive tooth wear seems to have been the norm in all ancient societies, with factors such as dietary habits, food composition and its preparation, and age being among its main contributory factors.[1,2] As a consequence of such widespread tooth wear in prehistoric populations, notable changes in dentoalveolar and craniofacial morphology occurred over a lifetime.[3] Compensatory mechanisms maintained the occlusal vertical dimension and facial height. Lingual tilting of anterior teeth towards a more "edge-to-edge" bite and an anterior rotation of the mandible occurred. All of these changes in craniofacial morphology supposedly had an important purpose, namely to create an efficient masticatory organ, which was vital for survival.

The effects on certain dentoalveolar morphologic features, including that of wear, of excessive function have been shown to be similar in modern humans and their ancestors (Fig 22-1).[4] It is generally felt that, in prehistoric populations, the extensive wear of molars was mainly the result of a coarser diet, and the more vigorous and lengthy masticatory activity required by such a diet. The wear of anterior teeth, in addition to being a consequence of mastication, may also reflect the effects of using the teeth as tools. Indeed, tooth wear was a more common cause of tooth damage, and consequent cause of tooth loss, than either dental caries or periodontal disease. In

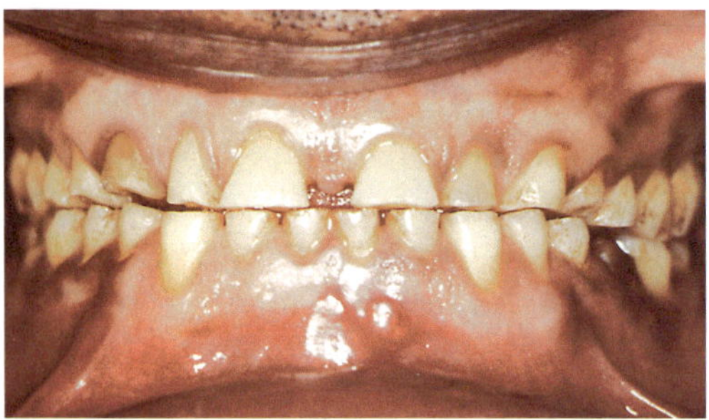

**Fig 22-1** Development of an "edge-to-edge" bite in a contemporary 50-year-old Saudi man. (Reprinted with permission from Johansson et al.[1])

Egyptian mummies, almost all abscesses in the jaws were ascribed to tooth wear and only a fraction to caries. Similarly high proportions of tooth wear as a cause of abscesses have been documented in much later historic materials, such as in medieval Britons. From this it would seem that the natural history of the human dentition in earlier times differed quite markedly from the one that prevails today.[5,6] Nevertheless, even though tooth wear in modern humans is usually far less extensive, its impact on patients' satisfaction with their dentition can be severe and affect their quality of life.[7]

In the anthropological literature, it has been assumed that tooth wear had a linear progression, so that it could be used for age determination in historic skull materials.[8] While not questioning the linearity of its progression, it has been emphasized that the use of the method should nevertheless be confined to a particular cultural period and diet, and not universally. In contrast to linear progression, modern humans more likely experience "bursts" of wear, coinciding with the presence of certain causative factors. Such an episode may comprise frequent acid regurgitation or vomiting as occurs in eating disorders or reflux diseases, frequent intake of acid-containing drinks during childhood or adolescence, or periods of extensive bruxism. Consequently, a relatively short period of exposure, rather than ongoing exposure, is most likely responsible for the widely differing severities and patterns of wear found in people today, even among those of the same age.[9]

The mechanisms by which teeth wear include attrition, erosion, and abrasion (see Chapter 9). These mechanisms seldom operate singly, and the overlap of two or more of them, often at different times, adds to the complexity of the phenomenon of wear.[10] In prehistoric humans, the cause of tooth wear was generally believed to be due to attrition and abrasion, with erosion seldom considered or even examined. Today, it is well established that dental erosion is a major cause of tooth wear,[11] yet the morphologic features of the wear show a remarkable similarity with those seen in our ancestors (Fig 22-2). In this light, it may be reasonable to hypothesize that dental erosion has been overlooked as a factor in the wear observed in skull materials. Such a hypothesis is supported by observations in medieval Icelanders as well as in ancient British populations.[1]

It is hardly surprising that there is no evidence that any specific treatment of a worn dentition was provided to our ancestors. Nevertheless, the anthropologic observations described may provide some insights into causation and progression, and thus be of some value in the way clinicians prescribe restorative therapies for today's patients with worn teeth.

## Epidemiology

The current scientific literature reports more frequently on the prevalence of dental erosion than of attrition and abrasion, and mostly in younger age groups. The wide variation in prevalence reported is striking and suggests that conclusions from prevalence studies should be treated with caution.

There are only a few studies on the prevalence of tooth wear in older individuals in contemporary populations, and the lack of consensus about methods of assessment makes comparison of results uncertain. In a UK study,[12] it was reported that the mean proportion of teeth with moderate wear (involving more extensive exposure of dentin) increased from a few percent in

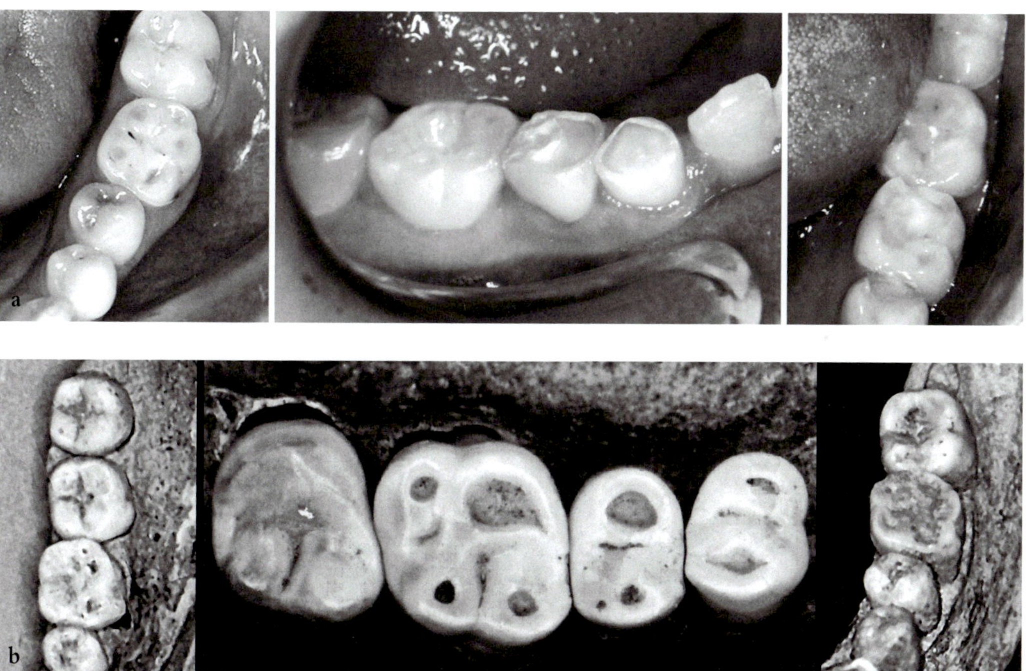


Fig 22-2 Severe tooth wear with "cuppings" in **(a)** a contemporary patient, and in **(b)** an ancient skull.[8] Note how closely the patterns and distributions of wear resemble each other. (Reprinted with permission from Johansson et al.[1])

adolescence to 9% in individuals over 65 years of age. In the same older age group, 2% of the teeth exhibited severe wear (complete enamel loss with exposure of pulp or secondary dentin). In a large German epidemiologic survey,[13] wear was scored according to a scale from 0 to 3 (extensive wear), with mean wear score increasing from 0.6 in 20–29-year-olds to 1.4 in 70–79-year-olds. A Swedish epidemiologic study[14] reported the prevalence of extensive tooth wear to be only 2%, but, not unexpectedly, increasing with age. The pattern of these results from current populations contrasts sharply with the near-universal, extensive occlusal wear found in historic skull materials. Even though the criteria for scoring wear that are used in different studies show wide variation, there seems to be a consensus that the prevalence of erosion-related tooth wear has increased in children and young adults over the past few decades.[15] Whether this applies to older generations is not known.

Notwithstanding the foregoing evidence about its seemingly increasing prevalence, the available literature on the need for rehabilitation of tooth wear comprises mainly case reports. Only one study could be found that attempted to assess treatment need in an epidemiologic context. A population study[16] in a northern Swedish county found advanced wear of maxillary anterior teeth in 14% of 35-year-old and 36% of 65-year-old subjects. The need for prosthetic treatment in these samples was estimated as 0.5% and 4%, respectively. Yet, the rate of treatment provided was even lower, confirming the different ways in which dentists and patients judge the need for treatment, as well as the differences that are known to exist between normative and subjective assessments of treatment need in general.

## Etiology of Tooth Wear

The terms "attrition", "erosion", and "abrasion" have widespread acceptance as descriptors of tooth wear. It has been suggested that the terms are not in themselves descriptive of the wear process, nor do they imply causation, but instead describe clinical outcomes of a number of underlying events. In this regard, the science of tribology, the study of objects in relative motion, may more accurately characterize the process of tooth wear (see Chapters 9, 10, and 19).

There is a tendency for concurrent action by the range of mechanisms that affect the teeth in the oral environment, which supports the multifactorial etiology ascribed to progressive tooth wear. Specific factors that have been implicated as being etiologic and/or associated with the processes of attrition, erosion, and abrasion include functional activity (i.e., chewing) or parafunctional habits (e.g., bruxism), and patterns of mandibular movement (i.e., canine guidance, anterior guidance, or group function). Similarly, diet (e.g., coarse and acidic substances), diseases (e.g., reflux diseases, eating disorders), salivary factors (e.g., buffering capacity, and quantity and quality of the saliva), occupational environment (e.g., airborne abrasives, acid), oral hygiene habits, and various aspects of the modern lifestyle have been found to be associated with tooth wear. In addition, reduced occlusal tactile sensitivity, high bite force and increased endurance time, all of which reflect muscle and functional proprioception, have been shown to be correlated with extensive wear. However, the current consensus is that dental erosion is a major contributory factor to tooth wear today. In younger groups, extrinsic factors such as excessive soft drink consumption, and in adults, intrinsic factors such as gastroesophageal reflux are among the causes considered to be the predominant ones.

### *Bruxism*

Some patients develop opposing matched wear facets that are believed to be associated with intense tooth grinding (Fig 22-3). However, such faceting may not be "typical" of bruxism alone, and is more likely the result of a combination of different factors. In addition, a diagnosis of bruxism is generally based on the clinician's opinion

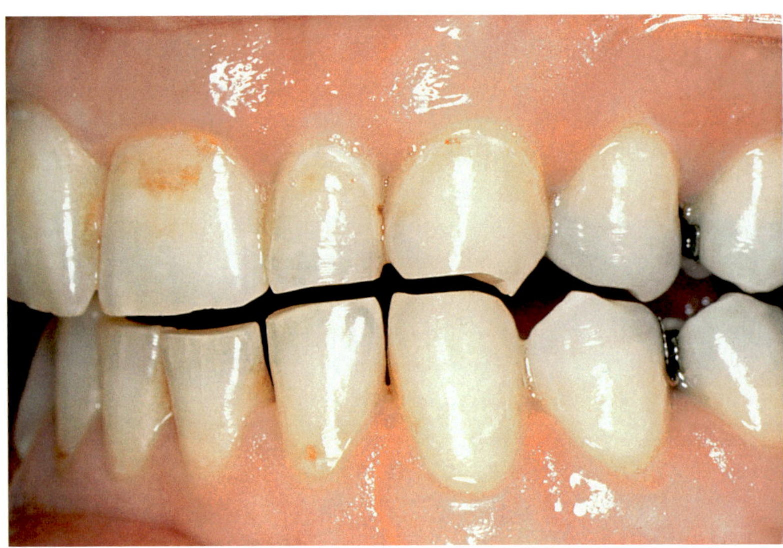

Fig 22-3 Well-matching opposing facets that are considered to be "typical" in patients with heavy bruxism. (Reprinted with permission from Johansson et al.[1])

and is seldom verified by an accurate diagnostic test, such as somnography or video/audio recordings. Even given a reliable diagnosis of bruxism, its frequency and intensity over time in that patient are seldom known. It is also the case that severe tooth wear almost always shows clinical signs of erosive damage, while "attrition-like", bruxing-induced wear as the sole feature is rare.

That bruxism is not the major cause of occlusal tooth wear has considerable documented support. A number of observations strengthen the theory of the multifactorial etiology of tooth wear. It may be fair to conclude that the overall significance of bruxism as a causative factor is not fully known, but it is even fairer to say that it is probably overestimated.[1]

***Tooth Brushing and Non-carious Cervical Lesions***
Tooth brushing has generally been held to be responsible for the development of buccal cervical lesions, currently often referred to as non-carious cervical lesions (NCCLs) (see Chapter 12). Such lesions are sometimes subgingivally located, beyond the influence of "toothbrush abrasion". They have also been observed in animals, especially in cats, as well as in other herbivorous and omnivorous species. NCCLs have also been observed in individuals who seldom brush their teeth, and in prehistoric populations before the toothbrush era. As an additional explanation for such defects it has been postulated that heavy stressing of the teeth (e.g., heavy chewing or bruxism) will result in strain microfractures along the buccal cementoenamel junction, possibly making the area more prone to substance loss. On the other hand, the theory has received some criticism owing to lack of robustness of the evidence.[17] A recent review concluded that tooth brushing, with or without dentifrice, only minimally contributes to the development of wear of enamel, whereas tooth brushing and an acidic diet may be linked to dentin wear and hypersensitivity. Other studies have consistently found significant correlations between the presence of erosive lesions and cervical defects.[1]

It is likely that NCCLs have a multifactorial etiology and that tooth brushing is not the only important factor but, in the presence of acid, may contribute to a more rapid development of cervical defects. It is clear that the etiology and natural history of such lesions must be considered when prescribing preventive measures and restorative options for the worn dentition.

## Principles and Management Strategies for Tooth Wear

Although a combination of factors is usually involved in the development of tooth wear, it is feasible in most cases to identify a perceived major factor. The importance of identifying such a cause in the eventual treatment opted for, and its prognosis, cannot be overemphasized. An assessment of possible causative factors should include a systematic history and a thoroughly methodical approach to the clinical examination to reduce diagnostic incompleteness or uncertainty (see Chapters 2, 9, and 20).

In order to quantify the severity and progression of wear, different techniques are available, ranging from sophisticated optical or laser scanning methods to relatively simple ordinal scales. The latter are designed for epidemiologic studies, but can be appropriately adapted for clinical use. Examples of such scales and their different purposes are shown in Tables 22-1 to 22-3. Besides the morphologic variations of tooth wear indicated in the first two tables, clinical symptoms may also appear (e.g., sensitivity or even pain initially), which can eventually grow in seriousness to affect eating, appearance, and the quality of life of the individual.

*Table 22-1*

**Ordinal scale used for grading severity of occlusal/incisal wear without reference to a presupposed cause (Carlsson et al[10]).**

| Grade | Criteria |
|---|---|
| 0 | No visible facets in enamel; occlusal/incisal morphology intact |
| 1 | Marked wear facets in enamel; occlusal/incisal morphology altered |
| 2 | Wear into dentin; dentin exposed occlusally/incisally and/or adjacent tooth surface; occlusal/incisal morphology changed in shape with height reduction of tooth |
| 3 | Extensive wear into dentin; larger dentin area (>2 mm$^2$) exposed occlusally/incisally and/or adjacent tooth surface; occlusal/ incisal morphology totally lost locally or generally; substantial loss of crown height |
| 4 | Wear into secondary dentin (verified by photographs) |

*Table 22-2*

**Ordinal scale used for grading severity of dental erosion on buccal and lingual surfaces of maxillary anterior teeth (Johansson et al[18]).**

| Grade | Criteria |
|---|---|
| 0 | No visible changes; developmental structures remain; macro-morphology intact |
| 1 | Smoothened enamel; developmental structures totally or partially vanished; enamel surface is shiny, matt, irregular, "melted", rounded, or flat; macro-morphology generally intact |
| 2 | Enamel surface as described in Grade 1; macro-morphology clearly changed; faceting or concavity formation within the enamel; no dentinal exposure |
| 3 | Enamel surface as described in Grades 1 and 2; macro-morphology greatly changed (close to dentinal exposure of large surfaces) or dentin surface exposed by up to one-third |
| 4 | Enamel surface as described in Grades 1, 2, and 3; dentin surface exposed by more than one-third, or pulp visible through the dentin |

Note: Approximal erosion, presence of "shoulder" and "cuppings" should be recorded.

*Table 22-3*

**Scale used for scoring the progression of occlusal/incisal wear (Johansson et al[19]).**

| Grade | Criteria |
|---|---|
| 0 | No visible change |
| 1 | Visible change, such as increase of facet areas, without measurable reduction of tooth length; occlusal/incisal morphology changed in shape compared to the first examination |
| 2 | Measurable reduction of tooth length <1 mm |
| 3 | Marked reduction of tooth length ≥1 mm |

### *General Management Strategies*

The literature on tooth wear provides very little scientific evidence that can be said to support unambiguous recommendations about its management. An article that endeavored to present some clinical guidelines cautioned: "There are no hard and fast rules and the need for treatment should be established after considering: the degree of wear relative to the age of the patient; the aetiology; the symptoms; the patient's wishes."[20] A recent systematic review also failed to find sound evidence supporting the superiority of one occlusion-based treatment over others for the management of attrition.[21] The account on management recommendations is therefore, of necessity, based on available literature of lower scientific strength than randomized controlled trials (RCTs) and on our own clinical experience.

In general terms, and based on the history, clinical examination, and diagnosis, management should be directed towards elimination of the etiologic factors and strengthening of modifying factors. It follows that the central tenet of management is the implementation of preventive measures, followed by, where necessary, restorative or prosthodontic corrective solutions. Since tooth wear is usually a relatively slow process, urgent restoration will, in many patients, not be necessary. Proceeding with caution is especially important for adolescents since the longevity of restorations is finite and frequently quite limited.[9] However, for a patient suffering from demonstrably progressive wear, it becomes important to hasten the investigatory phase in order to retard or prevent further deterioration.

### *Preventive Measures*

Prevention may at times involve making lifestyle changes, which in children would not solely involve the affected individual, but the whole family. In this regard, it has been shown that a child's dietary pattern commonly reflects their mother's dietary pattern.

The child with worn deciduous teeth presents a challenge but also an opportunity to prevent later involvement of the permanent dentition. Some advice and information about tooth wear at the right time may in some patients prevent further damage, while in others the situation may be more difficult. However, even in very severe cases, such as with eating disorders, it has been shown that information and prophylaxis is useful for the control of further progression of the tooth wear.

Preventing tooth wear is quite different from preventing dental caries. Well-structured dental caries preventive measures, especially those based on fluoride use, oral hygiene and organized dental examinations, regular recall, and even subsidized treatments, have long been available. The positive effect of fluoride in the prevention of dental caries is well established. Its role in the erosion process is considered to be far more limited, although a recent experiment performed in human volunteers reported that $TiF_4$ and $SnF_2$ both have significant protective effects against erosion-like lesions in situ.

Tooth wear, on the other hand, rather than being a community-based problem, is still perceived as a problem of individual patients even though it is increasing in prevalence. It is also difficult to predict, thus limiting the achievement of true prevention. Thus, a change in lifestyle is more effective for the prevention of tooth wear than "oral" measures such as topical fluoride application and the use of special dentifrice or dentin bonding agents. Such an approach may be valid at both the individual and the population level.

Even once wear is identified in a given patient, eradicating the causative factor(s) may not be a simple task. For example, preventing bruxing activity, treating gastrointestinal disorders that cause acid regurgitation, stopping frequent vomiting as in cases of alcoholism or eating disorders, are all fraught with extreme difficulties. In severe cases, consultation with the patient's physician, dietary counseling, prescription of medication, salivary data, etc., must be explored in the initial management of a patient's tooth wear. If nocturnal bruxism is confirmed, a full-coverage hard acrylic resin occlusal splint should be constructed for nighttime use (see Chapter 25). However, it may be difficult to motivate a patient in the long-term use of such an appliance, which would be necessary for the full benefit of the treatment to be realized. A long-term study of patients with extensively worn dentitions provided with stabilization splints showed that the splints were used on average for 2 years but with varying usage frequency.[10] As a cautionary note, however, if dental erosion is the main perceived cause of the wear, an occlusal splint may not be protective and could even worsen the situation by retaining acidic substances inside the mouth during sleep.

While it is possible to determine the major causative element in most cases of wear, occasionally the main cause will defy identification. Aside from such rare exceptions, the general rule for those cases where a causal phase of treatment has been implemented and its objectives accomplished, but esthetic, functional, or other demands remain, is that intervention is warranted.

### *Observation, Monitoring, and Palliative Strategies*

In addition to the identification of etiologic and modifying/aggravating factor(s), and before any definitive reconstructive procedures are carried out, the rate of progression of wear should be determined.[22] The rationale for such a step lies in the fact that wear is normally a slow process, with patients seldom complaining of overt symptoms. In the case of erosion, recognizing how the appearance of the affected teeth changes with wear can be helpful in assessing the activity. For example, a clean surface as well as hypersensitivity suggests activity while staining suggests inactivity.

It is recommended that serial investigations be performed, using study casts at approximately 6–12-monthly intervals (depending on the perceived rate of progression), and comparing the recordings. Based on an assessment of the rate (see Table 22-3), it would be possible to decide whether or not intervention is necessary. However, in cases in which a dominant and actively ongoing erosive influence has been clearly implicated, a very rapid deterioration of tooth structure may be expected; in such a case, reconstructive procedures should be carried out without delay. Equally, if there are severe symptoms of sensitivity, some form of immediate, active treatment may be warranted although other measures such as reducing "soft" drink intake or changing the drinking method might manage the sensitivity sufficiently.[23] If desensitizing treatment is deemed necessary, potassium-containing dentifrices are considered appropriate for at-home use, while fluorides such as sodium fluoride and stannous fluoride have been shown to be effective in-office treatments.[24] In a meta-analysis of seven blinded clinical studies[25] that compared variously 0.4% stannous fluoride gel, 0.7% fluoride solution, and placebos, the 0.7% fluoride solution showed virtually immediate and definable effect that seemed to continue for several months. The effect of 0.4% stannous fluoride was more gradual, and the authors concluded that an effective strategy involving the use of stannous fluoride gel should include the application of a 0.7% fluoride solution in-office followed by at-home application of stannous fluoride gel to achieve a long-term effect. Composites may be placed temporarily or semi-permanently overexposed areas, while dentin bonding agents may be effective in reducing sensitivity and possibly preventing further damage – although such measures may not last too long and have to be frequently repeated. Endodontic treatment is the last resort for extreme sensitivity that cannot be treated more conservatively.

If, on the basis of relevant objective and subjective criteria, the patient's appearance, function, and occlusal stability are satisfactory, the patient is monitored according to a customized recall schedule.

## Rehabilitative Strategies

A search of the dental literature on rehabilitation of tooth wear for the purpose of a critical review identified a large number of articles. However, only 24 (1.7%) were RCTs concerned with reconstructive procedures, and of these, 20 studied the restoration of NCCLs, two evaluated the esthetics of resin materials, one the restoration of chipped or worn incisal edges, and the last one the performance of posterior composite/compomer restorations.[1] Not a single paper with a RCT design was found that studied fixed or removable prosthodontic treatment of the worn dentition.

Based on this systematic search, it is evident that there is a stark absence of documented outcomes with regard to the rehabilitation of the worn dentition. Bearing this constraint in mind, the recommendations that follow are necessarily based on studies whose designs are conventionally regarded to be of less scientific rigour than RCTs, clinical experience, and opinions of respected authorities. While treatment recommendations that are based on these sources are not without merit, their less compelling scientific value must be noted.

Given that definitive restorative procedures should not be performed without identification of etiologic factors, in conjunction with adequate preventive measures and advice, the question of restoration arises when the patient's needs, the severity of the wear, and the potential for progression are of concern. The evidence that the presence of tooth wear will inevitably lead to severe wear is scant, and the factors that are important in progression are not well understood either. Costly conventional fixed and removable prosthodontics was, and still is, the mainstay of rehabilitation of the extensively worn dentition when treatment is indicated. Such treatment is also complex and generally highly invasive. The tendency has, therefore, been to defer its provision if at all possible, with the result that tooth wear was usually well advanced by the time definitive restorative treatment was commenced.

In discussing rehabilitative strategies, it would seem appropriate to cite some key concepts about tooth wear from a book[26] on temporomandibular disorders (TMD):

- "Tooth wear is a natural process that normally does not require specific treatment. Even patients with more extensive tooth wear do not necessarily require oral rehabilitation if the adaptation is good.
- In patients who are concerned about the rate of progression of the wear, registration of the dentition by means of casts and/or photographs should be taken for comparison after 6 months to 1 year.
- If and when prosthodontic restoration is indicated, there is plenty of time to carefully plan the treatment. Tooth wear that reaches the advanced stage has, with few exceptions, taken several years".

### *Dentoalveolar Compensation*

Shortening of the clinical crowns is an effect of wear that can have significant restorative implications. Extensive wear may result in changes to the occlusal vertical dimension (OVD), possibly with increased interocclusal space. However, it has been shown that dentoalveolar compensation may cause the OVD to remain relatively constant, or even increased, despite tooth wear. This would mean that any increase in OVD as part of the reconstruction would be unnecessary.

If restoration is necessary, the pertinent question will be whether the space required for restoration is available in the maximum intercuspal position (MIP), and whether retention and resistance will be adequate. If the answer to the question is in the affirmative, restoration in MIP is probably going to be relatively straightforward. If, on the other hand, there is not sufficient space, the next question will be whether the wear is localized or generalized. For localized wear, methods exist that can confine treatment to the worn teeth and avoid it being disproportionately broadened: planned placement of single or multiple bonded restorations at increased OVD according to the Dahl principle in anticipation of rapid re-establishment of full intercuspation has been described.[27]

Generalized wear, on the other hand, will require a reorganized approach, with or without an increase in OVD, and this will be discussed later.

### *Biomechanical Factors*

When conventional fixed prosthodontic rehabilitation is necessary, single crowns should be constructed whenever possible and fixed dental prostheses (FDPs) should be of minimal extension. Nevertheless, many restorations fail as a result of stress concentration from differential wear and poorly planned occlusal contacts, a risk that is greater if a heavy bruxing habit exists. Inadequate retention and resistance of crowns on short abutments can be improved in several ways:[28,29]

- extending the finish line apically
- preparing vertical grooves or boxes with parallel sides
- including parallel pins in the preparation
- preparing occlusal boxes with parallel walls.

An effective mechanical way to increase the retention and resistance to dislodgment of conventionally retained crowns on short, worn abutments that may also be subject to parafunctional load is to furnish the preparation with boxes and grooves or include parallel pins in the preparation.

An increase in the length of a short clinical crown and extension of the finish line apically can be achieved by surgical crown lengthening, which implies removal of parts of the gingival tissues with or without osseous recontouring (Fig 22-4).

Another method to provide retention on a too-short abutment is by elective devitalization of the tooth in order to place a post and core. However, the techniques of surgical crown lengthening and devitalization that were once popular seem to be abating as non-preparation, adhesive bonding techniques, as well as techniques that reverse the effect of alveolar compensation to produce vertical space are developed (Fig 22-5).[30,31]

Splinting should be avoided whenever possible, and is not recommended in cases of confirmed bruxism. Similarly, splinting additional abutments in order to compensate for a short, poorly retentive primary abutment is contraindicated: the chances of cementation failure, rather than being reduced, will probably be as great at the short abutment, irrespective of the inclusion of secondary abutments. These considerations apply particularly to cases of heavy bruxism: the extremely high risk of mechanical failure (e.g., porcelain and connector fractures, cementation failure followed by secondary caries) should, therefore, limit restorations to single crowns. In this way, physiologic tooth mobility will be unrestrained: torquing forces are minimized and, in case of cementation failure, the condition would be easily detected, and be more easily correctable.

It is often suggested that a full-coverage occlusal splint should be constructed overlaying the restored teeth. In spite of its frequent use in such a manner, there is no evidence about the effectiveness of occlusal splints to prevent future failure.

### *Rehabilitative Techniques*

#### *Anterior wear*

In many cases of wear, only the anterior segments will be involved. These are also the most commonly affected teeth particularly with erosive wear, and rarely would the complete dentition be equally affected. The problem of restoring worn anterior teeth when little available interocclusal space exists is apparent. In this regard, a less radical alternative to complete occlusal reconstruction, based on the principles of combined forced intrusion of anterior teeth and supra-eruption of posterior teeth, was first described by Dahl and co-workers[27] and subsequently used by others. To achieve this, an anterior cobalt–chromium splint can be utilized (Fig 22-6). Such an approach can greatly simplify and curtail treatment, obviating

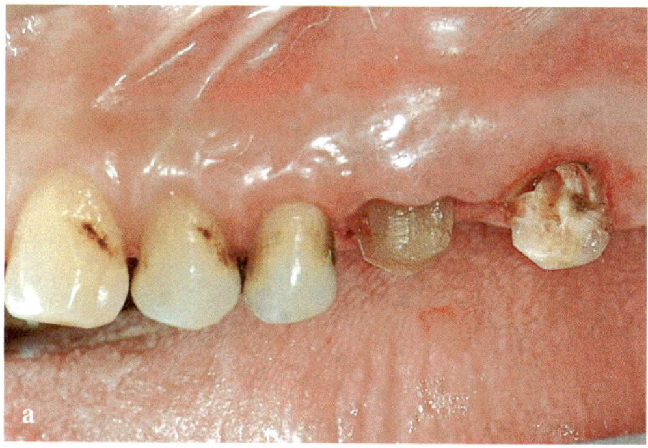

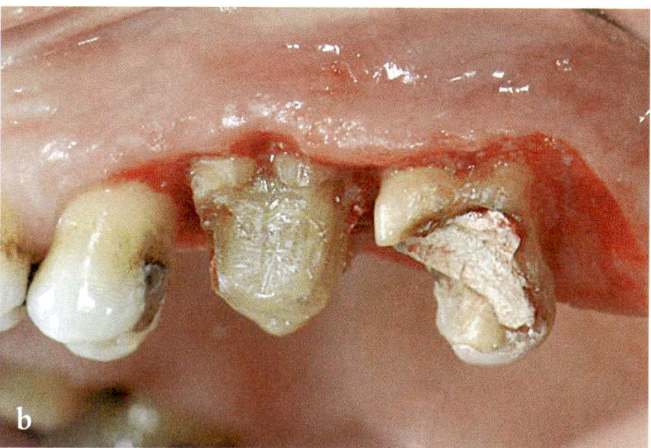

Fig 22-4 Surgical crown lengthening. **(a)** Short maxillary molars. **(b)** After removal of selected parts of the gingival tissues, the lengthened crowns will allow appropriate abutment preparation and restoration. (Reprinted with permission from Nor Tannlaegeforen Tid 2008;118:368–374.)

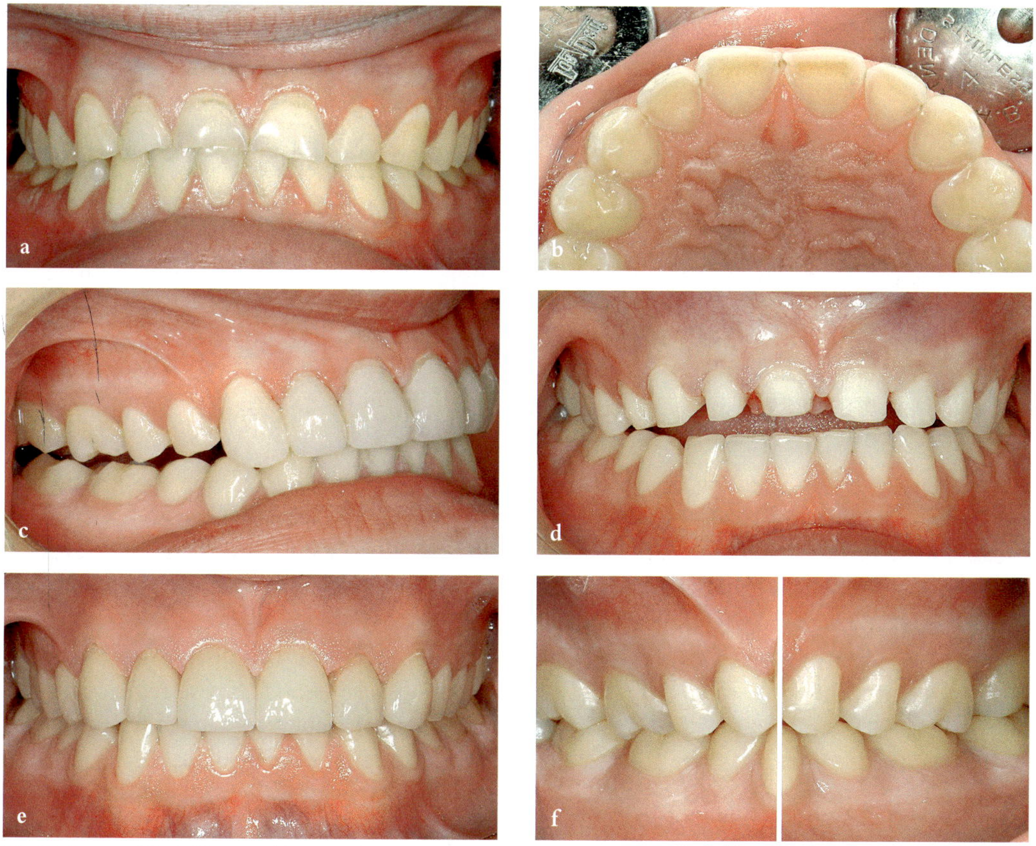

Fig 22-5 **(a and b)** A 20-year-old man with severe tooth wear affecting the whole dentition, caused by frequent "soft" drink consumption during his teenage years. **(c and d)** Anterior bite-raising temporary fixed dental prosthesis was placed for a period of 5 months in order to create space anteriorly and allow for increasing the crown height of the permanent restorations. **(e and f)** Empress crowns were bonded to 14–23. The patient has stopped drinking "soft" drinks, uses home-based fluoride prophylaxis, and attends regular check-ups. (Reprinted with permission from Johansson et al.[1])

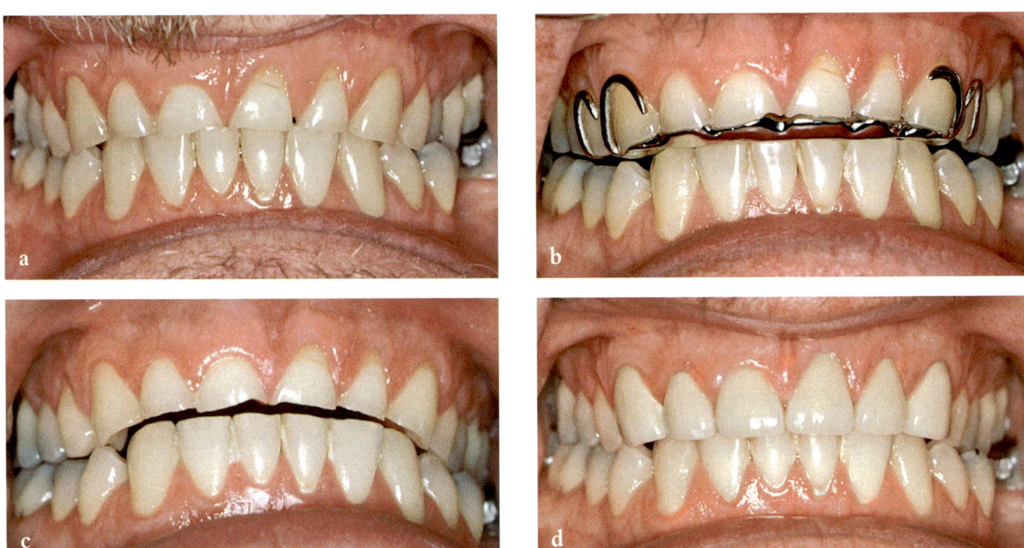

Fig 22-6 Swedish sailor (age 36 years) with a long history of frequent citrus fruit consumption. **(a)** His anterior maxillary teeth are extremely worn, with reduced buccolingual dimension and little available space for full-coverage restorations. **(b)** Cobalt–chromium splint providing anterior tooth separation of 2 mm and incorporating retentive clasps. **(c)** After 2 months' continuous use of the splint, adequate space had been created to provide anterior crowns (without undue tooth tissue sacrifice), and definitive reconstruction needs to be performed without delay. **(d)** Final metal–ceramic crowns on 13–23 after cementation. Although full posterior intercuspation posteriorly is not yet evident, there are posterior contacts. Note that the first premolar that had previously been clasped has reached occlusion in the short period following discontinuation of the splint. (Reprinted with permission from Johansson and Omar.[22])

the need for full-coverage restorations of frequently sound (albeit sometimes mildly worn) posterior teeth. Equally, relapse of the anterior interocclusal space so gained has been shown to be negligible in long-term follow-ups.[32] A recommendation of such a relatively conservative treatment modality is generally appropriate when severe wear affects the anterior segments only, and particularly so in the younger patient. The method has successfully withstood long-term scrutiny.[33]

A number of variations of the Dahl technique have been reported in the literature.[1] Instead of a metal splint, resin-bonded cast or composite palatal onlay build-ups or temporary crowns can be used with the same purpose (Fig 22-7). Several case reports have been published following the Dahl concept but substituting the metal splint with direct composite onlays (Fig 22-8). In a retrospective study, localized anterior tooth wear treated with direct composite restorations at an increased OVD of 1–4 mm posteriorly showed 90% servicing restorations, with good posterior occlusion, and patient satisfaction, at 30 months.[34] In another such follow-up, resin-bonded type III gold veneers cemented with Panavia Ex showed 89% survival at a mean of 60 months in 25 patients, irrespective of being cemented high or to correct the occlusion.[35]

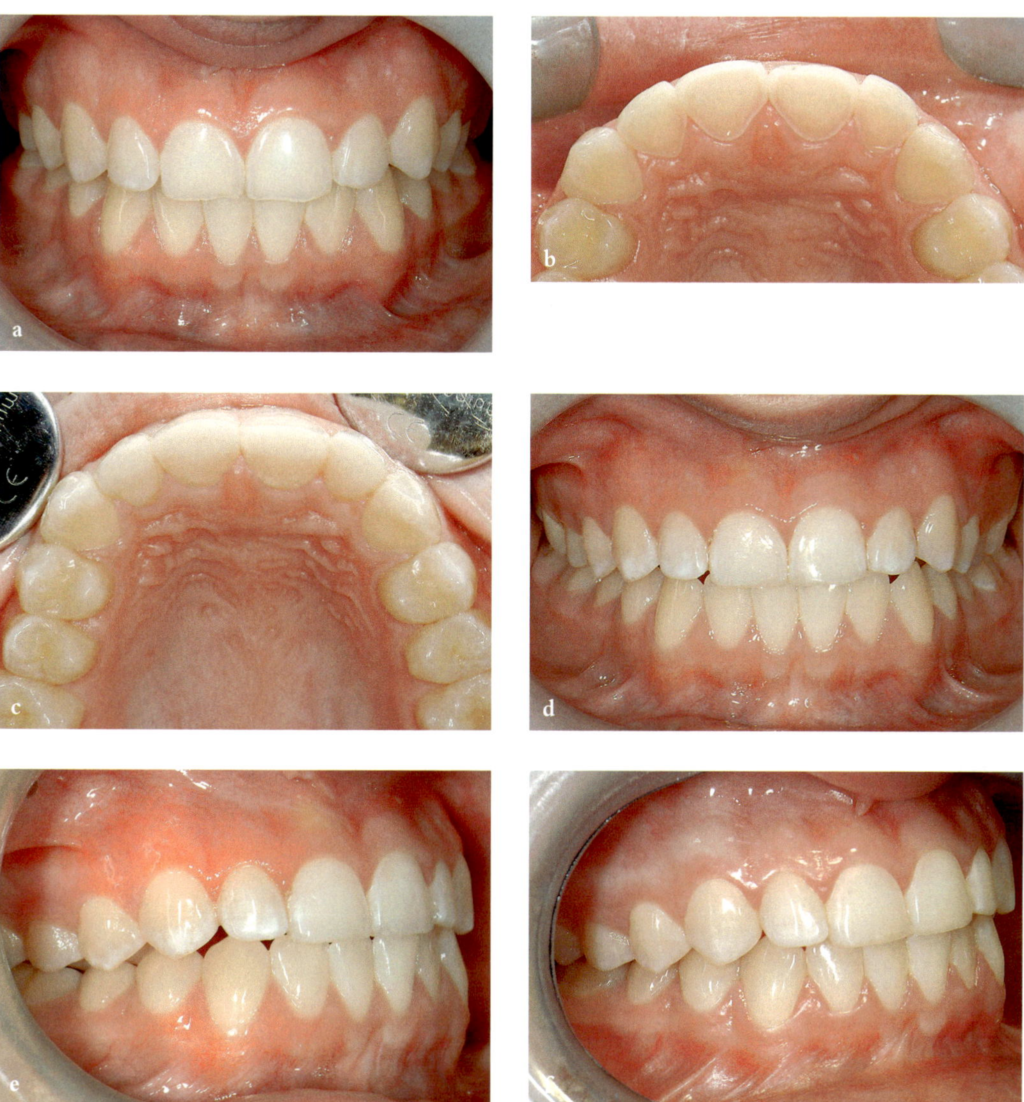

Fig 22-7 **(a and b)** A 15-year-old girl with "cola"-induced palatal erosion on the maxillary central and lateral incisors. **(c–e)** Palatal composite restorations initially produce a bilateral posterior open bite. **(f)** Six weeks later the occlusion has returned to normal through compensatory eruption of posterior teeth. (Reprinted with permission from Johansson et al.[1])

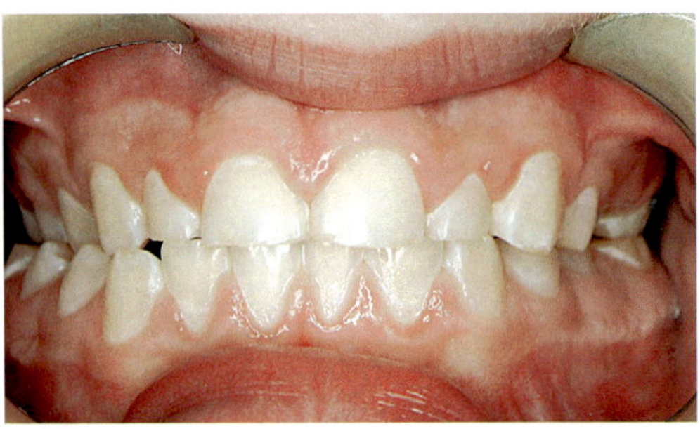

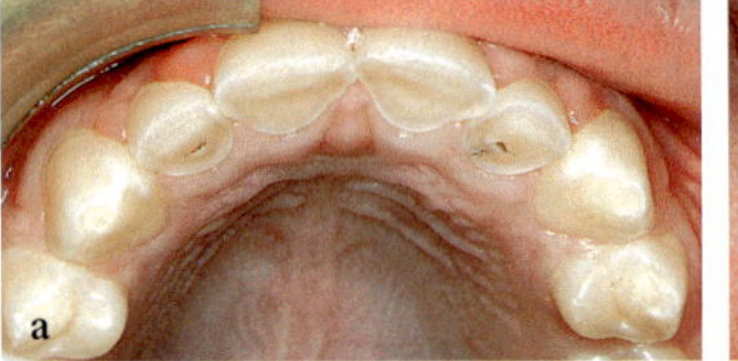

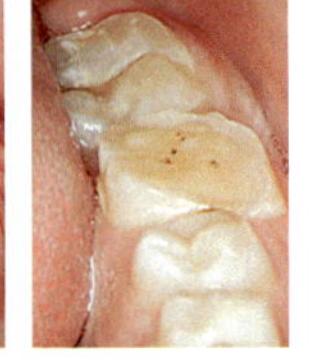

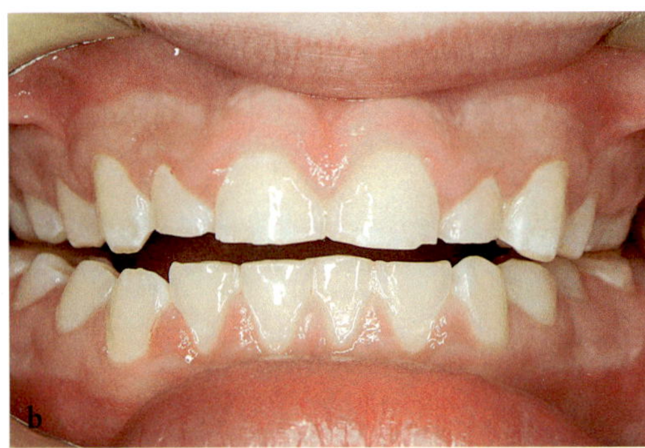

In addition to the aforementioned Dahl technique, space may also be gained, in certain cases, if occlusal analysis reveals a large horizontal discrepancy between centric relation (CR) and MIP, but with little vertical discrepancy; occlusal adjustment of such "centric interferences" will produce a significantly more distal MIP, and thus adequate palatal space for full-coverage anterior restorations to be constructed. In cases of extensive anterior wear, such an approach can maintain the original OVD, although, in cases that are planned for an increased OVD, the use of CR as the new reference maxillomandibular position is in any case implicit. The net space gained would in such cases have been achieved by a combination of the corrected CR–MIP slide and the increase in OVD (Fig 22-9).

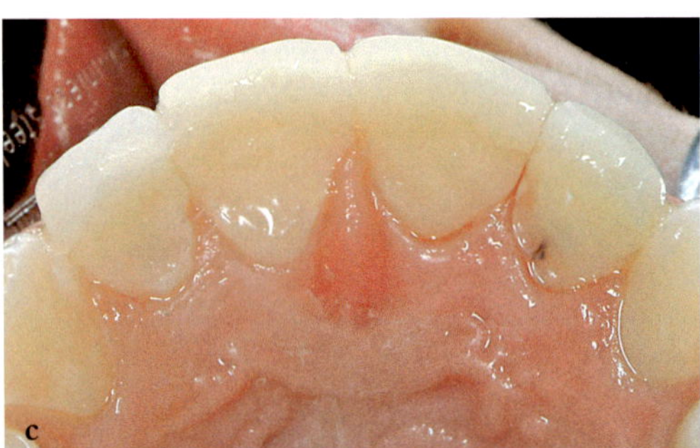

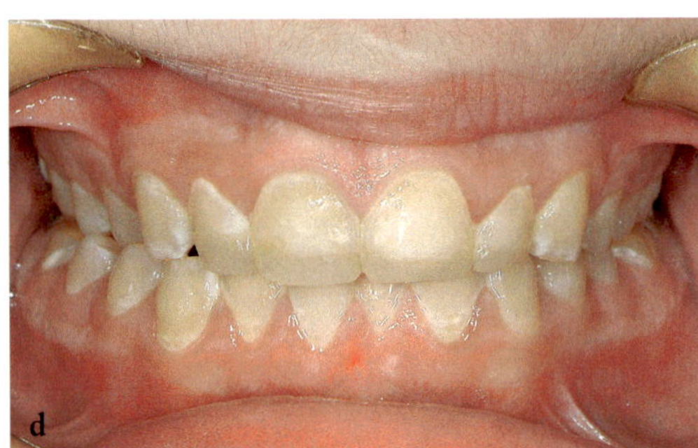

Fig 22-8 **(a)** A 12-year-old boy with "soft"-drink-induced erosion on the permanent maxillary incisors and all first permanent molars. **(b–d)** Composite restorations increasing the OVD have been placed on molars and maxillary incisors. Five years later the patient was offered permanent porcelain coverage free of charge, but he rejected it as he was happy with both esthetics and function. (Reprinted with permission from Johansson et al.[1])

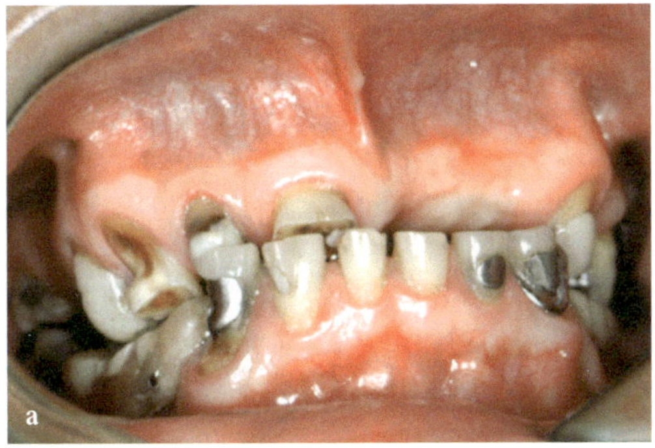

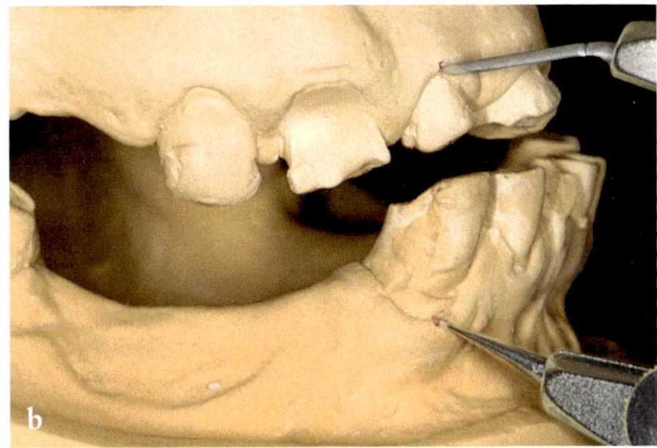

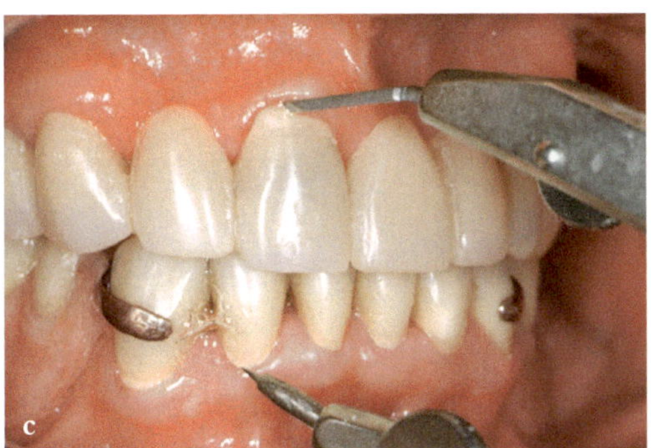

Fig 22-9 **(a)** A 50-year-old man with extensive generalized tooth wear resulting in dentoalveolar morphologic changes, manifesting as "edge-to-edge" bite and overclosure. **(b)** Treatment was extensive, including increasing the OVD, establishment of the new maxillomandibular relationship at a more distal mandibular position in CR, crown lengthening, and some elective endodontic treatments. **(c)** The acrylic provisional restoration phase (courtesy of Dr Tariq Abduljabbar, King Saud University). (Reprinted with permission from Johansson et al.[1])

*Generalized wear*

In cases of reduced OVD due to wear, it is generally recommended that it is so maintained. If possible, the patient's adapted "worn-in occlusion", in the absence of any functional problems, should be conformed to; increasing the OVD according to some predetermined "standard of normality" is not essential.

Increasing the OVD becomes necessary in those cases where interocclusal space problems or esthetic considerations are especially critical. In such instances, there need not be undue hesitation in increasing the OVD.[26] Conventional methods of determining the new OVD should be used, and there are seldom any adaptive problems. However, while there are hardly any difficulties involved in increasing the OVD in healthy individuals, a cautious approach is advocated with such procedures in patients exhibiting signs or symptoms of TMD. Such patients should first be treated with reversible methods to reduce the signs and symptoms of TMD and normalize function before any prosthodontic therapy is started.[36] As stated earlier, even if extensive tooth wear is present, the OVD could well be unaffected owing to compensatory eruption, which is an additional reason to leave it unchanged if possible.

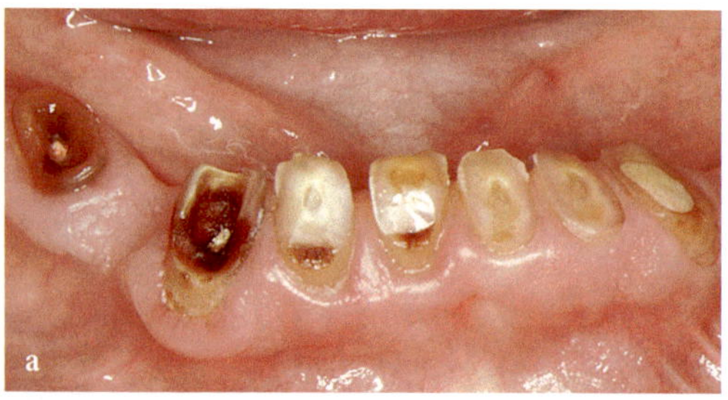

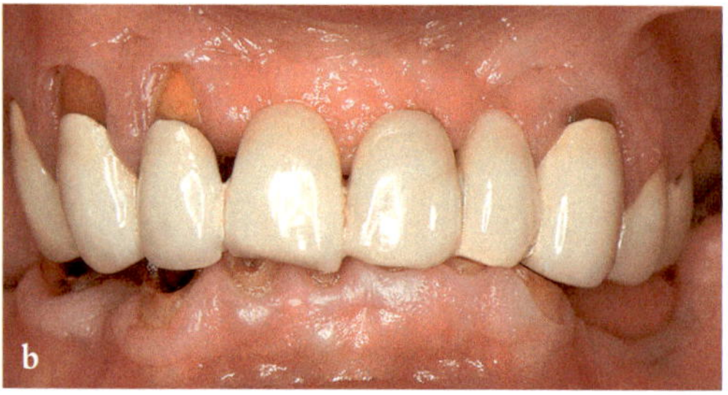

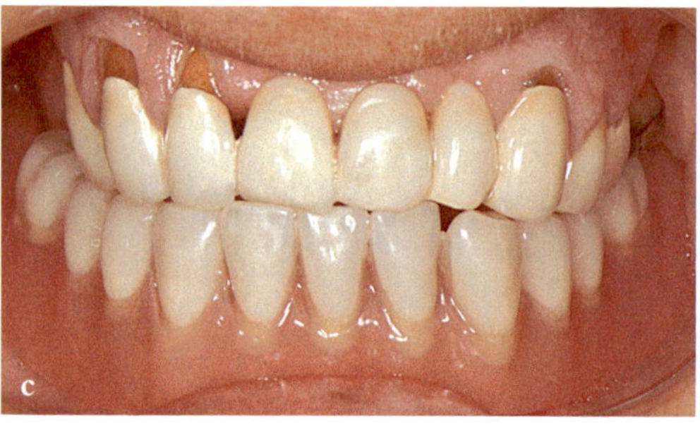

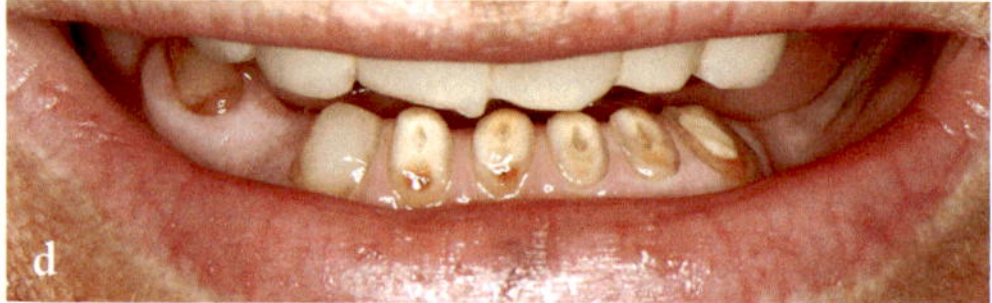

Fig 22-10 **(a and b)** A 66-year-old woman who has been on antidepressant medication for many years. She has pronounced xerostomia with documented hyposalivation and is a heavy bruxer. The risks in prescribing fixed prostheses are high, and which the patient cannot afford. **(c)** She was provided with an overdenture supported by remaining roots which have been restored with resin composite. A preventive regimen with fluoride gel inside the prosthesis was prescribed. **(d)** Follow-up after 1 year shows that the prosthesis has functioned well and there have been no further dental problems. (Reprinted with permission from Johansson et al.[1])

### *Removable Prosthodontic Strategies*

Fixed prostheses are expensive and not affordable for many patients who require treatment for tooth wear. In many countries where removable prostheses are common for reasons of tradition or economics, total extraction followed by complete dentures is the commonly suggested therapy for managing such patients' rehabilitative needs. Such treatment, however, can worsen residual ridge resorption (RRR) of the alveolar processes, leading to a deteriorating situation with regard to denture instability and poor retention. The possibility for future implant treatment also worsens. If single teeth or roots can be retained as overdenture abutments, the risk of progressive RRR is decreased.

If the patient can maintain good oral hygiene and the remaining teeth receive intensive fluoride prophylaxis regularly, a conventional overdenture is a relatively inexpensive option with a good prognosis (Fig 22-10). The use of gold copings on the abutment teeth supporting overdentures may produce surprisingly good long-term results. Removable partial dentures (RPDs) with occlusal overlays can also be used to re-establish OVD (Fig 22-11).[37]

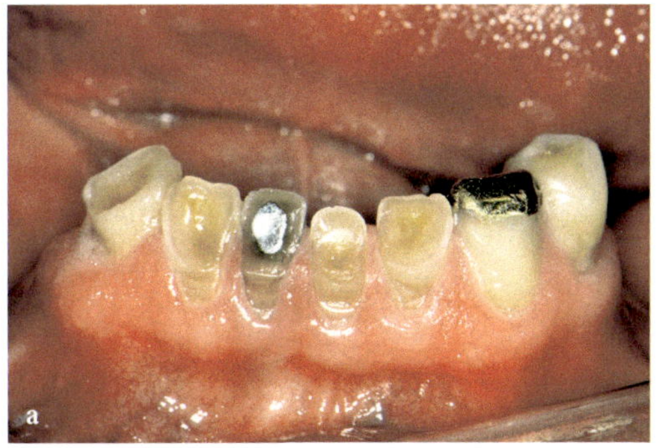

Fig 22-11 **(a–c)** A 65-year-old man with severe mandibular tooth wear treated with an overlay removable partial denture that provides the patient with increased occlusal vertical dimension.

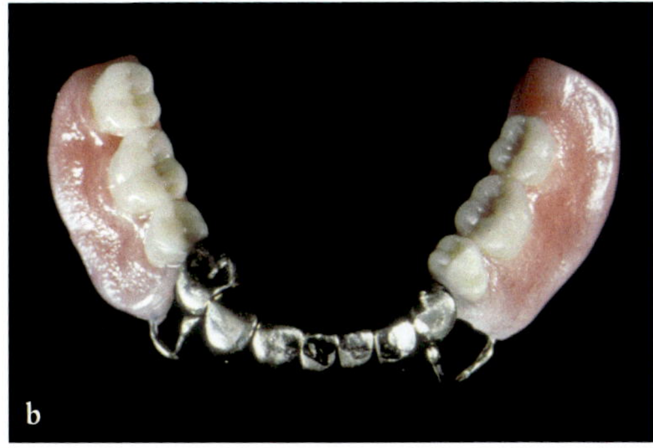

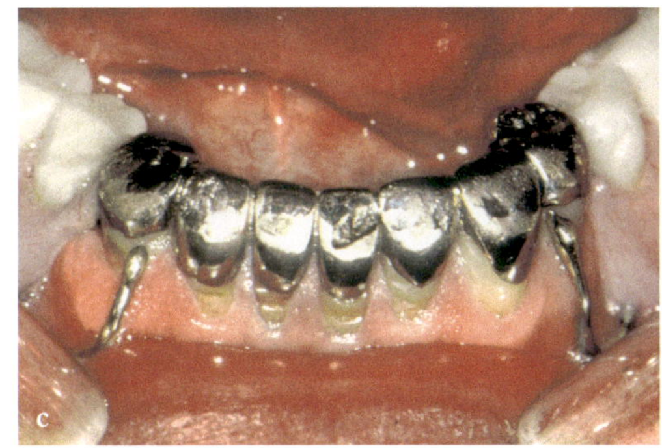

### *Materials*

The choice of material to be used for the restoration could be crucial, for example, if it is opposed by natural teeth or if the patient is a heavy bruxer. Studies on the wear process affecting restorative materials are almost always experimental, laboratory trials and extrapolating these results to the extremely variable conditions that apply clinically is very difficult. In cases of an opposing occlusion of tooth enamel, most clinicians and researchers agree that a metal occlusal surface, and preferably one of high noble-metal content, is preferred in order to minimize wear of the natural dentition. Unpolished ceramics could be detrimental to opposing natural teeth. However, there is lack of long-term clinical studies to support any strong conclusions regarding choice of material in restoration of worn teeth (see Chapter 19).

It is also very important to consider other factors that influence the wear resistance of natural teeth – erosive influences and salivary lubricatory factors, among others. In cases of heavy occlusal load (e.g., in bruxers) the situation becomes very complex as we need to consider not only the risk of wear of the restorative material itself and the opposing dentition, but also the demand for strength in all the components of the superstructure to be able to withstand the applied load. Besides the risk of mechanical failures under conditions of excessive load, biologic failures are even more likely (e.g., caries, marginal degradation, endodontic problems, and loss of retention).[38] Overall, metal or metal–ceramic restorations seem to be the safest choice in cases of high load conditions,[28] although under extreme conditions there is no material that will last for very long (Fig 22-12).

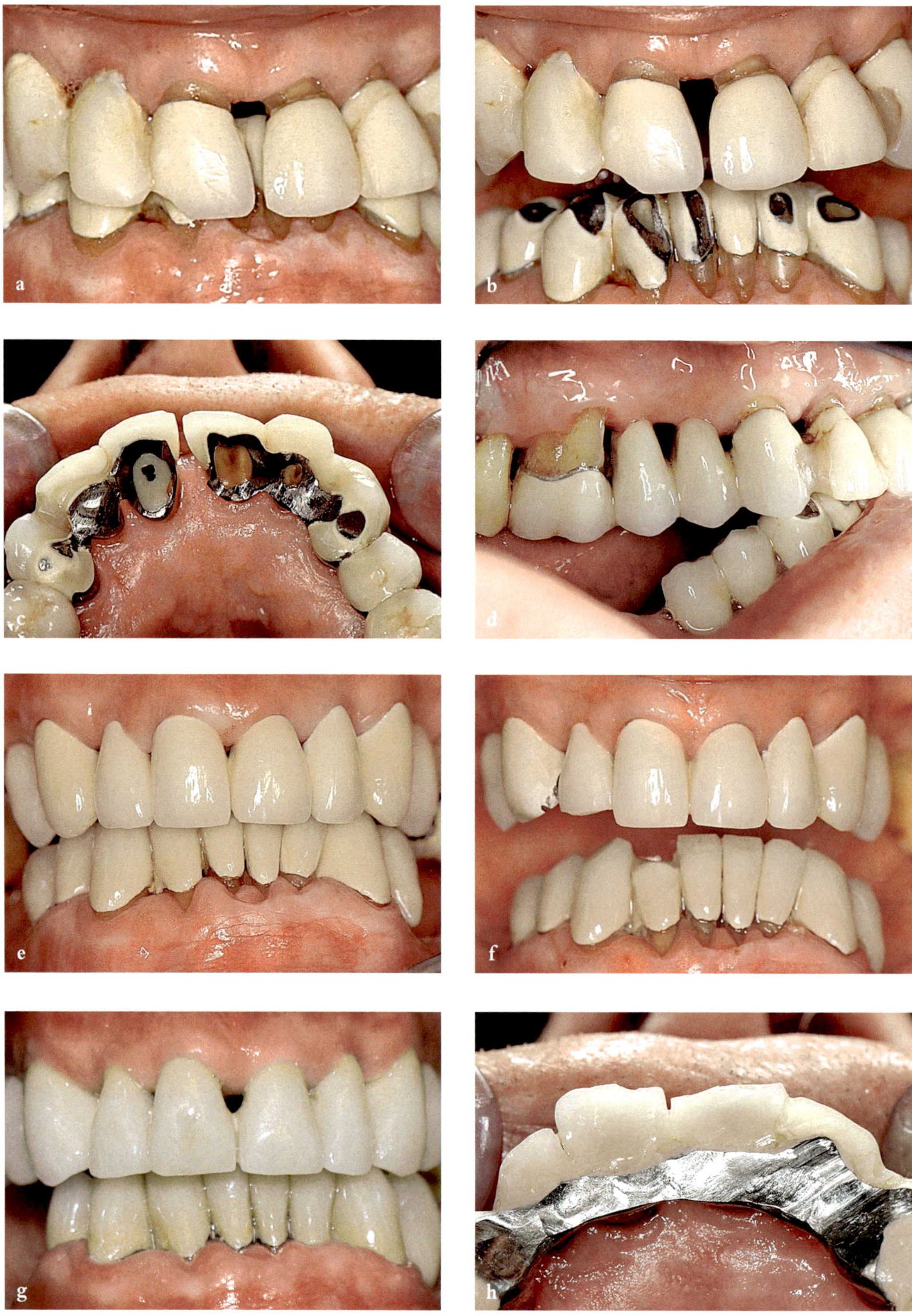

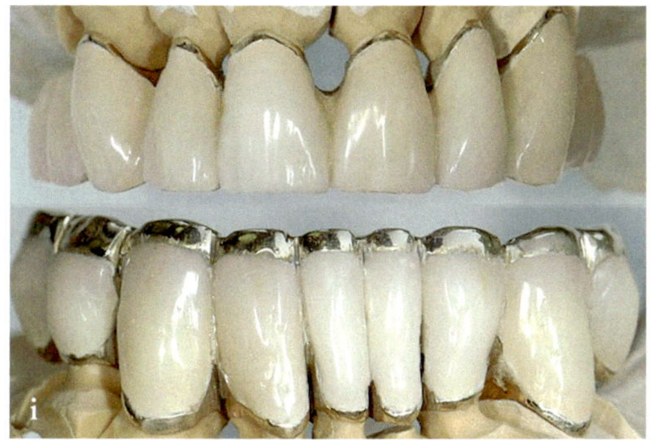

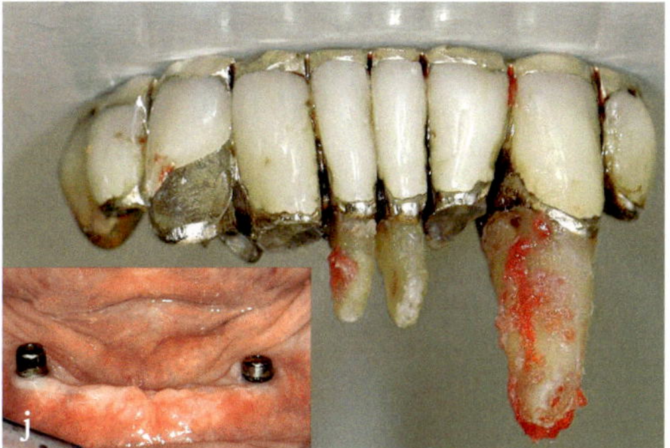

Fig 22-12 **(a–d)** A 60-year-old man with 10-year-old maxillary and mandibular metal–ceramic fixed dental prostheses (FDPs) and with a history of heavy chewing and bruxism which have resulted in fracture of the veneering porcelain. **(e and f)** New metal–ceramic FDPs were constructed but were again fractured after 2 years. **(g and h)** New FDPs were again constructed but fractured after a short time. **(i)** Acrylic-faced gold FDPs were provided with upper palatal and lower incisal metal surfaces. **(j)** After a further year, the mandibular FDP was totally dislodged with several of the abutments and a mandibular implant-retained overdenture was constructed. The prognosis is deemed extremely poor (courtesy of Dr Harald Gjengedal, University of Bergen, Norway). (Reprinted with permission from Johansson et al.[1])

Because of the risk of chipping of ceramic veneers in metal–ceramic reconstructions, many prosthodontists prefer gold–acrylic fixed dental prostheses for heavy bruxers. The few clinical studies published on wear of materials in bruxers indicate only small differences in wear resistance of gold and ceramic materials, whereas resin-based materials showed 3–4 times larger substance loss than gold or ceramics.[28]

### *Adhesive Strategies*

In children, and especially when wear affects permanent teeth in the mixed dentition, resin-based restorations are the restorative option of choice. These restorations may either be definitive or serve intermediately for later, more permanent reconstruction. The overwhelming majority of children with tooth wear have an erosive background and the restoration may serve several important functions: improve aesthetics, protect against further wear, reduce loss of OVD, and reduce dentin hypersensitivity, among others. The adhesive ability of resin-based materials also makes it the material of choice for restoring NCCLs and cuppings,[30] where they seem to perform reasonably well in a shorter term, although in the long-term the success rate falls dramatically.[39] However, in cases of active erosion they may have poorer prognosis. In general, however, excellent results from esthetic and biologic standpoints can be achieved (Fig 22-13; see also Figs 22-7 and 22-8).

In the older patient, too, the availability of increasingly reliable adhesive technologies and materials would seem to offer promise as a less invasive option for the treatment of the worn dentition. While clinical evidence for the efficacy of such technologies in restoring dentitions uncomplicated by tooth wear is appearing more and more, this is not the case for the worn dentition. For example, labial porcelain veneers are now established as a predictable long-term treatment option with a low failure rate, at least in controlled clinical settings.[40] In the worn dentition, direct resin-based composite restorations placed at an increased OVD when used to manage localized anterior tooth wear showed a median survival of 57 months for 225 restorations in 31 patients when all types of failures were considered; major failure requiring replacement was uncommon within the first five years, with the authors concluding the

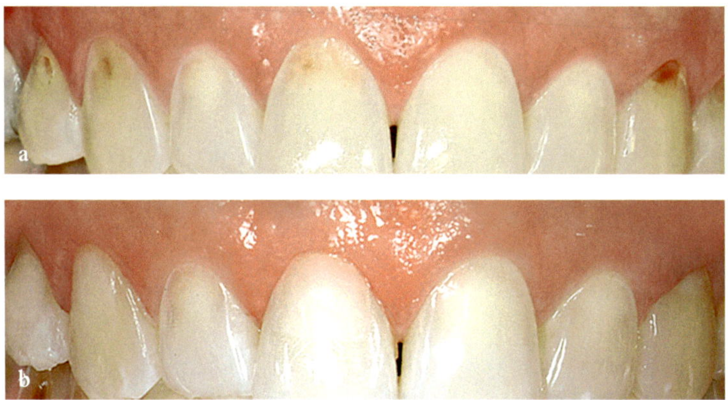

**Fig 22-13 (a and b)** A 40-year-old woman with severe buccal erosive damage, restored with resin composite restorations. (Reprinted with permission from Johansson et al.[1])

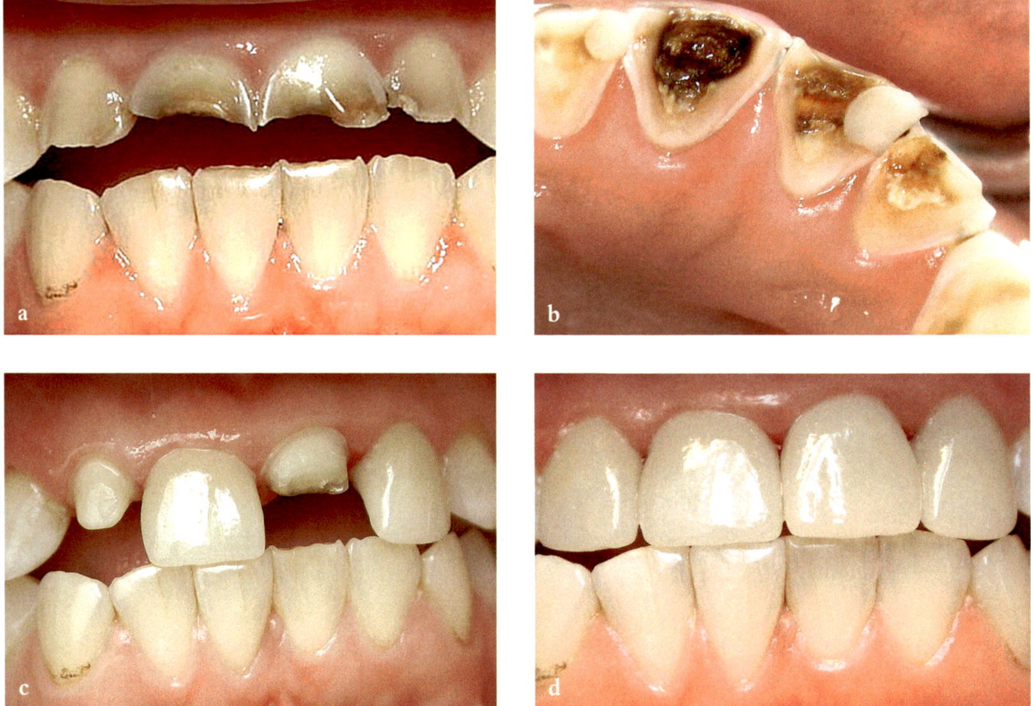

**Fig 22-14 (a and b)** Severe dental erosion localized to 12–22. **(c)** A crown is cemented on 11 using adhesive technique. Note the carefully, rounded line angles of the tooth preparations of 12 and 21. **(d)** Completed cementation of remaining crowns (courtesy of Dr Bo Sundh and Dr Peter Lingström, University of Gothenburg, Sweden).

method to be conservative, easily maintainable and with a good short- to medium-term survival.[41]

With regard to the adhesive bonding of indirect restorations in the worn dentition, evidence is even more sparse. A report of three case histories, each with one or more teeth with complete loss of the clinical crown, found one case to have survived 10 years, one failing at 6 years, and the third treated too recently to report on. While the suggestion that the method is a possible prosthodontic management strategy may be viewed as optimistic, it does illustrate the needs and demands of patients suffering from the effects of severe wear and the ongoing challenges that the rehabilitation of such dentitions will continue to pose for clinicians.

With regard to the perhaps less demanding partial-coverage indirect restorations, the use of bonded palatal porcelain veneers, in combination with initial orthodontic space creation, has been advocated, although clinical follow-ups on retention and effects on opposing tooth surfaces are limited. Long-term follow-ups of full-coverage bonded ceramic fixed dental prostheses are scant but show a higher failure rate compared to conventional fixed restorations. It seems that under such circumstances of limited information in even the unworn state, the more demanding conditions of restoring the worn dentition by these means suggests that much greater caution is needed in these situations.

Adhesively retained ceramic restorations are becoming almost routinely and exclusively practiced by some clinicians, but the procedures involved are technique-sensitive and the method is not yet suitable in the hands of all practitioners. For treatment of cases of tooth wear with an erosive background, there are no systematic studies and only case reports have been presented (Fig 22-14).[30] It is advisable to exercise some caution when it comes to restoring worn teeth with esthetic alternatives that rely solely on adhesive bonding until more reports on its clinical longevity have appeared. Conventional fixed prosthodontics, with its proven record of long service even if only in the context of the entirely lesser strategic demands of relatively unworn teeth (which these data relate to), would seem in many instances still to be the treatment of choice for extensively worn teeth (Fig 22-15).

An alternative rehabilitative strategy was recently proposed based on the principle of reversibility.[42] Because the worn dentition usually produces slow occlusal breakdown, it permits most patients to adapt to the changing situation until a level of unacceptable function or discomfort is reached. Contrasting with this, typical methods of reconstruction represent a sudden change that precludes proper evaluation of the patient's ability to readapt to changed oral conditions. Just as the pathway to the worn status may vary, so too does the reconstructive process need to be guided, and this is suggested by the authors to be best achievable through staged reconstruction using adhesive techniques wherever possible.[42] Even if the evidence for such a rationale is lacking, it seems possible that the all-too-frequent failures seen after traditional reconstructive efforts may be more controllable through a staged, reversible reconstruction that relies to a large extent on adhesive technology, including composite resin or similar materials.

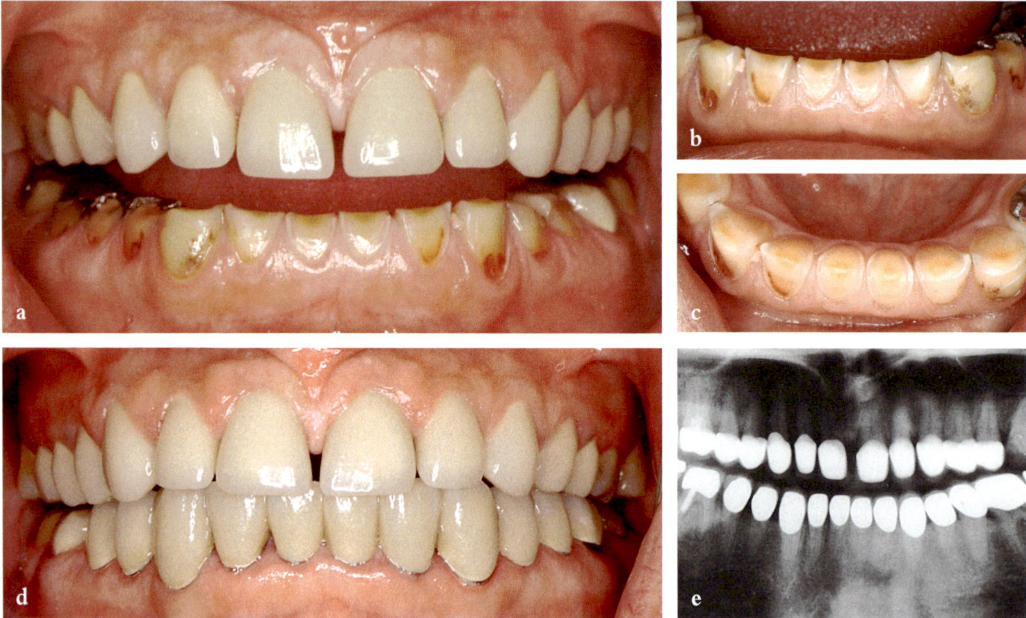

Fig 22-15 **(a–c)** A 32-year-old woman with long-standing bulimia nervosa which resulted in severe erosion. The maxillary teeth were treated 1 year previously in another clinic. **(d)** The extremely shortened and sensitive mandibular teeth were restored with conventional metal–ceramic single crowns. **(e)** Radiograph after 5 years. In a telephone check-up 17 years after treatment, the patient says that she had not had any relapse of the eating disorder and that her teeth had functioned well without problems throughout the period since her dental treatment. (Reprinted with permission from Johansson et al.[1])

## Maintenance Phase

Regular follow-up of reconstructions are necessary for several reasons. For example, a combination of short clinical crowns, differential wear, and bruxism, etc., increase the risks of cementation failure. Similarly, erosion-induced wear may continue even in the presence of teeth with full-coverage crowns and can progress cervical to the crowned tooth if causal factors have not been eliminated. In addition, occlusal splint treatment in combined attrition (bruxism) and erosion cases may not be successful. Cases should be reviewed at least annually when new study casts and photographs should be taken.

A careful clinical and radiographic examination of abutments should be performed: caries, failed retention, wear facets, porcelain integrity, etc., must be checked, recorded, and treated as necessary. Individually designed preventive regimens should be prescribed and carried out with an interval determined on the basis of the supposed etiology and future progression of the tooth wear. These could comprise topical fluoride application, dietary advice, and psychologic motivation for lifestyle changes, among others. The lack of knowledge of long-term results of restoration of tooth wear is a further reason for regular follow-ups.

## Conclusion

Tooth wear is a multifactorial process, which can make it difficult to identify a single cause at the individual patient level. Its progress is usually slow which characterizes it as a physiologic condition; when it threatens tooth survival or is of concern to the patient, it may be regarded as pathologic. Recognition of the early signs of wear, and especially erosion, could bring about timely prevention and improve the lifespan of teeth. The most obvious feature of wear is shortened clinical crowns, generally accompanied by dentoalveolar compensation. This may complicate definitive conventional rehabilitation, although research and newer technologies and materials offer broader possibilities for rationalization of treatment modalities.

Restoration of worn teeth will be needed in only some patients, and the measures with which need for treatment is assessed is one of the keys to successful outcomes. In broad terms, the decision to treat or not should be guided by the patient's stated and/or perceived need, the severity of the wear as determined by morphologic changes, and the potential for progression in the context of the patient's age. The decision will in most cases be tempered by the generally complex and expensive nature of rehabilitation of the worn dentition and the known risks of biomechanical failures. The striking lack of evidence regarding long-term outcomes of restorative treatment of tooth wear using different methods and materials also calls for caution in decision-making.

## References


1. Johansson A, Johansson AK, Omar R, Carlsson GE. Rehabilitation of the worn dentition. J Oral Rehabil 2008;35:548–566.
2. Molnar S. Tooth wear and culture: a survey of tooth function among some prehistoric populations. Curr Anthropol 1972;13:511–526.
3. Hylander WL. Morphological changes in human teeth and jaws in a high-attrition environment. In: Dahlberg AA, Graber TM (eds). Orofacial Growth and Development. Paris: Mouton, 1977:301–330.
4. Kiliaridis S, Johansson A, Haraldson T, Omar R, Carlsson GE. Craniofacial morphology, occlusal traits, and bite force in persons with advanced occlusal tooth wear. Am J Orthod Dentofacial Orthop 1995;107:286–292.
5. Johansson A. A cross-cultural study of occlusal tooth wear. Swed Dent J Suppl 1992;86:1–59.
6. Kerr NW. Dental pain and suffering prior to the advent of modern dentistry. Br Dent J 1998;184:397–399.
7. Al-Omiri MK, Lamey PJ, Clifford T. Impact of tooth wear on daily living. Int J Prosthodont 2006;19:601–605.
8. Wedel A, Borrman H, Carlsson GE. Tooth wear and temporomandibular joint morphology in a skull material from the 17th century. Swed Dent J 1998;22:85–95.
9. Johansson AK. On dental erosion and associated factors. Swed Dent J Suppl 2002;156:1–77.
10. Carlsson GE, Johansson A, Lundqvist S. Occlusal wear: a follow-up study of 18 subjects with extremely worn dentitions. Acta Odontol Scand 1985;43:83–90.
11. Bartlett DW. The role of erosion in tooth wear: aetiology, prevention and management. Int Dent J 2005;55(Suppl 1):277–284.
12. Nunn J, Morris J, Pine C et al. The condition of teeth in the UK in 1998 and implications for the future. Br Dent J 2000;189:639–644.
13. Bernhardt O, Gesch D, Splieth C et al. Risk factors for high occlusal wear scores in a population-based sample: results of the Study of Health in Pomerania (SHIP). Int J Prosthodont 2004;17:333–339.
14. Hugoson A, Bergendal T, Ekfeldt A, Helkimo M. Prevalence and severity of incisal and occlusal tooth wear in an adult Swedish population. Acta Odontol Scand 1988;46:255–265.
15. Jaeggi T, Lussi A. Prevalence, incidence and distribution of erosion. Monogr Oral Sci 2006;20:44–65.
16. Wänman A, Wigren L. Need and demand for dental treatment: a comparison between an evaluation based on an epidemiologic study of 35-, 50-, and 65-year-olds and performed dental treatment of matched age groups. Acta Odontol Scand 1995;53:318–324.
17. Bartlett DW, Shah P. A critical review of non-carious cervical (wear) lesions and the role of abfraction, erosion, and abrasion. J Dent Res 2006;85:306–312.
18. Johansson A-K, Johansson A, Birkhed D, Omar R, Baghdadi S, Carlsson GE. Dental erosion, soft-drink intake, and oral health in young Saudi men, and the development of a system for assessing erosive anterior tooth wear. Acta Odontol Scand 1996;54:369–378.
19. Johansson A, Haraldson T, Omar R, Kiliaridis S, Carlsson GE. A system for assessing the severity and progression of occlusal tooth wear. J Oral Rehabil 1993;20:125–131.
20. Davies SJ, Gray RJ, Qualtrough AJ. Management of tooth surface loss. Br Dent J 2002;192:11–23.
21. van't Spijker A, Keulen CM, Creugers NHJ. Attrition, occlusion, (dys)function, and intervention: a systematic review. Clin Oral Implants Res 2007;18(Suppl 3):117–126.
22. Johansson A, Omar R. Identification and management of tooth wear. Int J Prosthodont 1994;7:506–516.
23. Johansson AK, Lingstrom P, Imfeld T, Birkhed D. Influence of drinking method on tooth-surface pH in relation to dental erosion. Eur J Oral Sci 2004;112:484–489.
24. Orchardson R, Gillam DG. Managing dentin hypersensitivity. J Am Dent Assoc 2006;137:990–998

25. Thrash WJ, Dodds MW, Jones DL. The effect of stannous fluoride on dentinal hypersensitivity. Int Dent J 1994;44 (1 Suppl 1):107–118.
26. Carlsson GE, Magnusson T. Management of temporomandibular disorders in the general dental practice. Chicago: Quintessence, 1999.
27. Dahl BL, Krogstad O, Karlsen K. An alternative treatment in cases with advanced localized attrition. J Oral Rehabil 1975;2:209–214.
28. Dahl B, Øilo G. Wear of teeth and restorative materials. In: Öwall B, Käyser AF, Carlsson GE (eds). Prosthodontics: Principles and Management Strategies. London: Mosby-Wolfe, 1996:187–200.
29. Milleding P. Abutment preparation. In: Karlsson S, Nilner K, Dahl BL (eds). A Textbook of Fixed Prosthodontics: The Scandinavian Approach. Stockholm: Gothia, 2000: 151–172.
30. Carlsson GE, Johansson A, Milleding P. Rekonstruktiv behandling av erosionsskador. In: Johansson AK, Carlsson GE (eds). Dental Erosion: Bakgrund och Kliniska Aspekter. Stockholm: Gothia Förlag AB, 2006:163–180.
31. Toreskog S, Myrin C. A minimally invasive and esthetic bonded porcelain technique: the concept and the vision. Pt I. In: Schou L (ed). Nordic Dentistry 2003 Yearbook. Copenhagen: Quintessence, 2003:1–25.
32. Dahl BL, Krogstad O. Long-term observations of an increased occlusal face height obtained by a combined orthodontic/prosthetic approach. J Oral Rehabil 1985;12: 173–176.
33. Poyser NJ, Porter RW, Briggs PF, Chana HS, Kelleher MG. The Dahl concept: past, present and future. Br Dent J 2005;198:669–676.
34. Hemmings KW, Darbar UR, Vaughan S. Tooth wear treated with direct composite restorations at an increased vertical dimension: results at 30 months. J Prosthet Dent 2000;83:287–293.
35. Chana H, Kelleher M, Briggs P, Hooper R. Clinical evaluation of resin-bonded gold alloy veneers. J Prosthet Dent 2000;83:294–300.
36. De Boever JA, Carlsson GE, Klineberg IJ. Need for occlusal therapy and prosthodontic treatment in the management of temporomandibular disorders. II: Tooth loss and prosthodontic treatment. J Oral Rehabil 2000;27: 647–659.
37. Almog DM, Ganddini MR. Maxillary and mandibular overlay removable partial dentures for restoration of worn teeth: a three-year follow-up. N Y State Dent J 2006;72: 32–35.
38. Yip KH, Smales RJ, Kaidonis JA. Differential wear of teeth and restorative materials: clinical implications. Int J Prosthodont 2004;17:350–356.
39. van Dijken JW, Sunnegårdh-Grönberg K, Lindberg A. Clinical long-term retention of etch-and-rinse and self-etch adhesive systems in non-carious cervical lesions. A 13 years evaluation. Dent Mater 2007;23:1101–1107.
40. Layton D, Walton T. An up to 16-year prospective study of 304 porcelain veneers. Int J Prosthodont 2007;20:389-396
41. Redman CD, Hemmings KW, Good JA. The survival and clinical performance of resin-based composite restorations used to treat localised anterior tooth wear. Br Dent J 2003;194:566–572.
42. Creugers NH, van't Spijker A. Tooth wear and occlusion: friends or foes? Int J Prosthodont 2007;20:348–350.

Chapter 23

# Effects of Bruxism on Restorative Implant-assisted Prosthesis Treatments

*Jorge Mario Galante*

## Introduction

There is abundant literature on the care that should be taken when rehabilitating bruxers and on the terrible consequences this parafunctional activity has on the stomatognathic system. This automated habit has been related to temporomandibular disorders, natural dentition occlusal wear, cervical abfractions (Figs 23-1 and 23-2), crown fractures, tooth mobility from trauma, decementing, and fractures of individual or multiple fixed prostheses on natural teeth or implants (Figs 23-3 and 23-4).[1,2] In patients showing signs of bruxism, peri-implant bone loss and even implant integration loss from overload have been reported (Figs 23-5 and 23-6).[3,4] The objectives of this chapter are:

- to retrospectively evaluate the long-term effects of the treatments employed in the management of the general population with implant-assisted prostheses (IAPs)
- to evaluate the data reported in the literature on the complications shown by these patients, and to compare such data with the information obtained in our daily practice
- to classify the complications usually shown by patients treated with IAPs
- to relate the complications described or shown by the patients who underwent treatment to bruxism signs
- to identify high-risk patients
- to establish guidelines for the diagnosis, treatment, and prognosis of this group of patients and for the prevention of complications.

It has been demonstrated that, owing to the good results obtained in long-term clinical trials, the use of implants is the method of choice for the oral rehabilitation of patients who are partially or fully edentulous.[5] On the other hand, many complications have been described in patients with bruxism habits and/or tooth clenching habits who were treated with prosthetic rehabilitation.[3,4]

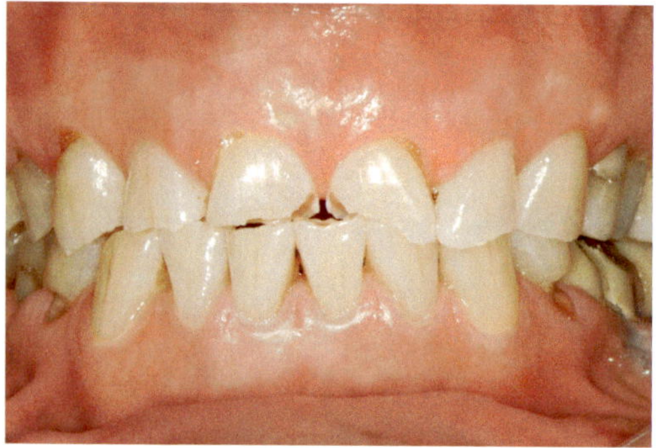

Fig 23-1 Frontal view of a bruxer showing tooth substance destruction aggravated by endogenous erosion.

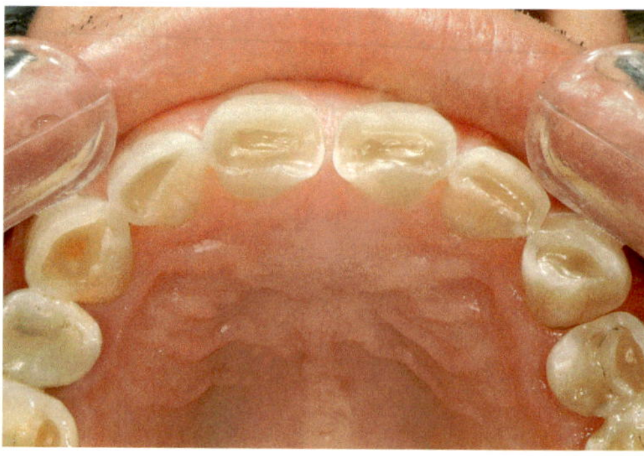

Fig 23-2 Occlusal view of patient showing enamel wear and dentin loss from the combined action of bruxism and erosion.

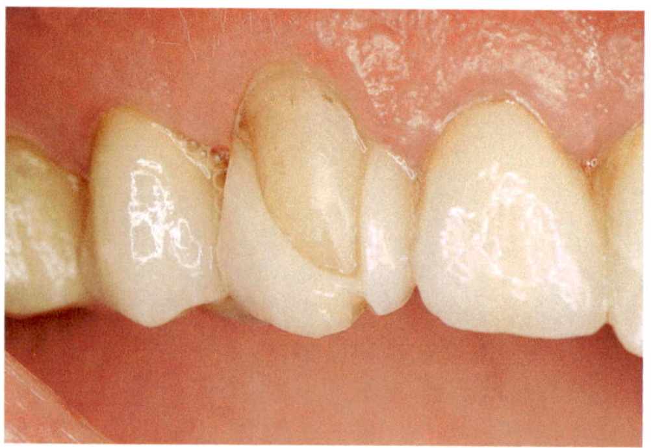

Fig 23-3 Bruxer rehabilitated with pure-porcelain crowns. Crown fracture and loss of porcelain is observed.

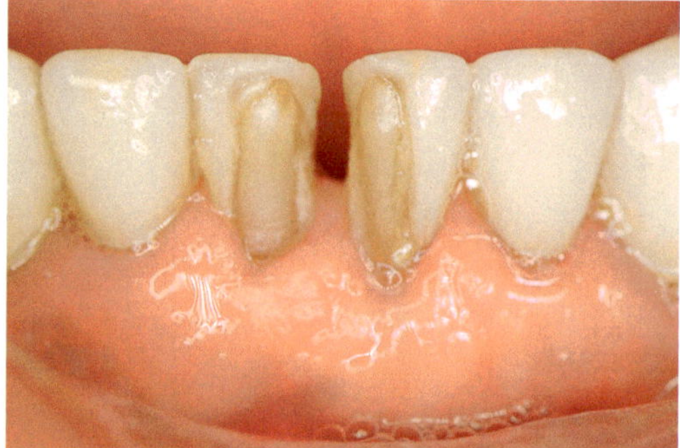

Fig 23-4 The same rehabilitated patient: view of his anterior guidance, with crown fracture of the incisors.

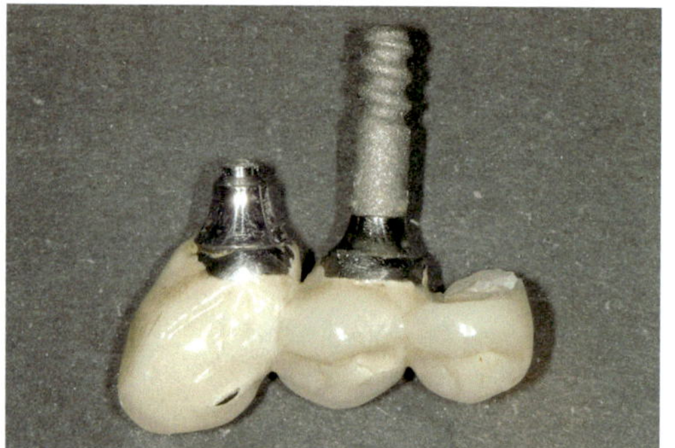

Fig 23-5 Implant/abutment set screw fracture and bone-integration loss in the adjoining implant.

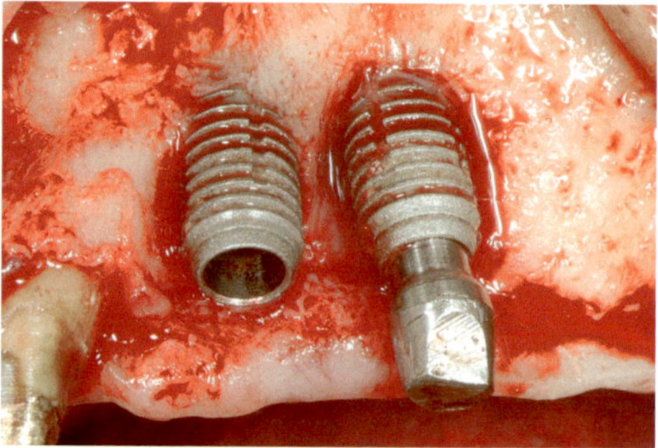

Fig 23-6 Adjoining implants, with severe marginal bone loss.

The many precautions that should be taken when employing IAP treatments for patients with signs and symptoms of bruxism are well known. This parafunctional habit is an exclusion criterion in most clinical trials on implants, so bruxers are not eligible for enrollment; many professionals will even consider apparent bruxism signs to be contraindications for implant rehabilitation.[6,7]

The effects of trauma and overocclusion on implant–bone integration are controversial. Although many reports exist on IAP treatment complications in bruxers, to date there is no evidence that implant integration loss is related to bruxism.[8] In the author's opinion, it is necessary to define the success criterion for implant–bone integration; for this purpose, we will follow Albrektsson and co-workers' suggestions, published in 1986 and summarized in five points:[9]

- On clinical monitoring, individual, independent implants should be immobile.
- No peri-implant radiolucency should be observed in the radiograph.
- Vertical bone-tissue loss should not be over 0.2 mm after the first year of functional activity.
- Individual implants should not show signs or symptoms such as pain, infection, neuropathy, or paresthesia.
- Success should be 85% after a 5-year monitoring period and 80% after 10 years.

For the purposes of the present chapter it is convenient to analyze specific peri-implant pathologies on the one hand and, on the other hand, the complications associated with restorations using implant-assisted prostheses.

## Peri-implant Pathology Classification

It is important to review the peri-implant pathology classifications existing in the literature. According to Chiapasco,[10] a good criterion for classifying these pathologies is their time of onset, according to which they can be divided into two categories: early peri-implantitis and late peri-implantitis.

### *Early Peri-implantitis*

Early peri-implantitis in patients treated with early-load implants or immediate-load implants occurs immediately or shortly after implant place-

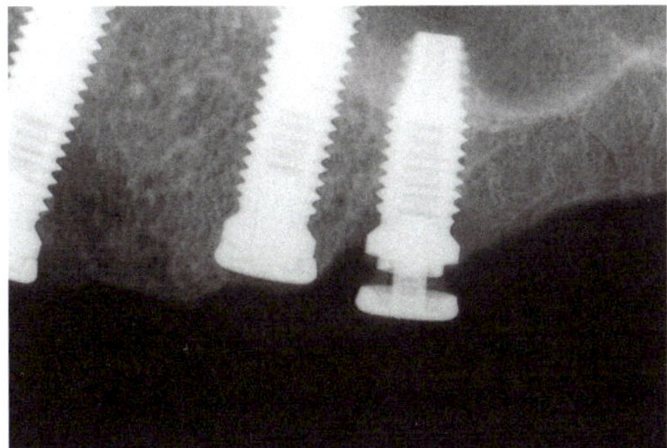

Fig 23-7 Implant placed according to protocol. The full removable prosthesis exerts pressure on the distal implant, causing the screw to loosen and resulting in its exposure to the oral environment and peri-implantitis.

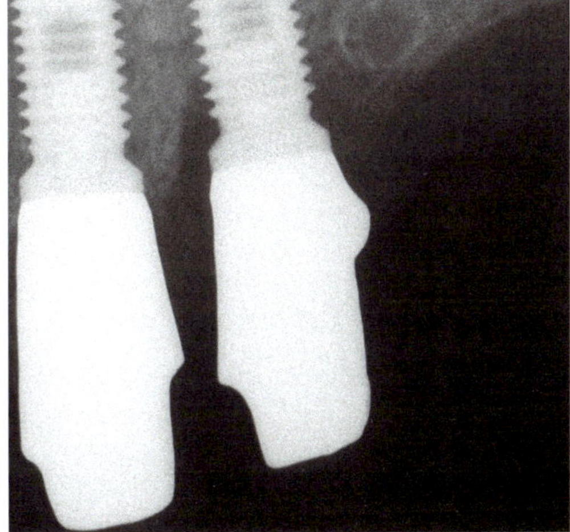

Fig 23-8 Biologic space re-establishment: post-restoration bone-margin migration to the third spiral.

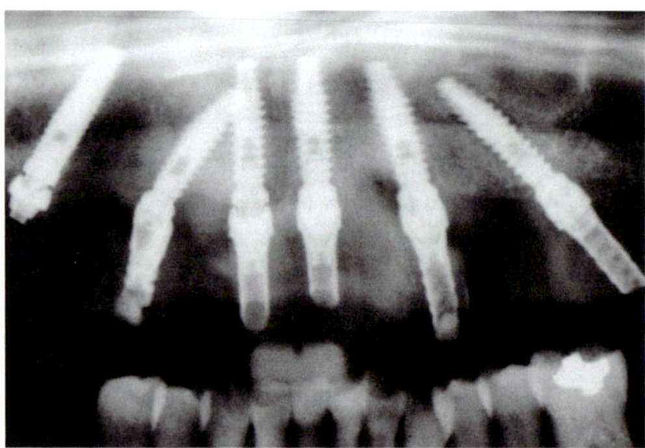

Fig 23-9 Panoramic radiograph taken 3 months after immediate loading of the maxilla. There is prosthetic overload causing loosening of the prosthetic retaining screws in 15, multiunit abutment loosening in 21, and integration loss in implant 25.

ment, between the first and the second surgical stage (in the first 6–8 weeks). The possible causes of early peri-implantitis include: wrong surgical-site preparation method; implant inserted in an infected or contaminated area; bacterial contamination of implant or instrumental set during surgery; and surgical or post-surgical wound contamination.

On contact with the affected peri-implant tissues, temporary removable prostheses may generate dislocating forces (Figs 23-7 and 23-8). Thus, excessive forces exerted by full fixed prostheses or immediate-load temporary partial fixed prostheses during the early stage of scar formation or during the implant integration period may be another cause of early peri-implantitis (Fig 23-9).

### *Late Peri-implantitis*

Late peri-implantitis occurs after the implant has been loaded and once it is integrated with its definitive prosthetic restoration. The possible causes of late peri-implantitis are plaque accumulation capable of producing bacterial colonization, and biomechanical overload from occlusal stress.

Peri-implant pathologies of bacterial etiology can be divided into *peri-implant mucositis*, which is a "reversible" inflammation affecting only the soft tissues adjacent to a bone-integrated implant; and *peri-implantitis*, which is an associated soft tissue inflammatory reaction responsible for progressive bone resorption and capable of causing loss of implant function.

There is disagreement regarding biomechanical overload caused by occlusal stress. We will analyze the biologic consequences of occlusion on bone-integrated implants. During the first year of function, a small marginal bone loss is observed around most of the implants; this is considered to be acceptable and within the ranges of normal or physiologic parameters. Such bone loss will eventually stabilize with time, and this will be seen even on long-term longitudinal follow-up.[5,11,12] This phenomenon was initially attributed to surgical problems, to trauma from countersink-bit use for subcrestal implant placement,[13] and to the concentration of forces in the implant-neck/threaded-body interface, that is, among other reasons, to an implant design deficiency[14,15] and to occlusal stress.[16–18]

Nowadays, there is clear evidence that peri-implant bone remodeling is ascribable to a biologic response that takes place when the implant has been exteriorized and is in contact with the oral environment. This phenomenon is known as "biologic width re-establishment"[19,20] (Figs 23-10 and 23-11). Bone margin apical migration approximately up to the standard-implant first spiral (with implants placed according to the protocol of the Swedish school: 1 mm subcrestal in two surgical procedures) will depend on the place where the implant shoulder is placed with respect to the bone crest in the crown-down direction.[5,11]

Based on animal experimental models, Hermann and co-workers[21] and Todescan and co-workers[22] claim that the bone level is always located approximately 2 mm apical to the implant/abutment gap in two-stage implants (Brånemark-type) and 2 mm from the limit of the polished portion with the treated surface in single-stage implants (Straumann-type), regardless of whether shoulder placement is juxtacrestal, subcrestal, or supra-

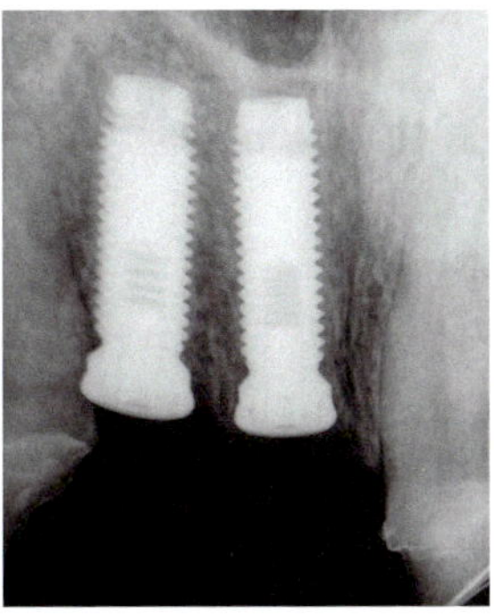

Fig 23-10 Post-extraction adjoining implant placed 1 mm subcrestal.

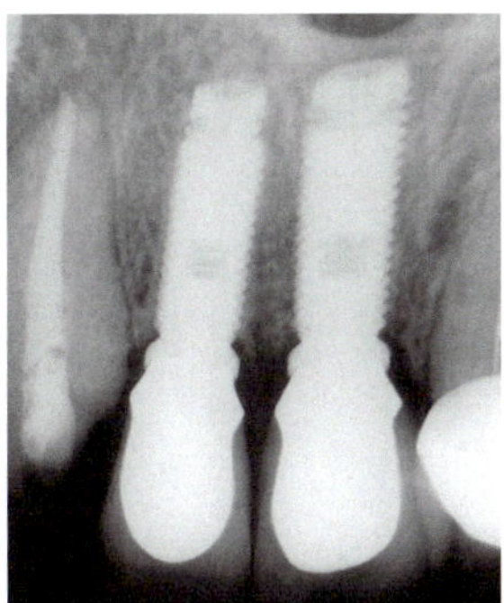

Fig 23-11 Implant with completed restoration: bone-margin migration to the first spiral.

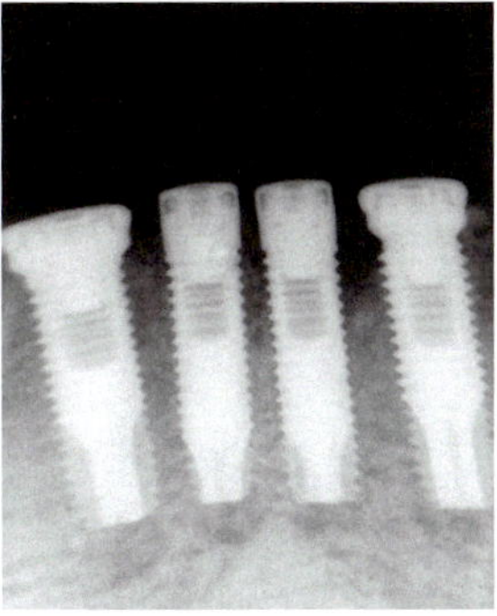

Fig 23-12 Minimally separated adjoining implants (separation is less than 2 mm), juxtacrestal.

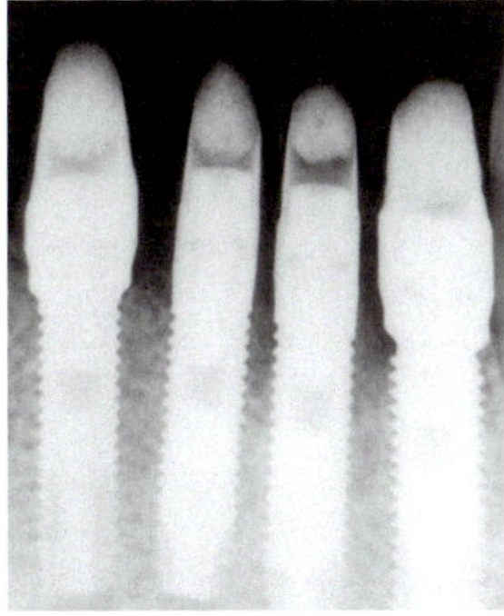

Fig 23-13 Abutment placement on the day of the opening, with the margins still preserved.

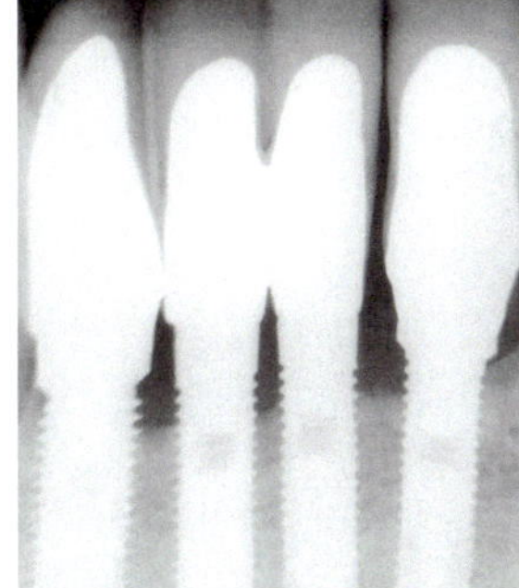

Fig 23-14 Once the definitive implant-assisted prostheses were placed, marginal bone resorption occured due to the establishment of the biologic width. Due to the fact that the proximity between implants is less than 2 mm, incremental bone resorption is observed.

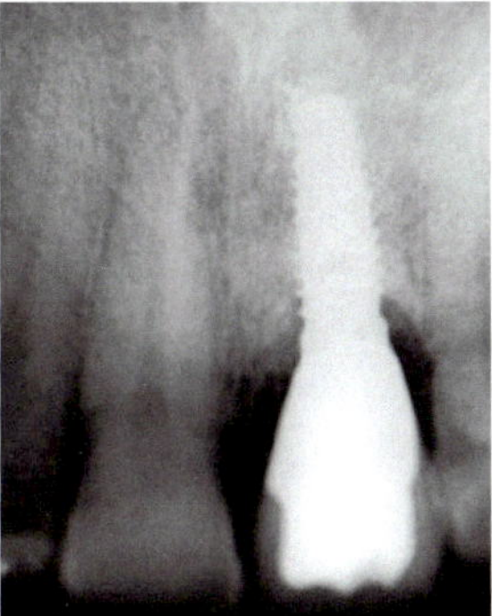

Fig 23-15 Crown on implant: bone loss up to the second spiral.

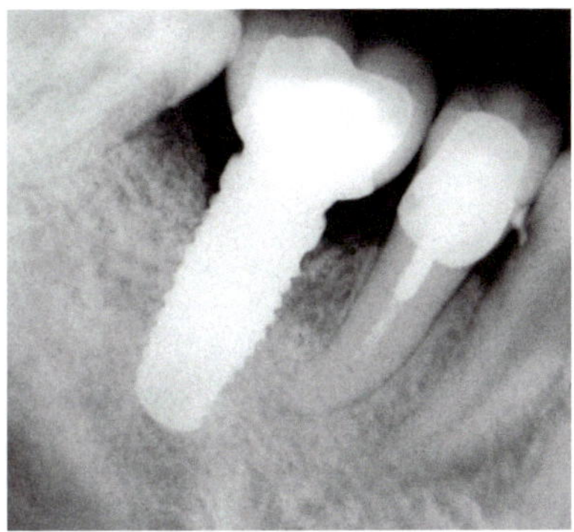

Fig 23-16 Crown on implant: though the platform has been changed, bone loss up to the second spiral may be observed.

crestal. For this reason, some authors suggest juxtacrestal or supracrestal implant placement whenever possible and esthetically viable, to minimize the effect of the apical migration of the peri-implant bone margin once the latter has been exteriorized or brought into function.[23] It must be remembered that bone-margin apical migration causes functional-load magnitude to progress geometrically, since the power arm increases and the resistance arm decreases with each millimeter lost. Grunder and co-workers[24] have shown that this biologic width re-establishment occurs three-dimensionally and affects the migration of the vestibular gingival margin, restorations on implants in the area of important esthetic involvement, and adjoining implants. Also in those cases of adjacent implants, the establishment of the biologic width on one implant is added to the contiguous implant, and this results in increased bone-margin apical migration between the implants. Tarnow and co-workers[25] suggest placing implants at least 3 mm apart to prevent bone crest resorption (Figs 23-12 to 23-14). Important bone loss beyond the above-mentioned 2 mm has been observed in some implants; such bone loss results from the biologic width re-establishment and is considered normal[5,11,26–28] (Figs 23-15 and 23-16).

Many clinical trials report a correlation between poor oral hygiene and marginal bone loss progression around the implants.[5,28–32] Experimental studies with animals have also shown that bacterial plaque accumulation may cause bone loss around bone-integrated implants.[33–39] Bacterial plaque accumulation produces inflammation of the peri-implant mucosa, and consequently induces peri-implant bone resorption. It has also been demonstrated that excessive occlusal forces exerted on bone-integrated implants may result in marginal bone loss or in full bone-integration loss, even when much function time has elapsed[5,40] (Fig 23-17).

Even though studies have been devised to evaluate the forces exerted during in-vivo function in patients, it is very difficult to clinically quantify the magnitude and direction of the occlusal forces exerted during biting.[41–43] Occlusal forces may exceed the mechanical capacity or the biologic load-bearing capacity and cause mechanical failure or bone-integration loss. When such is the case, the load may be defined as "overload".[16–18]

In-vivo studies carried out by Richter[44] have shown that vertical forces of around 60–120 Nmm (depending on the type of food) act on implants in the premolar area during mastication. During maximum tooth clenching on a metal paper, the load applied to the implant doubles. In another study, Richter[45] has shown that the horizontal component of the forces acting on the suprastructures of implants results in increased stress in the alveolar bone, with a maximum value of 6 MPa concentrated in the buccal area of the residual-ridge crest. For comparison, note that mesial–distal forces may cause a peak cervical stress of around 1 MPa. In other words, supposedly, mastication is a physiologic load for dental implants, while bruxism is an overload. When the term "overload" is used, implants are implicitly assumed to have failed or undergoing an ailing or failing process.[46]

In order to better understand the mechanisms by which overload produces excessive bone loss, we must understand that the mechanical loads acting on implants cause bone tissue adaptation and remodeling through a resorption and apposition process. When apposition and resorption rates are similar, the balance which characterizes the physiologic load acting on bone tissue is maintained[47,48] (Fig 23-18).

As for overload, the balance is broken and microfractures from fatigue occur around the implant and in the implant–bone interface.[47] These fractures are repaired through a resorption process and the resulting growth of connective tissue and epithelium, which invade the defective area instead of forming new bone (Fig 23-19).

Overload in patients with peri-implantitis of bacterial etiology is another controversial factor.

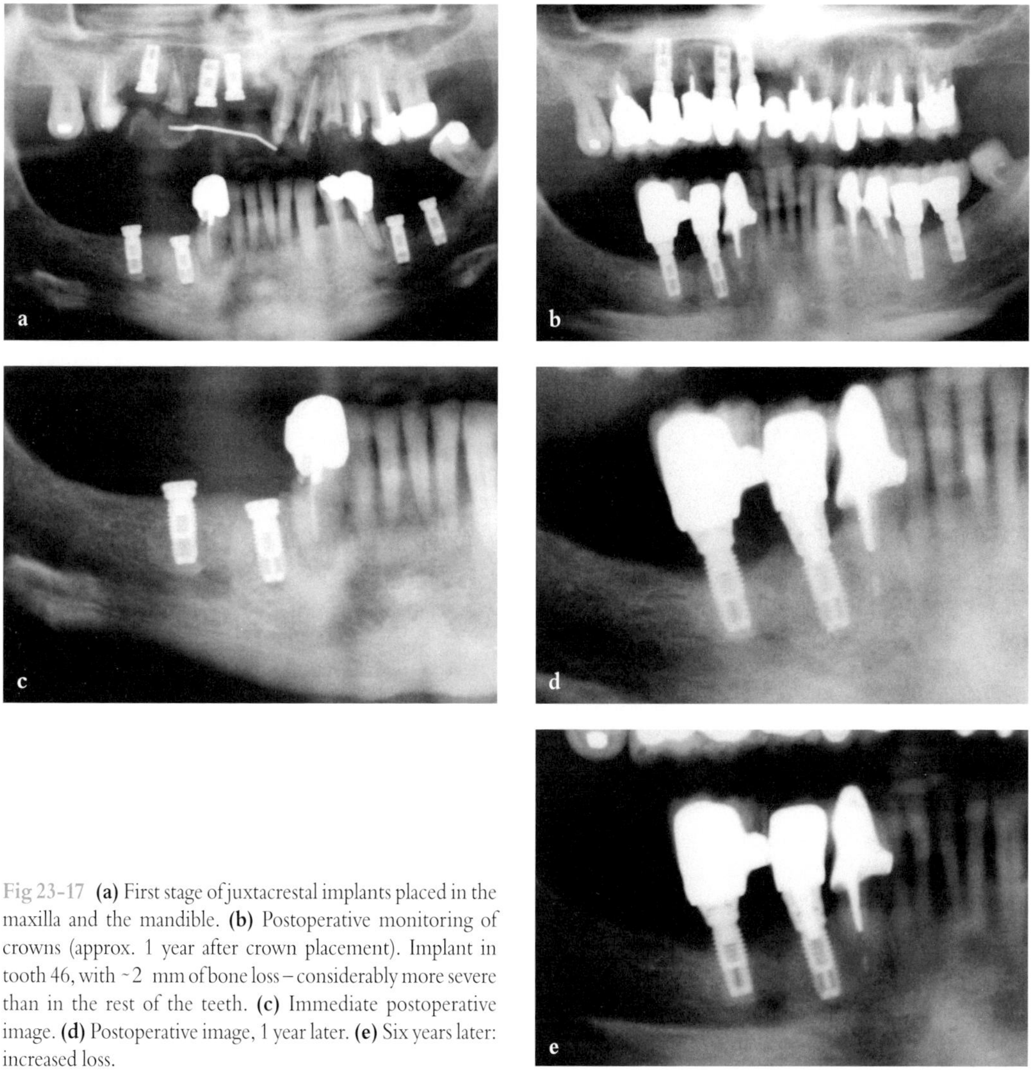

Fig 23-17 **(a)** First stage of juxtacrestal implants placed in the maxilla and the mandible. **(b)** Postoperative monitoring of crowns (approx. 1 year after crown placement). Implant in tooth 46, with ~2 mm of bone loss – considerably more severe than in the rest of the teeth. **(c)** Immediate postoperative image. **(d)** Postoperative image, 1 year later. **(e)** Six years later: increased loss.

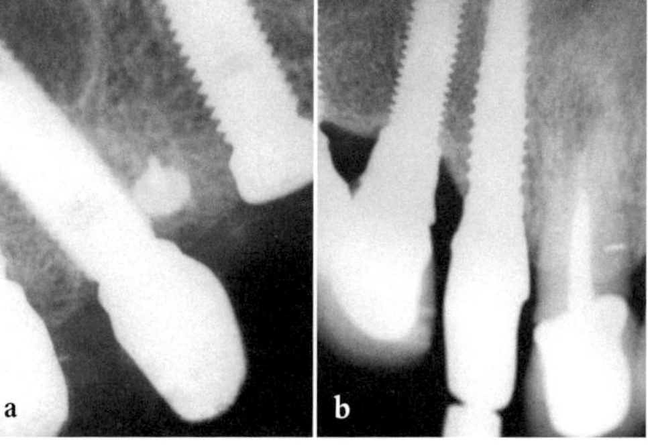

Fig 23-18 **(a)** Post-extraction implant in 13. **(b)** Implant follow-up 10 years later, when another implant was placed in 12. There is a stable, healthy interface, with the cortical bone showing increased thickness (sign of a good balance between function and biologic response).

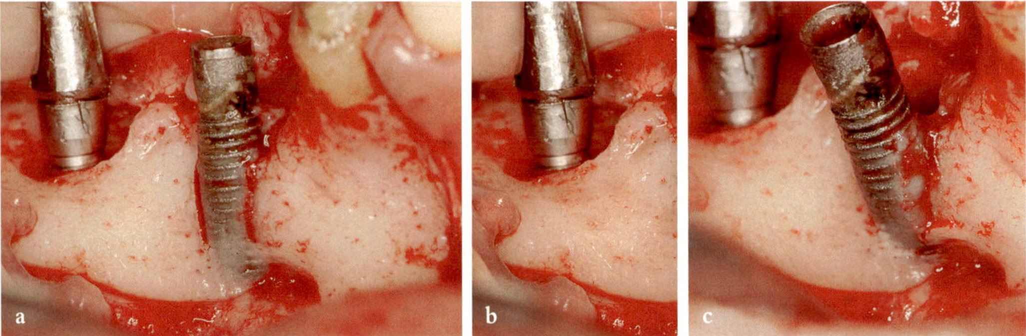

Fig 23-19 **(a)** Implants in 45 and 46. In 46, infundibuliform marginal-bone loss can be observed, probably caused by peri-implantitis of bacterial origin. In 45, three-dimensional coarse bone loss of the whole crown position can be observed; there is vestibular deficiency and fracture of the implant's crown wall. **(b)** Periimplantitis lesion, magnified view of 46. **(c)** Extraction of implant 45. Implant 45 must be regenerated and a new implant should be placed in the future. Note how the implant's apex comes into contact with the mental canal.

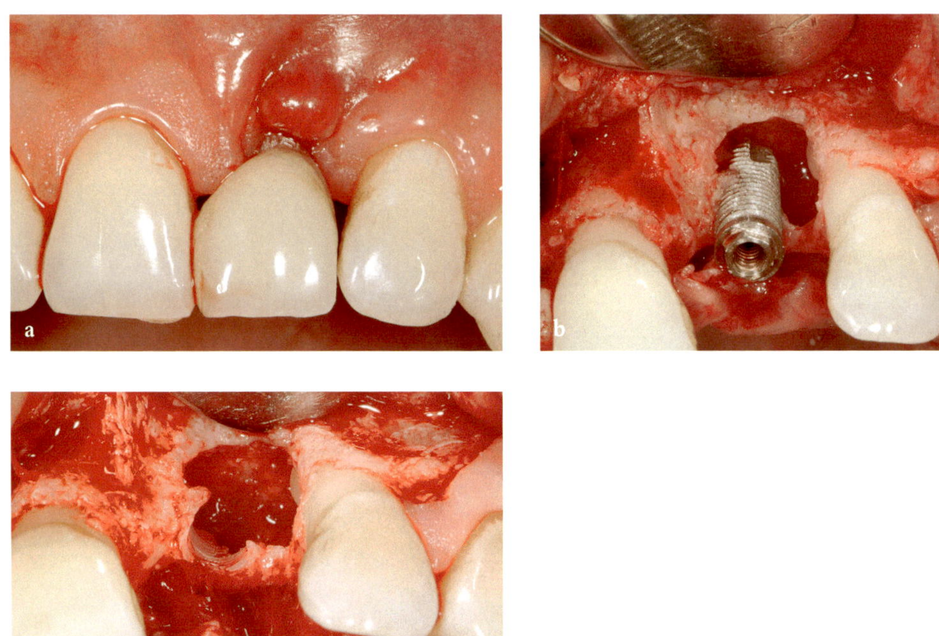

Fig 23-20 **(a)** Peri-implantitis in 21. **(b)** Surgical approach for treatment of the peri-implant lesion: the implant is held from its wall only. **(c)** Implant explantation and residual lesion.

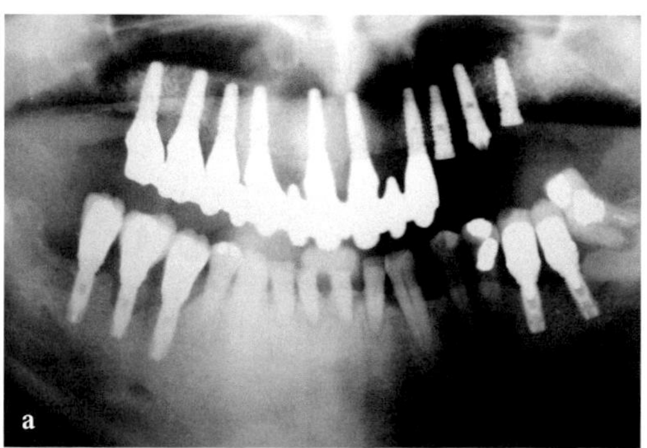


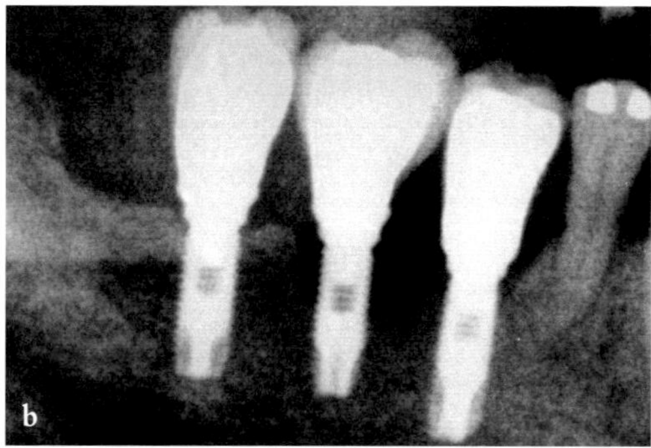


Fig 23-21 **(a)** Patient with upper implant-assisted prosthesis: crowns on implants in mandibular posterior pieces. Note the marginal-bone tissue loss in 46. **(b)** An increased peri-implant lesion: biologic complication, possibly overload combined with bacterial peri-implantitis.

Experimental models were used in studies with animals, and occlusal stress was applied to implants in monkeys by means of devices especially designed to produce trauma whenever the animal closed its mouth; models with healthy peri-implant tissues and models with ligature-induced bacterial peri-implantitis were used.

With this experimental model it was not possible to demonstrate that repetitive trauma has a greater histologic effect on healthy patients than in patients with peri-implantitis, and vice versa. Probably, the trauma produced in this experimental model was within physiologic tolerance ranges. On the other hand, an experimental model recently used in a study with dogs has shown that, when overload is applied on an implant with ligature-induced peri-implantitis, it may increase implant deterioration.[50] Evidently, if overload is capable of damaging a healthy implant, when the area is reduced due to marginal bone loss, the lever arm will increase the effect of the load and there will be increased risk of further resorption or implant integration loss[50] (Figs 23-20 and 23-21).

It is important to take into account the deformation of the jaw during mouth opening and tooth clenching movements.[51–53] This deformation can stress implants out not only during function, but also during opening movements in patients with a fully edentulous mandible, in whom implants are distributed in both the posterior and anterior areas and splinted with a rigid metal supra-structure. The rigidity of the structure prevents the natural flexion of the jaw and exerts a stress on the distal implants.[54–58] For this reason, in patients with a fully edentulous mandible, some schools suggest placing implants in the symphysis area, between the origins of the mental nerves, and extending prosthetically towards the distal aspect. When it is preferred to place implants in molar areas, it would be advisable to make definitive prostheses in two midline separate sections, to minimize trauma to posterior implants. With the aim of discussing this subject in depth, we will analyze the complications shown by patients treated with IAP and the causes of implant failure.

The differences observed in the biomechanical behavior of natural teeth and implants have been widely discussed among dental professionals. Implants show absence of, or decrease in, the tactile perception or proprioception mediated by the periodontal ligament mechanoreceptors.

The absence of these periodontal ligament mechanoreceptors allows for eventual peri-implant problems to occur and progress without accurate, well-defined symptoms and with a subclinical presentation that is very difficult to diagnose in early stages.[59] A compensatory phenomenon known as "osseoperception" has been described which, to a certain extent, occurs in patients who lost a limb, for example, a leg.[60] This phenomenon allows for the transmission of neurological stimuli that are necessary for controlling a prosthesis. This transmission of the tactile perception through the bone marrow has also been described in dental implants.[59,61] On the other hand, teeth, which have the periodontium as insertion mechanism, have micro-movement, intrusion, and adaptation capabilities that implants do not have.

The way in which occlusion should be harmonized in patients treated with implants – especially patients who are partially edentulous or those with a single tooth – in order to compensate for the difference in behavior between both entities has been much discussed.[62–66] Naturally, restorative treatments attempt to harmonize occlusion by following the principles of organic occlusion, trying to have as many simultaneous contacts as possible on both sides of the posterior sectors during mandibular closure, and, at the same time, to keep anterior teeth as close as possible to each other but without contacts.[67] Once this mandibular closure position has been achieved, any eccentric movement, either protrusive or lateral–protrusive, will have to be supported by the anterior teeth – called "anterior guidance" – and a mutually protective system will have to be established because the posterior segment protects the anterior segment during mandibular closure. The anatomic configuration of molars and premolars is biologically meant to absorb this load; owing to their design, canines and incisors are not prepared to perform this task. The anterior segment or anterior guidance protects the posterior segment against loads during excursive movements, since it is anatomically meant to allow soft sliding movements through the contacts of mandibular incisor and canine incisal edges against the palatal surfaces of their upper homonyms. On doing this, a trajectory known as "initial disclusion" is described in which the posterior teeth separate; final disclusion, which causes the posterior teeth to separate fully, allows for the apprehension and tearing movements during the masticatory function. Also, the mechanism of action of the anterior guidance prevents the posterior segment from receiving lateral occlusal loads. Several studies have been carried out with the aim of analyzing this cycle in detail.

Two further very interesting details about anterior guidance are its anatomic location (away from muscle forces), and the neuromuscular connection through proprioception, which, on contact between the anterior teeth, prevents the powerful medial masticatory muscles, masseter muscles, and pterygoid muscles from reaching their maximum contraction.[68] It is important to bear in mind that when a healthy patient whose tooth 46 has been rehabilitated with an IAP closes into occlusion without applying a significant load, there will be no problem; but during maximum tooth clenching the natural teeth may give way or intrude, causing the implant to be the only tooth that comes into contact or over-contact. If the rehabilitated piece belongs to the anterior group, the risk of overloading the implant is even higher.[59] In a periodontally healthy patient the consequences of this overload are minimal, but aggravation may occur if the patient develops inflammatory periodontal disease, which leads to increased tooth mobility and significantly increased implant overload. For this reason, some authors suggest that restorations on implants should be active only during maximum tooth clenching in order to prevent further damage.[59]

In general, the concepts applied in IAP rehabilitation derive from prosthodontics. Among other factors, it is these principles that have led to confusion, because implantology incorporates a microengineering mechanized system that is not always compatible with biology.

For these reasons, it may be inferred that it is necessary to incorporate into the general classification of complications what occurs in the implant itself, in the peri-implant tissue, in the structures connected to the implant, and in the corresponding prosthetic restoration.

## Classification of Complications of IAP Restorative Treatments

The complexity of the masticatory system is a challenge when an attempt is made at restoring function, health, and esthetics that have been affected by the loss of one, several, or all of the teeth owing to some specific pathology – caries, periodontal disease, trauma, or previous failed dental treatments. On proceeding to rehabilitating treatment with IAP, it is wise to bear in mind that, despite all the efforts made, problems and complications may arise in some part of the system treated. It is necessary to identify the possible causes of such complications in order to make a correct diagnosis and find a suitable solution.

Complications can be divided into two groups: those stemming from biologic causes, and those stemming from biomechanical causes (also called "prosthetic"). Complications stemming from biologic causes concern the interrelationship between the implant and the live tissues surrounding it. Complications occurring in the structures connected to the implant – the prosthetic meso-structure or supra-structure – are frequently reported; these are biomechanical complications.

### *Biologic Causes of Complications*

According to el Askary and co-workers,[49,69] such complications may be divided into three categories:

- *ailing* implant (mucositis)
- *failing* implant (peri-implantitis)
- *failed* implant (loss of integration).

The terms "ailing implant" and "failing implant" may be considered to be synonymous with "mucositis" and "peri-implantitis", respectively, not only from the point of view of the specific implant condition, but also from a rehabilitation or prosthetic point of view – that is, considering the impact the IAP has on the implant and the consequences of the overall loads applied to the implant by the prosthesis.

*Ailing implant – mucositis*

This is a reversible inflammation affecting only soft tissues, and it is usually caused by bacterial accumulation. The IAP may play a role owing to a poor design or to poorly adjusted prosthetic structures that create bacterial plaque-retentive areas.

*Failing implant – peri-implantitis*

Bacterial plaque accumulation from poor hygiene or from a maladjusted implant-assisted prosthesis or a prosthesis with an excessively plaque-retentive design will cause an inflammation of the peri-implant mucosa that, consequently, will induce peri-implant bone resorption. It has also been demonstrated that excessive occlusal forces exerted by IAPs with poor occlusal adjustment on bone-integrated implants may result in marginal bone loss or in full bone-integration loss, even when much function time has elapsed.[5,40]

*Failed implant*

The inflammation caused by peri-implantitis results in peri-implant bone resorption, and, eventually, in the loss of implant integration. Regardless of whether or not there is inflammation, overload may be responsible for a failed implant. Depending on the time of presentation of integration loss or implant failure, integration loss can be described as "early", "late", or "delayed".

- *Early integration losses* occur in the period following implant placement, during the scar formation period before activation. They are

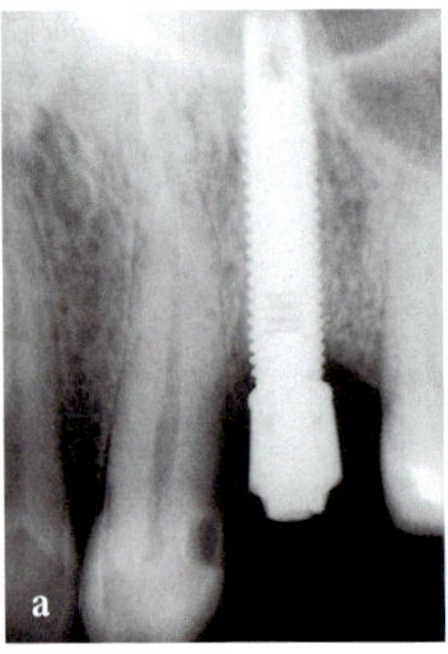
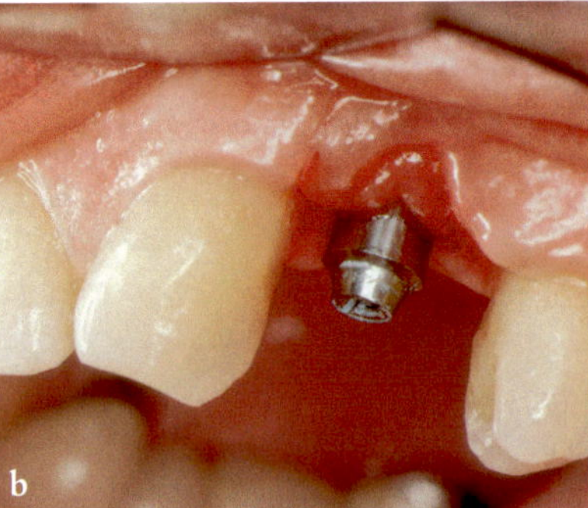
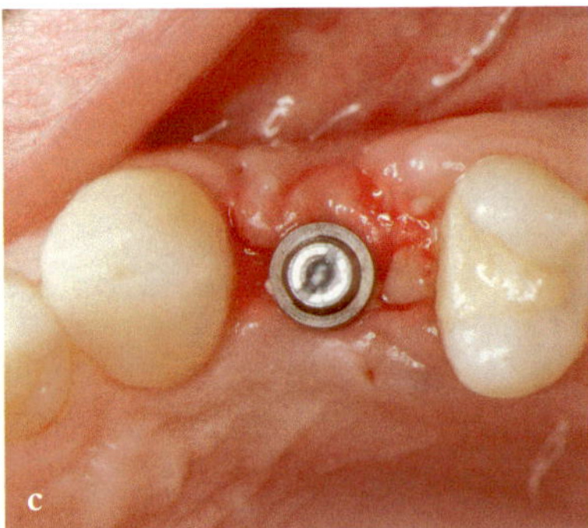

Fig 23-22 **(a)** The most frequent mechanical complication: implant in 24, with screwed abutment; crown loosening; misadjustment. **(b)** Buccal view. **(c)** Occlusal view.

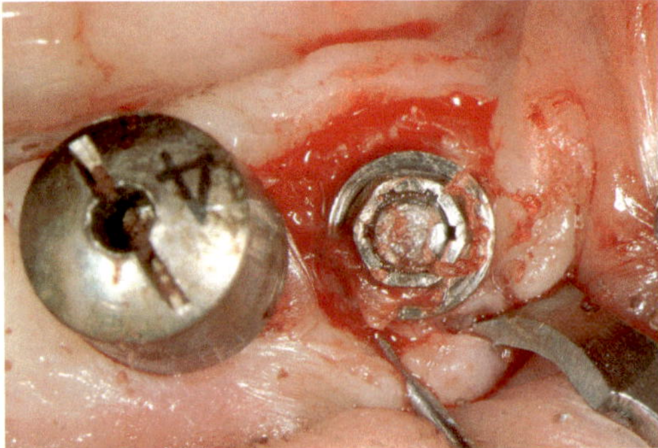

Fig 23-23 Fracture of an abutment/implant fitting screw.

spontaneous avulsions of the implants that are not yet osseointegrated. Their etiology is considered to be related to surgical complications, overtreatment, improper maneuvers, postoperative infections, undetected deficiency in the area, a patient with poor healing, or overload. Early-load implants and immediate-load implants are included in this category.

- *Late integration losses* occur mostly during the second stage. They are ascribed to the same causes as mentioned for early integration losses, as well as to prosthetic or functional traumatic factors during the scar formation period which lead to fibrous repair instead of bone regeneration.
- *Delayed integration losses* are those occurring in already integrated and prosthetically restored implants. Their causes include inflammatory processes of bacterial origin, occlusal factors related to an unsuitable IAP design, and extreme parafunctional activities.

### *Biomechanical/Prosthetic Causes of Complications*

Biomechanical complications occur in the structures connected to the implant – the prosthetic mesostructure or supra-structure. Six different scenarios can be identified. In order of frequency they are:

- crown decementing
- loosening of the IAP retaining screw (Fig 23-22)
- crown fractures
- IAP retaining screw fracture
- loosening of the set screw of the abutment (Fig 23-23)
- fracture of the set screw of the abutment
- implant fracture (Figs 23-24 and 23-25).

Usually, temporary cements are used in the early stage of definitive prosthesis placement, so as to have access to the implant and solve any problems that may arise. The professional should be aware of prostheses decementing, which is common. Abutment loosening is a very unpleasant problem

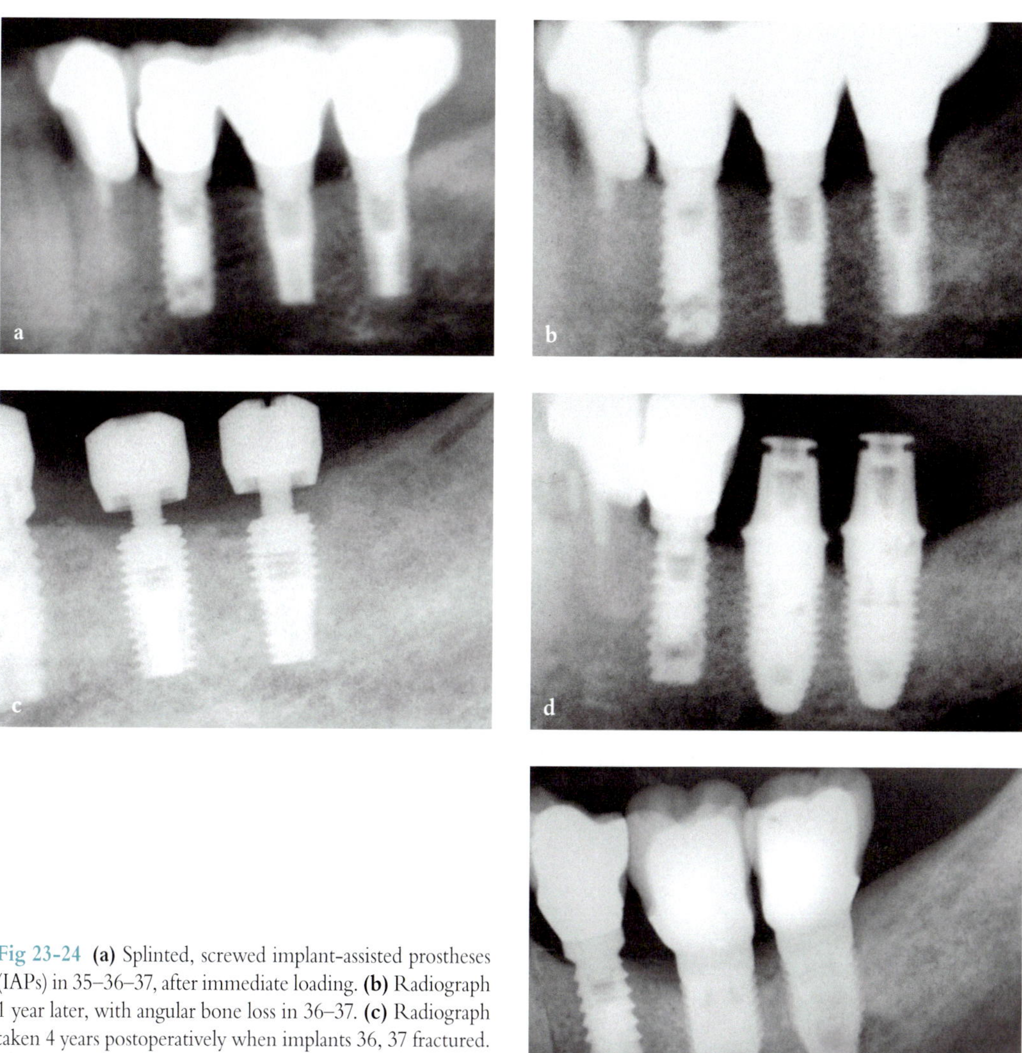

Fig 23-24 **(a)** Splinted, screwed implant-assisted prostheses (IAPs) in 35–36–37, after immediate loading. **(b)** Radiograph 1 year later, with angular bone loss in 36–37. **(c)** Radiograph taken 4 years postoperatively when implants 36, 37 fractured. **(d)** Fractured implants replaced by 2 large-diameter implants. **(e)** Definitive IAP.

whenever a prosthesis has been cemented with a strong cement, because it is very difficult to remove the prosthesis from the moving abutment by using impact extractors, since these may cause permanent damage to the implant's inner spirals. In most cases, the safest way to solve the problem is to sacrifice the prosthesis and perforate the occlusal face of the crown in order to have an access tunnel for the set screw of the abutment; another option is to cut the crown. In both cases, the screw should later be replaced and a new prosthesis should be fabricated.

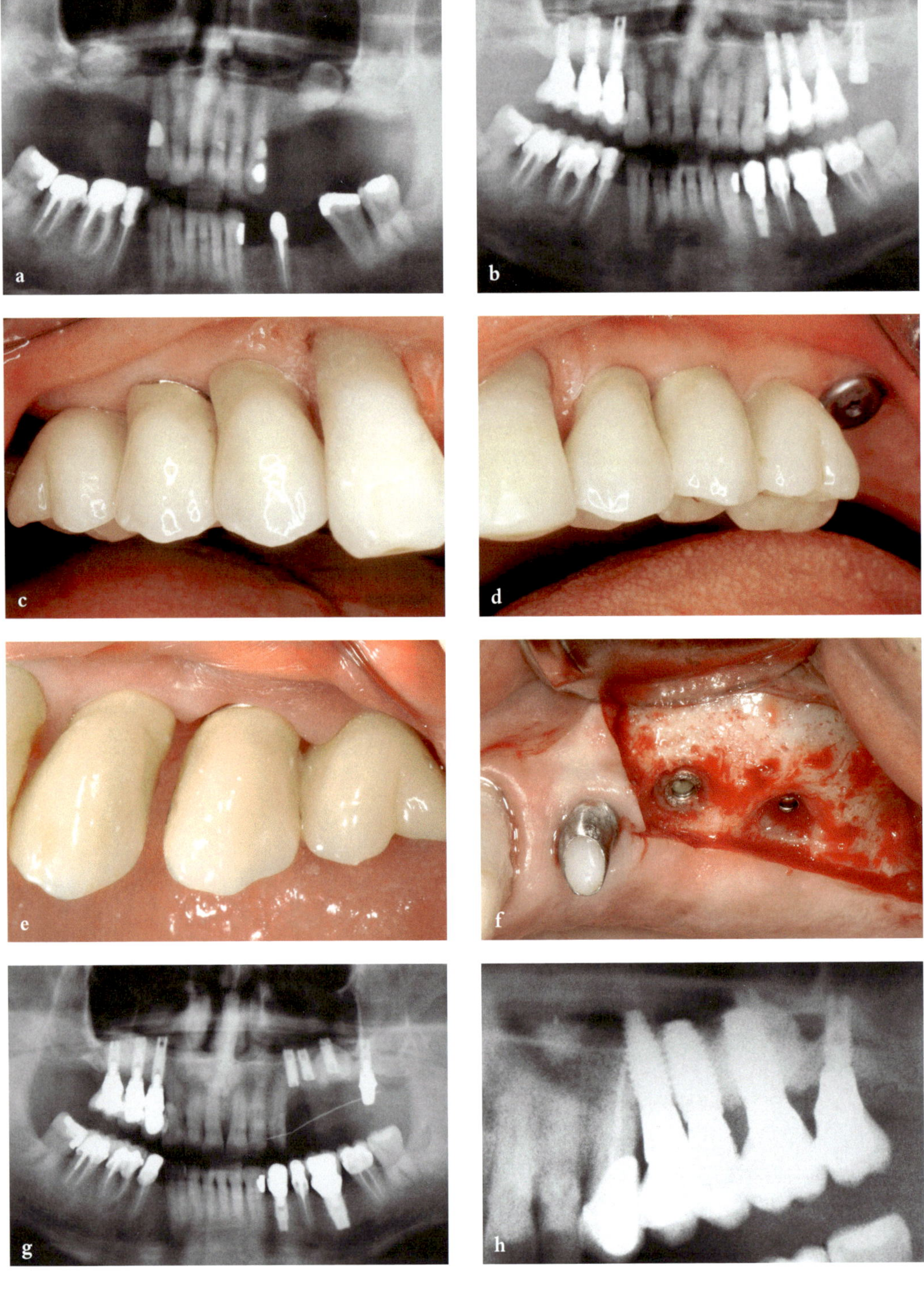
a
b
c
d
e
f
g
h

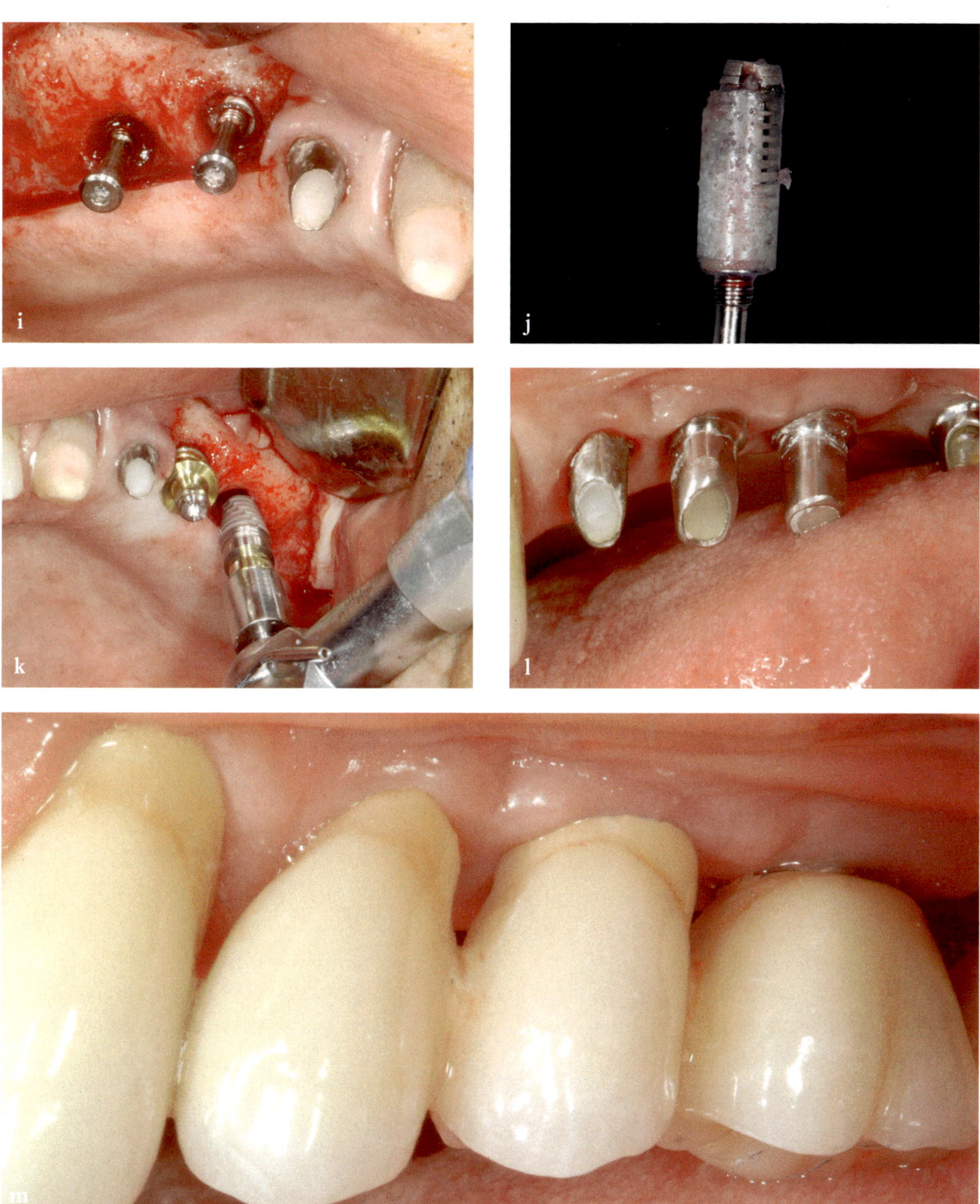

Fig 23-25 **(a)** Postoperative panoramic radiograph showing bilateral sinus elevation. **(b)** Radiograph after implant-assisted prosthesis (IAP) placement: splinted crowns in 14–15–16–24–25–26; crowns on implants in 45–46–47–34–36; crown on 35. **(c)** Right lateral view. **(d)** Left lateral view. **(e)** Fixed prosthesis showing mobility on fractured implants. **(f)** Surgical approach to fractured implants. **(g)** Fractured implants in 24, 25, and 26. **(h)** Postoperative monitoring radiograph. Explantation and implants of wider diameter and splinted IAP, with previous implant, inactive, in 27. **(i)** Fractured implants with explantation guides. **(j)** Removed implant. **(k)** Placement of new implants. **(l)** Definitive abutments. **(m)** Lateral view of splinted IAP in 24–25–26–27 and crown in 23.

In the recognized implant systems, resistance decreases progressively from the implant to the crown restoration. Therefore the implant is the most resistant factor, and ideally there are two increasing fuses: the set screw of the abutment, and the retaining screw of the prosthesis. The first fuse is the IAP's gold screw; the professional should be on the alert to recurrent loosening of this fuse, since it indicates the existence of some factor that is exceeding the functional capacity of the system.

Preventing this situation by using materials that are more resistant in the manufacturing of screws, or by cementing them with older-generation adhesives, will only cause the problem to be transferred to the next link, and it will be even more complicated to loosen or break the set screw of the abutment.

The most commonly reported complication is the loosening of the retaining screws of individual IAPs. In order to solve this problem, a company developed a gold set screw with a seating for a square-section driver that allows for increased tightening torque by using a special instrument called a "torque meter". It is advisable to tighten these screws to 32 Ncm, because with such load, the tension applied to the screw will produce higher tightening force between the abutment and the implant, preventing the common problem of individual IAP loosening.

With improvements to older-generation technology , the machining of prosthesis components has been optimized, tolerance ranges have been adjusted, and the adjustment between teeth has been improved. The new technology allows for a decrease in the number of set-screw and retaining-screw loosenings, but other complications have been reported. When component immobility was achieved, two prosthetic problems started to arise: cantilever acrylic breakage in hybrid fixed prostheses, and ceramic fracture (especially in metal–ceramic crowns). In patients showing overload, the stability of the prosthetic components transfers the fuse effect to the last link of the system and causes a higher number of implant fractures.[70,71] This is the most unpleasant complication for patients. The clinician will be forced to repeat the treatment, but this time with an even worse starting point. In most cases it will be necessary to surgically remove the remainder of the fractured implant by using a trephine, an instrument that produces a bony defect that prevents the placement of a new replacement implant in the best position – making it necessary to resort to guided bone regeneration procedures and to wait until the tissues are in perfect condition.

## Prosthetic Rehabilitation with Implants in Bruxers

The implant–prosthetic rehabilitation of patients showing signs of parafunction requires dental professionals to take some precautions to prevent unpleasant situations in the following scenarios:

- patients with a single implant
- patients who are partially edentulous
- patients with one edentulous jaw (maxilla or mandible)
- patients who are without teeth.

### *Patients with a Single Implant*

Figures 23-26 to 23-28 demonstrate some principles. Figure 23-29 shows a case study.

In patients with a single implant in the posterior segment, it is advisable to use implants of wider diameter, with a wide prosthetic platform and internal connection. The indirect system should be used (abutment screwed to the implant and crown screwed or cemented to the abutment) instead of using systems that are directly screwed to the implant. This allows for increased system flexibility. Though accepted and used in the dental population worldwide, the external connection is the least stable of implant–abutment connections. It is advisable to use a single implant and prosthetic abutment system, and to avoid combining different systems even if they are compatible, because it

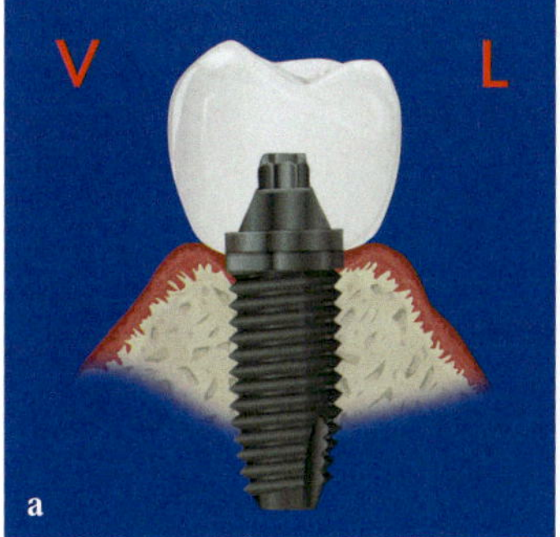


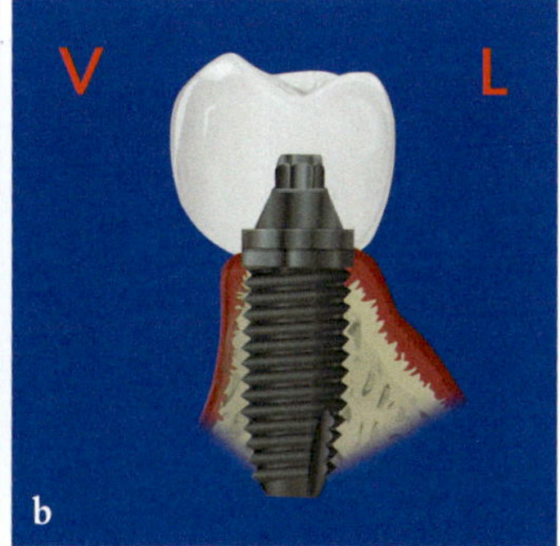


Fig 23-26 **(a)** The ideal position of the implant with respect to the tooth in the axis plane of the central fossa of the tooth to be replaced. **(b)** A common situation in which, owing to the increased resorption of the vestibular table of the alveolar ridge, the implant must be placed more towards the lingual aspect, which results in a cantilever of the crown towards the vestibular aspect.

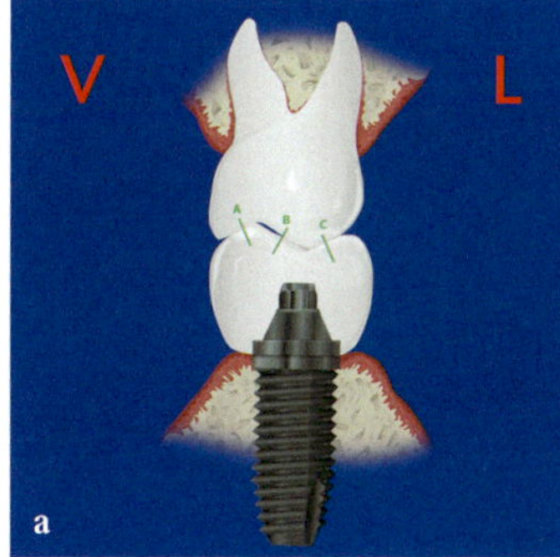


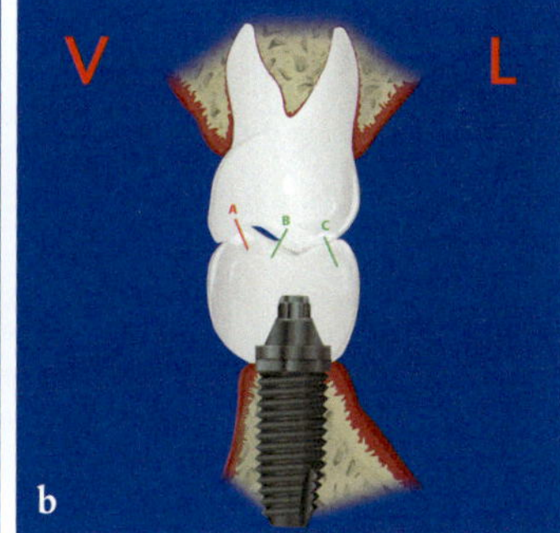


Fig 23-27 **(a)** Frontal vestibular–palatal view. Note the relationship of the antagonist teeth with an implant placed in the ideal position; the implant will absorb the loads without any problems. **(b)** A similar situation, but with the implant placed more towards the lingual aspect. Note how A contacts, between the buccal slope of the mandibular buccal cusp and the palatal slope of the maxillary buccal cusp, produce a force moment which is harmful for the implant.

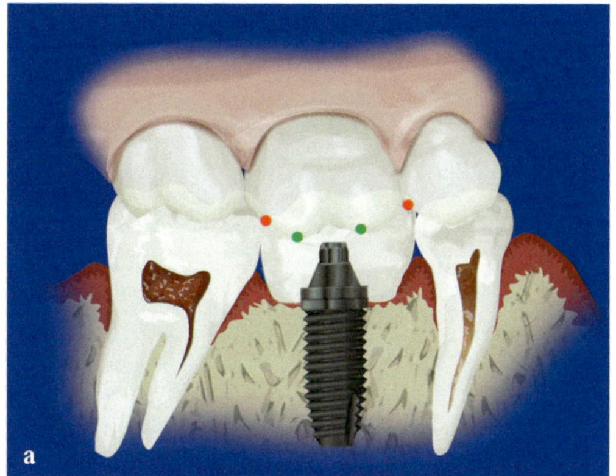


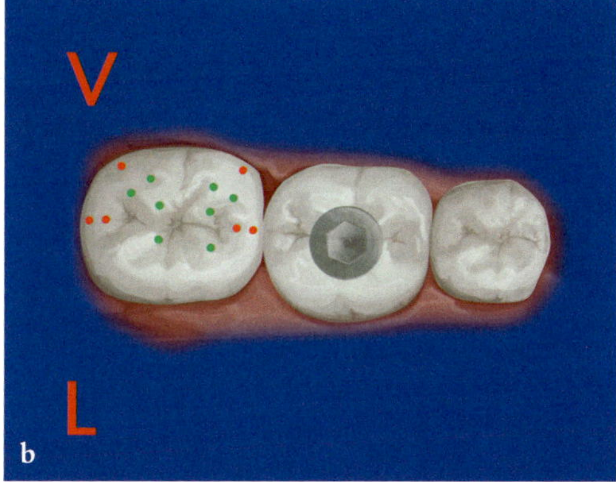


Fig 23-28 **(a)** Mesial–distal view showing how the mesial and distal marginal ridge contacts are outside the implant axis projection, which produces force moments that are harmful for the implant. This is centric contact which, in fact, is eccentric for the implant. **(b)** Occlusal view showing the projection of an implant placed as replacement for a single molar; undoubtedly, implants of wider diameter reproduce the natural dimension of a molar better. The contacts that should be eliminated in the occlusal adjustment are shown in red – for example, the marginal ridges and the contacts in the buccal slopes of the mandibular buccal cusps.

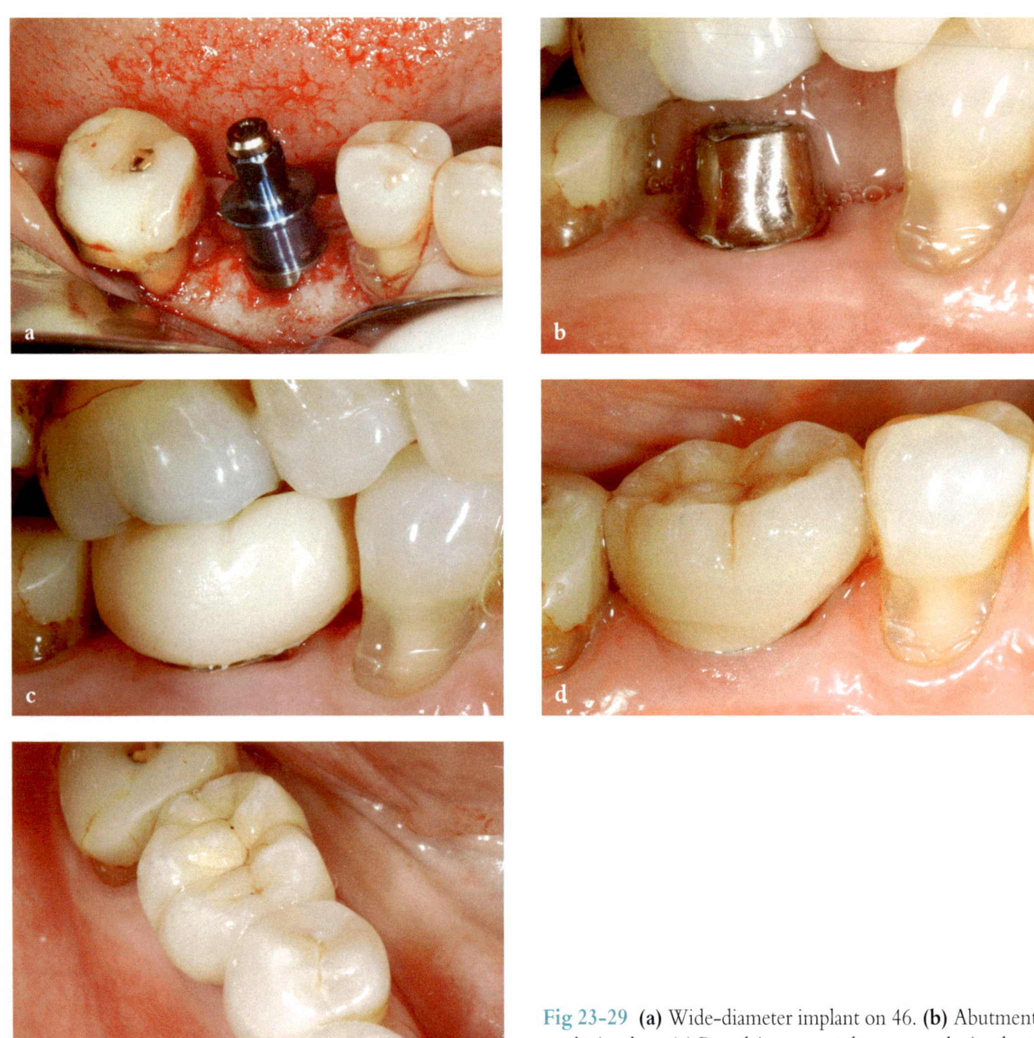

Fig 23-29 **(a)** Wide-diameter implant on 46. **(b)** Abutment on the implant. **(c)** Porcelain-on-metal crown on the implant. **(d)** The crown in occlusion. **(e)** Occlusal view of the crown.

is very difficult to control adjustment tolerance ranges.[72]

A thorough occlusal adjustment should be carried out; the implant should not be brought into function during maximum tooth clenching, and it must be remembered that, in crown restorations on implants, contact in centric may be eccentric. For example, a contact in a marginal, mesial, or distal ridge, or a contact on the buccal slope of the buccal cusp of a mandibular molar, will be outside the implant axis projection and will generate a force moment that will cause an increased load to be applied on the implant; in turn, in individual implants, such increased load is counteracted by the implant–abutment set screw in the first place, which frequently causes the screw to loosen. The occlusal adjustment should keep active contacts in centric as close as possible to the axis projection, and should prevent or reduce outlying contacts between vestibular cusps – such as marginal ridges and type-A occlusal contact. No contact at all should occur in the restorations during excursive movements.

In the case of anterior-segment individual implants, during the closure movement the implant should come into contact only during maximum tooth clenching. Ideally, during eccentric movements, only group-function soft contacts should occur.

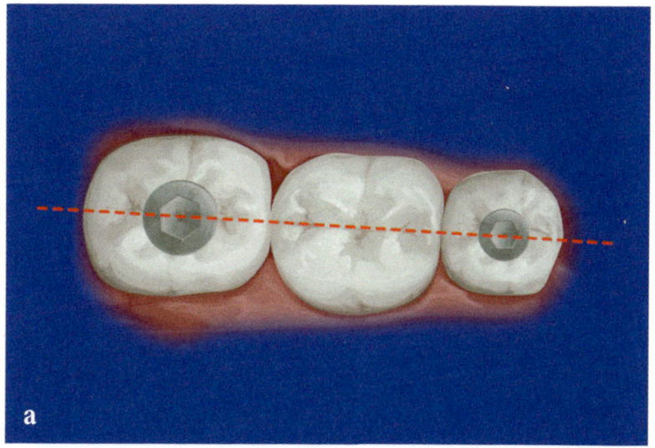

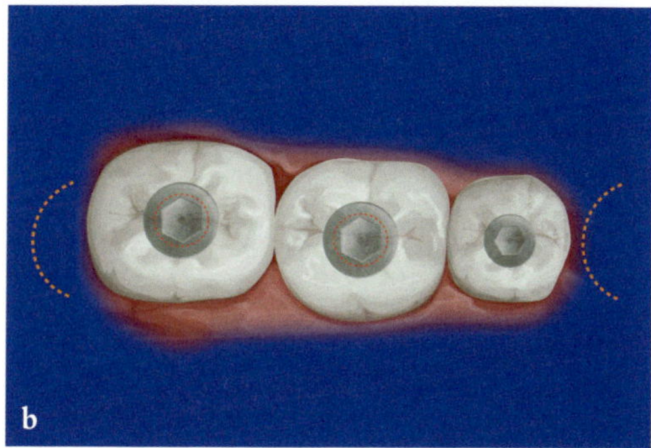

Fig 23-30 **(a)** Occlusal view of two implants as replacement for three teeth; a vestibular–lingual fulcrum is produced. **(b)** Occlusal view of three implants as replacement for three teeth. Implants of greater diameter were used for the molars to create a larger support area and to counteract vestibular–lingual dislocation forces.

### *Patients who are Partially Edentulous*

Figure 23-30 demonstrates some principles. Figure 23-31 is a case study.

In patients who are partially edentulous, if adjoining implants are placed, splinted restorations should be used to maintain structural rigidity. In these patients, it is also advisable to place one implant per tooth to be replaced, provided the distances between teeth respect the biologic width; a biomechanical protection criterion should prevail. The support area should be increased to the maximum in order to counteract the effect of the potential overload.

Whenever possible, fixed prostheses with long sections supported on their ends only by implants should be avoided, to eliminate a vestibular–palatal or bucco-lingual fulcrum axis. Preferably, a third implant that is axis-displaced should be used, so as to create a tripod support area as recommended by the Swedish school in the original designs. Another option is to use implants of wider diameter to make the support area larger.[73,74]

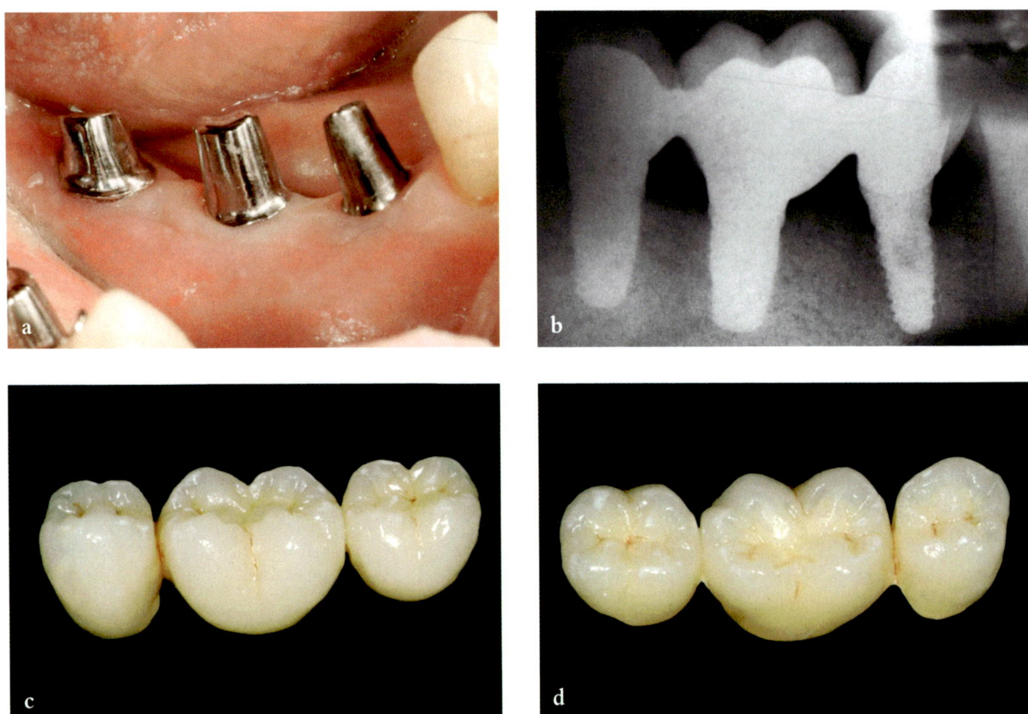

Fig 23-31 **(a)** Multiple implants, on 45 with regular diameter and with greater diameter on 46 and 47. **(b)** Periapical radiograph in which a favorable ratio of implant to crown diameters can be seen. **(c)** Lateral view: crowns on implants for 34 and 36, and a crown on 35. **(d)** Occlusal view.

### *Patients with One Edentulous Jawbone*

In bruxers with fixed prostheses, at least six implants (ideally, eight) should be strategically distributed in the arch, trying to create the largest support area possible. When eight implants are placed, their ideal locations are teeth 16, 14, 13, 11, 21, 23, 24, and 26. This allows simplification of the prosthetic restoration by having four fixed-partial prosthesis sections (16–14, 13–11, 21–23, and 24–26), as suggested by the Swiss school.[75] Bearing in mind that potential conflicts may arise, this disposition allows for a rapid resolution of problems such as porcelain fracture, screw loosening, etc.

When a poor bone availability does not allow placement of eight implants, the alternative is to distribute six in a radiate way, as recommended by the Brazilian school[76] (Figs 23-32 to 23-34). The implants should be distributed in the 15, 13, 11, 21, 23, and 25 areas. Implants 15 and 25 should be positioned to face the distal aspect, following the anterior wall of the maxillary antrum and emerging, approximately, at the level of the first molars. Implants 13 and 23 should follow the canine abutment, and the two central implants (11 and 21) should be slightly positioned to face the vestibular aspect. This design enables the placement of very long implants (15 mm and, in some cases, 18 mm long) in areas of good anchorage with high bone quality. The prosthesis can comprise only one section and be fully splinted; it can be cemented to individual abutments screwed to the implants, or it can be divided into two sections in the midline and screwed to intermediate multi-unit or conical abutments.

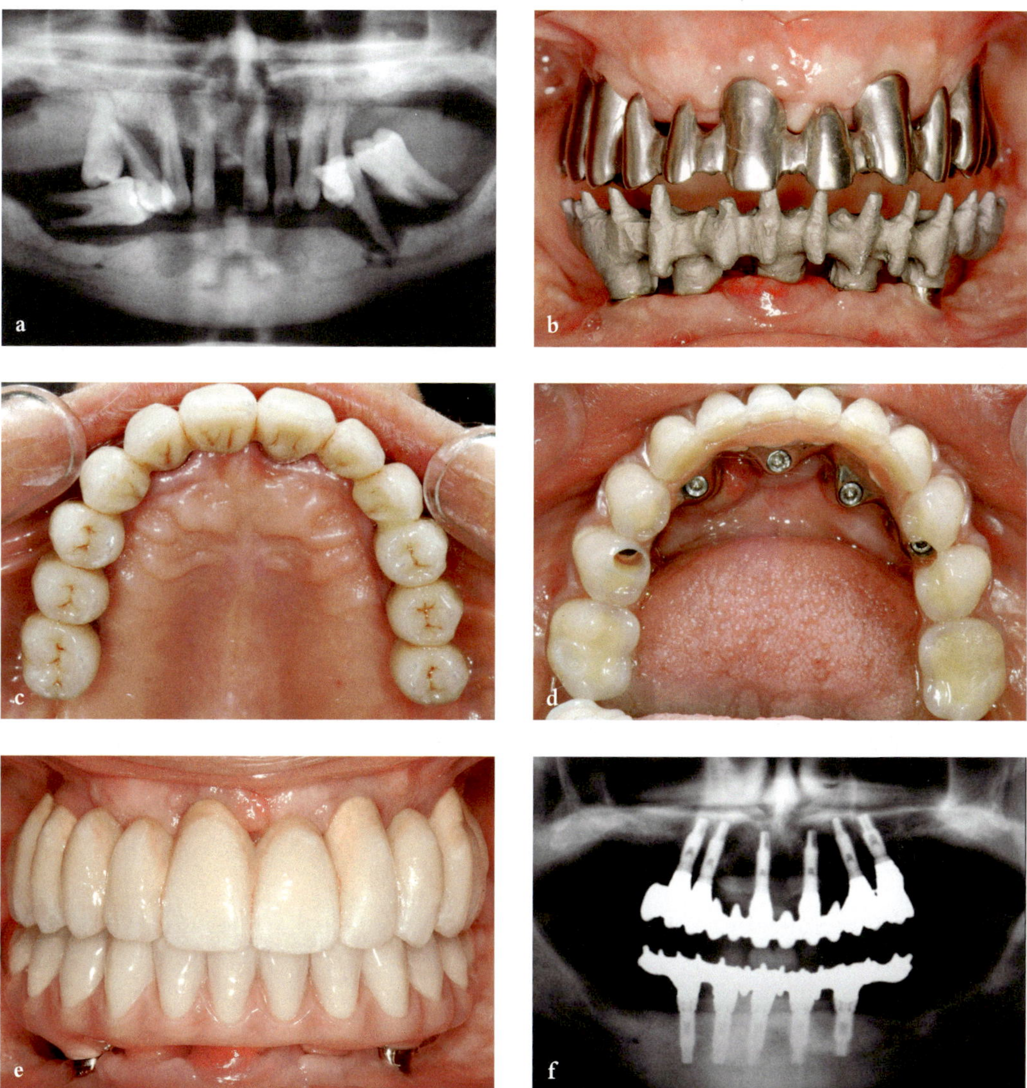


Fig 23-32 **(a)** Preoperative radiograph showing severe end-stage periodontal disease. **(b)** Upper prosthetic structures for ceramic-on-metal implant-assisted prosthesis (IAP) and lower hybrid IAP. **(c)** IAP: upper is porcelain, lower is hybrid. **(d)** Occlusal view of lower hybrid prosthesis. **(e)** Occlusal view of upper porcelain-on-metal IAP. **(f)** Panoramic radiograph.

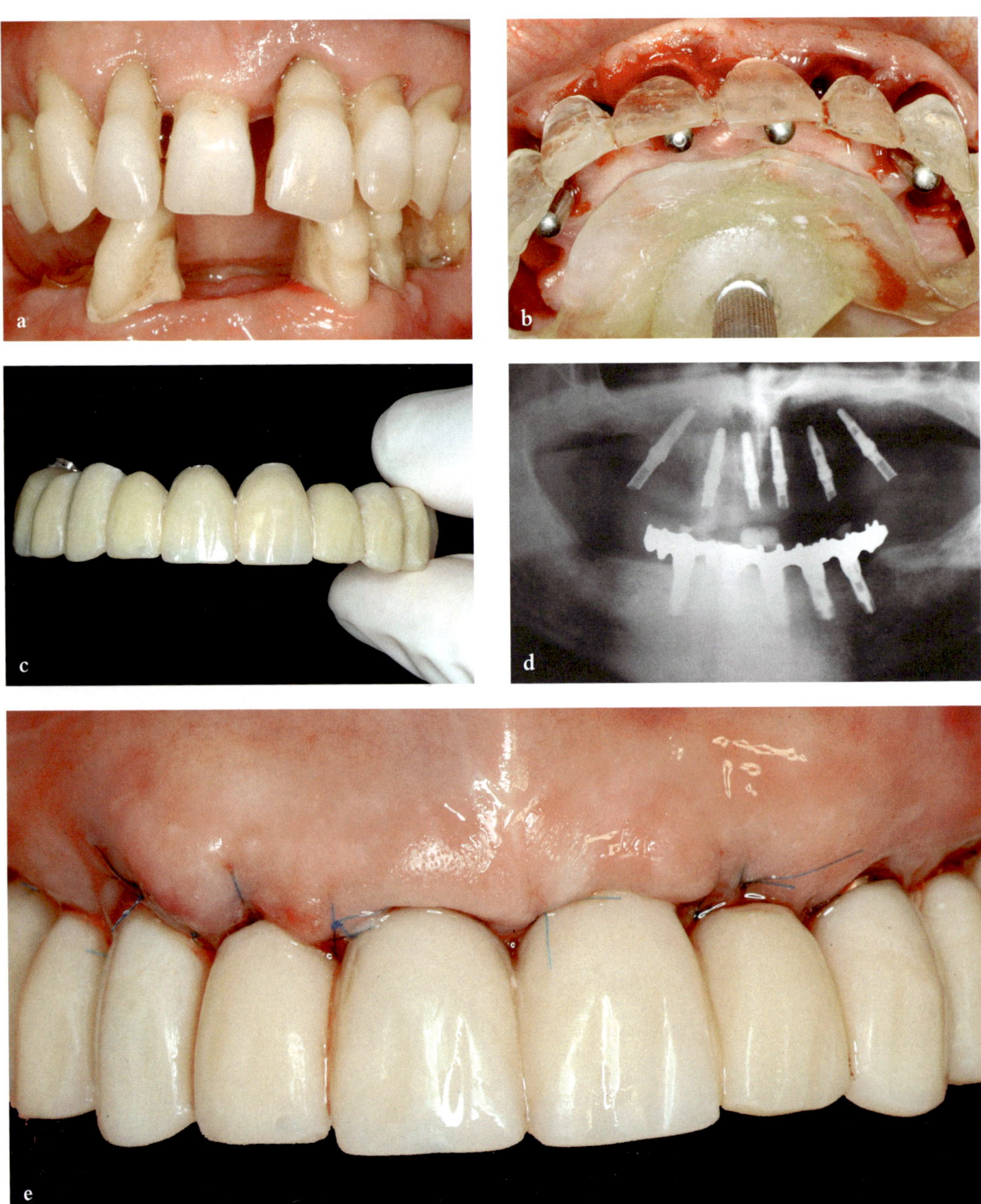

Fig 23-33 **(a)** Preoperative front view of patient with severe periodontal disease. **(b)** Surgical guide with indicators in position. **(c)** Immediate-load fixed prosthesis in the maxilla, ready to be placed. **(d)** Radiograph after immediate load: implants placed in a radiating fashion in the maxilla; mandible – hybrid of medium complexity. **(e)** Immediate-load fixed prosthesis in place.

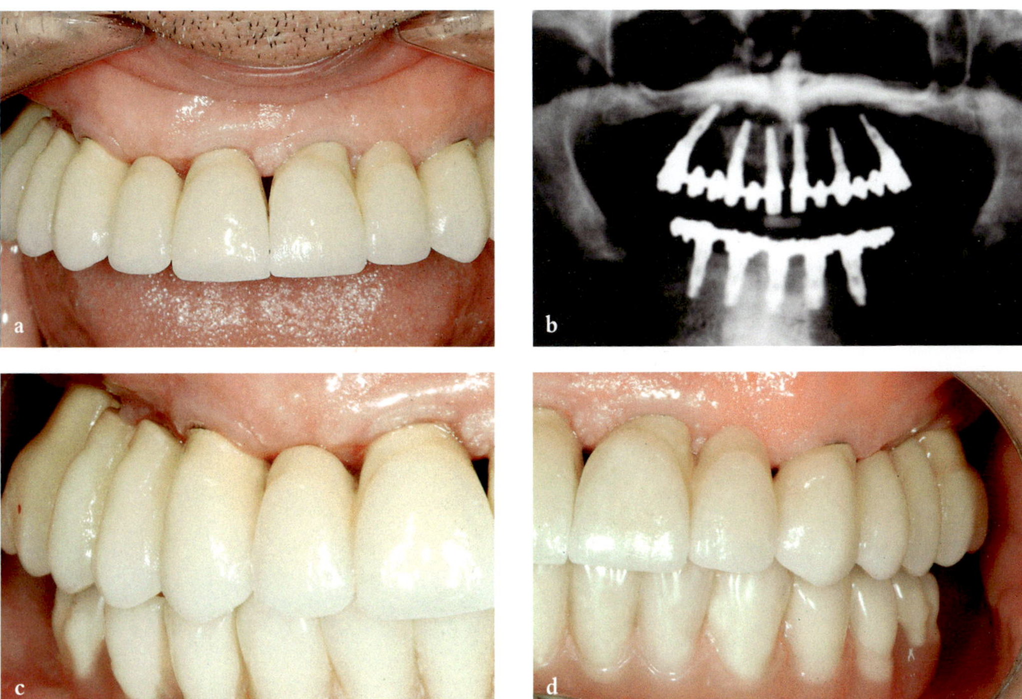

Fig 23-34 **(a)** Upper porcelain-on-metal fixed prosthesis, screwed in two separate sections in the midline. **(b)** Right and left half views of the maxilla and mandible in occlusion. **(c and d)** Postoperative radiograph: maxillary implants – porcelain-on-metal screwed fixed prosthesis; mandibular implants – hybrid fixed prosthesis with metal meso-structure and resin dental supra-structure.

In patients with a fully edentulous mandible, the Swedish school protocol is the ideal choice: five or six implants in the symphysis area, distributed between the mental foramens and rehabilitated with a removable hybrid fixed prosthesis. In those cases in which the remainder of the alveolar ridge is preserved, with minimal or zero bone loss, implants can be placed either in the posterior segments or in the anterior segment. Ideally, they should be distributed as follows: the implants, in the 46, 44, 43, 33, 34, and 36 areas; the definitive fixed prosthesis may be divided into three small sections (46 to 44, 43 to 33, and 34 to 36) and cemented to abutments screwed to the implants.

In fully edentulous patients with overdentures, although the removable prosthesis will generally be the fuse, contrary to what is widely believed (i.e., that overdentures will protect implants), there is a good chance of applying excessive torque to the implants. It is necessary to differentiate between implant-retained/mucosa-supported prostheses and implant-retained/implant-supported prostheses.

The least harmful prostheses for treating bruxers with implant-retained mucosa-supported dentures are those that use magnet-type components, since magnets will activate only when an attempt is made at dislocating the prosthesis and not during functional loads; on the other hand, they are the

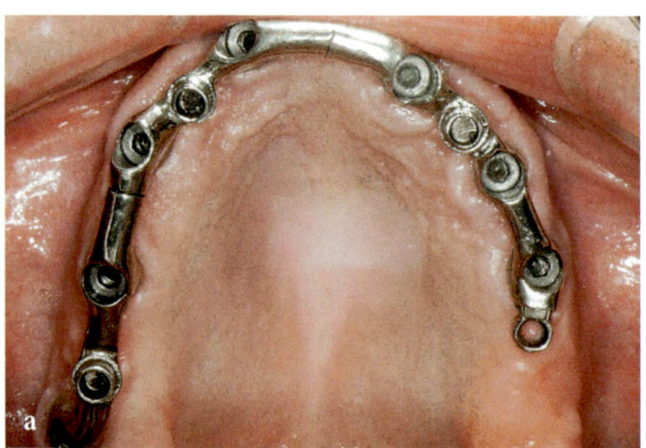

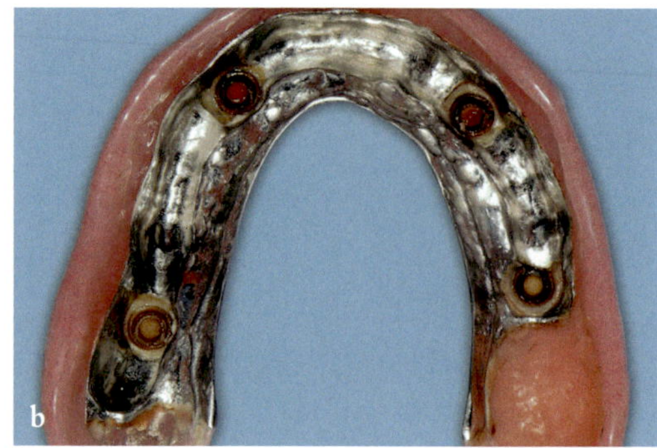

Fig 23-35 **(a)** Overdenture bar on seven implants. **(b)** Full prosthesis on denture with ERA-type retentive elements.

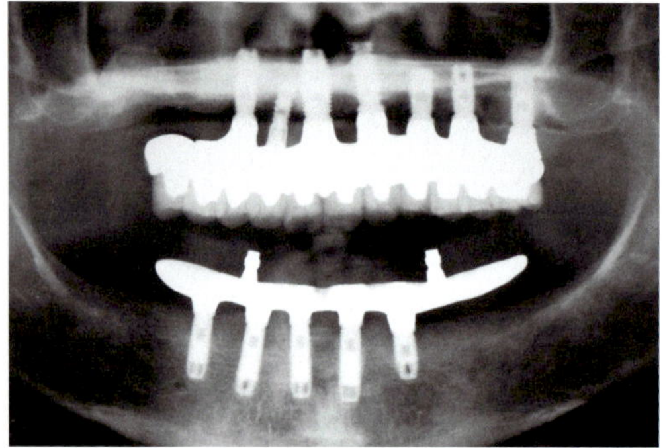

Fig 23-36 **(a)** Panoramic radiograph: maxilla- metal-ceramic fixed prosthesis; mandible – hybrid fixed prosthesis with resin occlusal faces.

least effective. Retention systems of the plug-and-socket type with interchangeable accessories (Era, Locator, O-Ring, Dalro, etc.) can be used in non-splinted implants in the mandible only. Within this category, the systems of choice for bruxers are those having the socket in the component which is fixed to the implant, and the plug in the prosthesis. In this way, less lever arm and torque are applied to the implant.

In high-risk patients, implant-retained and implant-supported prostheses require the same number of implants as fixed prostheses, because the retention and the load are absorbed by the implants. The proper therapeutics for the maxilla is at least six implants (ideally, eight) splinted to each other by means of a bar, with retention systems between implants (Fig 23-35).

In the mandible, four to six implants are splinted to each other, with retention systems between implants. Once the treatment is completed, the patient should wear a rigid night guard and attend periodic control and maintenance visits.

### *Bruxers without Teeth*

In bruxers with fully edentulous maxilla and mandible who wear fixed prostheses, in one of the jaws (preferably, the maxilla) we suggest using a ceramic-on-metal fixed prosthesis cemented to abutments screwed to the implants, and a screwed hybrid composite-resin-on-metal fixed prosthesis in the mandible. The mandible is the fuse, since the resin on the occlusal surfaces wears away, thus preventing implants from suffering irreversible damage. It can be periodically and easily repaired by dismounting the supra-structure of the prosthesis and renewing the teeth in the laboratory (Figs 23-36 and 23-37).

### *Note on Materials*

There is a need for materials that are able to absorb impact and which, to a certain extent, are less hard than dental enamel. Avoidance of materials such as ceramic and use of composite-resin materials have been recommended. The disadvantages of ceramic

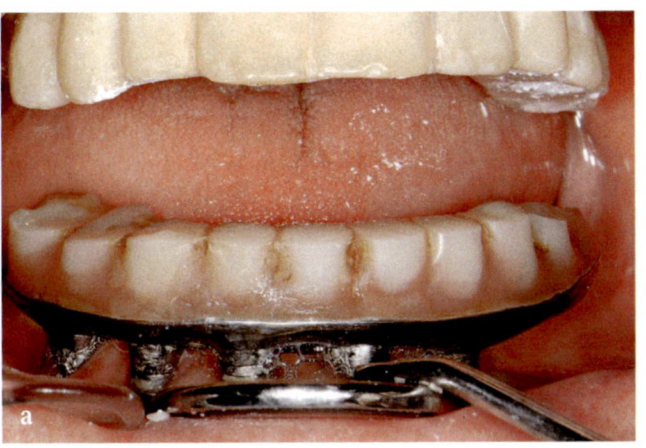

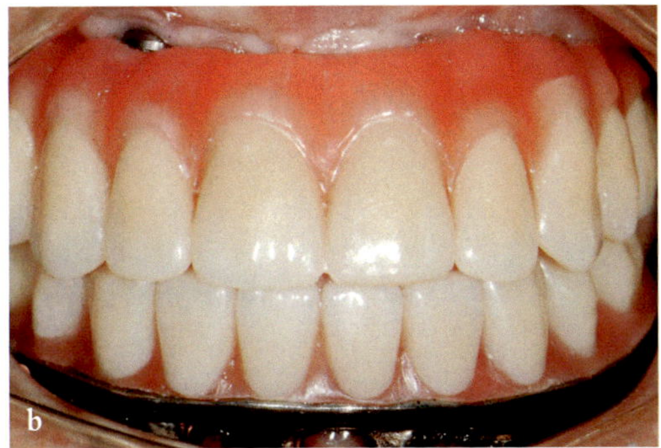

Fig 23-37 **(a)** Fully worn lower occlusal surfaces. **(b)** Supra-structure replacement with teeth.

are its rigidity and fragility, which may result in ceramic fractures, and potential implant overload, and may cause the occlusal surfaces of the antagonist teeth to wear out.

Composite resins are less hard than ceramic, and they are even slightly less hard than dental enamel. In bruxers, this disadvantage turns into a protection factor for implants, since the restoration material will now be the system fuse. Whenever composite resins are used for fixed implant-assisted prostheses in partially or multiple long-section edentulous patients, it is essential that they have an internal metal structure to provide structural rigidity. If the prosthesis material bends during function, a tangential load will be exerted on the implants that will result in peri-implant tensions which are much greater than axial loads; this may produce overload. It is important to bear this in mind during temporization procedures in fully or partially-multiple edentulous patients (especially in immediate-load cases, and to a lesser extent in delayed-load cases) when acrylic resins are used, because these resins may bend and apply harmful tension to implants.

### *Screws or Cement?*

Another controversial factor is the use of screwed or cemented fixed prostheses. Undoubtedly, a detachable and recoverable system is more advantageous, especially when compared with biomechanical complications like the loosening of one of the retaining screws of the prosthesis, the loosening of one of the set screws of the abutment, or the need to renew the whole prosthesis. Also, it is well known that the manufacturing of screwed fixed prostheses in the laboratory is a very complex technical process, since maintaining accuracy and adjustment passivity on implants is difficult. When there are biologic complications, detachable systems allow dental professionals to dismount the prosthesis, treat peri-implantitis, even immerse the implant again, and, once the complication has been solved, mount the prosthesis again or fabricate a new one. Also, the technical and clinical procedures involved in the fabrication of cemented fixed prostheses are very simple, and components and laboratory fees are cheaper.

In the author's practice, we follow the guidelines of the Swiss school and Gallucci's works in the combination of both techniques for immediate-load treatment of patients with a fully edentulous maxilla and mandible.[75] During the implant-integration process, we use screwed devices for the temporization which, in case a problem arises, allow us to remove the prosthesis without damaging the device. Once the implants are integrated, we prefer fixed prostheses cemented to screwed abutments in partial sections.

## Conclusion

This chapter has compiled and analyzed the published material available on the effects of bruxism in patients rehabilitated with IAPs. Although bruxism is generally considered to be a contraindication for dental implant treatments, there is no conclusive evidence that bruxism is responsible for implant failure. Specific, prospective, random-controlled trials will need to be carried out in order to collect more data about the results obtained in treated patients, and to establish guidelines and parameters that allow identifying risk situations and reducing or minimizing the damage bruxism may cause to the masticatory system. This chapter has provided some suggestions and guidelines for the treatment of bruxers; as a general rule, all the necessary precautions should be taken and extreme caution and care should be used in the resolution of highly complex situations. As a preventive measure, whenever rehabilitating patients with implants we should bear in mind that all of them may be bruxers.

## References


1. Lavigne GJ, Rompre PH, Montplaisir JY, Lobbezoo F. Motor activity in sleep bruxism with concomitant jaw muscle pain: a retrospective pilot study. Eur J Oral Sci 1997;105:92–95.
2. Lobbezoo F, Van der Zaag J, Visscher CM, Naeije M. Oral kinesiology: a new postgraduate programme in the netherlands. J Oral Rehabil 2004;31:192–198.
3. Lundgren D, Laurell L. Oclusal aspects in fixed bridgework supported by endosseous implants. In: Lang NP, Karring T (eds). Proceedings of the 1st European Workshop in Periodontology. London: Quintessence, 1994: 326–327.
4. Palmer RM, Smith BJ, Howe LC, Palmer PJ. Complications and maintenance: single tooth and fixed bridge. In: Implants in Clinical Dentistry. London: Martin Dunitz, 2002:241.
5. Adell R, Leckholm U, Rockler B, Brånemark PI. A 15-year study of osseointegrated implants in the treatment of the edentulous jaw. Int J Oral Surg 1981;10: 387–416.
6. Becker W, Becker BE. Replacement of maxillary and mandibular molars with single endosseous implant restorations: a retrospective study. J Prosthet Dent 1995; 74:51–55.
7. Vanden Bogaerde L, Pedretti G, Dellacasa P, Mozzati M, Rangert B. Early function of splinted implants in maxillas and posterior mandibles using Brånemark system machined-surface implants: an 18-month prospective clinical multicenter study. Clin Implant Dent Relat Res 2003;5(Suppl 1):21–28.
8. Lobbezoo F, Brouwers JE, Cune MS, Naeije M. Dental implants in patients with bruxing habits. J Oral Rehabil 2006;33:152–159.
9. Albrektsson T, Zarb G, Eriksson AR. The long-term efficacy of currently used dental implants: a review and proposed criteria of success. Int J Oral Maxillofac Implants 1986;1:11–25.
10. Chiapasco M, Romeo E. La Riabilitazione Implantoprotesica nei Casi Complessi. Torino, Italy: Unione Tipografico-Editrice Torinese, 2006.
11. Brånemark PI, Hansson BO, Adell R et al. Osseointegrated implants in edentulous jaws: experience from a 10-year period. Scand J Plast Reconstr Surg Suppl 1977; 16:1–132.
12. Quirynen M, Naert I, Van Steenberghe D, Nys L. A study of 589 consecutive implants supporting complete fixed prostheses. I: Periodontal aspects. J Prosthet Dent 1992;68:655–663.
13. Lindquist LW, Rockler B, Carlsson GE. Bone resorption around fixtures in edentulous patients treated with mandibular fixed tissue-integrated prostheses. J Prosthet Dent 1988;59:59–63.
14. O'Mahony A, Bowles Q, Woolsey G, Robinson SJ, Spencer P. Stress distribution in the single-unit osseointegrated dental implant: finite element analyses of axial and off-axial loading. Implant Dent 2000;9:207–218.
15. Geng JP, Tan KBC, Liu GR. Application of finite element analysis in implant dentistry: a review of the literature. J Prosthet Dent 2001;85:585–598.
16. Hoshaw SJ, Brunski JB, Cochran GVB. Mechanical overloading of Brånemark implants affects interfacial bone modeling and remodelling. J Oral Surg 1994;9:345–360.
17. Isidor F. Loss of osseointegration caused by occlusal load of oral implants: a clinical and radiographic study in monkeys. Clin Oral Implants Res 1996;7:143–152.
18. Isidor F. Histological evaluation of peri-implant bone at implants subjected to occlusal overload or plaque accumulation. Clin Oral Implants Res 1997;8:1–9.
19. Berglundh T, Lindhe J. Dimension of the peri-implant mucosa: biologic width revisited. J Clin Periodontol 1996;23:971–973.
20. Cochran DL. Biologic width around titanium implants: a histometric analysis of the implant–gingival junction around unloaded and loaded non-submerged implants in the canine mandible. J Periodontol 1997;68:186–198.

21. Hermann JS, Cochran PV, Buser D. Crestal changes around titanium implants: a radiographic evaluation of unloaded nonsubmerged and submerged implants in the canine mandible. J Periodontol 1997;68:1117–1130.
22. Todescan F, Pustiglioni F, Imbronito A, Albrektsson T, Gioso M. Influence of the microgap in the peri-implant hard and soft tissues: a histomorphometric study in dogs. Int J Oral Maxillofac Implants 2002;17:467–472.
23. Davarpanah M, Martinez H, Tecucianu JF. Apical coronal implant position: recent surgical proposals. Int J Oral Maxillofac Implants 2000;15:865–872.
24. Grunder U, Gracis S, Capelli M. Influence of the 3-D bone-to-implant relationship on esthetics. Int J Periodontics Restorative Dent 2005;25:113–119.
25. Tarnow DP, Cho SC, Wallace SS. The effect of inter-implant distance on the height of inter-implant bone crest. J Periodontol 2000;71:546–549.
26. Cox JF, Zarb GA. The longitudinal clinical efficacy of osseointegrated dental implants: a 3-year report. Int J Oral Maxillofac Implants 1987;2:91–100.
27. Malmqvist JP, Sennerby L. Clinical report on the success of 47 consecutively placed Core-Vent implants followed from 3 months to 4 years. Int J Oral Maxillofac Implants 1990;5:53–60.
28. Astrand P, Almfeldt I, Brunell G et al. Non-submerged implants in the treatment of the edentulous lower jaw: a 2-year longitudinal study. Clin Oral Implants Res 1996;7:337–344.
29. Becker W, Becker BE, Newman MG, Nyman S. Clinical and microbiologic findings that may contribute to dental implant failure. Int J Oral Maxillofac Implants 1990;5: 31–38.
30. Lindquist LW, Carlsson GE, Jemt T. A prospective 15-year follow-up study of mandibular fixed prostheses supported by osseointegrated implants: clinical results and marginal bone loss. Clin Oral Implants Res 1996;7: 329–336.
31. Rosenberg ES, Torosian JP, Slots J. Microbial differences in two clinically distinct types of failures of osseointegrated implants. Clin Oral Implants Res 1991;2:135–144.
32. Teixeira ER, Sato Y, Akagawa Y, Kimoto T. Correlation between mucosal inflammation and marginal bone loss around hydroxyapatite-coated implants: a 3-year cross-sectional study. Int J Oral Maxillofac Implants 1997; 12:74–81.
33. Brånemark PI, Adell R, Breine U, Hansson BO, Lindström J. Intra-osseous anchorage of dental prostheses: experimental studies. Scand J Plast Reconstr Surg 1969;3: 81–100.
34. Hanisch O, Tatakis DN, Boskovic MM, Rohrer MD, Wikesjö UM. Bone formation and reosseointegration in peri-implantitis defects following surgical implantation of rhBMP-2. Int J Oral Maxillofac Implants 1997;12: 604–610.
35. Hickey JS, O'Neal RB, Scheidt MJ et al. Microbiologic characterization of ligature induced periimplantitis in the microswine model. J Periodontol 1991;62:548–553.
36. Lang NP, Brägger U, Walther D, Beamer B, Kornman KS. Ligature induced periimplant infection in cynomolgus monkeys. I: Clinical and radiographic findings. Clin Oral Implants Res 1993;4:2–11.
37. Marinello CP, Berglundh T, Ericsson I et al. Resolution of ligature-induced peri-implantitis lesions in the dog. J Clin Periodontol 1995;22:475–479.
38. Tillmanns HW, Hermann JS, Cagna DR, Burgess AV, Meffert RM. Evaluation of three different dental implants in ligature-induced peri-implantitis in the beagle dog. I: Clinical evaluation. Int J Oral Maxillofac Implants 1997;12:611–620.
39. Tillmanns HW, Hermann JS, Tiffee JC, Burgess AV, Meffert RM. Evaluation of three different dental implants in ligature-induced peri-implantitis in the beagle dog. II: Histology and microbiology. Int J Oral Maxillofac Implants 1998;13:59–68.
40. Jemt T, Lekholm U, Adell R. Osseointegrated implants in the treatment of partially edentulous patients: a preliminary study on 876 consecutively placed fixtures. Int J Oral Maxillofac Implants 1989;4:211–217.
41. Duyck J, Van Oosterwyck H, Vander Sloten J et al. Magnitude and distribution of occlusal forces on oral implants supporting fixed prostheses: an in-vivo study. Clin Oral Implants Res 2000;11:465–475.
42. Guichet DL, Yoshinobu D, Caputo AA. Effect of splinting and interproximal contact tightness on load transfer by implant restorations. J Prosthet Dent 2002;87:528–535.
43. Duyck J, Van Oosterwyck H, Vander Sloten J et al. In-vivo forces on oral implants supporting a mandibular overdenture: the influence of attachment system. Clin Oral Investig 1999;3:201–207.
44. Richter EJ. In-vivo vertical forces on implants. Int J Oral Maxillofac Implants 1995;10:99–108.
45. Richter EJ. In-vivo horizontal bending moments on implants. Int J Oral Maxillofac Implants 1998;13:232–244.
46. El Askary AS, Meffert RM, Griffin T. Why do dental implants fail? Pt I. Implant Dent 1999;8:173–185.
47. Brunsky JB. In-vivo bone response to biomechical loading at the bone–dental implant interface. Adv Dent Res 1999;13:88–119.
48. Duyck J, Ronold HJ, Van Oosterwyck H et al. The influence of static and dynamic loading on marginal bone reactions around osseointegrated implants: an animal experimental study. Clin Oral Implants Res 2001;12:207–218.
49. Hürzeler MB, Quinones CR, Kohal RJ et al. Changes in peri-implant tissues subjected to orthodontic forces and ligature breakdown in monkeys. J Periodontol 1998;69: 396–404.
50. Kozlovsky A, Tal H, Laufer BZ et al. Impact of implant overloading on the peri-implant bone in inflamed and non-inflamed peri-implant mucosa. Clin Oral Implants Res 2007;18:601–610.

51. Jiang T, Ai M. In-vivo mandibular elastic deformation during clenching on pivots. J Oral Rehabil 2002;29: 201–208.
52. Picton DC. Distortion of the jaws during biting. Arch Oral Biol 1962;7:573–580.
53. Koriot TWP, Hannam AG. Deformation of the human mandible during simulated tooth clenching. J Dent Res 1994;73:56–66.
54. Hobkirk JA, Schwab J. Mandibular deformation in subjects with osseointegrated implants. Int J Oral Maxillofac Implants 1991;6:319–328.
55. Hobkirk JA, Havthoulas TK. The influence of mandibular deformation, implant numbers, and loading position on detected forces in abutments supporting fixed implant superstructures. J Prosthet Dent 1998;80:169–174.
56. Abdel-Latif HH, Hobkirk JA, Kelleway JP. Functional mandibular deformation in edentulous subjects treated with dental implants. Int J Prosthodont 2000;13:513–519.
57. El-Sheikh AM, Abdel-Latif HH, Howell PG, Hobkirk JA. Midline mandibular deformation during nonmasticatory functional movements in edentulous subjects with dental implants. Int J Oral Maxillofac Implants 2007;22: 243–248.
58. Al-Sukhun J, Kelleway J. Biomechanics of the mandible. II: Development of a 3-dimensional finite element model to study mandibular functional deformation in subjects treated with dental implants. Int J Oral Maxillofac Implants 2007;22:455–466.
59. Misch CE, Bidez MW. Implant-protected occlusion. Pract Periodontics Aesthet Dent 1995;7:25–29.
60. Brånemark PI. Osseoperception and musculo-skeletal function. In: Williams E, Rydevik B, Johns R, Brånemark PI (eds). Osseoperception and Musculoskeletal function. Gothenberg: Institute of Applied Biotechnology, 1999: 6–10.
61. Hämmerle CH, Wagner D, Brägger U et al. Threshold of tactile sensitivity perceived with dental endosseous implants and natural teeth. Clin Oral Implants Res 1995;6:83–90.
62. Lundgren D, Laurell L. Occlusal aspects of fixed bridgework supported by endosseous implants. In: Lang NP, Karring T (eds). Proceedings of the 1st European Workshop in Periodontology. London: Quintessence, 1994: 326–327.
63. Strazzeri AJ. Applied harmonious occlusion and plaque prevention most important in implant success. Oral Implantol 1975;5:369–377.
64. McCoy G. Occlusion and implants. Dent Today 1997;16: 110–111.
65. McCoy G. Recognizing and managing parafunction in the reconstruction and maintenance of the oral implant patient. Implant Dent 2002;11:19–27.
66. Misch CE. The effect of bruxism on treatment planning for dental implants. Dent Today 2002;21:62.
67. McCollum BB, Evans RL. The gnathological concepts of Charles E. Stuart, Beverly B. McCollum and Harvey Stallard. Georgetown Dent J 1970;36:12–20.
68. Williamson EH, Lundquist DO. Anterior guidance: its effect on electromyographic activity of the temporal and masseter muscles. J Prosthet Dent 1983;49:816–823.
69. el Askary AS, Meffert RM, Griffin T. Why do dental implants fail? Pt II. Implant Dent 1999;8:265–277.
70. Rangert B, Krogh PHJ, Langer B, Van Roekel N. Bending overload and implant fracture: a retrospective clinical analysis. Int J Oral Maxillofac Implants 1995;10:326–334.
71. Piattelli A, Piattelli M, Scarano A, Montesani L. Light and scanning electron microscopic report on four fractured implants. Int J Oral Maxillofac Implants 1998;13:561–564.
72. Binon PP. Evaluation of machining accuracy and consistency of selected implants, standard abutments, and laboratory analogs. Int J Prosthodont 1995;8:162–178.
73. Brånemark R, Skalak R. An in-vivo method for biomechanical characterization of bone-anchored implants. Med Eng Phys 1998;20:216–219.
74. Brånemark R, Ohrnell LO, Skalak R, Carlsson L, Brånemark PI. Biomechanical characterization of osseointegration: an experimental in-vivo investigation in the beagle dog. J Orthop Res 1998;16:61–69.
75. Gallucci GO, Bernard JP, Belser UC. Treatment of completely edentulous patients with fixed implant-supported restorations: three consecutive cases of simultaneous immediate loading in both maxilla and mandible. Int J Periodontics Restorative Dent 2005;25:27–37.
76. Bezerra F, Vasconcelos L, Azoubel E. Tilting implants technique, for the treatment of the edentulous maxillae. Brasil 3I Innovations Jl 2002;6:31–35.

Chapter 24

# Botulinum Toxin in the Treatment of Bruxism

*Daniele Manfredini and Luca Guarda Nardini*

## Introduction

Botulinum toxin is a neurotoxin produced by *Clostridium botulinum*, a Gram-positive spore-forming anaerobic bacterium, which is responsible for botulism. Botulism is a potentially lethal disease, whose signs include limb paralysis, facial weakness, ophthalmoplegia, dysphagia, dysarthria, constipation (progressing to ileus), dyspnea (progressing to respiratory arrest), and urinary retention.[1] Botulism can occur following ingestion of contaminated food, from colonization of the infant gastrointestinal tract, or from a wound infection. Fortunately, both prevalence and mortality of botulism have markedly decreased in recent years.[2]

Research studies have identified seven neurotoxic types (BTX-A, B, C1, D, E, F, G) of botulinum toxin, of which the first two are primarily responsible for human intoxications.[3]

Botulinum toxins cause a prolonged inhibition of neurotransmitter release at peripheral cholinergic nerve terminals at both neuromuscular junctions and autonomic sympathetic and parasympathetic nerve terminals. The discovery of these properties has been the basis for hypotheses involving therapeutic use of botulinum toxin and, nowadays, this potentially dangerous poison has been transformed into a widely used drug that is useful for the management of several muscle disorders associated with an excessive cholinergic activity.[4]

Indeed, the purification of botulinum toxin at basic research levels has allowed its adoption in the treatment of spasticity,[5] blepharospasm,[6,7] spasmodic dysphonia,[8–10] and cervical dystonia.[11–13]

## History of Botulinum Toxin as a Therapeutic Drug

Botulinum toxins are produced by *C. botulinum*, an anaerobic bacterium whose spores are commonly located within the soil. The bacterium grows in a pin-like form within the food only if the contact between the food and the spore occurs under determined conditions (absence of oxygen, temperature <10°C, acidic conditions). In such an environment, *C. botulinum* can grow and release new spores; ultimately it implodes, thus destroying the cell membrane and releasing its powerful neurotoxins. The seven types of botulinum toxins are actually the most powerful and dangerous among known neurotoxins; and even though they probably have different biochemical properties, they share similar effects on muscle activity – which have been described in detail for the serotype BTX-A.

Studies on BTX-A biochemistry date back to the 1920s, with the first attempts at purifying the toxin. The efforts of Sommer and other pioneering researchers laid the basis for successive studies from Schantz who, in 1946, obtained a purified crystalline form of botulinum toxin, thus improving the quality of future research. Later in the 1950s, Brooks described a temporary paralysis following BTX-A injection in a hyperactive muscle. This effect was described as a consequence of the inhibition of acetylcholine release at motor nerve terminals, and obviously led to a growing interest in the potential therapeutic use of botulinum toxin. A decade later, Scott provided animal experimental models supporting the usefulness of a purified version of BTX-A to correct strabismus (an ophthalmic dystonia) in monkeys. In 1978, Scott obtained US Food and Drug Administration (FDA) approval to begin studies on the effects of botulinum toxin on strabismus in human volunteers. In 1989, botulinum toxin was definitively introduced in the market under the trade name Oculinum, with FDA-labeled indications in the treatment of strabismus and blepharospasm; also included was facial nerve paralysis. Later, a pharmaceutical company, Allergan, bought the BTX-A licence, and changed its trade name to Botox, which is now currently used for a number of muscle hyperactivity disorders. In 2000, both BTX-A and BTX-B (MyoBloc) were approved by the FDA for cervical dystonia; and in 2002 Botox was approved by the FDA for the treatment of glabellar lines, and most recently for primary axillary hyperhydrosis. Thus, from the time of its clinical debut, reports on the indications of BTX have been growing in number and fields of application.

The type-A botulinum toxin has high affinity for the neuromuscular junction and causes a long-lasting inhibition of neurotransmitter release at peripheral cholinergic nerve terminals at both neuromuscular junctions and autonomic sympathetic and parasympathetic nerve terminals.

Like many other biologic and pharmaceutical agents, Botox is produced via a process of fermentation and purification, and available information about its structures and properties will be discussed here.

## Mechanism of Action

The size of the structural complex of the different botulinum toxins varies among serotypes, ranging from 300 to 900 kDa. The purified BTX-A has a molecular weight of 900 kDa and includes three proteins: the neurotoxin (made up of a heavy and a light chain for a total 150 kDa molecular weight), a non-hemagglutinin protein, and a hemagglutinin protein (associated with the toxin with the aim to protect it from degradation and combining for about 750 kDa).[14]

The heavy chain of the BTX-A is responsible for binding to its serotype specific receptor/acceptor on the target cell and mediates translocation, allowing for the expression of the light chain outside of the cholinergic vesicle, while the effect of BTX-A depends on the enzymatic action of the light chain (very specific peptidase with a specific target – this region is unique for each serotype).

Once active, the toxin produces a muscle relaxant effect that is local – effective within a predictable radius at the site of injection, and temporary – lasting up to 3–6 months. Muscle relaxation is the result of the block of acetylcholine release at the endplate of the motor neuron.[15]

From a molecular viewpoint, the current hypothesis for its motor mechanism of action in skeletal muscle provides that, at the nerve terminal, botulinum toxin type A induces a temporary chemodenervation through the following steps.[16,17]

- The toxin binds to acceptors (yet to be identified) on cholinergic terminals.
- The molecule is internalized into the nerve ending by endocytosis.
- Once inside the nerve ending, botulinum toxin interferes with the exocytosis of cholinergic vesicles. This leads to chemo-denervation and reduced muscular contractions.
- Over time, terminal sprouting occurs.
- Finally, the original functional endplate is re-established and sprouts regress. At this point symptoms may return in some patients.

## Fields of Application

In 1990, the National Institutes of Health Consensus Development Conference Statement recommended that botulinum toxin therapy was safe and effective for treating strabismus, blepharospasm, hemifacial spasm, adductor spasmodic dysphonia, jaw-closing oromandibular dystonia, and cervical dystonia;[18] it also stated that BTX is not curative in chronic neurologic disorders. Since that time, clinical and research experience of the use of BTX to treat these disorders has been intense, and BTX-A is currently available under the trade names Botox (Allergan, Irvine, CA, USA) and Dysport (Speywood Pharmaceuticals, Maidenhead, UK) in the USA and Europe, respectively. A purified version of BTX-B has been approved for the treatment of cervical dystonia and is available on the market under the names Neurobloc (Elan Pharmaceuticals, Shannon, Co. Clare, Ireland) and MyoBloc (Elan Pharmaceuticals, San Diego, CA, USA).

A National Library of Medicine's PubMed database search performed with the keyword "botulinum toxin" identified over 8,000 articles, more than half of which regarded the clinical use of botulinum toxin as a therapeutic drug. Along with studies lending support to the above-described indications, research were performed on the use of botulinum toxin in a number of minor disorders related to muscular hyperactivity.

Those so-called emerging applications included treatment for conditions associated with pain (e.g., tension headache, migraine headache, cervicogenic headache, cluster headache, myofascial pain, chronic low back pain, tennis elbow), hypersecretion of glands (e.g., hyperhydrosis, sialorrhea, crocodile tear syndrome, intrinsic rhinitis), excessive or dyssynergic muscle contraction (e.g., myokymia, bruxism, anal fissure, anismus, vaginismus, detruso-sphincter dyssynergia, sphincter of Oddi dysfunction, esophageal spasm, laryngeal and pyloric spasm, achalasia), and for cosmetic use.[19,20]

Promising data have emerged for all of these indications and, even though the quality of published papers has not been excellent so far, thus needing to be consistently improved before definitive confirmation of results, it appears that botulinum toxin may find increasing application in the future.

## Safety of Botulinum Toxin Treatments

Botulinum toxin therapy is effective for several of the disorders described above, and has a good safety level. The only absolute contraindications to its use are allergy to the drug and infection/inflammation at the site of the injection; safety for use during pregnancy, lactation, and childhood has not been assessed. Diseases of neuromuscular transmission, coagulopathy, and inability of the patient to cooperate are relative contraindications.[18]

Nonetheless, therapeutic administration of botulinum toxin must be performed by skilled practitioners, possibly within a skilled interdisciplinary team, owing to the risk of side-effects and complications.

Side-effects are usually transitory and well tolerated. They are mainly related to diffusion of the drug into the nearest muscular groups, thus being different in dependence of the target muscles and the type of the treated disorder. Systemic complications and side-effects, such as generalized weakness or severe electromyographic abnormalities, are rare.

A small percentage of patients develop antibodies to the toxin and, even though the mechanism leading to the development of antibodies is unknown, this may be a main reason to explain therapeutic failure.

## Orofacial Pain Relief

Once the use of botulinum toxin was settled as a possible therapeutic approach to muscle hyperactivity-related disorders, research began to support its use as a pain relief drug as well. Indeed, in most patients pain relief exceeded the benefits related to the reduction of muscle activity, as observed with electromyographic (EMG) recordings. These observations were mostly valid for cervical dystonia[21,22] and were the basis for successive studies on the usefulness of botulinum toxin in the treatment of orofacial painful disorders.

There is a limited amount of literature suggesting that the analgesic effect of BTX-A is related to reduction of the local release of nociceptive neuropeptides from either cholinergic neurons or from other nerve terminals in vivo, which would prevent the local sensitization of nociceptors and thus reduce the perception of pain.[23,24] This mechanism of action appears to be independent of the reduction of muscular hyperactivity, and is in line with current theories supporting a non-linear relationship between pain and EMG signs of neuromuscular activity.[25,26] BTX-A hence found applications in a number of orofacial pain disorders, such as various types of headache and temporomandibular disorders.

Botulinum toxin was introduced in the treatment of tension-type headache owing to the supposed role of muscle activity in its pathogenesis.[27] Nonetheless, there is a paucity of literature on this issue, and findings are not consistent among the different studies.[28–31] This suggests that larger sample investigations are needed, with a well-defined and homogeneous study protocol with regard to the dose and site of BTX-A injections in these patients.[20]

In contrast, botulinum toxin has been found effective in the treatment and prophylaxis of migraine headache, as measured on subjective rating scales, on the basis of currently available clinical trials.[32,33] With regard to cervicogenic and cluster headaches, only pilot data have been published so far, and they are mainly based on case reports, so they need to be further assessed.[34,35]

## Temporomandibular Disorders

Interestingly, botulinum toxin has shown good therapeutic efficacy in the approach to some forms of chronic myofascial pain, a term which is used here in its wide definition of being a localized musculoskeletal pain with tenderness in association with trigger points. Given the inconsistent findings reported by the literature on the use of non-steroidal anti-inflammatory drugs, steroids, antidepressants, and other drugs in the treatment of these disorders – and considering that corticosteroids, which are the currently adopted first-choice drugs to treat chronic myofascial pain, may produce undesired systemic and side-effects – some trials have assessed the analgesic efficacy of BTX-A in such patients.[36–38]

Literature findings are generally supportive of an efficacy of botulinum toxin in the treatment of these disorders, being superior to both placebo saline solution and methylprednisolone injections. However, all the research on the therapeutic use of botulinum toxin has a common limitation – the difficulty in patient recruitment and selection for studies of "off-label" drug use, to the point that this basic consideration must be kept in mind before generalizing positive results from preliminary small-sample studies. Nonetheless, it seems that the potential of BTX for achieving muscle relaxation and analgesic effects in many muscular disorders is well-evidenced, and this led to a search for new therapeutic applications.

The adoption of botulinum toxin in temporomandibular disorder (TMD) patients is a consequence of these considerations, given the high rate of comorbidity of TMD with some forms of headache[39,40] and the common uncertainties about the pathophysiology of both disorders, which force clinicians and researchers to adopt a symptomatic therapeutic approach in both cases.[41–43]

In 2004, at the time of a systematic review of the literature on the usefulness of BTX-A in the treatment of head and neck muscle disorders,[44] only one study satisfied the authors' qualitative criteria to be included in the review. In that study, which tested a small sample of highly selected patients with muscular TMD treated with a crossover protocol (BTX-A vs. placebo), the dropout rate was up to one-third of participants, due to either pain increase (treatment inefficacy) or muscle paralysis (side-effect of the treatment). No significant differences in pain improvement were observed between the two treatments, thus not providing support for the efficacy of BTX-A in muscular TMD.[45]

Similar conclusions emerged from a systematic review in 2007 on the potential therapeutic effects of botulinum toxin in orofacial pain disorders, which claimed that literature findings are not so promising for orofacial pain, except for migraine prophylaxis.[46] In contrast, two other reviews, one descriptive[47] and one systematic,[48] partly revisited the earlier conclusions and tried to provide a rationale for using BTX-A in TMD patients. Nonetheless, there is a general consensus that the quality of the literature on the therapeutic effects of botulinum toxin in TMD patients is currently poor, and further studies are strongly needed.

A PubMed search performed with the key terms "botulinum toxin" and "temporomandibular disorders" yielded 36 references many of which were single-patient case reports on off-label uses of BTX-A within the orofacial region, such as in the case of masseter hypertrophy,[49] TMJ anterior disc displacement,[50] TMJ disc disfigurement,[51] and chronic or recurrent TMJ dislocation.[52–56] Apart from studies on these particular applications, most clinical data on the use of type-A botulinum toxin to treat facial pain has come from case series on TMD patients.

An uncontrolled preliminary investigation by Freund and co-workers[57] found that the injection of 150 units of BTX-A (50 U within each masseter and 25 U within each temporalis muscle) provided a significant reduction in both objective (mouth opening) and subjective (pain, function, tenderness) jaw function in a sample of 15 subjects with non-homogeneous TMD over an 8-week period. Similar findings were reported by the same group of researchers in a successive case series study on a larger sample,[58] and by Von Lindern,[59] who reported encouraging findings with the injection of 200 U of BTX-A per side in a sample of 41 patients with muscular TMD over a 6-month span.

## Botox and Bruxism

Myofascial pain of the masticatory muscles has a strong epidemiologic relevance, affecting from 38% to 75% of patients with signs and symptoms of TMD in Caucasian populations[60,61] and about 30% Asian patients.[62] Therefore, despite the fluctuating and self-limiting nature of these disorders,[63] efficacious first-step symptomatic therapies are requested to reduce their psychosocial impact. There is a complex pathogenesis which is often the expression of a multifactorial etiology, with a number of systemic and local risk factors.[64]

Some similar epidemiologic and psychosocial characteristics have been described for bruxism as well, which is a parafunctional activity strongly detrimental for all the stomatognathic structures.[65] In particular, despite a lack of demonstration of its causal role for TMD,[66] and doubts existing about the etiology of both awake and sleep bruxism,[67–70] a clinical association between bruxism and myofascial pain has been reported in several works.[71,72] Many therapies have been proposed to treat bruxism-related muscle hyperactivity, but published data have not been conclusive so far.[73–76]

Similarly, uncertainty about the etiopathogenesis of myofascial pain has led to the proposal of several treatment approaches for this condition, among which are occlusal splints,[77,78] physical therapy,[79] behavioral and physical treatments,[80] and drugs.[81–83]

These considerations, which support the need for a symptomatic management approach to these disorders in the absence of a specific causal therapy to achieve muscle relaxation, along with the above-described attempts of introducing botulinum toxin in the treatment of myofascial TMD, have led to hypotheses on the possible efficacy of BTX-A to reduce muscle activity in bruxers. However, studies are complicated by the difficulty of obtaining objective data on the severity of bruxism and on the different patterns of parafunctional activity (clenching or grinding).

At the time of writing there are no studies assessing the polysomnographic activity of bruxers before and after a botulinum toxin injection, and the simplest approach to the evaluation of a treatment for bruxism appears to be clinical assessment.

Tan and Jankovic[84] assessed the efficacy of BTX-A injections (25–100 MU per masseter muscle) in a sample of 18 subjects with severe long-term bruxism. The efficacy of treatment was assessed with a combination of patients' self-perception of improvement and their partners' interviews. The mean duration of response was about 6 months, and the mean peak effect was 3.4 on a scale of 0 to 4, in which 4 is equal to total abolishment of grinding. Only one subject (5.6%) reported having experienced dysphagia.

Self-report perception of efficacy was also reported by a patient affected by amphetamine-induced bruxism treated with BTX-A,[85] and clinical improvement was shown in a 7-year-old child who exhibited teeth clenching and grinding as a consequence of a post-traumatic brain injury.[86]

At present, the only available randomized clinical trial on the use of botulinum toxin in bruxers is a preliminary double-blind, placebo-controlled investigation with a 6-month follow-up period, aiming to assess the efficacy of type-A botulinum toxin to treat myofascial pain symptoms and to reduce muscle hyperactivity in bruxers.[87] Twenty subjects with a clinical diagnosis of bruxism and with myofascial pain of masticatory muscles were randomly enrolled and included either within a treatment group (BTX-A injection) or a control group (saline placebo injections). A number of objective and subjective clinical parameters were assessed at baseline, and at 1-week, 1-month, and 6-month follow-up appointments. The parameters were: pain at rest and at chewing; mastication efficiency; maximum unassisted and assisted mouth opening, protrusive, and laterotrusive movements; functional limitation during usual jaw movements; subjective efficacy of the treatment; and tolerability of the treatment. Interestingly, improvements in both objective and subjective clinical outcome variables were higher in Botox than in placebo patients. Besides, patients treated with BTX-A reported a higher subjective improvement with time in their perception of treatment efficacy than did the placebo patients. According to the authors, the differences were not significant in some cases owing to the small sample size. Nonetheless, the findings supported the efficacy of BTX-A to reduce myofascial pain symptoms in bruxers, thus providing pilot data that have to be confirmed by further research on larger samples.

Taken together, this scarce literature suggests that BTX-A studies in bruxers have suffered from the same methodologic concerns as other investigations on bruxism, such as the issues of clinical evaluation and quantification of the disorder. The study by Guarda-Nardini and co-workers[87] is an example of the difficulties of identifying which part of a patient's symptoms improved. Is pain relief a direct consequence of bruxism reduction, or is it due to the analgesic/muscle relaxant properties of botulinum toxin?

## Conclusion

The reliability of clinical diagnostic criteria for bruxism is much debated.[88,89] When assessing the efficacy of a therapeutic modality, the clinician must be conscious that pain in the masticatory muscles might be a spurious outcome variable, being the expression of concurrent disorders as well.

Evidence-based knowledge on bruxism characteristics and effects is mostly based on findings from studies of sleep bruxism, which is more suitable for a reliable diagnosis in a scientific research setting. Unfortunately, PSG studies are expensive and adequately equipped sleep laboratories are not numerous. The problem of patient recruitment affects experimental studies on bruxism treatments, including investigations on botulinum toxin efficacy.

Nonetheless, the generally positive findings suggesting that botulinum toxin may provide potential for minor neuromuscular conditions, along with the number of neuromuscular disorders for which BTX-A represents a first-choice option (e.g., blepharospasm, cervical dystonia, and several other focal dystonias), seem to justify further investigations of its efficacy in bruxers.

## References


1. Cai S, Singh BR, Sharma S. Botulism diagnostics: from clinical symptoms to in-vitro assays. Crit Rev Microbiol 2007;33(2):109–125.
2. Isturiz RE, Torres J, Besso J. Global distribution of infectious diseases requiring intensive care. Crit Care Clin 2006;22:469–88,ix.
3. Horowitz BZ. Botulinum toxin. Crit Care Clin 2005;21: 825–39,viii.
4. Davis LE. Botulinum toxin: from poison to medicine. West J Med 1993;158:25–29.
5. Simpson DM. Clinical trials of botulinum toxin in the treatment of spasticity. Muscle Nerve 1997;6:169–175.
6. Silveira-Moriyama L, Goncalves LR, Chien HF, Barbosa ER. Botulinum toxin A in the treatment of blepharospasm: a 10-year experience. Arq Neuropsiquiatr 2005;63(2A):221–224.
7. Bhidayasiri R, Cardoso F, Truong DD. Botulinum toxin in blepharospasm and oromandibular dystonia: comparing different botulinum toxin preparations. Eur J Neurol 2006;13(1):21–29.
8. Adler CH, Bansberg SF, Krein-Jones K, Hentz JG. Safety and efficacy of botulinum toxin type B (Myobloc) in adductor spasmodic dysphonia. Mov Disord 2004;19: 1075–1079.
9. Adler CH, Bansberg SF, Hentz JG et al. Botulinum toxin type A for treating voice tremor. Arch Neurol 2004;61: 1416–1420.
10. Damrose JF, Goldman SN, Groessl EJ, Orloff LA. The impact of long-term botulinum toxin injections on symptom severity in patients with spasmodic dysphonia. J Voice 2004;18:415–422.
11. Benecke R, Jost WH, Kanovsky P et al. A new botulinum toxin type A free of complexing proteins for treatment of cervical dystonia. Neurology 2005;64:1949–1951.
12. Comella CL, Jankovic J, Shannon KM et al. Comparison of botulinum toxin serotypes A and B for the treatment of cervical dystonia. Neurology 2005;65:1423–1429.
13. Oleszek JL, Chang N, Apkon SD, Wilson PE. Botulinum toxin type A in the treatment of children with congenital muscular torticollis. Am J Phys Med Rehabil 2005;84: 813–816.
14. Huang W, Foster JA, Rogachefsky AS. Pharmacology of botulinum toxin. J Am Acad Dermatol 2000;43:249–259.
15. Humeau Y, Doussau F, Grant NJ, Poulain B. How botulinum and tetanus neurotoxins block neurotransmitter release. Biochimie 2000;82:427–446.
16. Schiavo G, Matteoli M, Montecucco C. Neurotoxins affecting neuroexocytosis. Physiol Rev 2000;80: 718–766.
17. dePaiva A, Meunier FA, Molgo J, Aoki KR, Dolly JO. Functional repair of motor endplates after botulinum neurotoxin type A poisoning: biphasic switch of synaptic activity between nerve sprouts and their parent terminals. Proc Natl Acad Sci U S A 1999;96:3200–3205.
18. NIH Panel. Clinical Use of Botulinum Toxin (NIH Consensus Statement 1990) 12–14 Nov;8:1–20.
19. Jankovic J, Brin M. Therapeutic uses of botulinum toxin. N Engl J Med 1991;324:1186–1194.
20. Thant ZS, Tan EK. Emerging therapeutic applications for botulinum toxin. Med Sci Monit 2003;2:40–48.
21. Tsui JK, Eisen A, Stoessl AJ, Calne S, Calne DB. Double-blind study of botulinum toxin in spasmodic torticollis. Lancet 1986;2:245–247.
22. Jankovic J, Schwartz K. Botulinum toxin injections for cervical dystonia. Neurology 1990;40:277–280.
23. Aoki KR. Pharmacology and immunology of botulinum toxin serotypes. J Neurol 2001;248(Suppl 1): 3–10.

24. Aoki KR. Review of a proposed mechanism for the antinociceptive action of botulinum toxin type A. Neurotoxicology 2005;26:785–793.
25. Svensson P, Graven-Nielsen T, Matre D, Arendt-Nielsen L. Experimental muscle pain does not cause long-lasting increases in resting electromyographic activity. Muscle Nerve 1998;21:1382–1389.
26. Svensson P, Wang K, Sessle BJ, Arendt-Nielsen L. Associations between pain and neuromuscular activity in the human jaw and neck muscles. Pain 2004;109:225–232.
27. Carruthers A, Langtry JA, Carruthers J, Robinson G. Improvement of tension-type headache when treating wrinkles with botulinum toxin A injections. Headache 1999;39:662–665.
28. Schulte-Mattler WJ, Wieser T, Zierz S. Treatment of tension-type headache with botulinum toxin: a pilot study. Eur J Med Res 1999;4:183–186.
29. Rollnik JD, Tanneberger O, Schubert M, Schneider U, Dengler R. Treatment of tension-type headache with botulinum toxin type A: a double-blind, placebo-controlled study. Headache 2000;40:300–305.
30. Schmitt WJ, Slowey E, Fravi N, Weber S, Burgunder JM. Effect of botulinum toxin A injections in the treatment of chronic tension-type headache: a double-blind, placebo-controlled trial. Headache 2001;41:658–664.
31. Silbertstein SD, Gobel H, Jensen R et al. Botulinum toxin type A in a prophylactic treatment of chronic tension-type headache: a multicentre, double-blind, randomized, placebo-controlled, parallel-group study. Cephalalgia 2006;26:790–800.
32. Brin MF, Swope DM, O'Brain C. Botox for migraine: double-blind, placebo-controlled region-specific evaluation. Cephalalgia 2000;421–422.
33. Binder WJ, Brin MF, BlitzerA, Schoenrock LD, Pogoda JM. Botulinum toxin type A (Botox) for treatment of migraine headaches: an open-label study. Otolaryngol Head Neck Surg 2000;123:669–676.
34. Wheeler AH, Goolkasian P, Gretz SS. A randomized, double-blind, prospective pilot study of botulinum toxin injection for refractory, unilateral, cervicothoracic, paraspinal, and myofascial pain syndrome. Spine 1998;23:1662–1666.
35. Freund BJ, Schwartz M. Treatment of chronic cervical-associated headache with botulinum toxin A: a pilot study. Headache 2000;40:231–236.
36. Acquadro M, Borodic G. Treatment of myofascial pain with botulinum A toxin. Anesthesiology 1994;80:705–706.
37. Cheshire WP, Abashian SW, Mann JD. Botulinum toxin in the treatment of myofascial pain syndrome. Pain 1994;59:65–69.
38. Porta M. A comparative trial of botulinum toxin type A and methylprednisolone for the treatment of myofascial pain syndrome and pain from chronic muscle spasm. Pain 2000;85:101–105.
39. Ciancaglini R, Radaelli G. The relationship between headache and symptoms of temporomandibular disorder in the general population. J Dent 2001;29(2):93–98.
40. Freund BJ, Schwartz M. Relief of tension type headache symptoms in subjects with temporomandibular disorders treated with botulinum toxin-A. Headache 2002;42:1033–1037.
41. Stohler CS, Zarb GA. On the management of temporomandibular disorders: a plea for a low-tech, high-prudence therapeutic approach. J Orofac Pain 1999;13:255–261.
42. Krymchantowski AV, Rapoport AM, Jevoux CC. The future of acute care and prevention in headache. Neurol Sci 2007;28(Suppl 2):S166–178.
43. Grazzi L, Usai S, Bussone C. Chronic headaches: pharmacological and non-pharmacological treatment. Neurol Sci 2007;28(Suppl 2):S134–137.
44. Sycha T, Kranz G, Auff E, Schnider P. Botulinum toxin in the treatment of rare head and neck pain syndromes: a systematic review of the literature. J Neurol 2004;251 (Suppl 1):I19–30.
45. Nixdorf DR, Heo G, Major PW. Randomized controlled trial of botulinum toxin A for chronic myogenous orofacial pain. Pain 2002;99:465–473.
46. Clark GT, Stiles A, Lockerman LZ, Gross SG. A critical review of the use of botulinum toxin in orofacial pain disorders. Dent Clin North Am 2007;51:245–261,ix.
47. Song PC, Schwartz J, Blitzer A. The emerging role of botulinum toxin in the treatment of temporomandibular disorders. Oral Dis 2007;13:253–260.
48. Ihde SK, Konstantinovic VS. The therapeutic use of botulinum toxin in cervical and maxillofacial conditions: an evidence-based review. Oral Surg Oral Med Oral Pathol Oral Radiol Endod 2007;104:e1–11.
49. Al-Ahmad HT, Al-Qudah MA. The treatment of masseter hypertrophy with botulinum toxin type A. Saudi Med J 2006;27:397–400.
50. Bakke M, Moller E, Werdelin LM et al. Treatment of severe temporomandibular joint clicking with botulinum toxin in the lateral pterygoid muscle in two cases of anterior disc displacement. Oral Surg Oral Med Oral Pathol Oral Radiol Endod 2005;100:693–700.
51. Karacalar A, Yilmaz N, Bilgici A et al. Botulinum toxin for the treatment of temporomandibular joint disk disfigurement: clinical experience. J Craniofac Surg 2005;16:476–481.
52. Daelen B, Thorwirth V, Koch A. Treatment of recurrent dislocation of the temporomandibular joint with type A botulinum toxin. Int J Oral Maxillofac Surg 1997;26:458–460.
53. Moore AP, Wood GD. Medical treatment of recurrent temporomandibular joint dislocation using botulinum toxin A. Br Dent J 1997;183:415–417.
54. Ziegler CM, Haag C, Maehling J. Treatment of recurrent temporomandibular joint dislocation with intramuscular botulinum toxin injection. Clin Oral Investig 2003;7:52–55.
55. Aquilina P, Vickers R, McKellar G. Reduction of a chronic bilateral temporomandibular joint dislocation with intermaxillary fixation and botulinum toxin A. Br J Oral Maxillofac Surg 2004;42:272–273.

56. Martinez-Perez D, Garcia Ruiz-Espiga P. Recurrent temporomandibular joint dislocation treated with botulinum toxin: report of three cases. J Oral Maxillofac Surg 2004; 62:244–246.
57. Freund B, Schwartz M, Symington JM. The use of botulinum toxin for the treatment of temporomandibular disorders: preliminary findings. J Oral Maxillofac Surg 1999; 57:916–920.
58. Freund B, Schwartz M, Symington JM. Botulinum toxin: new treatment for temporomandibular disorders. Br J Oral Maxillofac Surg 2000;38:466–471.
59. Von Lindern JJ. Type A botulinum toxin in the treatment of chronic facial pain associated with temporo-mandibular dysfunction. Acta Neurol Belg 2001;101:39–41.
60. List T, Dworkin SF. Comparing TMD diagnoses and clinical findings at Swedish and US TMD centers using Research Diagnostic Criteria for Temporomandibular Disorders. J Orofac Pain 1996;10:240–253.
61. Manfredini D, Chiappe G, Bosco M. Research diagnostic criteria for temporomandibular disorders (RDC/TMD) axis I diagnoses in an Italian patients population. J Oral Rehabil 2006;33:551–558.
62. Yap AJU, Dworkin SF, Chua EK et al. Prevalence of temporomandibular disorders subtypes, psycologic distress and psychosocial dysfunction in Asian patients. J Orofac Pain 2003;17:21–28.
63. McNeill C. History and evolution of TMD concepts. Oral Surg Oral Med Oral Pathol Oral Radiol Endod 1997;83:51–60.
64. Greene CS. The etiology of temporomandibular disorders: implications for treatment. J Orofac Pain 2001;15: 93–105.
65. Bader G, Lavigne GJ. Sleep bruxism: overview of an oromandibular sleep movement disorder. Sleep Med Rev 2000;4:27–43.
66. Lobbezoo F, Lavigne GJ. Do bruxism and temporomandibular disorders have a cause-and-effect relationship? J Orofac Pain 1997;11:15–23.
67. Lobbezoo F, Naeije M. Bruxism is mainly regulated centrally, not peripherally. J Oral Rehabil 2001;28:1085–1091.
68. De Laat A, Macaluso GM. Sleep bruxism is a motor disorder. Mov Disord 2002;17(2):S67–69.
69. Lavigne GJ, Kato T, Kolta A, Sessle BJ. Neurobiological mechanisms involved in sleep bruxism. Crit Rev Oral Biol Med 2003;14:30–46.
70. Manfredini D, Landi N, Romagnoli M, Cantini E, Bosco M. Etiopathogenesis of parafunctional activities of the stomatognathic system. Minerva Stomatol 2003;52: 339–349.
71. Ciancaglini R, Gherlone E, Radaelli G. The relationship of bruxism with craniofacial pain and symptoms from the masticatory system in the adult population. J Oral Rehabil 2001;28:842–848.
72. Manfredini D, Cantini E, Romagnoli M, Bosco M. Prevalence of bruxism in patients with different Research Diagnostic Criteria for Temporomandibular Disorders (RDC/TMD) diagnoses. Cranio 2003;21:279–285.
73. Treacy K. Awareness/relaxation training and transcutaneous electrical neural stimulation in the treatment of bruxism. J Oral Rehabil 1999;26:280–287.
74. Wieselmann-Penkner K, Janda M, Lorenzoni M, Polansky R. A comparison of the muscular relaxation effect of TENS and EMG-biofeedback in patients with bruxism. J Oral Rehabil 2001;28:849–853.
75. Alvarez-Arenal A, Junquera LM, Fernandez JP, Gonzalez I, Olay S. Effect of occlusal splint and transcutaneous electric nerve stimulation on the signs and symptoms of temporomandibular disorders in patients with bruxism. J Oral Rehabil 2002;29:858–863.
76. van der Zaag J, Lobbezoo F, Wicks DJ et al. Controlled assessment of the efficacy of occlusal stabilization splints on sleep bruxism. J Orofac Pain 2005;19:151–158.
77. Dao TT, Lavigne GJ. Oral splints: the crutches for temporomandibular disorders and bruxism? Crit Rev Oral Biol Med 1998;9:345–361.
78. Raphael K, Marbach JJ. Widespread pain and the effectiveness of oral splints in myofascial face pain. J Am Dent Assoc 2001;132:305–316.
79. Nicolakis P, Erdogmus B, Kopf A et al. Effectiveness of exercise therapy in patients with myofascial pain dysfunction sindrome. J Oral Rehabil 2002;29:362–368.
80. De Laat A, Stappaers K, Papy S. Counseling and physical therapy as treatment for myofascial pain of the masticatory system. J Orofac Pain 2003;17:42–49.
81. Dionne RA. Pharmacologic treatment of acute and chronic orofacial pain. Oral Maxillofac Surg Clin North Am 2000;12:309–320.
82. Plesh O, Curtis D, Levine J, McCall WD. Amitriptyline treatment of chronic pain in patients with temporomandibular disorders. J Oral Rehabil 2000;27:834–841.
83. Manfredini D, Romagnoli M, Cantini E, Bosco M. Efficacy of tizanidine hydrochloride in the treatment of myofascial face pain. Minerva Med 2004;95:165–171.
84. Tan EK, Jankovic J. Treating severe bruxism with botulinum toxin. J Am Dent Assoc 2000;131:211–216.
85. See SJ, Tan EK. Severe amphethamine-induced bruxism: treatment with botulinum toxin. Acta Neurol Scand 2003;107:161–163.
86. Pidcock FS, Christensen JR. Treatment of severe post-traumatic bruxism with botulinum toxin-A: case report. J Oral Maxillofac Surg 2002;60:115–117.
87. Guarda-Nardini L, Manfredini D, Salamone M et al. Efficacy of botulinum toxin in treating myofascial pain in bruxers: placebo-controlled pilot study. Cranio 2008;26: 126–135.
88. Lavigne GJ, Romprè PH, Montplaisir JY. Sleep bruxism: validity of clinical research diagnostic criteria in a controlled polysomnographic study. J Dent Res 1996;75: 546–552.
89. Marbach JJ, Raphael KG, Janal MN, Hirschkorn-Roth R. Reliability of clinician judgements of bruxism. J Oral Rehabil 2003;30:113–118.

Chapter 25

# Clinical Treatment of Bruxism

*Daniel A. Paesani and Fernando Cifuentes*

## Canine Guidance in the Control of Bruxism Effects

### *Why Canine Guidance?*

Natural occlusion guidance is traditionally divided into two categories: canine guidance and group function. In its glossary of prosthodontic terms, the American Academy of Prosthodontics defines canine guidance as "a form of mutually protected articulation in which the vertical and horizontal overlap of the canine teeth disengage the posterior teeth in the excursive movements of the mandible".[1] In the same glossary, group function is defined as "multiple contact relations between the maxillary and mandibular teeth in lateral movements on the working side whereby simultaneous contact of several teeth acts as a group to distribute occlusal forces".

A great number of studies aimed at determining which guidance is better have focused on the prevention and/or the resolution of temporomandibular dysfunction (TMD). These studies neither objectively measured parafunction modifications nor determined whether such modifications were or were not successful; they were based on the objective and subjective variations of the signs and symptoms of TMD. Thus, this chapter will review only the information available from studies carried out on normal subjects which evaluated the performance of the different occlusal guidance by "objectively" measuring bruxism.

A long time ago, Gysi and Bonwill, pioneers in dentistry, advocated tripodization of the occlusion as a resource aimed at increasing the stability of full dentures. This theory, which is well known in the full-prosthesis field as "bilateral balanced occlusion", states that there are at least three contact points in mandibular movements. Later, McLean suggested applying these principles to natural occlusions in order to reduce occlusal trauma.[2]

In 1935, Schuyler[3] warned about the potential destructive forces generated by balanced occlusion contacts, and suggested avoiding them in natural dentitions in order to prevent tooth wear.

This author advocated the replacement of bilateral balanced occlusion with unilateral balanced occlusion or "group function", which consists of:

- an occlusion scheme with full contacts in centric relation
- posterior segment disclusion during protrusion
- during lateral movements, simultaneous contact of anterior and posterior teeth on the working side and no contacts at all on the non-working side.

This occlusal theory is supported by many; unfortunately, they have not provided any scientific evidence on its effects.[4–7]

The canine-protection occlusion scheme was first proposed by D'Amico[8] who, in view of the significant tooth wear shown by prehistoric populations, suggested preventing it by means of canine protection. This author also suggested controlling horizontal movements by means of a canine-generated guidance; such guidance would prevent the contact between posterior teeth. D'Amico's suggestion was supported by Stuart and Stallard,[9] who made it one of the pillars of the gnathologic school they founded. Later, D'Amico's theory was also supported by others, who emphasized the advantages of resorting to canines – that is, canine roots are longer than the roots of the adjacent teeth, and thus have a greater number of sensory receptors;[10] the crown/root ratio of canines is very favorable and allows for any force exerted on the crown to be transmitted to the periodontium without any intensification; and canines are the teeth that tend to be lost last.[11] Canines are located at the end of the arm of a class-3 lever, away from the power arm of the powerful levator muscles.[12]

In a survey conducted on 1200 American soldiers aged below 25, Scaife[13] found that most of the soldiers showed canine disclusion, either unilateral or bilateral. They also pointed out that tooth wear increases in inverse proportion to canine disclusion. From this it may be inferred that, as canine attrition develops, the resulting group function becomes the factor that boosts tooth wear. In a review of the literature, Woda and coworkers[14] conclude that "pure canine protection or pure group function rarely exists and balancing contacts [on the non-working side (balance side)] seem to be the general rule in the population of contemporary civilization".

Belser and Hannam[15] studied 12 bruxers who showed occlusion with attrition and group function on the working side during lateral movement. Their original group function occlusions were transformed into canine disclusion, and this resulted in lower electromyographic (EMG) readings. Later, another team of researchers conducted a similar trial and obtained similar results.[16] However, these researchers pointed out that the decrease in EMG activity from canine disclusion was not as significant as the one in Belser and Hannam's trial. Another trial compared the EMG readings of two groups of healthy individuals – one group showing group function and the other one showing canine guidance – during lateral movement.[17] Canine guidance was shown to reduce EMG activity more than group function.

From a strictly mechanical point of view, we should prefer a canine guidance scheme to a group function scheme. When there is canine guidance, only two teeth will be subject to wear from eccentric bruxism: the canines. The scenario is different when there is group function, since between eight and 10 teeth may be interacting. Undoubtedly, the fact that more teeth are involved during tooth grinding boosts tooth hard-tissue loss.

Fig 25-1 **(a–d)** Patient showing major signs of attrition in his anterior teeth. **(e and f)** Canine attrition boosts wear of the posterior teeth (posterior group function). **(g and h)** Acid-etched right maxillary canine; a strip of acetate protects adjacent teeth from the action of the acid.

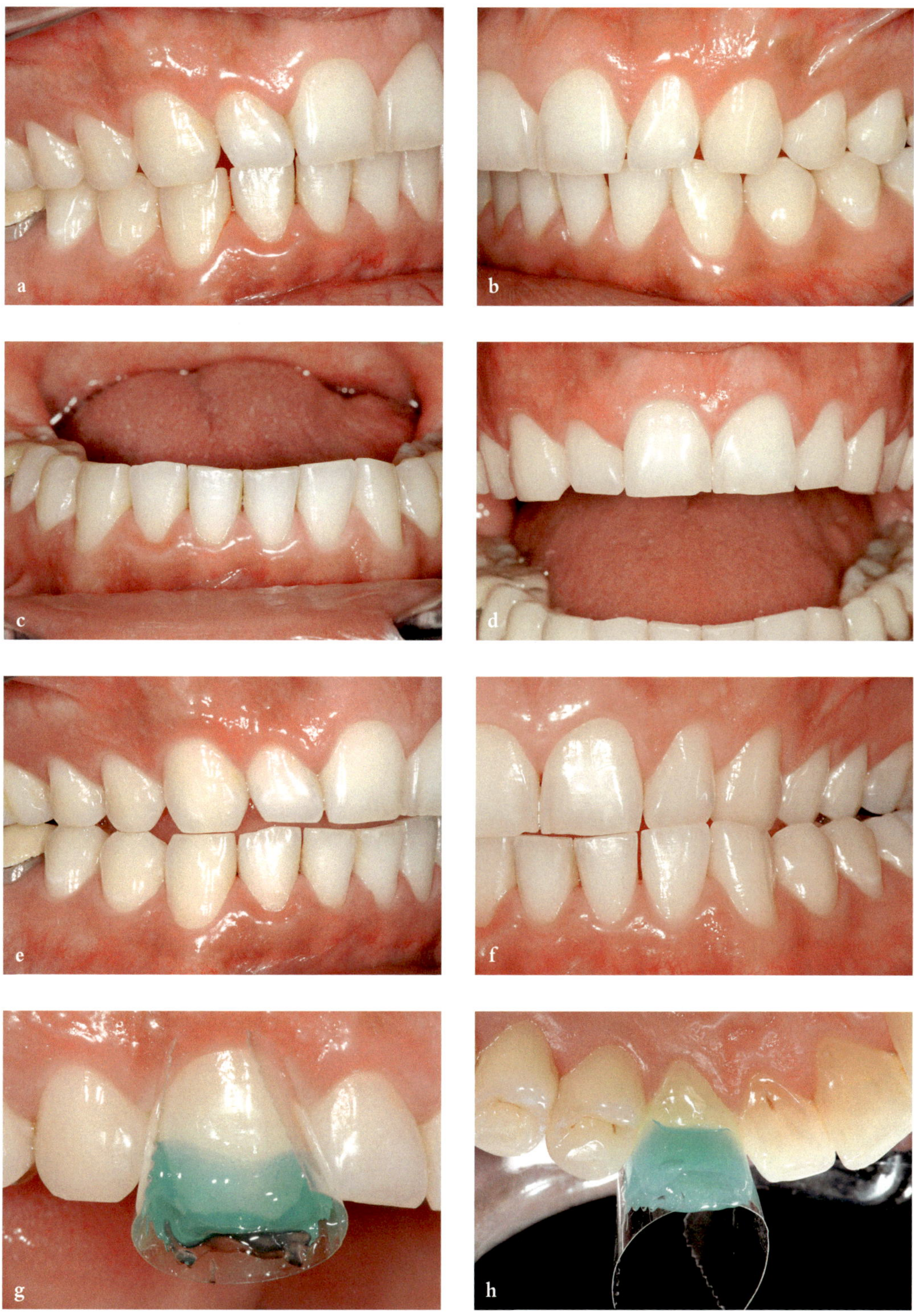
a
b
c
d
e
f
g
h

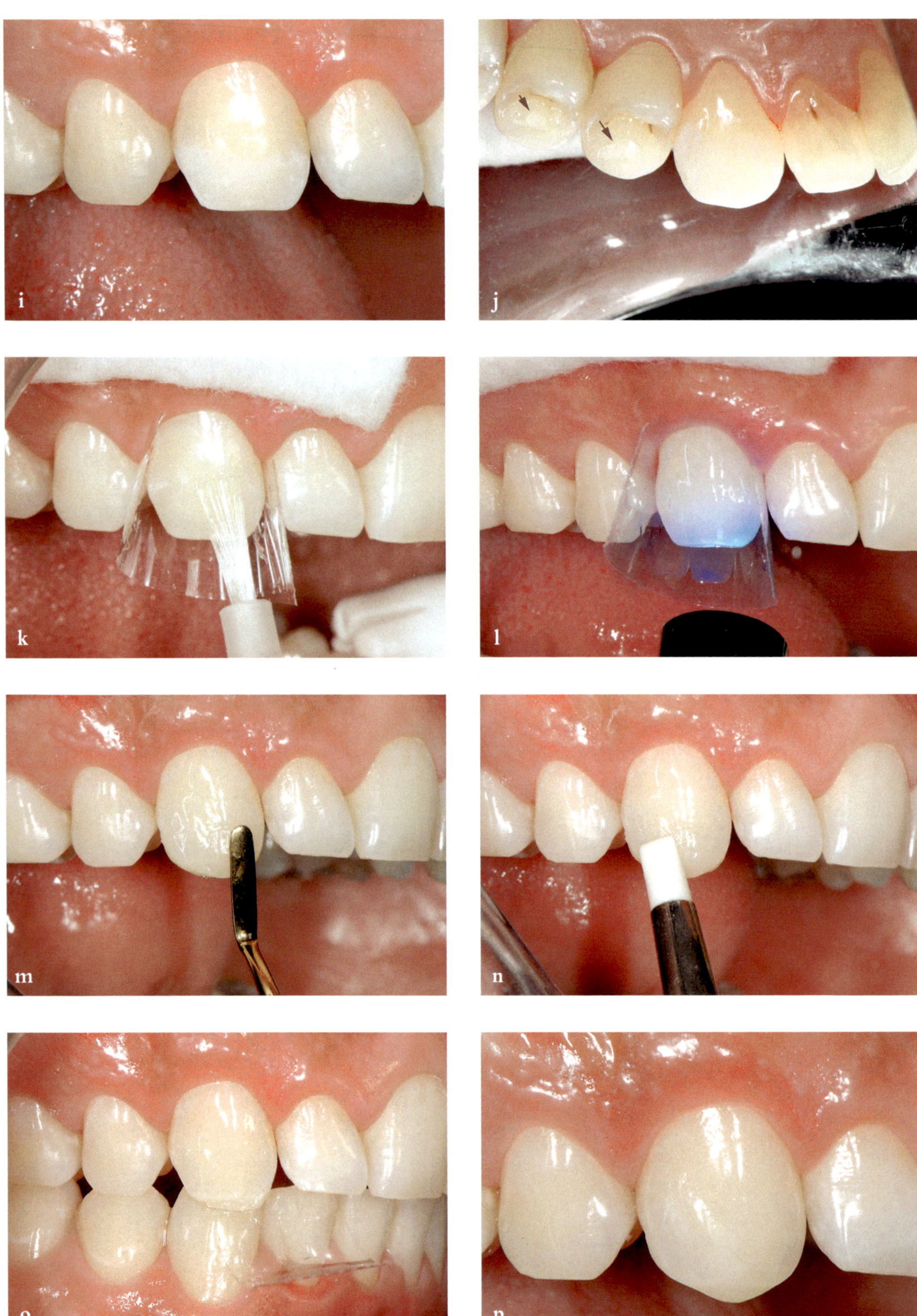
i
j
k
l
m
n
o
p

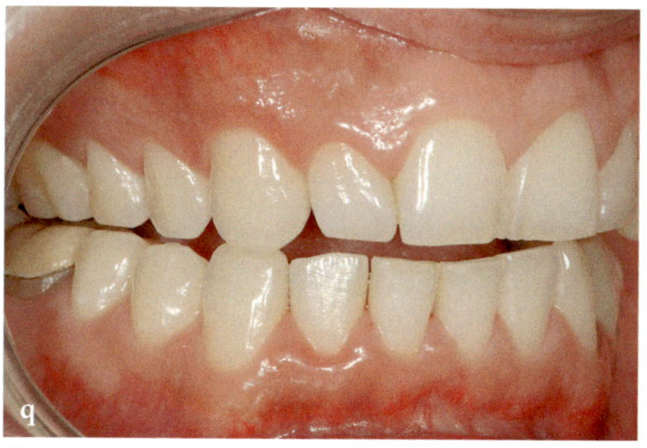


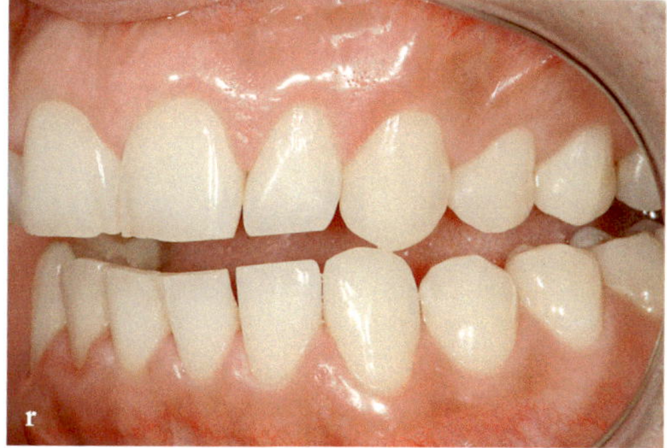


Fig 25-1 **(i and j)** Acid-etched surfaces extending widely to increase the resin anchoring area; the arrows indicate premolar attrition. **(k and l)** Bonding placement and subsequent light polymerization. **(m and n)** Composite molding. **(o)** Before proceeding to light polymerization, the patient is requested to bite over an acetate strip to prevent future composite overocclusion. **(p)** Reconstructed canine. If needed, the same procedure is repeated in the other canines. **(q and r)** Both lateral movements are controlled by canine guidance. The next step is to fabricate a bruxism splint.

### *Why is Canine Guidance Reconstructed before Splint Wearing?*

Since almost all individuals who grind their teeth will usually do it during sleep, we should wonder whether wearing a night guard is enough to protect teeth. Also, not all patients tolerate night guards or accept the wearing of them; the ones who do will usually not do it conscientiously – they will not systematically put the splint inside their mouth when they are going to sleep. The reasons are many: they will fall asleep while watching TV; they are embarrassed to wear the splint in front of "occasional bed partners"; they do not take the splint with them when they go on a journey for fear that it might get lost; or, simply, they are not consistent.

Irregularity in the use of splints is common. A study carried out in Sweden showed that the frequency of use of splints is variable, and after 2 years patients will stop wearing them.[18] Although the reasons have not been reported, lack of motivation may be inferred to be one of them – in other words, lack of health education. Dental practitioners have the responsibility of explaining to each patient who is diagnosed a bruxer how to prevent its harmful effects. Some clinicians will "present" their patients with bruxism splints on finishing treatment, especially if such treatment entailed long occlusal rehabilitation. The true goal behind such kindness is to protect the supposed durability guarantee implicitly demanded by patients after spending a great amount of money on the treatment. In this regard, it is important to point out that giving a splint as a gift does not guarantee that it will be worn. The following example will better illustrate this idea. If one buys a luxury car, the insurance is not included nor given as a gift by the dealer; it must be bought separately, and the insurance premium will usually be accordingly expensive. Coming back to dentistry, we consider that it is the patient who should freely decide to "buy" a splint after receiving a detailed "bruxism lesson" from the clinician and if feeling motivated to protect themselves from the effects of bruxism.

It is also true that, nowadays, bruxism splints are made for all patients as a routine, often including patients who are not bruxers. This may be another reason why patients will usually stop wearing the splints – in this case, it is a justified

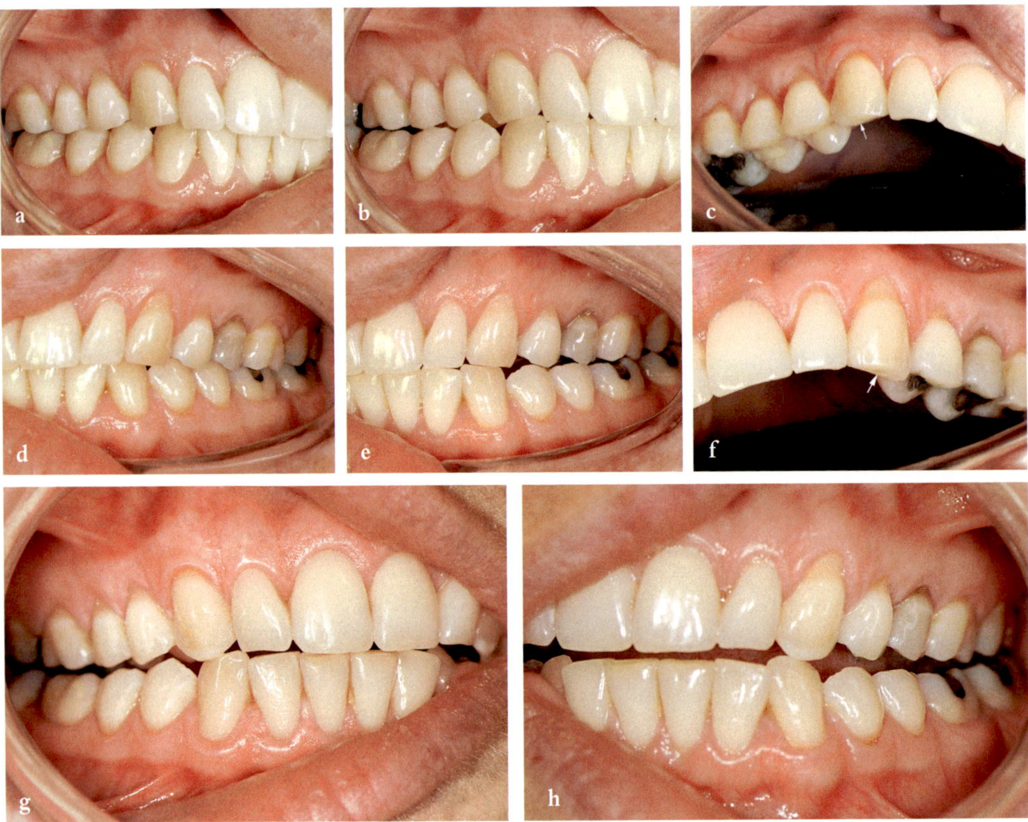

Fig 25-2 **(a and b)** Patient with tender non-carious cervical lesions in his posterior teeth. Such lesions may possibly be related to the group function which results from canine guidance wear due to bruxism. **(c)** Canine attrition, with exposed dentin (arrow). **(d–f)** The same is observed on the left side. **(g and h)** Resultant canine protection after composite reconstruction.

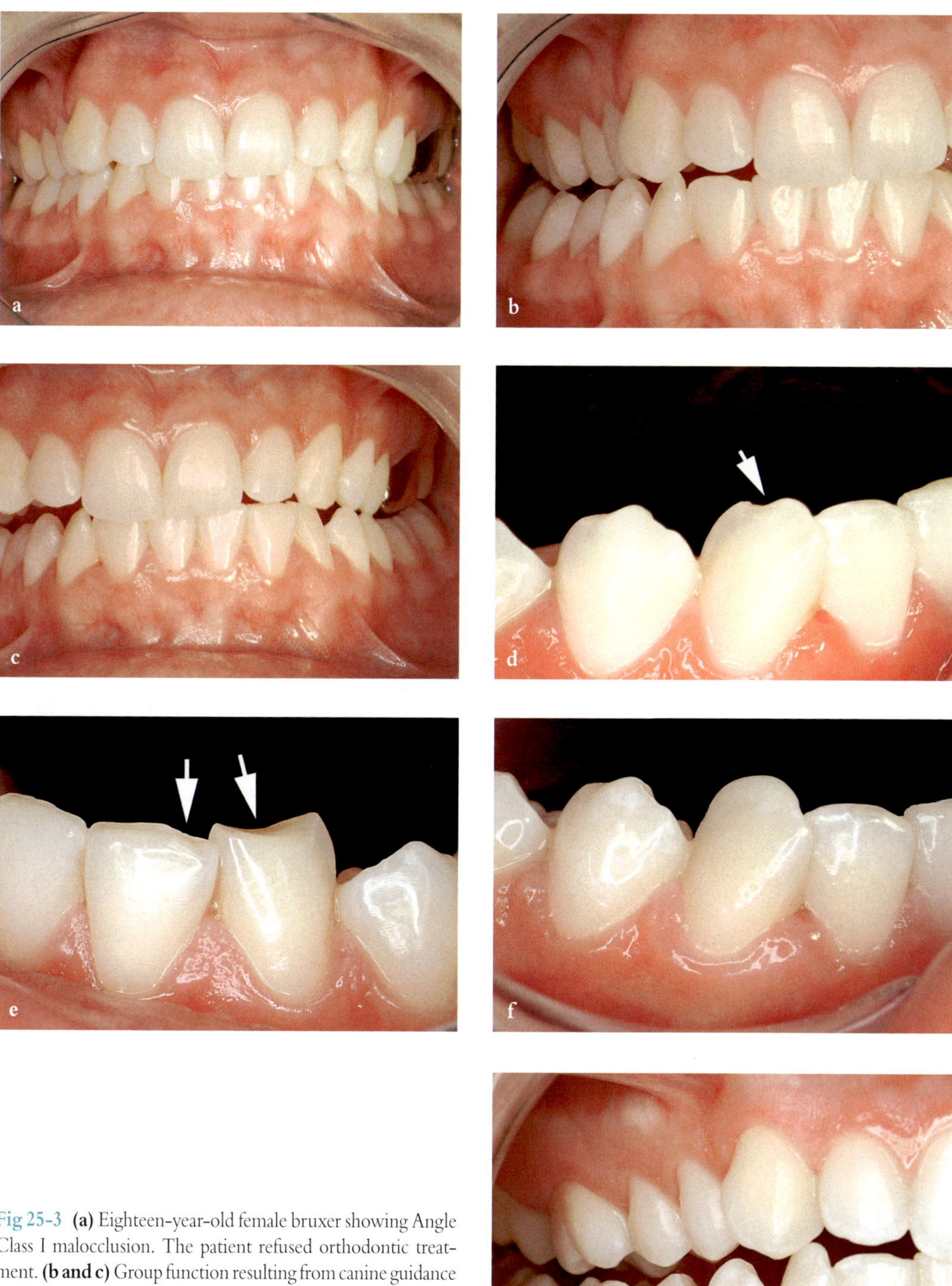


Fig 25-3 **(a)** Eighteen-year-old female bruxer showing Angle Class I malocclusion. The patient refused orthodontic treatment. **(b and c)** Group function resulting from canine guidance attrition: presence of fresh non-carious cervical lesions. **(d and e)** Major dental tissue loss (arrow). **(f and g)** Mandibular right canine reconstruction restores the correct functioning of the canine guidance.

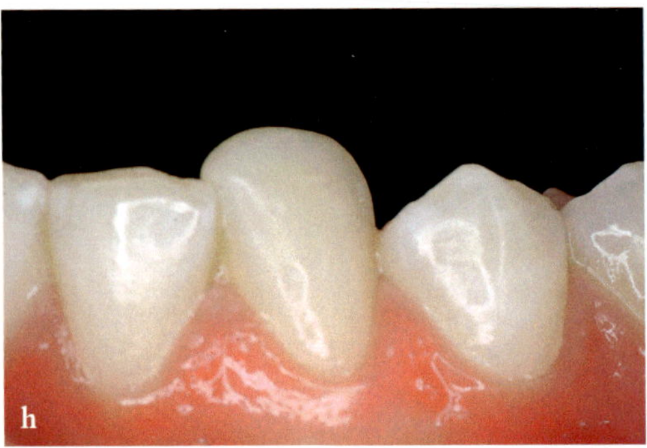

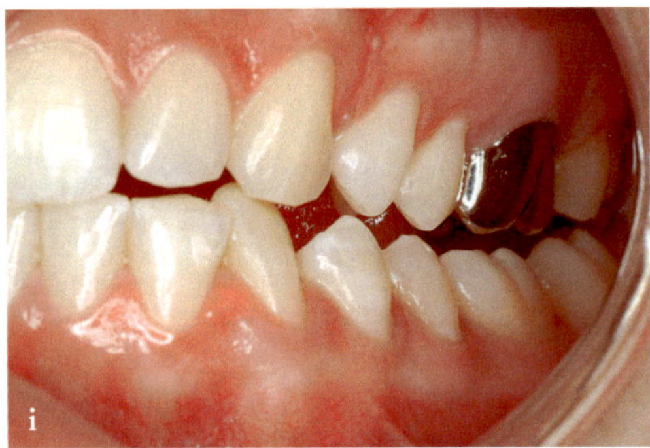

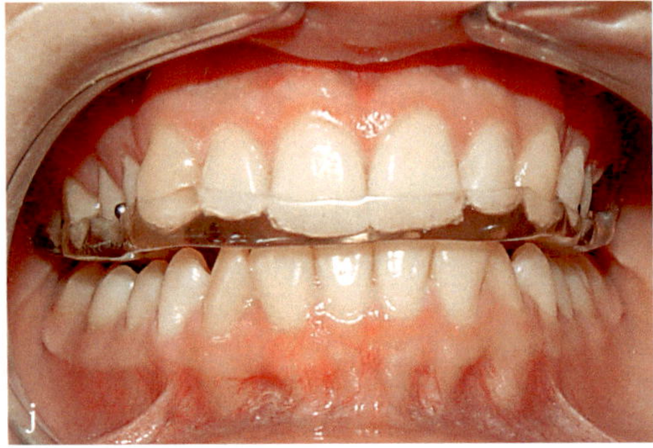

Fig 25-3 **(h and i)** The left side was treated similarly. **(j)** This simple, minimal treatment is completed by a bruxism splint which the patient will wear during sleep.

reason, simply because these subjects are not bruxers, and thus they do not need to wear a splint.

For all the above reasons, and whenever there is doubt or uncertainty about the consistency of the patient regarding splint wear and about the amount of time the splint will need to be worn, we think it advisable to restore canine guidance before prescribing a splint. This does not entail the necessity of sophisticated treatment; it just involves restoring the guidance that has been lost. The treatment consists of simple, non-aggressive procedures using composite and the acid-etching technique. A treatment plan involving a more significant prosthetic development can be decided on only when the patient demands esthetic and/or functional satisfaction.

Canine protection can also help reduce the loss of tooth hard tissue in some diurnal tooth grinding cases. Though this is rare, there are patients who grind their teeth during wakefulness – they will even grind their teeth without noticing it while we are questioning them.

The clinical series in Figs 25-1 to 25-4 show simple canine guidance reconstructions performed with light-cured composites.

## Bruxism Splints

As discussed in Chapter 20, splints effectively protect teeth against the action of bruxism. Fabricating a bruxism splint is much easier than other tasks performed by dental practitioners in their offices. However, in their visits to craniomandibular dysfunction or bruxism specialists, many patients will complain that they were never able to wear the

Fig 25-4 **(a and b)** Female bruxer suffering from significant tenderness at the cervical level of the teeth in the posterior segment; fresh non-carious lesions are present. **(c and d)** Canine attrition caused group function to occur in posterior teeth during tooth grinding. **(e and f)** Canine reconstruction restored right-side guidance. **(g and h)** The left side was treated similarly.

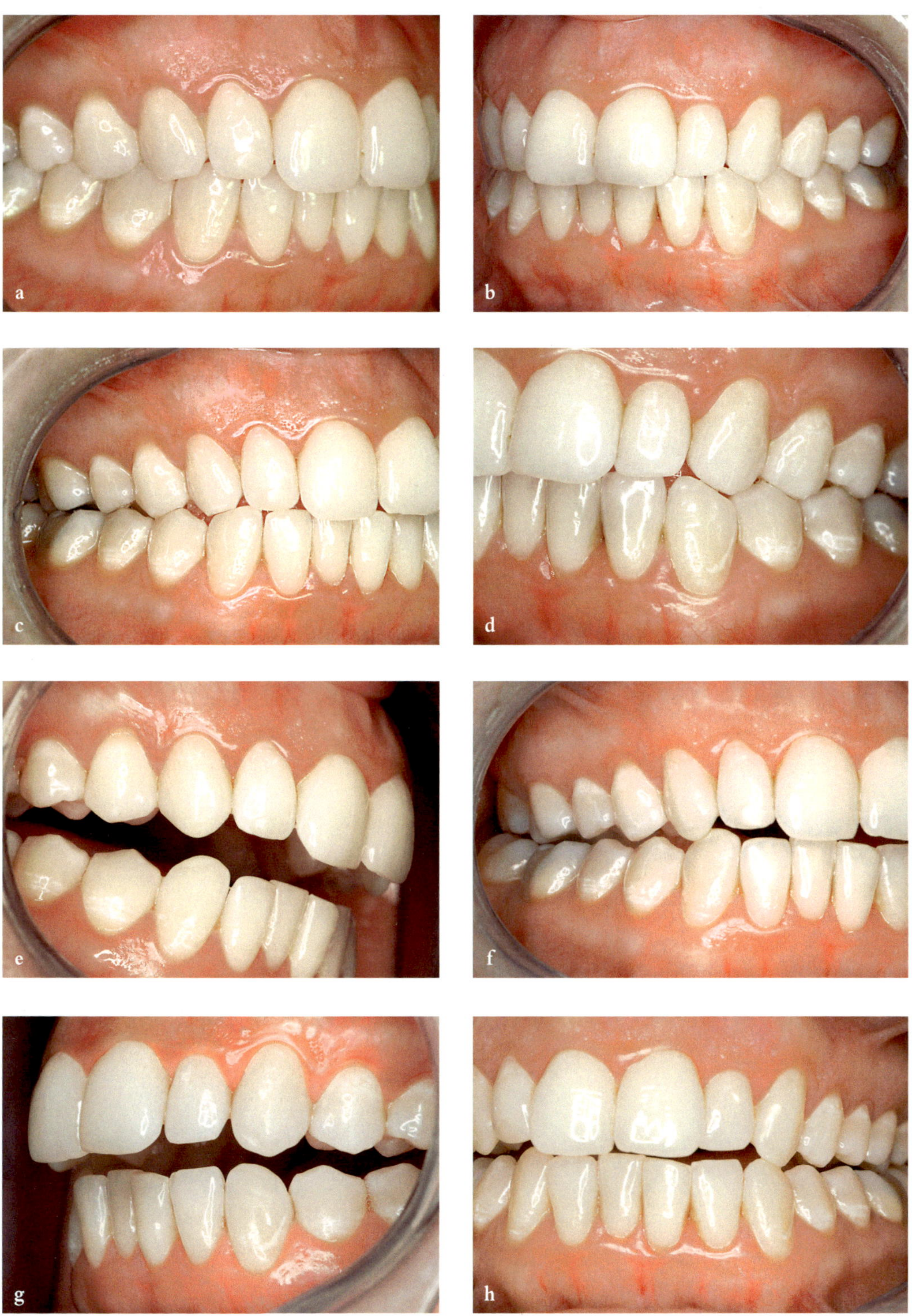
a
b
c
d
e
f
g
h

splints fabricated for them. Although no data on this subject are available in the literature, this situation is common in clinical practice. Clearly, clinicians do not always take into consideration all the details necessary to make a splint acceptable to a patient.

The human mouth is much more than just a door through which food comes into the body. Its exquisite sensitivity is the product of the sum of innumerable sensory receptors, each contributing to its components. The tongue, the teeth, soft tissues, muscles, and temporomandibular joints coexist in harmony from birth and throughout the different growth and development stages. When a splint is incorporated into the oral cavity, it will immediately be detected as a foreign body by the components of the mouth, and it will have to coexist in harmony with them. If details like size, texture, etc. are taken care of when fabricating a splint, the device will be well-accepted by the demanding oral environment.

This has not been the case with the design of some experimental splints that were recently used.[19,20] Splints without occlusal coverage and "extra thick" palate will reduce EMG activity but will not fully eliminate bruxism. In our opinion, it is not advisable to use these splints, for several reasons. First, they do not protect teeth, and although they have been shown to have some degree of effectiveness, they do not eliminate bruxism. Second, no reports are available on the degree of patient acceptance of these splints. Besides, the study population was composed of dental practitioners and dental students, who show a high degree of cooperation. The characteristics of the study population are not representative of real patients and their demands.

### *Requirements to be Met by Splints*

Splints should meet some requirements tending to promote patient acceptance and to prevent iatrogenic effects.

*Requirements for good patient acceptance*

In summary:

- A reasonable balance should exist between thickness and resistance.
- They should be smooth, soft and well-polished.
- In order to prevent them from moving, they should be attached by means of clasps.
- They should not cause any pain; the patient should feel comfortable.
- The patient should feel comfortable when occluding; simultaneous contact of all the antagonists should occur.

Balance should be sought between the thickness and resistance of a splint. Thick splints guarantee greater durability, but coexistence with the components of the oral environment will be difficult. Initially, in the 1980s, thick splints (around 10 mm thickness) were thought to produce a greater decrease in muscle activity.[21] However, this was called into question, since such decrease in EMG activity, though immediate, has not been shown to persist.[22] In a biomechanical study carried out to demonstrate the balance of normal force vectors transmitted into the masticatory system by a splint, Dos Santos and De Rijk[23] warn about the potential risk of wearing thick splints. These researchers recommend wearing thin splints, which exert less force at the articular level. On the other hand, though thin splints take less space in the mouth and will be better tolerated, they will be affected by the forces to which they are subjected. One of the drawbacks of thin splints is that they can break easily. If this should happen during sleep, the patient might swallow some pieces (Fig 25-5). This can be prevented by embedding a stainless steel mesh inside the acrylic in the posterior segments (Fig 25-6). The esthetic appearance of night guards is usually not taken into consideration, but it should be, since many patients have bed partners and they will often request that we do not neglect esthetics.

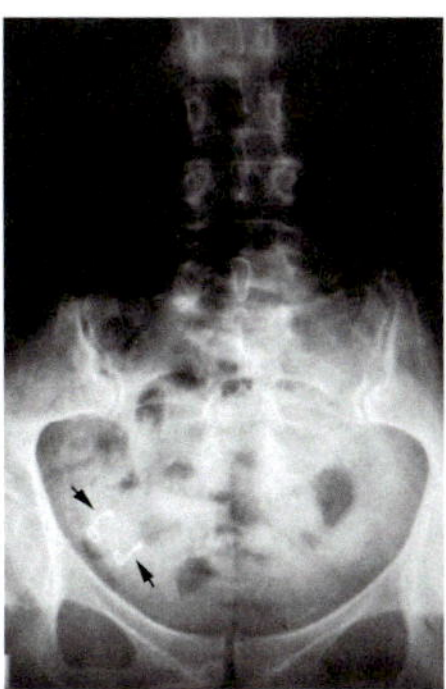

Fig 25-5 Radiograph showing a piece of splint in the intestine. Arrows indicate the metallic retainers.

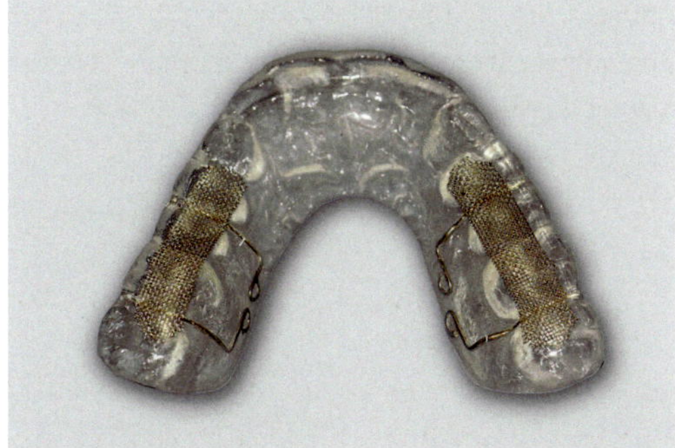

Fig 25-6 Bruxism splint with a stainless steel mesh embedded in the acrylic. If the splint breaks while it is being worn, the pieces will not be swallowed by the patient.

Splints should be smooth, well-polished, and well-finished in order not to cause an unpleasant feeling when they come into contact with soft tissues, and to prevent quick pigmentation and the bacterial accumulation typically resulting from the coexistence with oral fluids. Also, bad smell and bad taste – which may lead the patient to reject the splint – will be prevented. Clinicians should have a polisher in the dental office, because after making all the necessary occlusal adjustments that splints usually require, such splints must be polished.

Though involuntarily, many individuals will take the splint off in their sleep. Adding properly tightened retainers to the splint will solve this problem. Splints should act as a block element that is perfectly adjusted to the anatomy of the dental arch, and they should not move at all; this will prevent the exertion of orthodontic-type forces that might cause some teeth to move. Retainers should not produce morning pain from over-tightness or from being in decubitus position against oral soft tissues. Splints should remain steady, but they should not cause a feeling of pressure or pain. Sometimes, defects from wrongly taken impressions cause splints to fit poorly and exert pressure on a tooth or soft tissue. This should be corrected in the first try-in visit, to prevent the patient from rejecting the splint from the very beginning.

It is essential that the patient feels that there is simultaneous occlusion of all the antagonist teeth. Heavy occlusal contacts between some isolated pieces may cause traumatic periodontitis, and the patient will be forced to take the splint off in order to relieve the pain. The occlusion should be adjusted before the splint is delivered to the patient. Two pieces of information are essential in order to successfully adjust occlusion: data provided by articulating paper, and the feeling perceived by the patient on closing their mouth. Usually, patients themselves will cause the initial occlusal adjustment to fail: though they perceive that the occlusion is not perfectly balanced, they ascribe this to the fact that they have "a new element in the mouth", and they will say "I'm sure that I will get used to it soon". But we know too well that this will not happen, and, as hours go by, the patient will have increased periodontal perception caused by the lack of occlusal adjustment.

*Requirements to prevent iatrogenic effects*

To prevent irreversible effects on dental occlusion, certain requirements should be met when fabricating a bruxism splint:

- There should be coverage of all the teeth of the jaw.
- The splint should control the contacts of all antagonist teeth.

- The splint should hold the vestibular third of teeth.
- The splint should be of the proper size, in order to prevent swallowing or broncho-aspiration.

Dental occlusion is a dynamic system; teeth tend to extrude and antagonist teeth are their natural control mechanism. Thus, failure to cover all the teeth may cause the bruxism splint to act as an orthodontic appliance. This unwanted effect is common whenever the splint does not reach the third molars, so that they are free to extrude and produce an open bite (Fig 25-7).

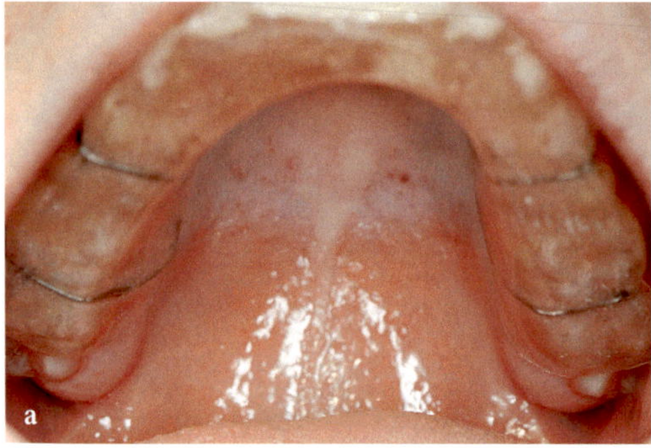

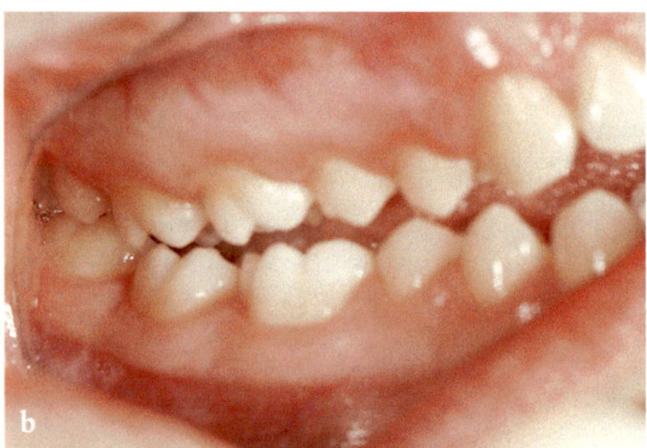

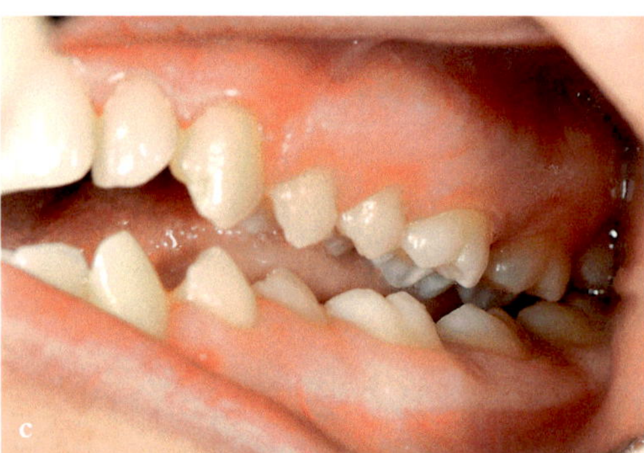

Fig 25-7 **(a)** Bruxism splint that does not cover the third molars. **(b and c)** Malocclusion from wearing this splint.

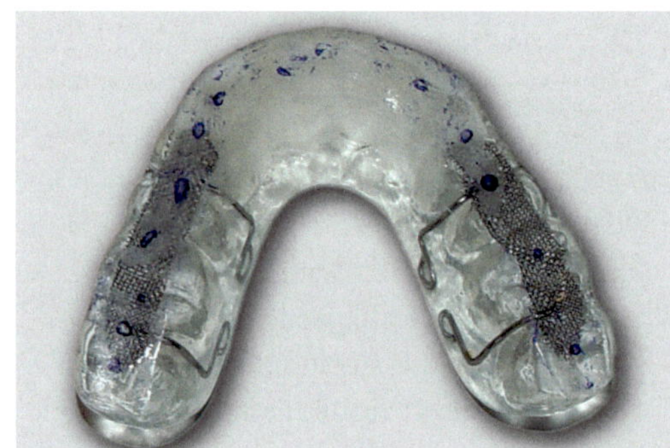

Fig 25-8 A flat occlusal surface helps to control occlusion on the splint.

This effect is an important resource that can be used therapeutically to treat a bruxism sequel: tooth wear. In 1975, Dahl and co-workers[24] described the use of a removable anterior splint that creates a posterior interocclusal space in patients showing loss of tissue in their anterior teeth. The technique is described in detail in Chapter 20.

Occlusal control from antagonist teeth is very important. Teeth that do not come into contact with the splint may soon extrude. In contrast, those in premature occlusal contact may undergo intrusion. Controlling occlusion is very easy when the surface of the splint is smooth and flat; this allows the clinician to clearly visualize where the opposite cusps rest (Fig 25-8). In contrast, when splints with occlusal "geography" are made, adjustment is tedious and hard to monitor (Fig 25-9).

Is it advisable to "encircle" the incisal-vestibular edges of teeth with acrylic (Fig 25-10) to prevent potential vestibularization of the teeth – especially of the maxillary central and lateral incisors, which are more prone to mobility (Fig 25-11). Eventually, some patients may have the fantasy that the splint has caused some tooth to move, and they will complain about this. A minimal encirclement of cusp tips and incisal edges will prevent this situation. It is also advisable to keep photographs and/or previous casts as evidence, and to compare the current status of teeth with the status they had before the arches were treated. This will prevent unpleasant conflicting situations with patients.

A splint should cover all the teeth of the jaw. This will prevent accidents that may even put a patient's life at risk. On no account should "partial" splints be prescribed for wear during sleep because they are very easy to swallow. Even worse, they may enter the respiratory tract. Some have reported that wearing the so-called "mandibular deprogrammer" or "anterior jig" is beneficial.[25] This device consists of a small piece of acrylic that covers the maxillary incisors. It was introduced by Lucía in 1964 (Lucía's jig) as a tool for removing

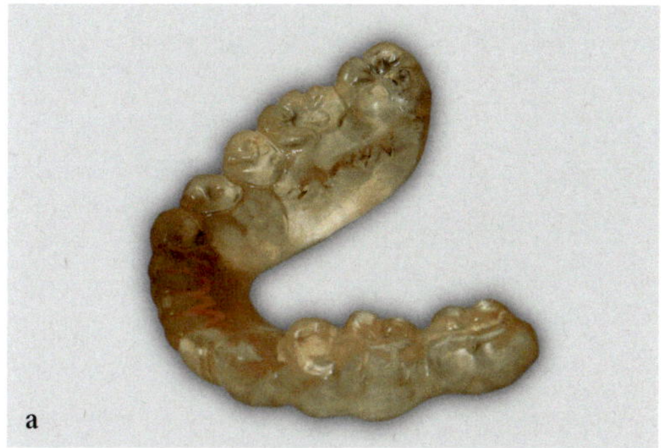


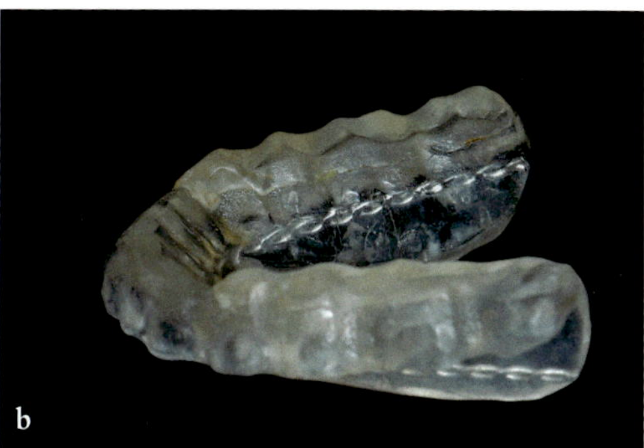


**Fig 25-9 (a and b)** Splints with occlusal "geography" are not suitable, since occlusion adjustment is very difficult.

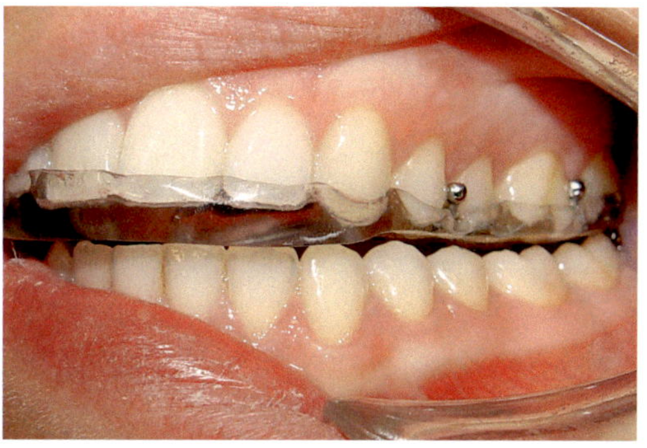

**Fig 25-10** The splint should "encircle" the incisal-vestibular edges of teeth in order to prevent them from moving.

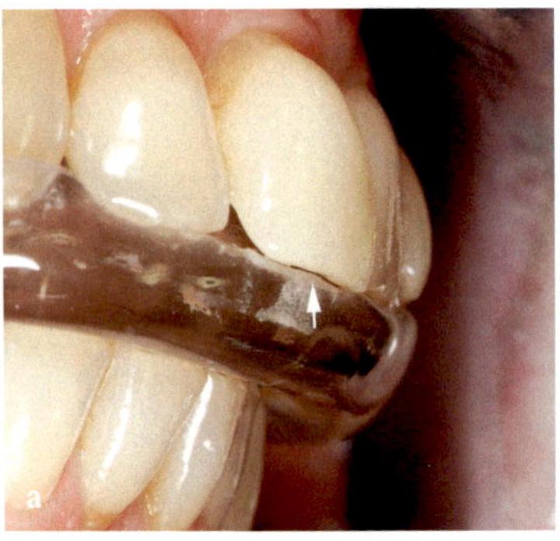


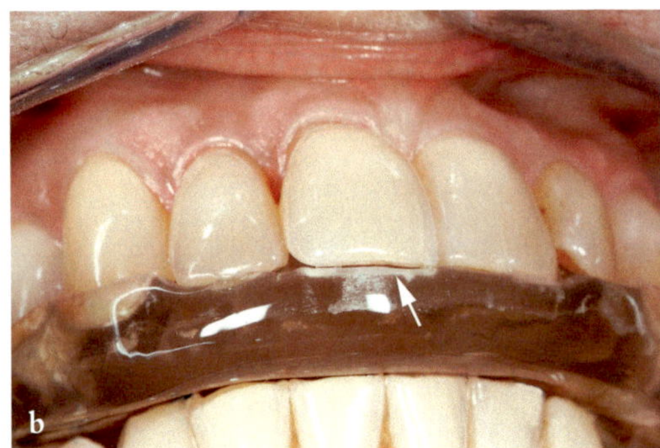


Fig 25-11 **(a and b)** This splint has an unsuitable design, since it does not "encircle" teeth. The arrow indicates a space between the splint and the incisor; this space has resulted from the movement of the tooth.

muscle engrams, and thus for being able to establish the centric relationship.[26] Although it was designed to be used in clinical maneuvers with the patient awake, many dental practitioners currently prescribe it for sleep wear. Regardless of the potential therapeutic benefits of this device (which we will not discuss here), in view of the above-mentioned risks, under no circumstances do we approve its use.

## Fabrication of the Bruxism Splint

Based on the requirements set out above and on the concepts developed in Chapter 21, this section will describe ways to fabricate splints. Although there is no evidence showing that the maxilla is any better than the mandible for splint wear, and vice versa, it seems that clinicians favor maxillary splints. In view of that predilection, and for didactic purposes, we will describe maxillary splint fabrication. Regardless of the method used, the final goals are the same.

- When closing the mouth, simultaneous occlusion of all the vestibular cusps (premolars and molars) and lower incisal edges (incisors and canines) should occur on the surface of the splint.
- During lateral movements, contact should exist only at the level of the canine on the working side (canine guidance). During protrusion, only contact in the anterior segment of the splint (incisors and canines) should occur.

Splints can be fabricated in two ways: (a) by using a muffle-up technique, and (b) by using a vacuum-stamping technique. They involve different manufacturing processes.

### *Muffled-up Bruxism Splints*

Though it involves a greater number of clinical and laboratory steps, the muffle-up technique will provide superior quality splints that are more resistant to wear. Whenever necessary, and for the reasons already discussed, we recommend that canine guidance reconstruction be performed before taking the impressions (Figs 25-12 and 25-13).

#### *Impressions*

Taking impressions in a proper way is a vital clinical step. If mistakes are made at this initial point in treatment – when capturing the oral anatomy – they will reveal themselves once the splint has been finished. It will be poorly adjusted to the mouth, it will possibly move and/or be unsteady, and the patient will find it difficult to wear.

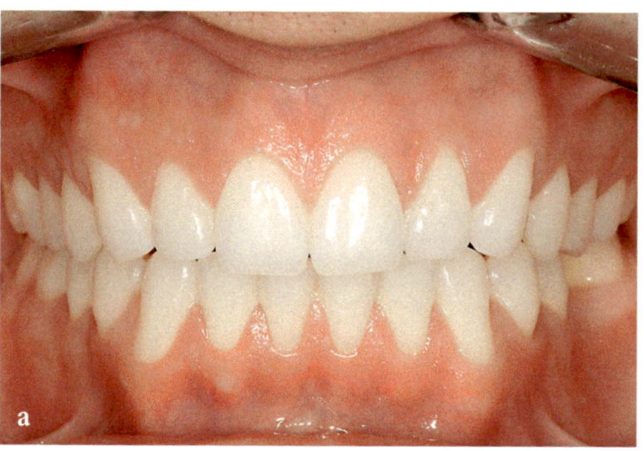


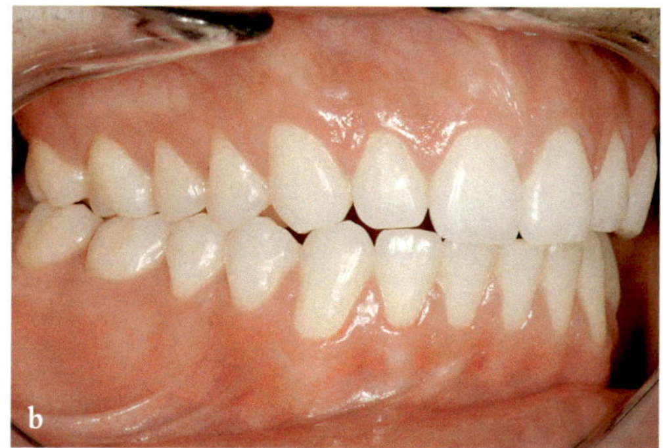


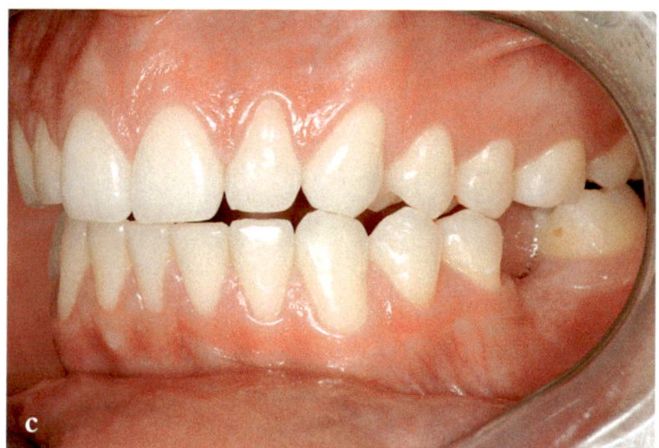


Fig 25-12 **(a–c)** Bruxer showing canine attrition which results in posterior group function during lateral movements.

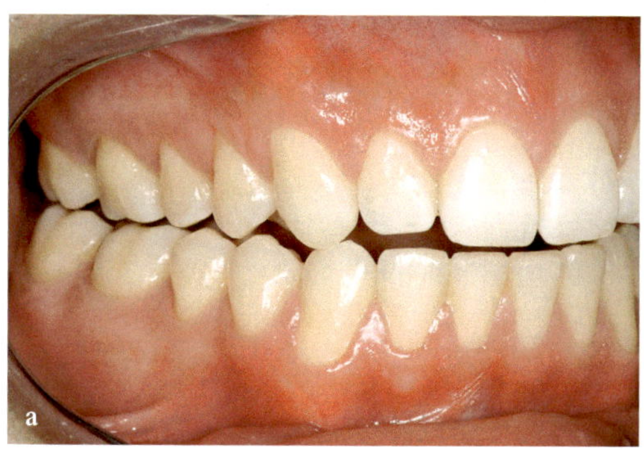


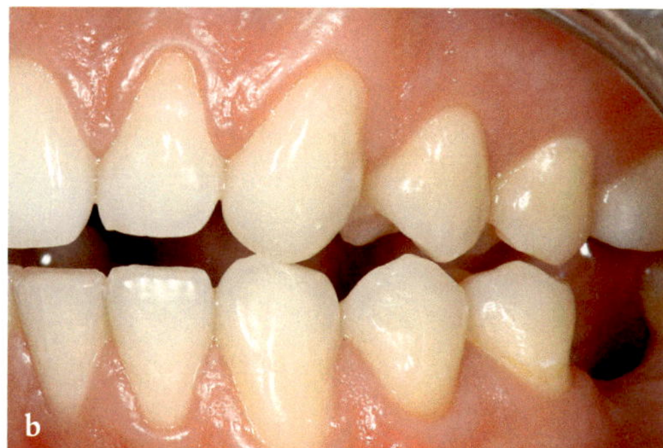


Fig 25-13 **(a and b)** Before taking the impressions for splint fabrication, canine guidance is reconstructed.

Although improved-fidelity impression materials are available, we recommend using the traditional sodium alginate. To fabricate splints, impressions are taken in patients who usually have full (though worn) dentitions. In a full dental arch, there are more than 10 interdental contact points with their corresponding gingival embrasures, into which the impression material will penetrate. Later, significant retention will occur in these areas, which will make it difficult to remove the material from the mouth. Since it can be broken easily and it has acceptable elastic recovery, the material of choice for this type of procedure is alginate.

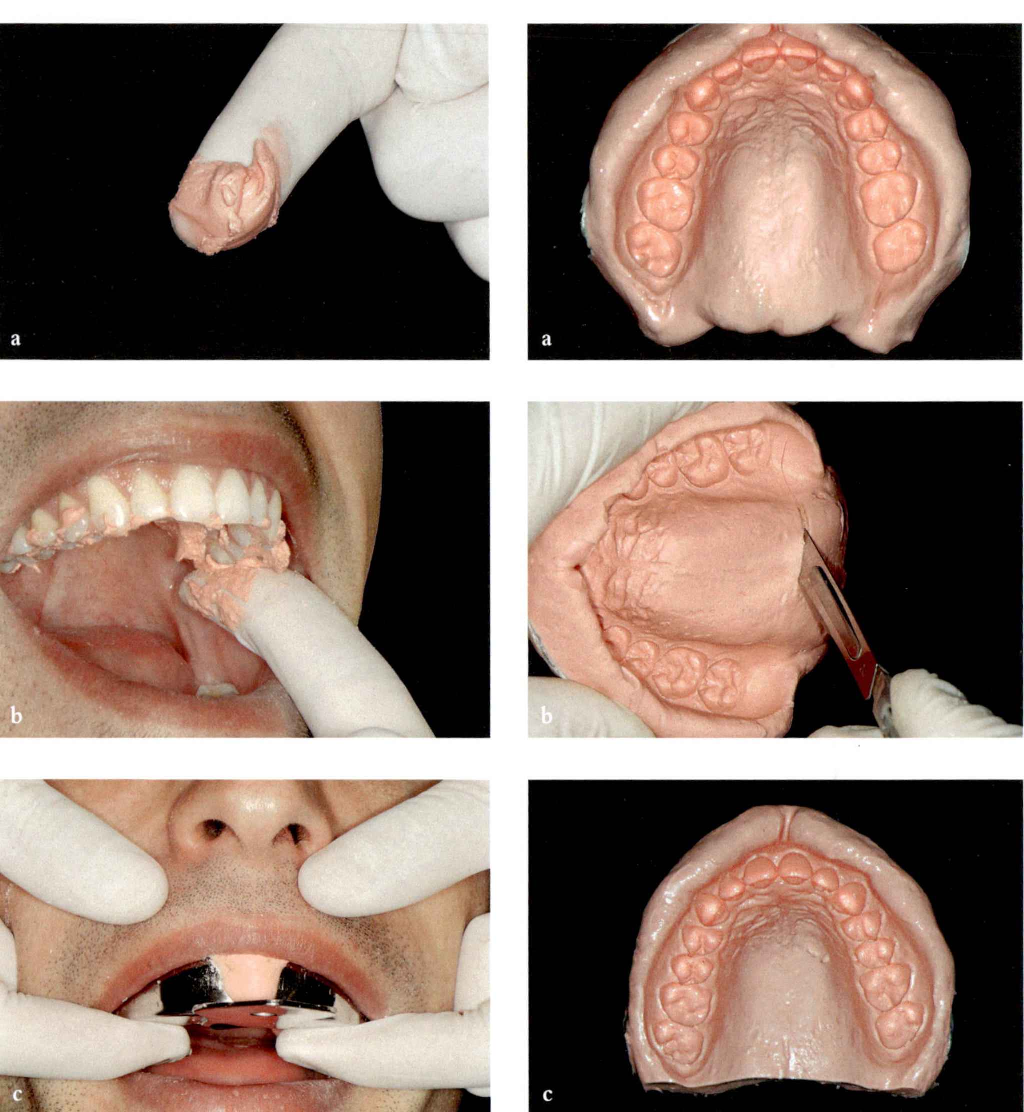

Fig 25-14 **(a and b)** Making the impression: with the forefinger tip covered with alginate, pressure is exerted on the occlusal surfaces and gingival embrasures. **(c)** The impression tray is introduced into the mouth and held with both thumbs.

Fig 25-15 **(a)** Maxilla impression. **(b)** The excess of material in the posterior segment is cut with a scalpel to prevent distortions during impression pouring. **(c)** Impression ready to be poured.

It is essential that the impressions obtained faithfully reproduce dental structures, since the splint will be in a decubitus position on them. As illustrated in Fig 25-14, before introducing the impression tray in the mouth, a good tip is to apply alginate with the forefinger in all areas that are difficult to reach, forcing the material to penetrate into interproximal spaces, cavities, and occlusal surface grooves.

When the impression tray has been removed from the mouth, it is important to cut the excess of alginate from the areas behind molars to prevent potential deformation during plaster pouring (Fig 25-15). For impression pouring, it is advisable to use high-resistance plaster (e.g., Densita plaster) which guarantees better cast integrity preservation in later stages, during laboratory work.

*Clinical registrations*

Three registrations are necessary for splint fabrication: facebow registration (to mount the upper cast); registration of the interjaw relationship (to mount the lower cast); and finally, mandibular lateral movement registration (to reproduce these movements on the articulator). Though we have already described these procedures in Chapter 21, they are illustrated once again in Figs 25-16 to 25-23.

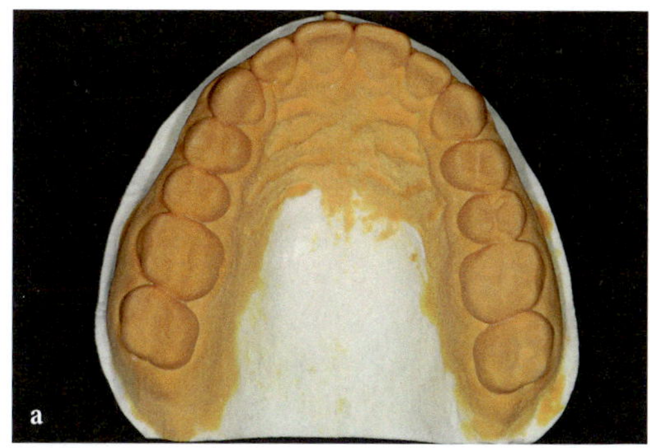
a

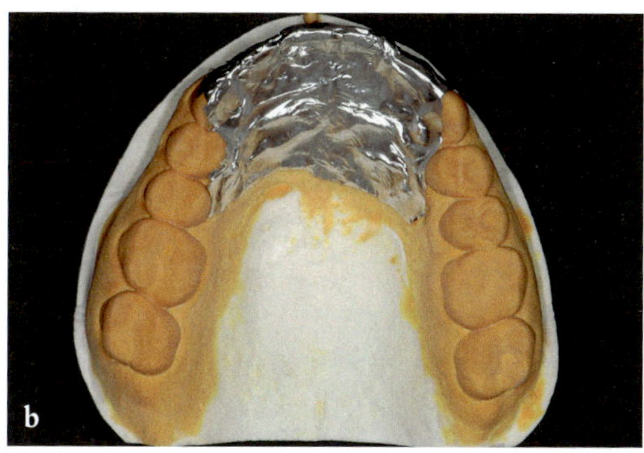
b

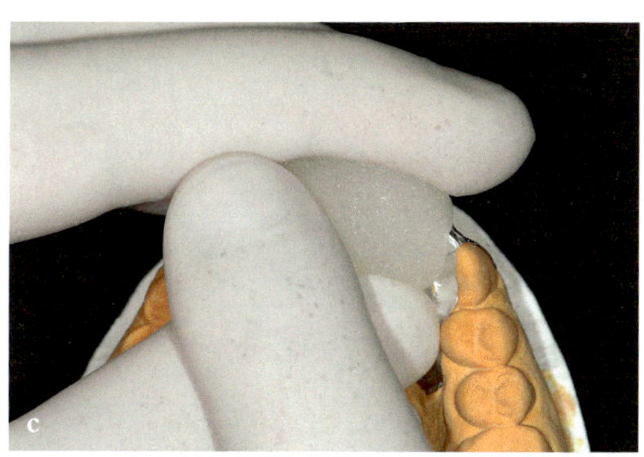
c

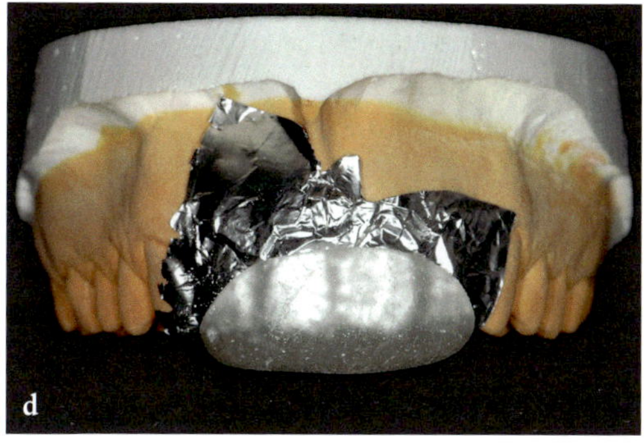
d

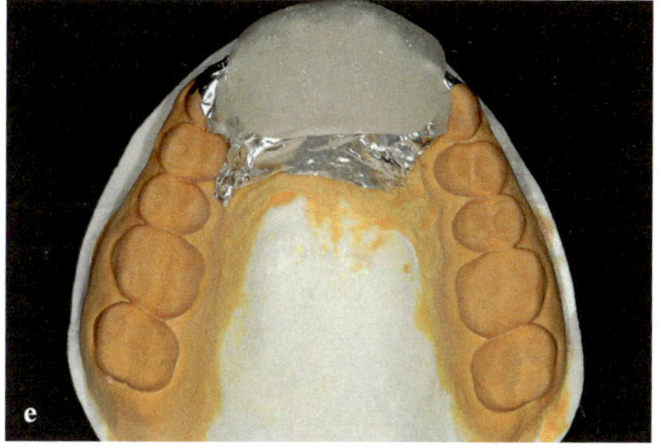
e

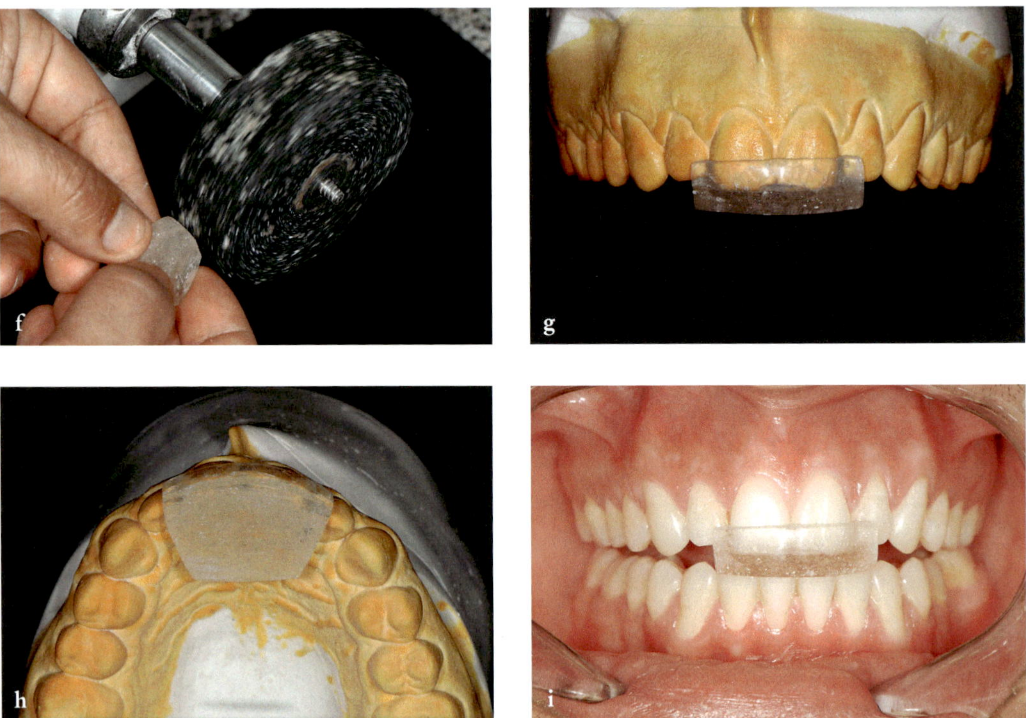

Fig 25-16 **(a–i)** Anterior bite plane fabrication. A piece of aluminum paper is adapted over the anterior teeth of the cast. Acrylic is molded with the fingers over the incisors. After acrylic polymerization, any excess material is removed and the bite plane is tried in the mouth.

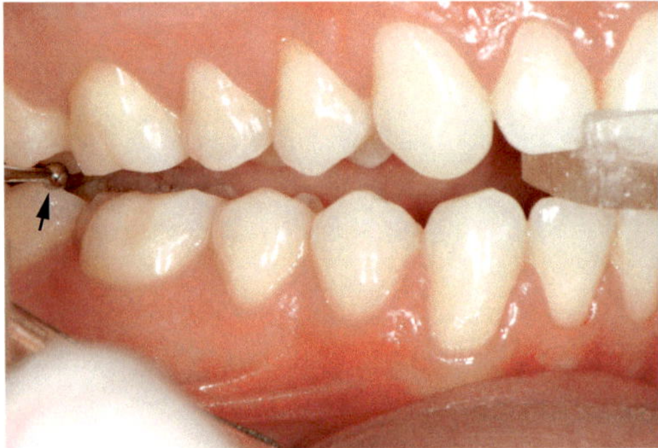

Fig 25-17 The anterior bite plane is worn down until a 2 mm lumen is obtained at the level of the second molar. Using a tool of matching size is helpful (arrow).

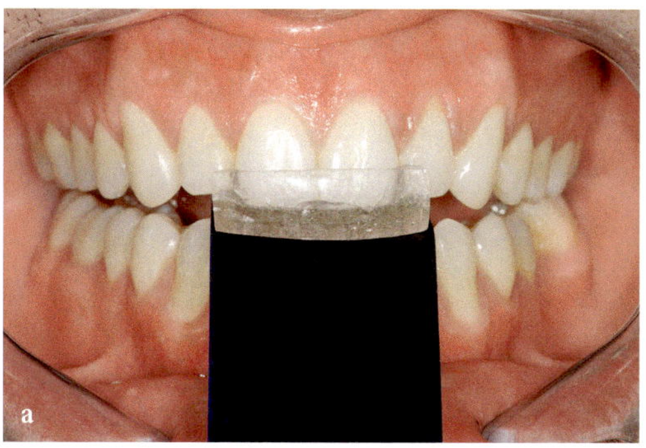

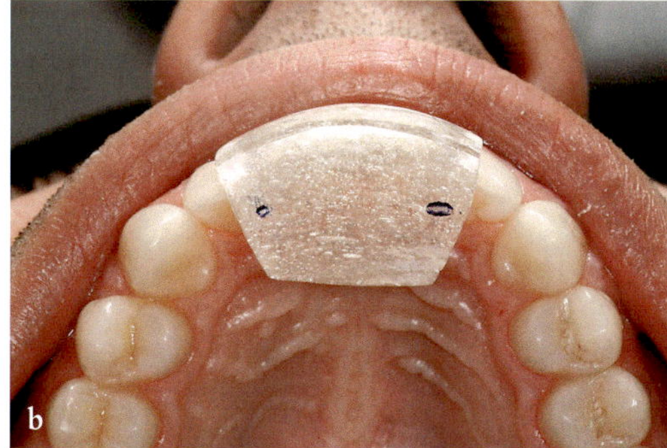

Fig 25-18 **(a)** To achieve the therapeutic position, the patient is requested to give a series of taps (3 or 4 per second) with their teeth on the surface of the platform, as the operator places articulating paper between them (as described in detail in Chapter 21). **(b)** The bite plane shows the obtained therapeutic position (blue).

Fig 25-19 Reference position. With the thumb, the operator gently manipulates the jaw into a more retrusive position, from which several taps are given on the bite plane. At the same time, the operator places articulating paper of another color in between the teeth.

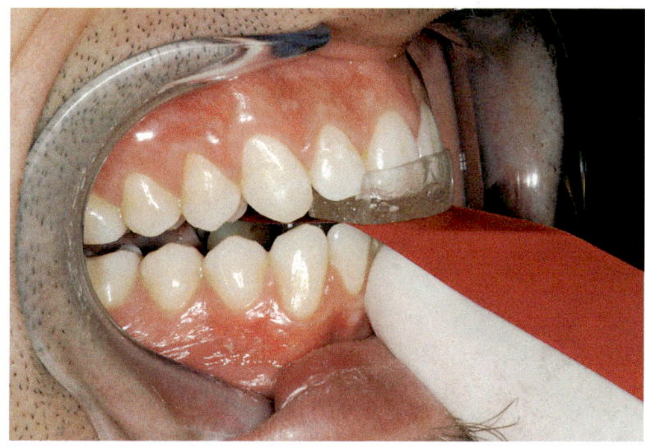

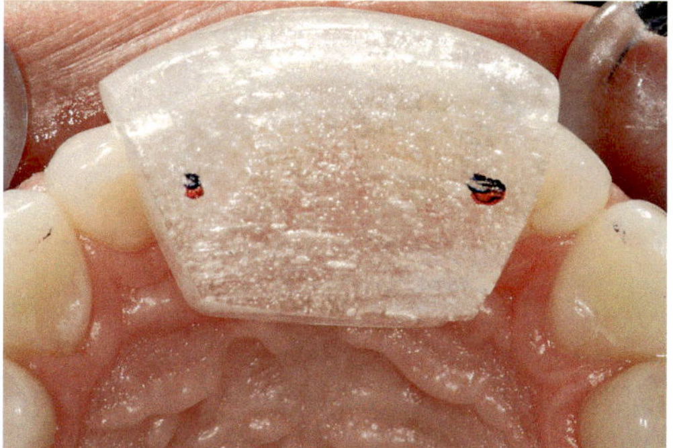

Fig 25-20 Behind the therapeutic position (blue), the retrusive position (red) used as reference can be observed. The distance between them is within an acceptable range.

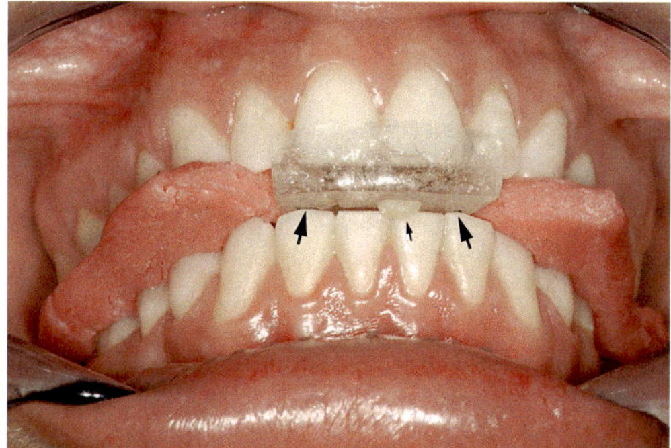

Fig 25-21 Interjaw registration by using two pieces of wax. An acrylic bite key was previously made (small arrow) while having the patient maintain their bite in the therapeutic position (big arrows).

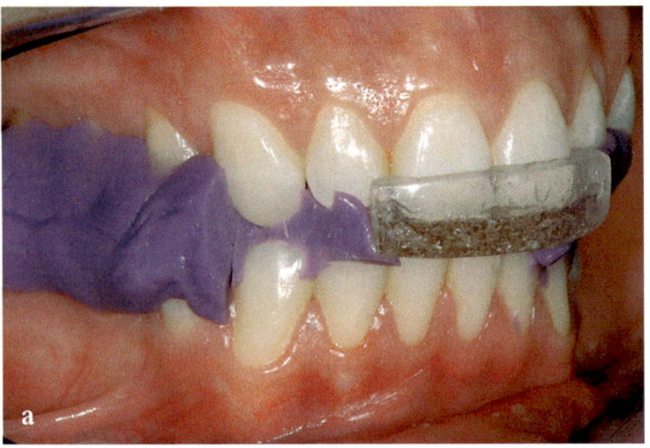
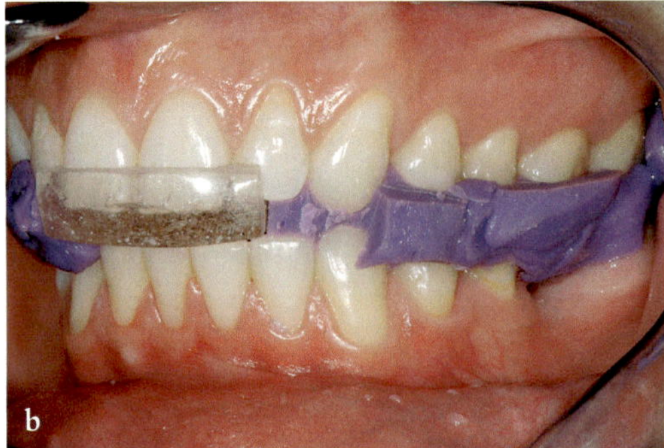

Fig 25-22 **(a and b)** Lateral movement registration by using silicone. Note the extent of the lateral movement of the jaw: canine cusp tips face each other.

*Laboratory procedures*

Although as a routine many dental practitioners will send the casts mounted on an articulator to a dental prosthesis laboratory, delegating the fabrication of the splint to them, we will describe some laboratory steps that we consider important from a didactic point of view (Fig 25-24 and 25-25).

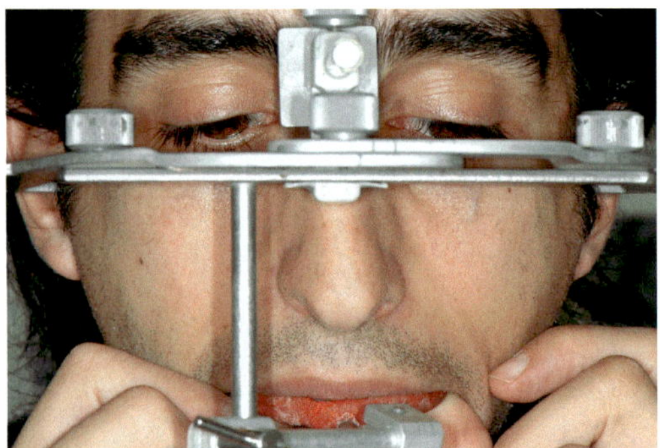

Fig 25-23 Facebow registration, which will later determine the position of the upper model on the articulator.

*Splint demarcation*

With a graphite pencil, the limits of the splint are drawn on the cast. On the vestibular surfaces, as already mentioned above, the splint should encircle the incisal edges and the cusp tips by approximately 2 mm. On the palatal surfaces, the limit should be approximately 10 mm away from the cervical region; the inactive portion of the retainers should be contained within such perimeter (Fig 25-26a–c).

*Retainer construction process*

It is essential to use metallic retainers to retain the bruxism splint in place. The strong forces of bruxism will cause the splint to progressively loosen. Being able to periodically tighten these retainers guarantees permanent anchorage of the splint to the dental arch. This can be achieved perfectly by using 0.9 mm ball clasps. Four retainers should be used, the active portions of which will be placed in the gingival embrasures, between the premolars and molars on both sides. The adjustment on the cast model is shown in detail in Fig 25-26d, e. Special care must be taken not to extend the active portion (ball) too much; this will prevent gingival papillae trauma. Once the clasps have been forged, they are attached in place to the cast by means of melted wax.

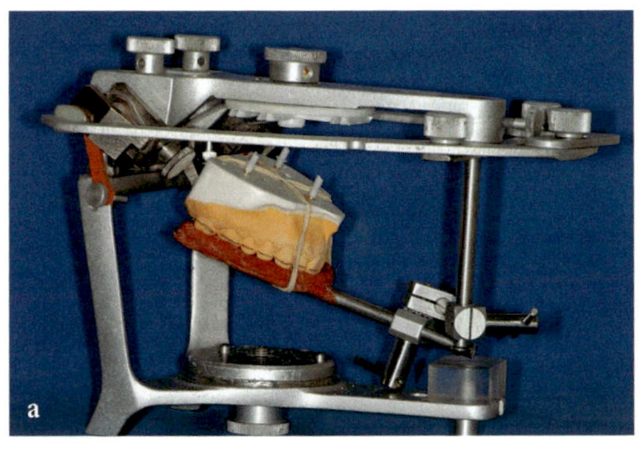

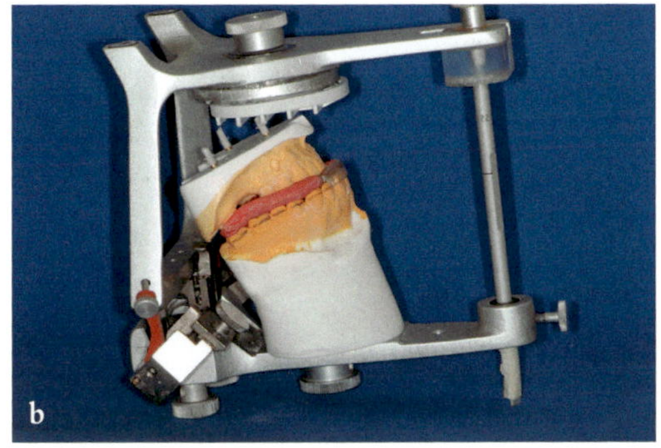

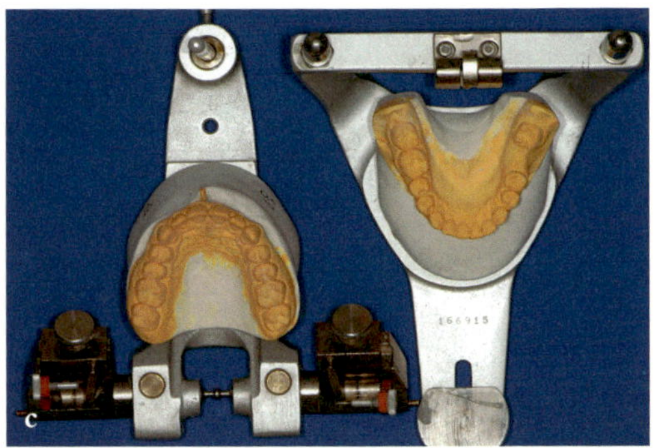

**Fig 25-24 (a–c)** Mounting of the models on the articulator.

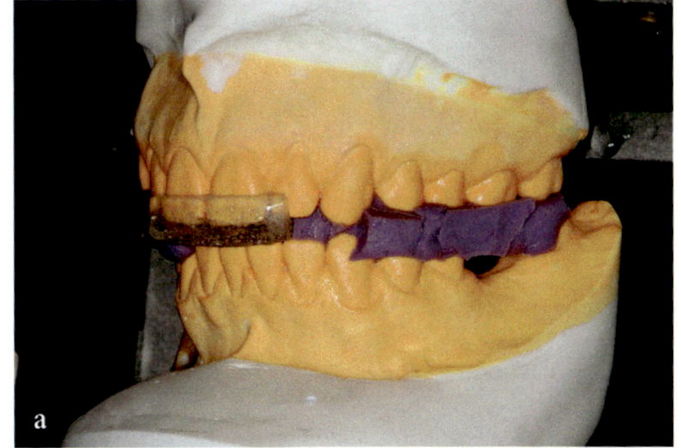

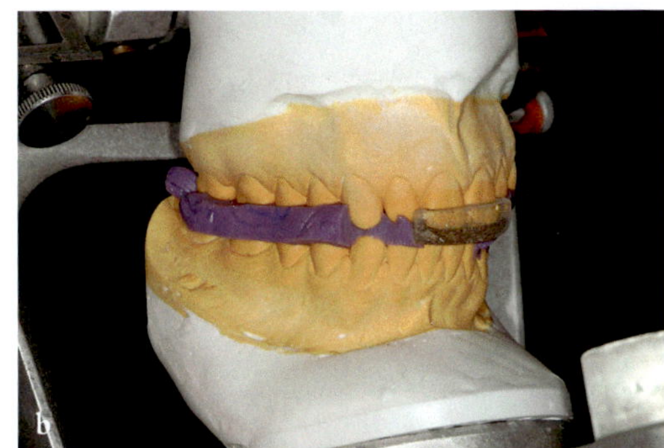

**Fig 25-25 (a and b)** Lateral-movement registrations are placed in order to program lateral movement on the articulator. **(c)** Cast mounted; the separation between models corresponds to the final thickness of the splint.

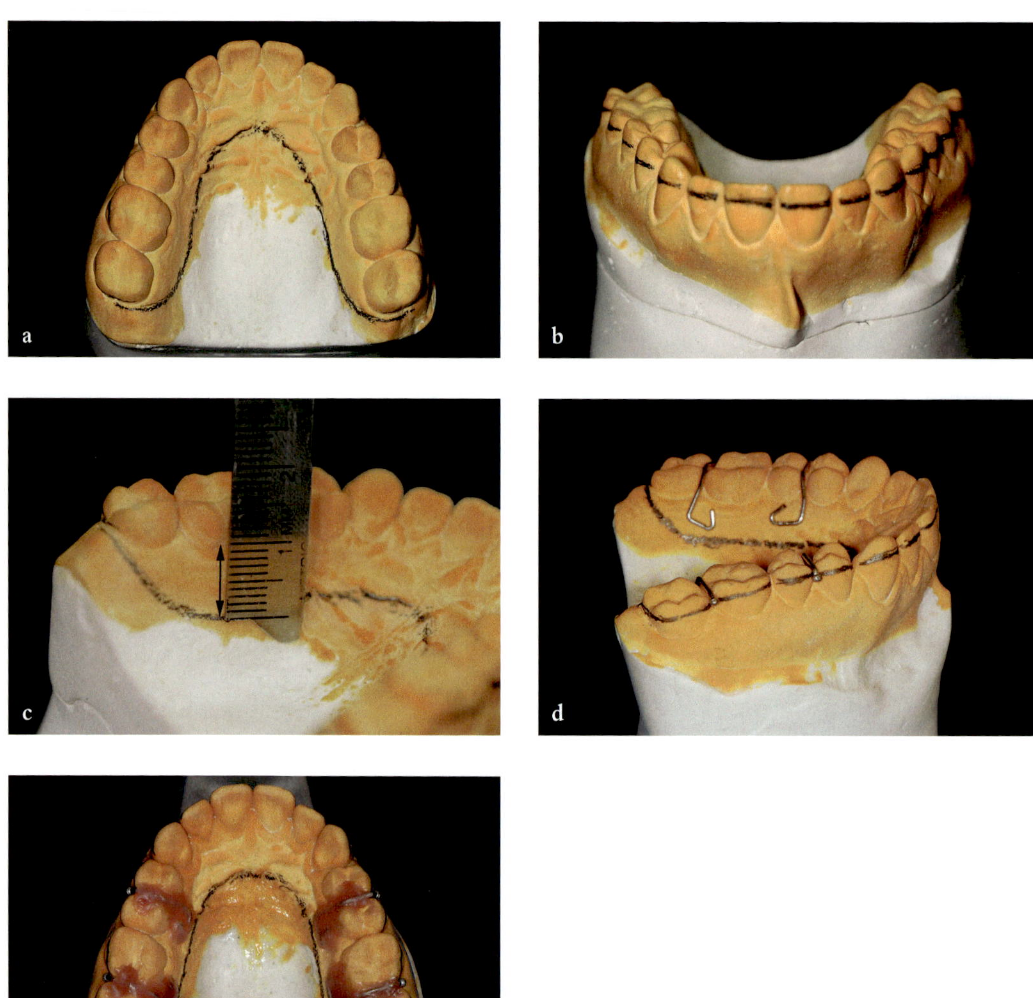

Fig 25-26 **(a–c)** Splint demarcation: approx. 10 mm in the palatal surface and 2 mm in the vestibular surface. **(d and e)** Once adapted, the retainers are stuck with wax on the cast.

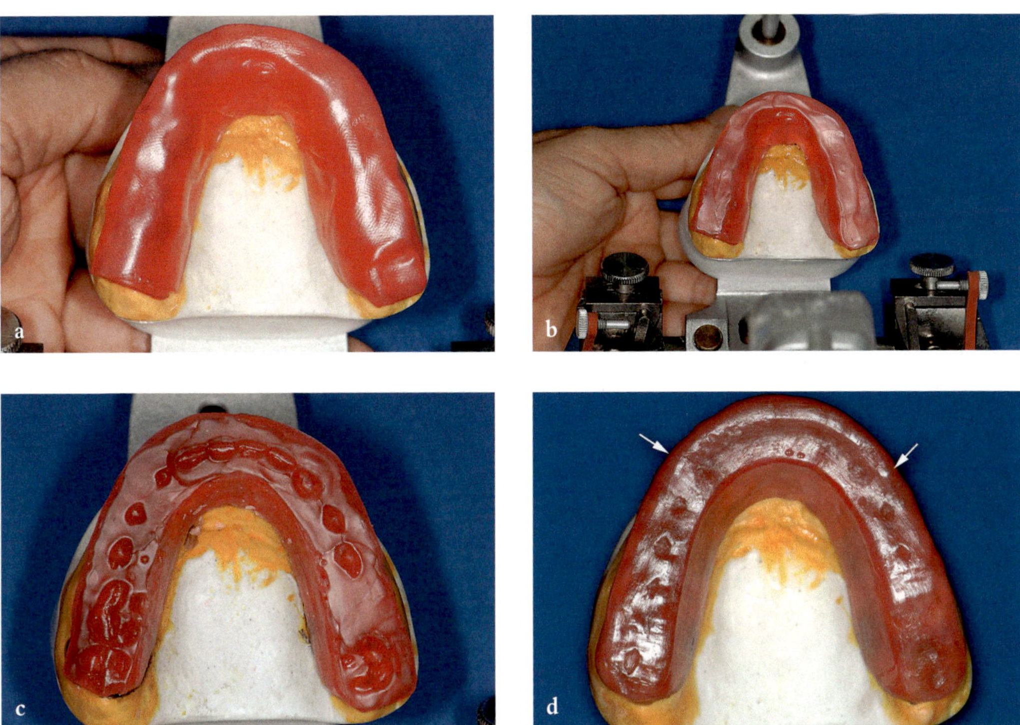

Fig 25-27 **(a–d)** Splint wax-up. Two layers of pink wax are molded; their surfaces are softened over a flame, and the articulator is closed in order to obtain the impressions of the mandibular cusps. Then the wax is tidied up. Finally, the anterior guidance (between arrows) is enhanced with wax.

*Splint wax-up*

The splint is waxed-up according to the occlusal design principles already described (Figs 25-27 and 25-28). Two layers of pink wax are softened over a flame; with aid of the fingers, the wax is immediately and carefully molded over the cast. Using a laboratory scalpel, the excess of wax that goes beyond the set limits is cut. After passing the surface of the wax over the flame, opening and closing movements are made with the articulator arms in order to record the impressions of the mandibular antagonist teeth. If needed, wax is added on the occlusal surface, until all the vestibular cusps of the posterior teeth and the edges of antagonist incisors and canines come into contact with this surface. Then, any wax excess is removed until a flat occlusal surface is obtained which prevents cusp tips from interfering with the posterior surface of the splint during lateral and protrusive movements.

Anterior guidance wax-up is made by adding wax on the vestibular surfaces, using the impressions left by the anterior teeth as a guide; this will create an inclined plane or ramp that will guide the trajectory of the lateral and protrusive movements. This last step is made easier by the use of a semi-adjustable articulator that has been programmed to reproduce the patient's lateral movements. Later, the wax-up is tidied up with aid of an alcohol torch, and it is then sent to the laboratory to be replaced by heat-cured acrylic.

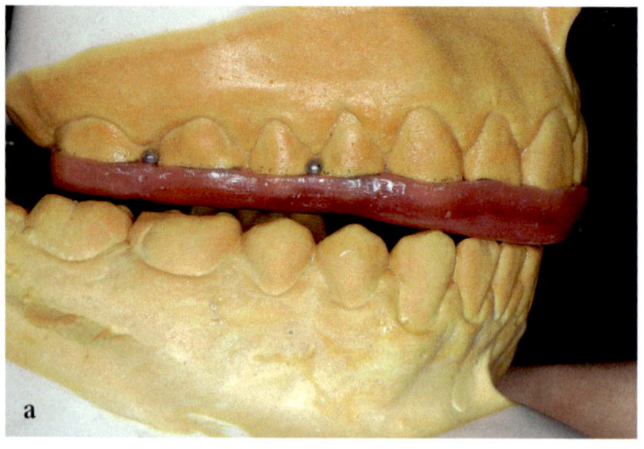

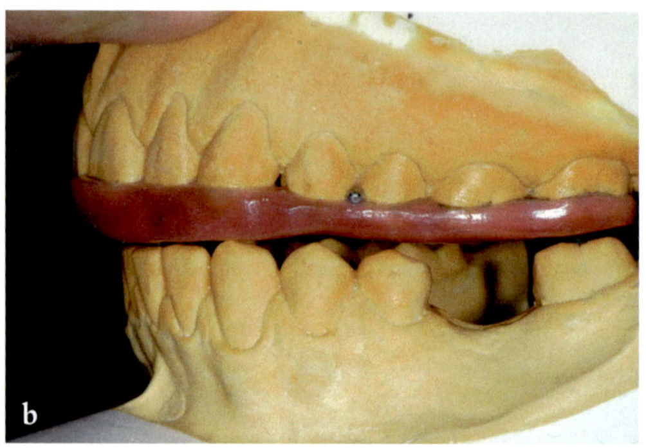

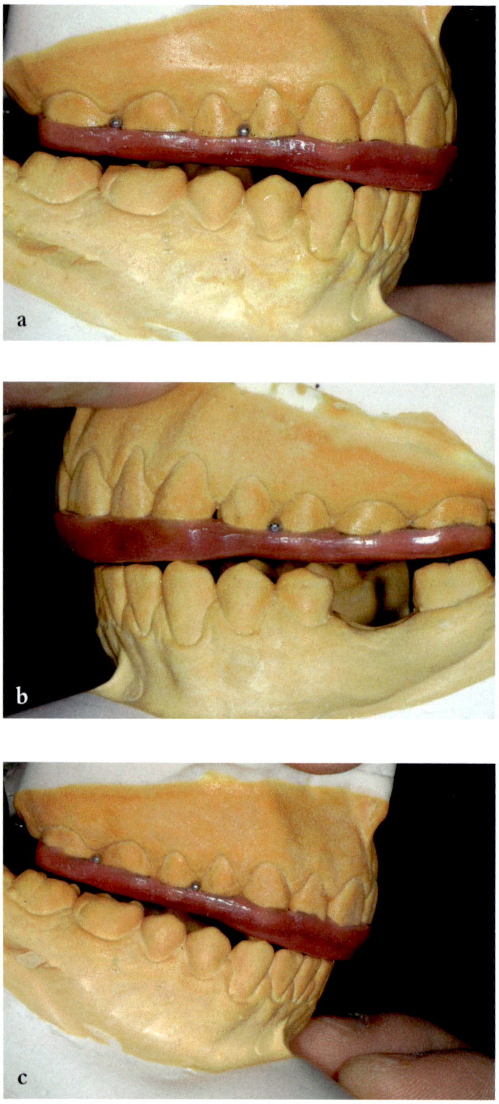

Fig 25-28 **(a–c)** Splint already waxed and ready to be muffled-up and replaced with acrylic. Note the functioning of the anterior guidance during lateral movements and protrusion.

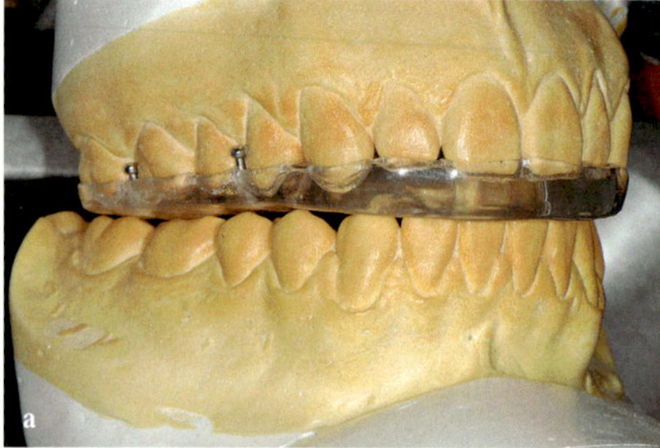

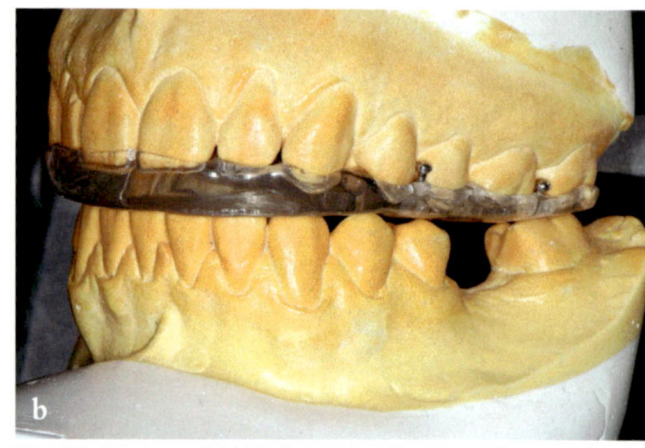

Fig 25-29 **(a and b)** Before it is taken into the mouth, the acrylic splint is tested on the articulator.

*Splint try-in and adjustment in the mouth*

Before the acrylic splint is tried in by the patient, it can be placed on the articulated cast and a preliminary occlusal adjustment can be performed (Fig 25-29). Then it is ready for clinical work: it is tried in the patient's mouth, and its stability and proper attachment are checked (Fig 25-30). It is essential that these two latter requirements be satisfactorily met before proceeding to occlusal adjustment. The splint may have poor stability and

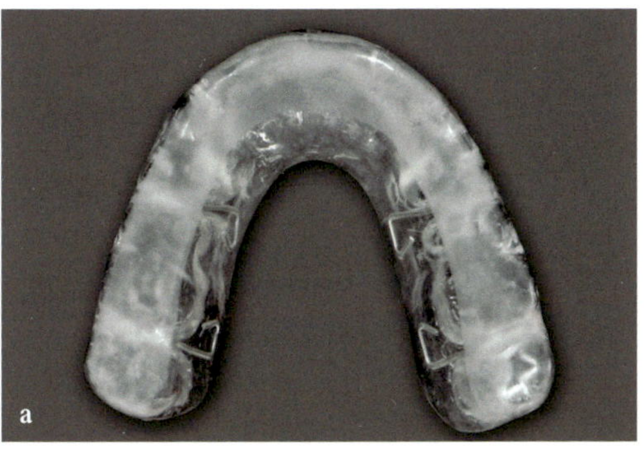

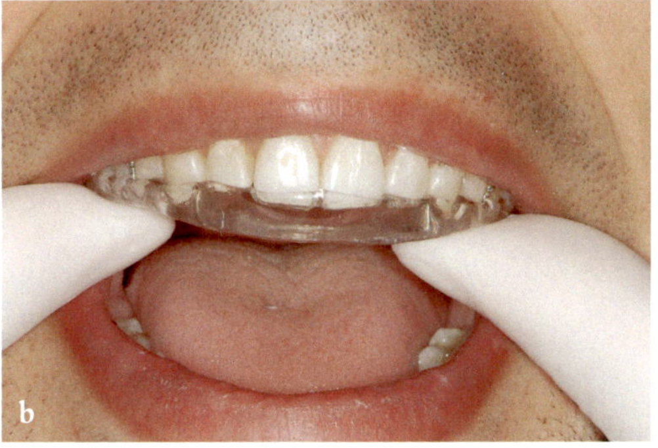

Fig 25-30 **(a)** Splint ready for clinical try-in. Note the coarse occlusal surface, which will render the visualization of occlusal contacts easier. **(b)** Splint settling is tested by exerting pressure with both thumbs.

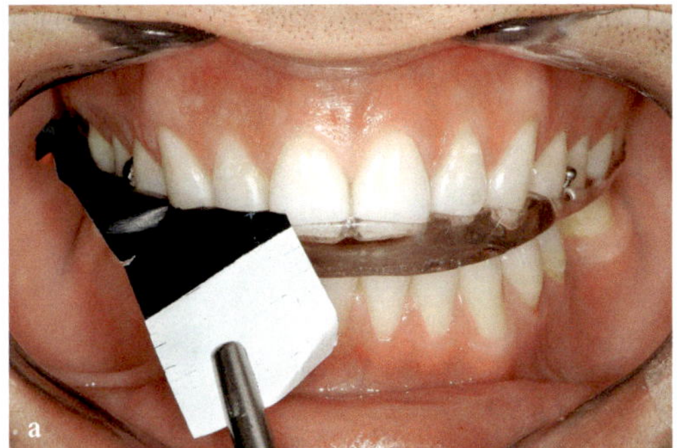

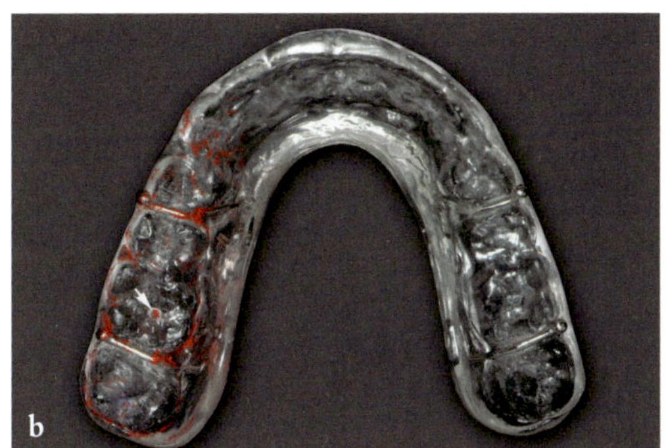

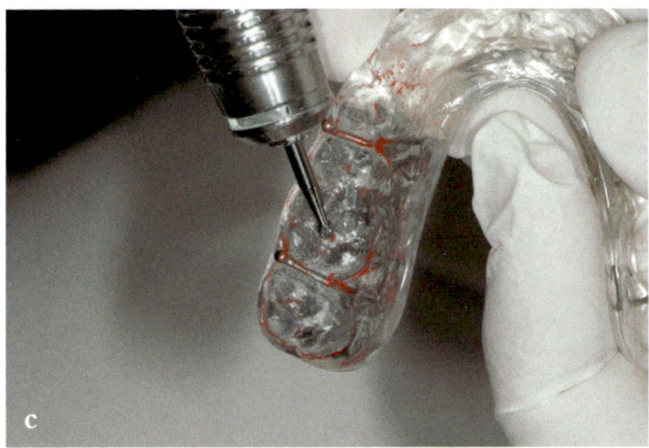

Fig 25-31 **(a)** If an adjustment problem arises, articulating paper of two colors is placed between the splint and the teeth to identify the premature contact point. **(b and c)** The arrow indicates a small area preventing the splint from settling correctly; this area can be removed by using a round bur.

swing over a tooth, so it is essential to resolve this issue before proceeding to occlusal adjustment. The problem may be due to some impression distortion or to acrylic entering into an air bubble in the plaster cast. When this happens, a piece of extra-thin articulating paper should be placed between the splint and the teeth to identify the area preventing the splint from settling correctly; once identified, that area should be removed by using a small bur (Fig 25-31).

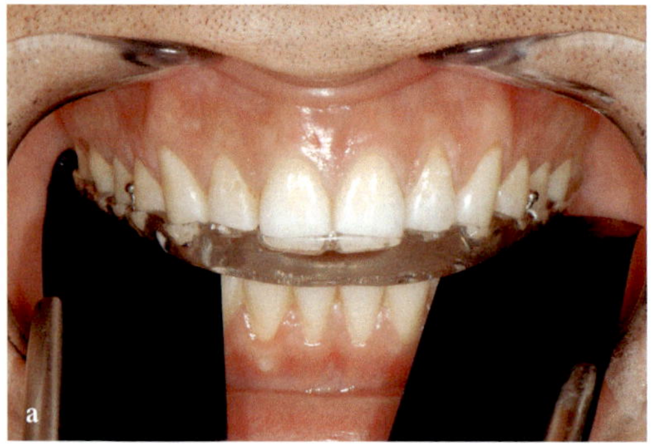

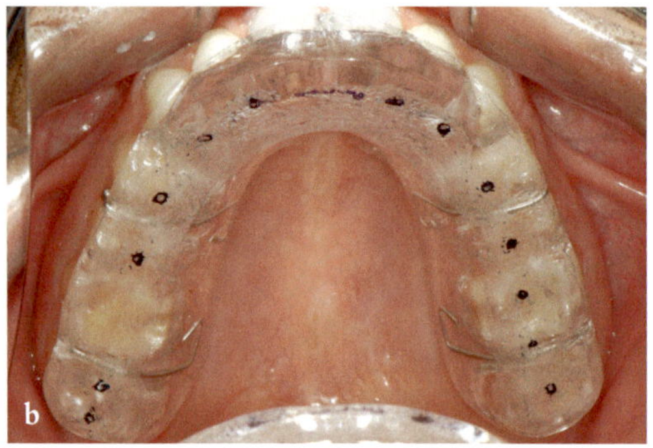

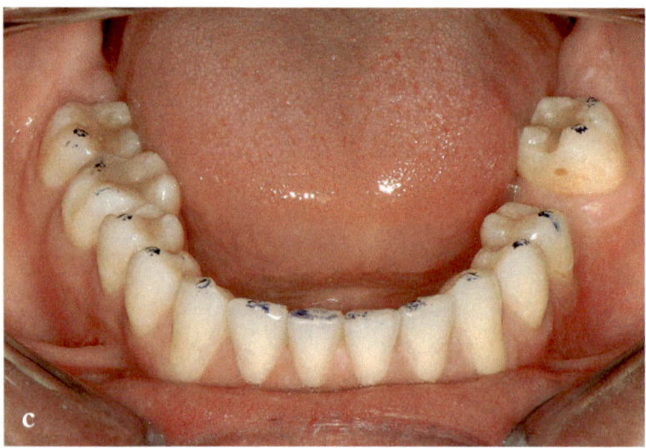

**Fig 25-32** Occlusal adjustment of the splint. **(a)** Ask the patient to close their mouth repeatedly and give a series of taps with their teeth on the splint, while articulating paper is placed between the splint and the teeth. **(b and c)** The aim is to obtain one contact point per cusp or antagonist incisal edge.

Splint attachment problems are much simpler to solve, since only retainer tightening is required.

In order to perform splint occlusal adjustment, it is advisable not to polish the surface of the splint fully. Another option is to request the laboratory to deliver the splint with a coarse surface, or to remove the splint's gloss by using thin sandpaper in order to better visualize occlusal contacts. Once the patient is in the dorsal recumbent position, they are requested to give a series of quick taps with their teeth on the splint, while articulating paper is made to come between splint and teeth (Fig 25-32). An acrylic bur is used to wear out all the premature contact points. This procedure is repeated as many times as necessary, until all the vestibular cusps and incisal edges simultaneously occlude on the surface of the splint. The simultaneous contacts obtained during mouth closure are comparable to maximum intercuspation at a dental level. Thus, each of these points (closure stops) will be responsible for the stability of its respective antagonist tooth. Also, the combined action of all of them guarantees a steady position of the jaw during mouth closure and, especially, during tooth clenching episodes while the bruxer is wearing the splint.

Next, the aim is to make anterior guidance harmonious (Figs 25-33 and 25-34). To do this, it is advisable to use articulating paper of a different color. Articulating paper is placed between the teeth and the splint while having the patient make lateral and protrusive movements. Any contact in the posterior segment should be carefully removed, with the exception of those contacts matching the ones obtained in the previous step (closure stops). In short, during closure, one contact per cusp or lower incisal edge should occur in the splint; during eccentric movements (lateral movement and protrusion), the anterior guidance should prevent premolar and molar cusps from coming into contact with the surface of the splint.

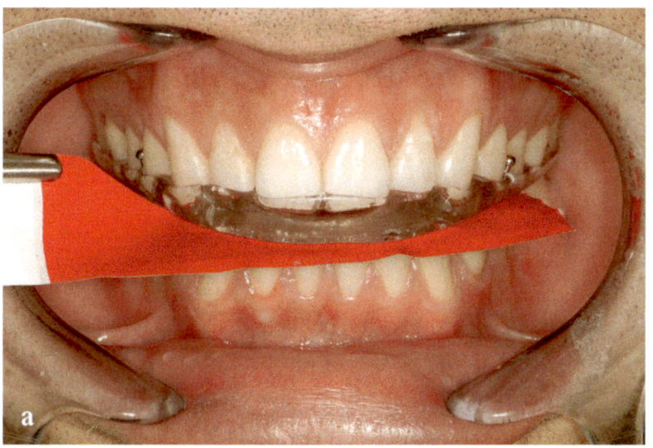

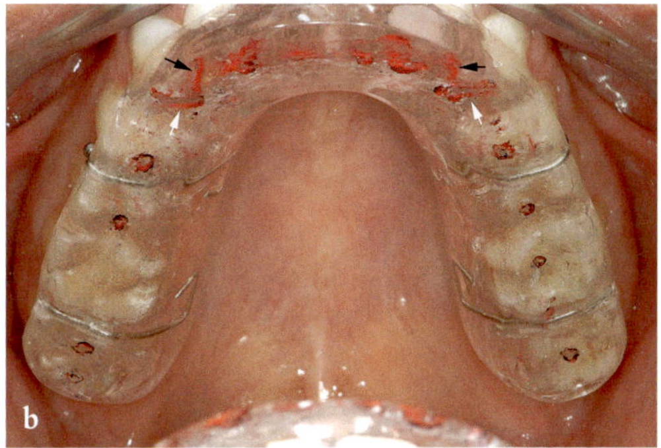

Fig 25-33 **(a)** With articulating paper of a different color, anterior guidance functioning is tested. **(b)** The white arrows indicate the trajectories created during lateral movements; the black arrows indicate protrusive movement trajectories.

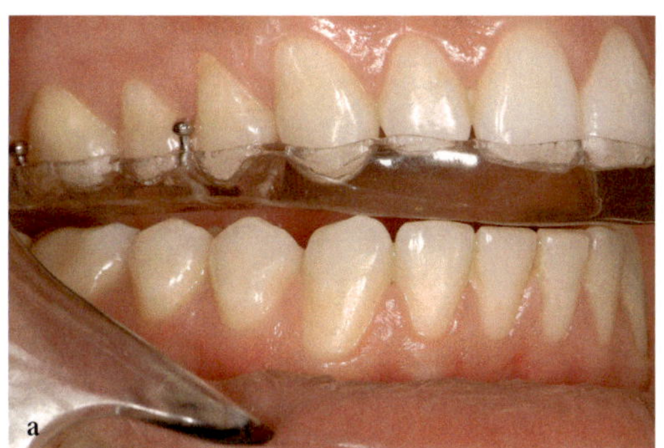

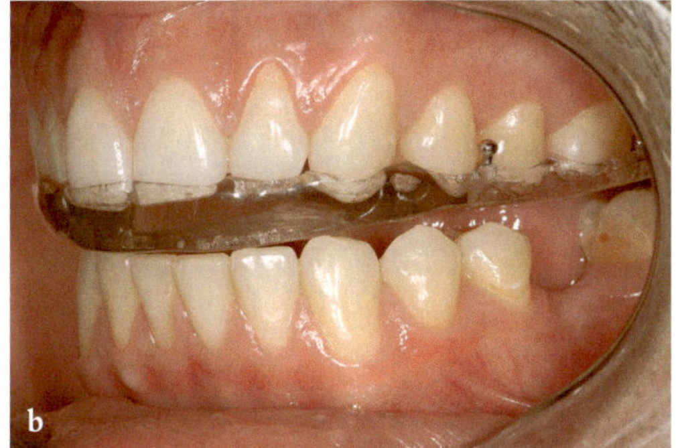

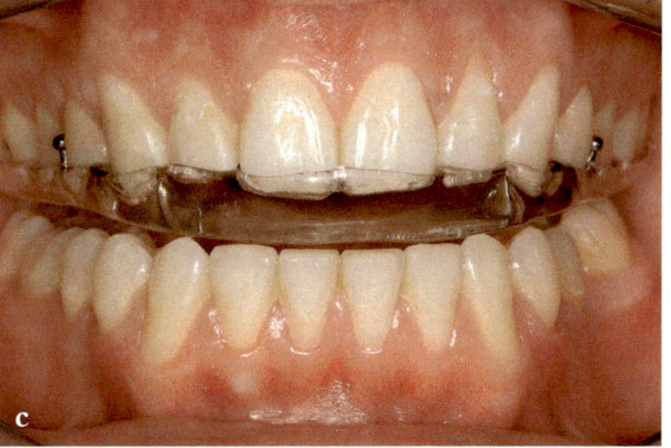

Fig 25-34 **(a–c)** Correct functioning of the anterior guidance of the splint causes the posterior segments to separate and protects them against premature wear during tooth grinding episodes.

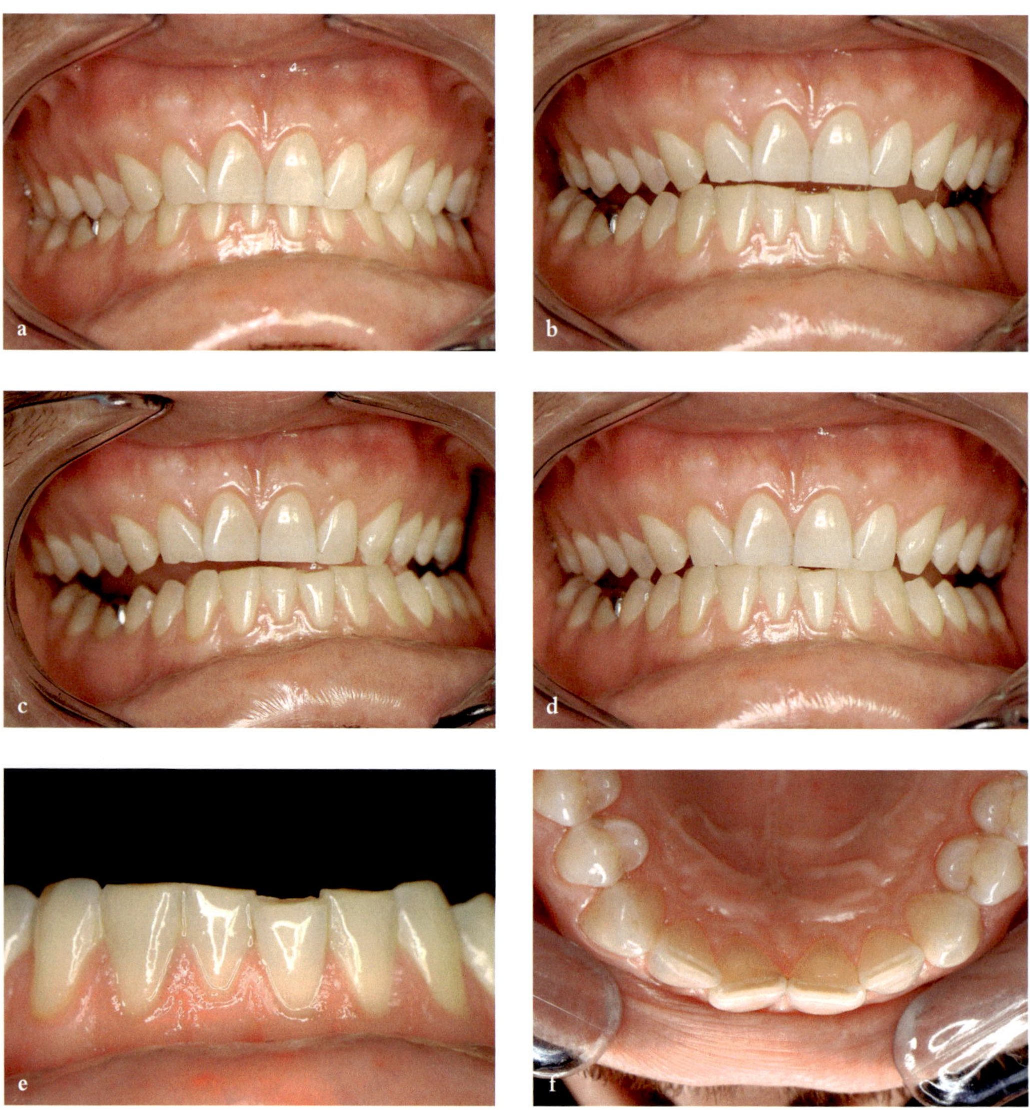

**Fig 25-35 (a–f)** Patient suffering from sleep tooth grinding in the protrusive direction. During lateral movements, canine guidance functioning is optimum. Bruxism has resulted in significant incisor attrition.

*Final polishing*

The splint is carefully polished to remove any roughness generated during the occlusal adjustment. First it is polished by means of a mounted abrasive rubber tool; then it is polished in the traditional way by using a lathe.

## *Vacuum-stamped Bruxism Splints*

Many clinicians are reluctant to use semi-adjustable articulators. For this reason, our postgraduate students sometimes ask us to describe a fabrication technique in which this valuable tool need not be used. Although we respect such refusal

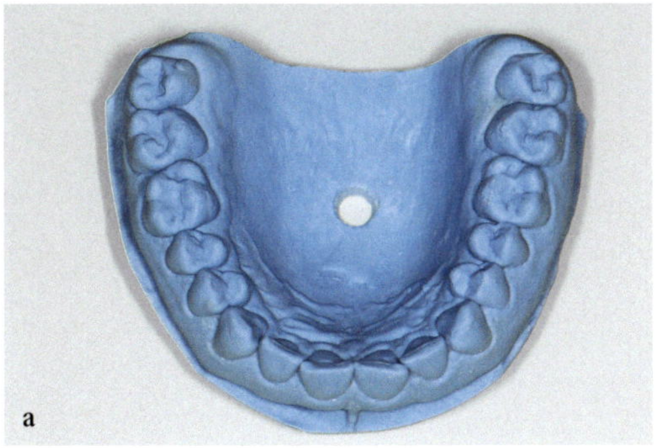

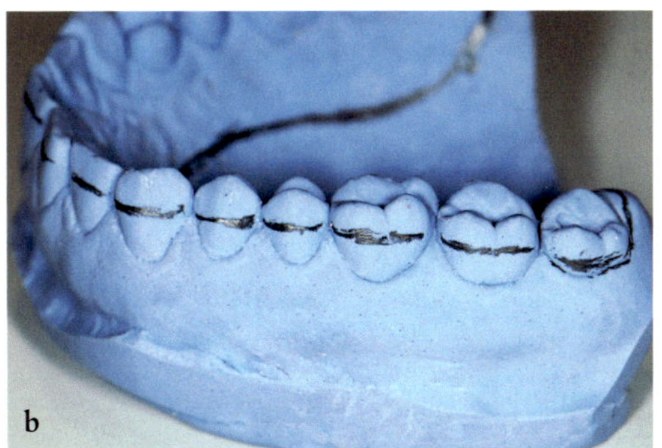

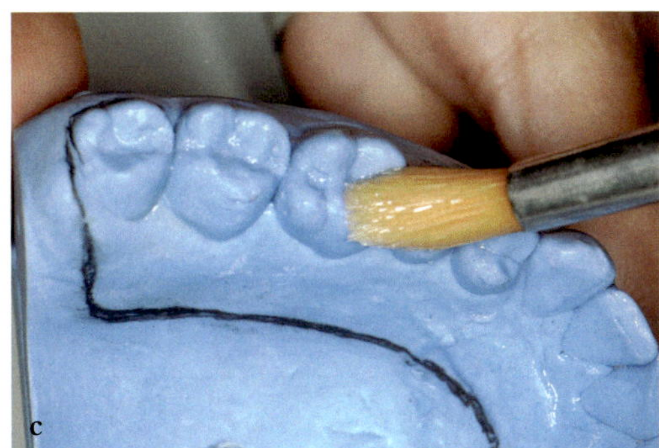

Fig 25-36 **(a–c)** Upper cast of a patient for whom a vacuum-stamped bruxism splint will be fabricated. The splint perimeter is drawn and painted with plaster spreader.

to use articulators, we deem it to be just a prejudice, since, far from making treatment more complex, articulators will simplify it. An articulator that is correctly programmed with a patient's registrations allows one to fully delegate splint fabrication to a lab; this reduces clinical time since one then has only to deal with impression-taking, registrations, and occlusal adjustment of the splint. Nevertheless, this section will describe a technique that requires neither the use of the articulator nor sending the material to a prosthesis laboratory.

We will use the clinical case shown in Fig 25-35 as an example. The procedure has three stages (two clinical and one in the lab): impression taking, hybrid splint fabrication, and occlusal surface shaping.

*Impression taking*

When fabricating a splint, the first step is to obtain impressions of the jaw. Any mistakes made during this step will invariably affect the final result. In a similar way to muffled-up splints, the impression of the maxilla should be a faithful reproduction of the maxilla, free from bubbles and distortions. Since the shaping of the occlusal surface will be performed directly in the patient's mouth, an impression of the mandible need not be taken.

*Splint stamping*

As shown in detail in the series of images in Figure 25-36, the perimeter of the device is drawn on the cast by using a graphite pen, and then it is painted with plaster separator. Then, four retainers are adapted and their ends (balls) are attached to the model by using plastic filler (Fig 25-37). A 2 mm thick Biocryl sheet (Buffalo Dental, Brooklyn, NY) is placed in a vacuum and temperature shaping machine (Fig 25-38). When the Biocryl sheet starts to lose its shape (a convexity is generated), crystal autopolymerizing acrylic is prepared and applied to

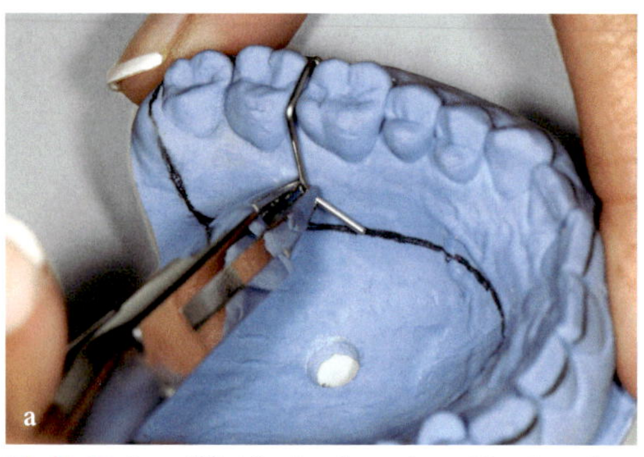
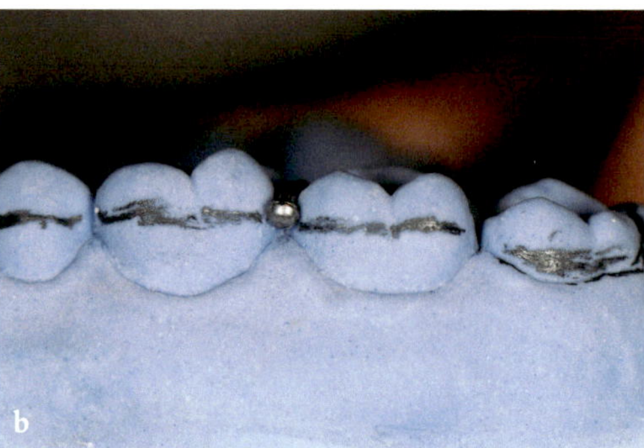

Fig 25-37 **(a and b)** Adapting the retainers. Note how the active portion (ball) should not affect the gingival papilla.

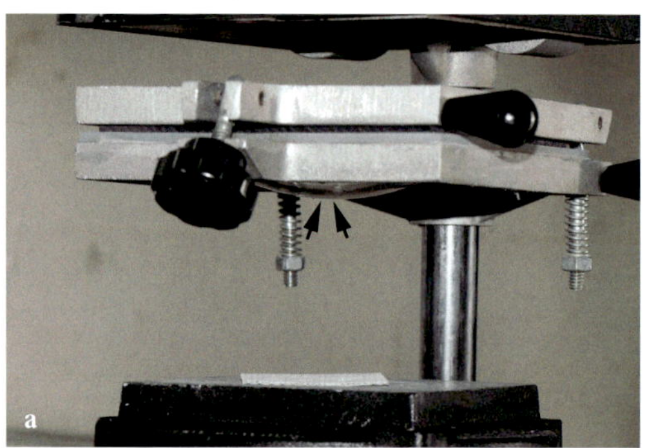
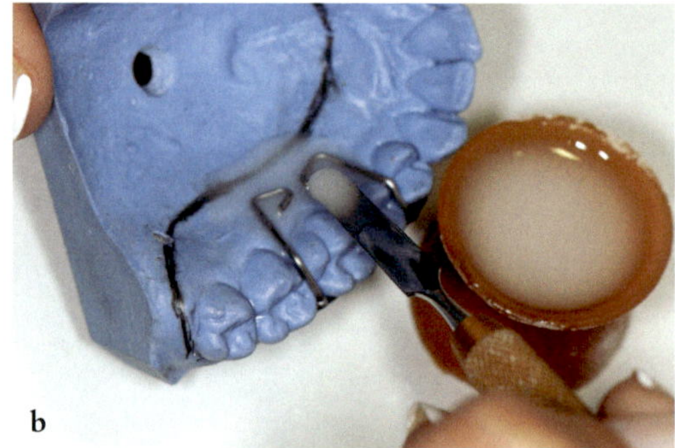
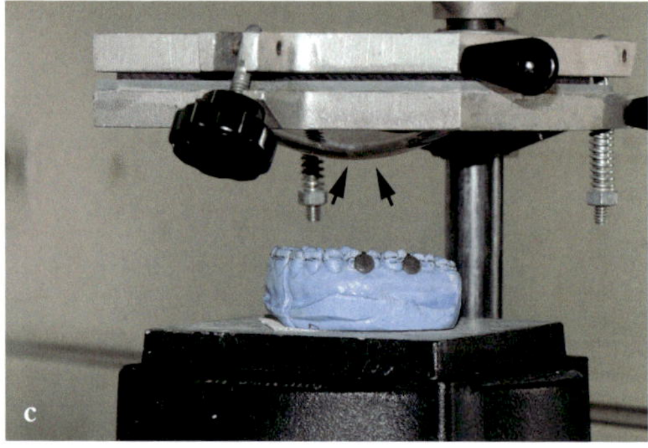
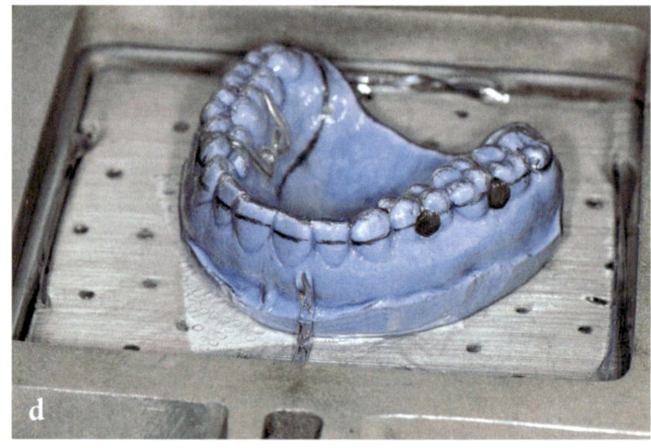

Fig 25-38 **(a–d)** A Biocryl sheet is placed in a thermo-shaping machine. When a convexity starts to appear (arrows), autopolymerizing acrylic is applied to the palatal end of the retainers and the set is immediately placed on the machine and stamped, and the vacuum machine is operated.

the inactive ends of the retainers (in the palatal area), and the sheet is immediately stamped on the cast while the suction mechanism is operated. Chemical combination of the acrylic and the splint occurs, and the ends of the retainers are contained within the splint. Later, the splint is cut with a disk by following the marks of the previous design, removed from the cast and its edges tidied up (Fig 25-39).

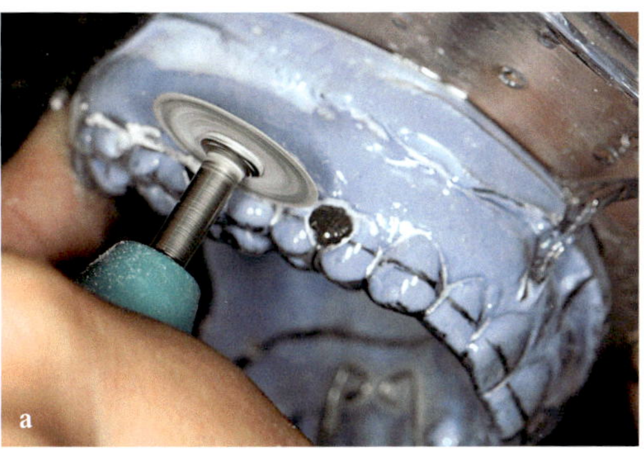

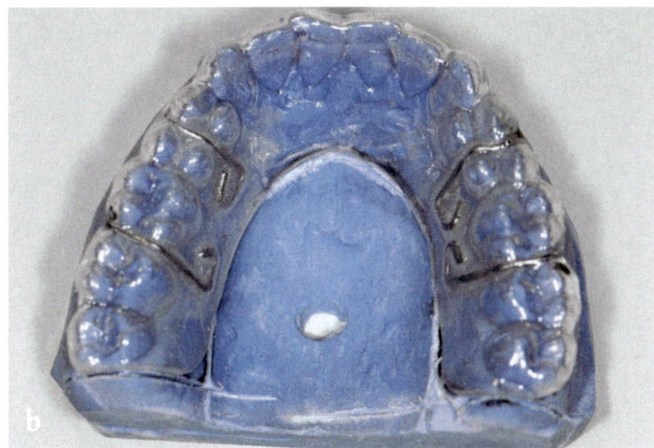

Fig 25-39 **(a and b)** The splint is cut with a disc by following the outline marks.

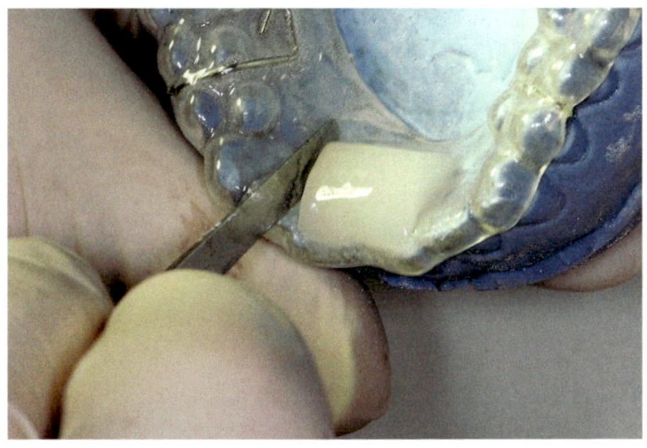

Fig 25-40 An anterior bite plane intended for thickness regulation and interjaw relationship registration is made with autopolymerizing acrylic.

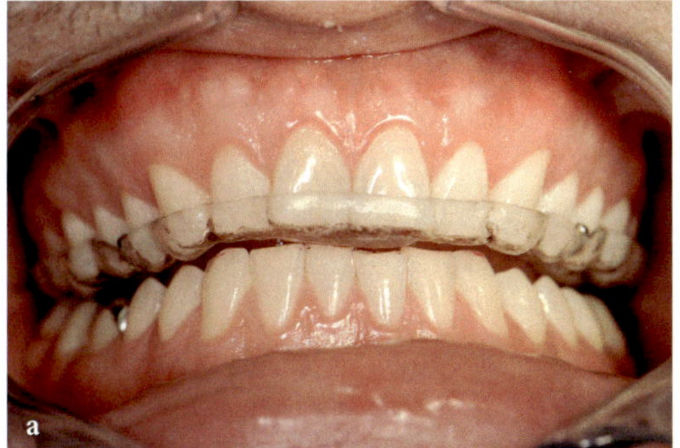

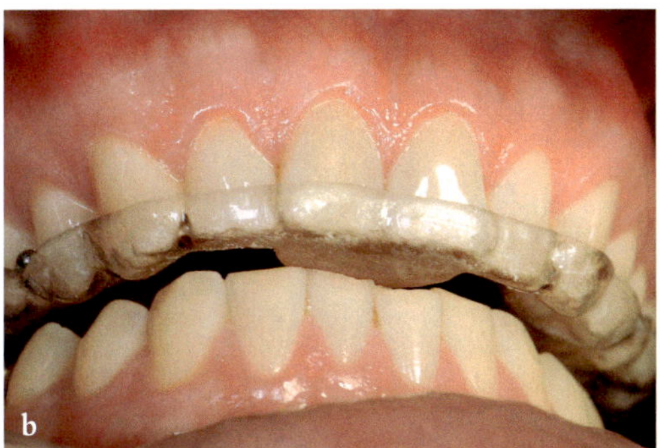

Fig 25-41 **(a and b)** Splint try-in, with anterior bite plane included. Note how a suitable thickness has been deliberately left for the future occlusal surface.

*Occlusal surface shaping*

So far, we have a hybrid splint, and attention has mostly been paid to its adjustment and attachment to the maxilla. The next step concerns the shaping of the splint's occlusal surface. In accordance with the concepts developed in Chapter 21, an anterior bite plane will be created on the splint that will allow establishment of a repeatable

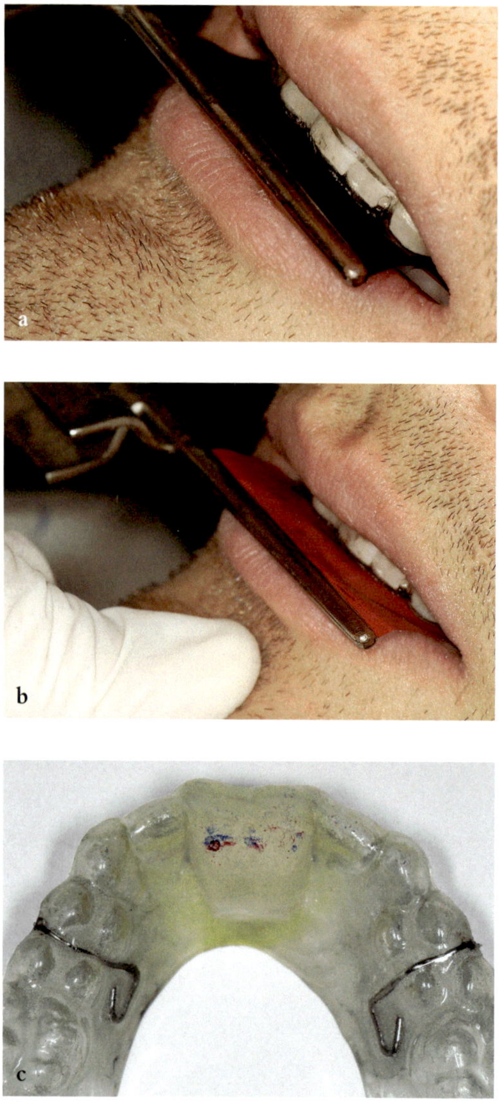

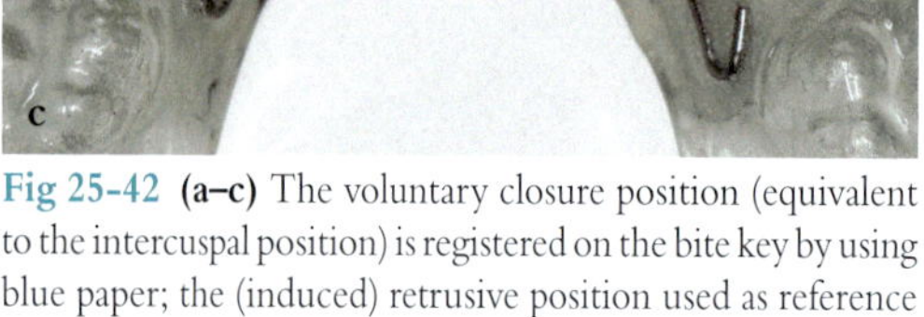

Fig 25-42 **(a–c)** The voluntary closure position (equivalent to the intercuspal position) is registered on the bite key by using blue paper; the (induced) retrusive position used as reference is registered with red paper.

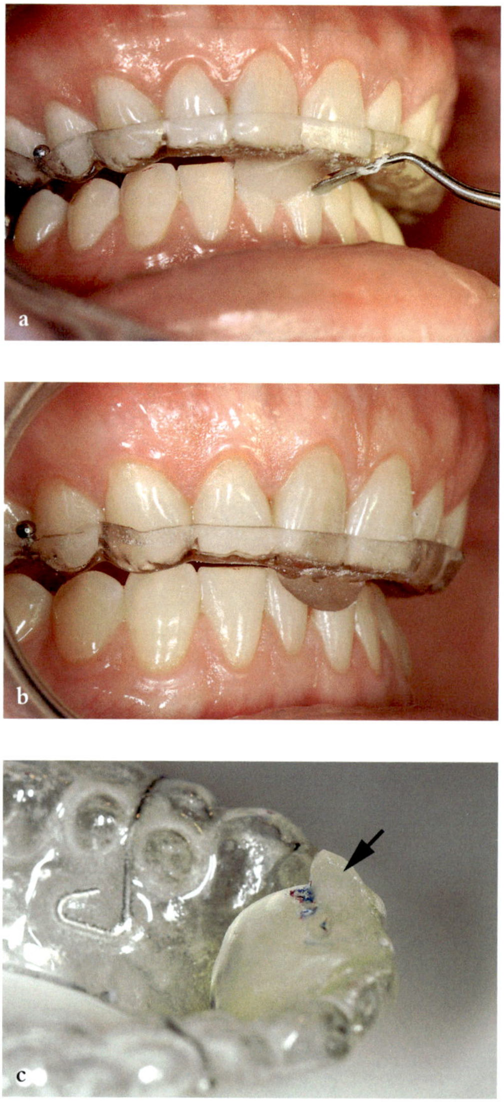

Fig 25-43 **(a–c)** Bite key fabrication. While having the patient occlude in the therapeutic position obtained before, autopolymerizing acrylic is applied to the angle formed by the vestibular surface of the mandibular incisors and the splint. The arrow indicates the key already fabricated.

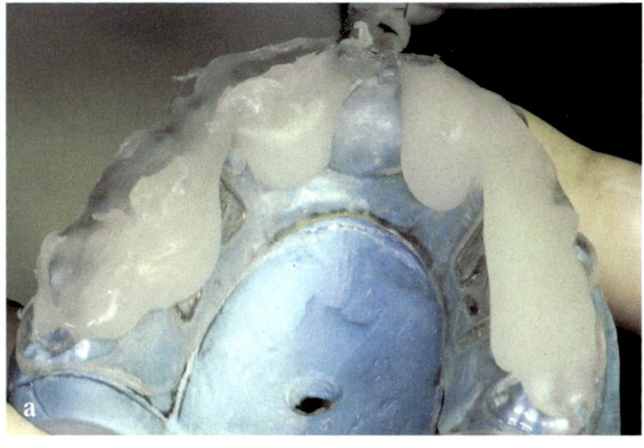
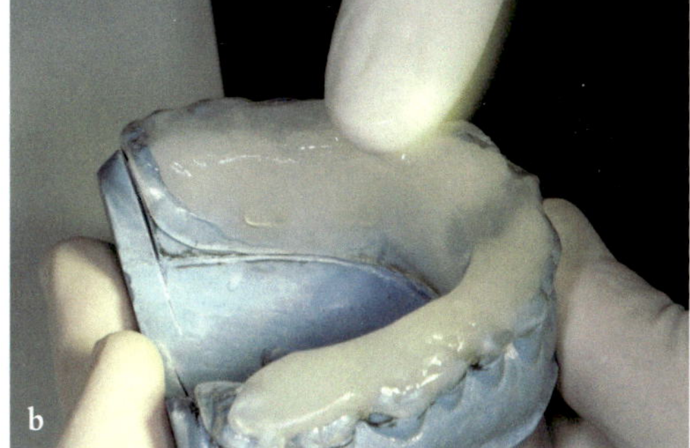
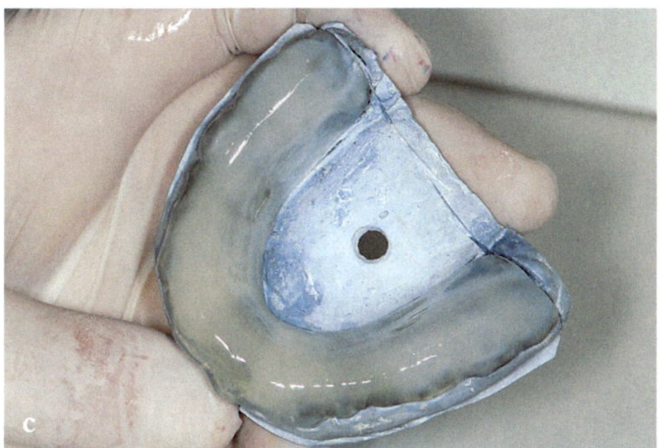

**Fig 25-44** **(a–c)** Occlusal surface fabrication: Acrylic is placed on the splint and it is molded with a monomer-moistened forefinger until a homogeneous surface is obtained.

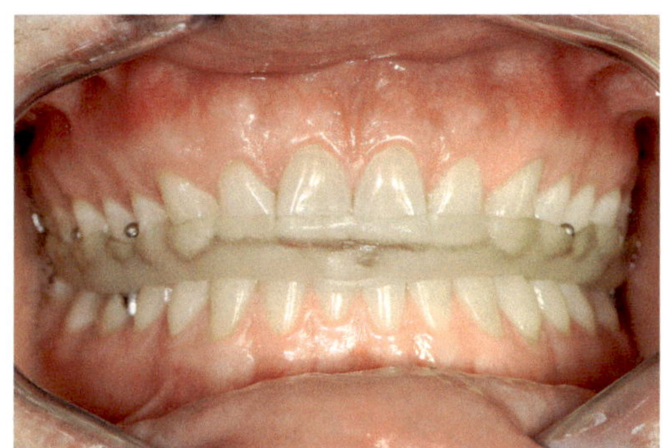

**Fig 25-45** The patient occludes before acrylic polymerization. The position is determined by the bite key.

closure position that is similar to the intercuspal position and that will be checked against the retrusive position used as reference.

Anterior bite plane fabrication details are shown in Figs 25-40 and 25-41. The subsequent establishment of the repeatable closure position and its corroboration against the retrusive position are shown in Fig 25-42. Since the occlusal surface will be made of acrylic that will fully cover the platform, and in order not to run the risk that the patient might occlude in a different position from the one obtained in the previous step, an acrylic bite key will be fabricated first, as shown in Fig 25-43.

Acrylic in the plastic state is placed on the splint's occlusal surface, and it is molded with a monomer-moistened forefinger until it is homogenized into the rest of the splint (Fig 25-44). This procedure should be done quickly, since the set must be taken to the mouth before acrylic polymerization starts; such polymerization should occur while the patient keeps their arches in occlusion (Fig 25-45). The splint is washed with running water, and having the impressions left by the antagonist teeth as reference, the surplus acrylic is removed by means of a bur, until a flat surface is obtained that facilitates the fabrication of a platform on which antagonist cusps will simultaneously come into contact (Fig 25-46).

Next, optimization of the anterior guidance is performed (Fig 25-47). By using articulating paper of different colors, the posterior segment areas coming into contact during eccentric move-

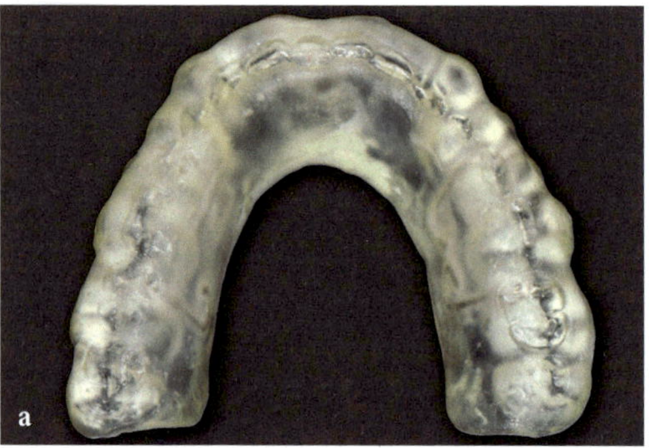

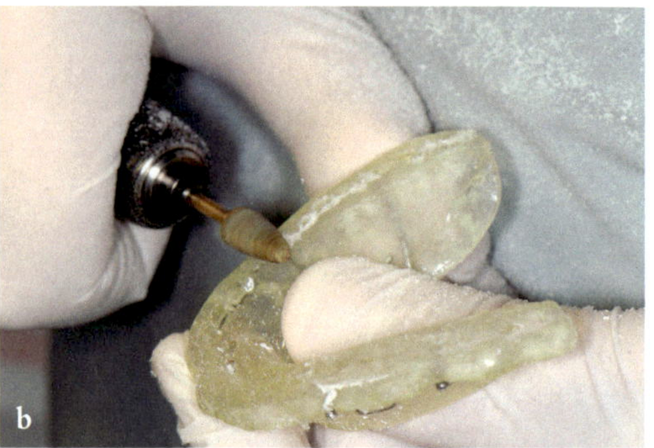

**Fig 25-46** **(a and b)** The splint is removed from the mouth and acrylic excess is eliminated with a bur.

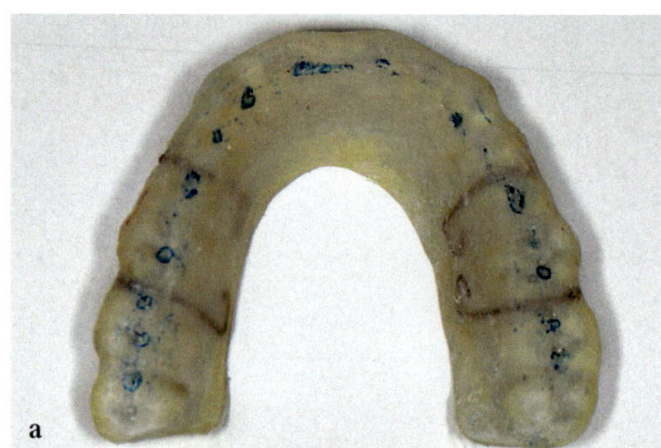

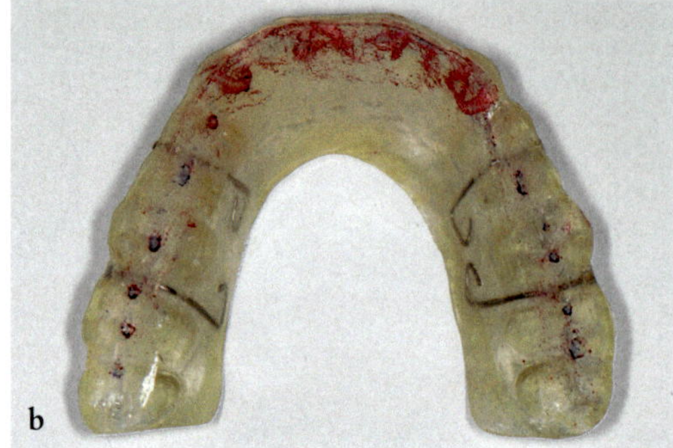

**Fig 25-47** **(a and b)** Occlusal adjustment of the splint. First, simultaneous contact of all the vestibular cusps and antagonist incisal edges (in blue) is achieved. Then, the anterior guidance is adjusted by using paper of another color (red), until contacts during protrusion and lateral movements occur only in the anterior guidance.

ments are worn out, and only the stops obtained during closure are kept. The last step is to meticulously polish the splint surface sequentially by means of abrasive rubbers and pumice to a high-gloss finish (Fig 25-48).

### *Splints with Metallic Canine Guidance*

Some patients will brux so heavily on their splints that the latter must be fixed frequently (Fig 25-49). Although this should not be considered a negative effect, since it confirms that the splint is effectively protecting teeth, the making of metallic canine guidances with silver amalgam has been suggested in order to extend the lifespan of the splint[27] (Figs 25-50 to 25-53).

There is no harm in pointing out that, when a metal guidance is added to the splint, it should have a low wear coefficient. In this regard, another option is to use gold. This precious metal allows for a more comprehensive anterior guidance that includes both canines and incisors and has a longer lifespan without affecting the integrity of antagonists. However, using gold is expensive and requires a complex manufacturing technique (Fig 25-54).

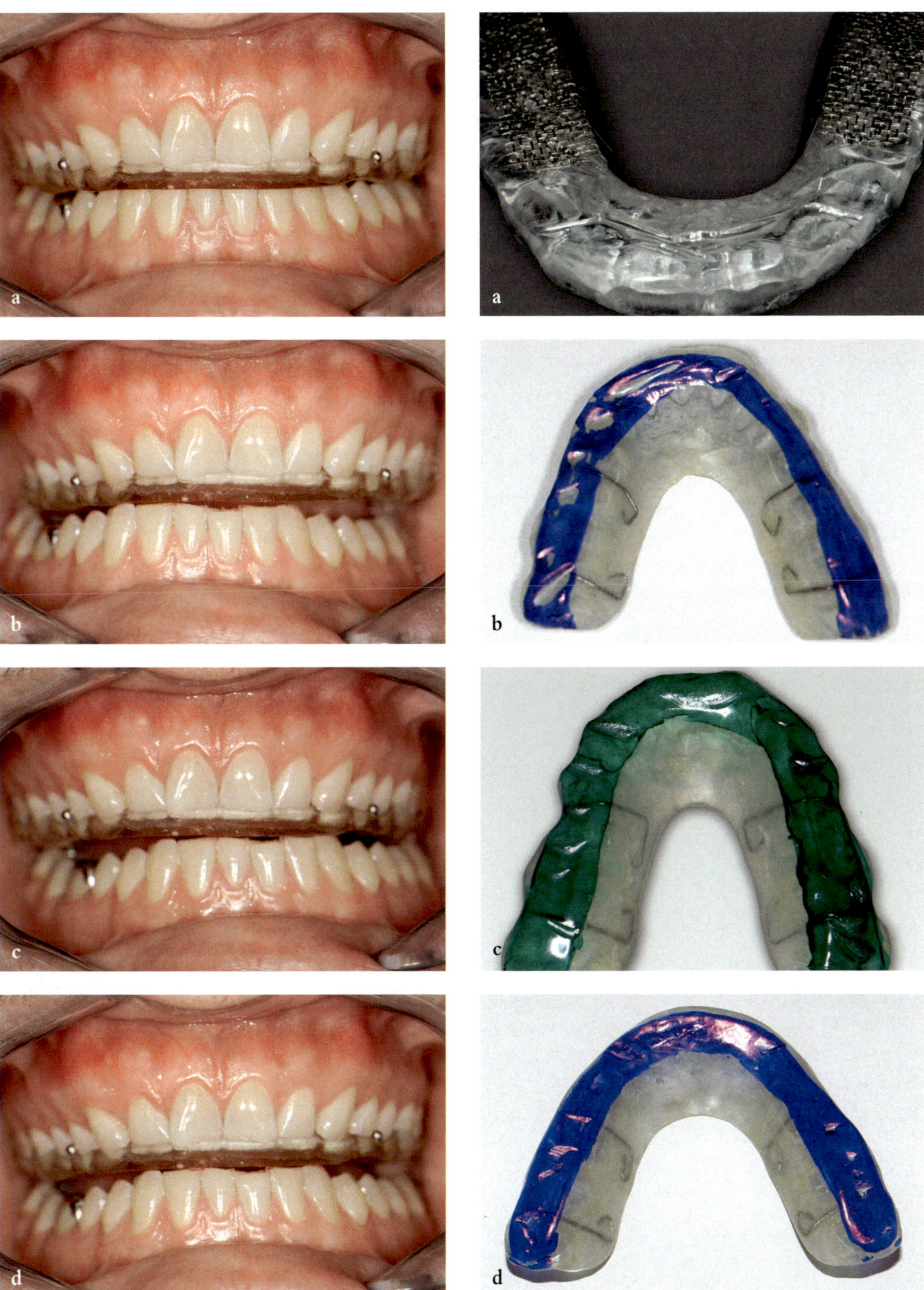

Fig 25-48 **(a–d)** Splint already polished, inside the mouth. Optimum anterior guidance during protrusion and lateral movements.

Fig 25-49 **(a–d)** Splints belonging to heavy bruxers. Anterior guidance wear causes the posterior segments to deteriorate quickly.

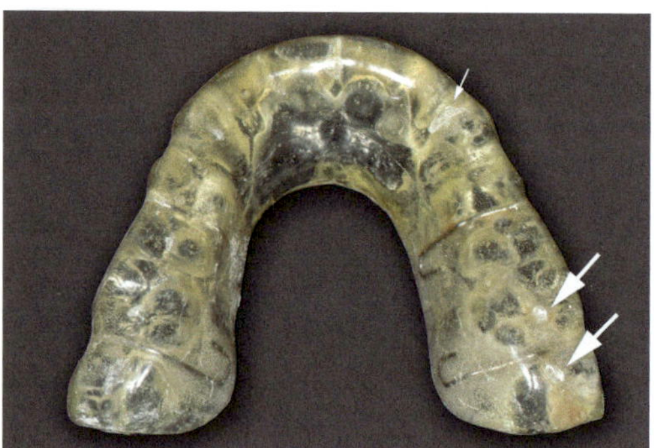

Fig 25-50 Splint belonging to a patient showing a left unilateral bruxism pattern. Canine guidance premature wear (small arrow) boots posterior segment wear (big arrows).

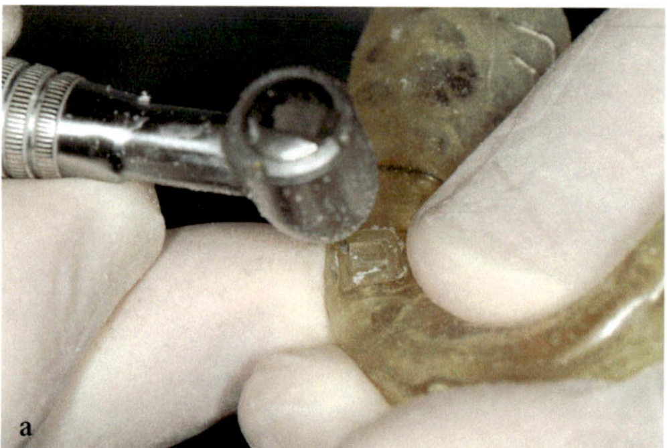

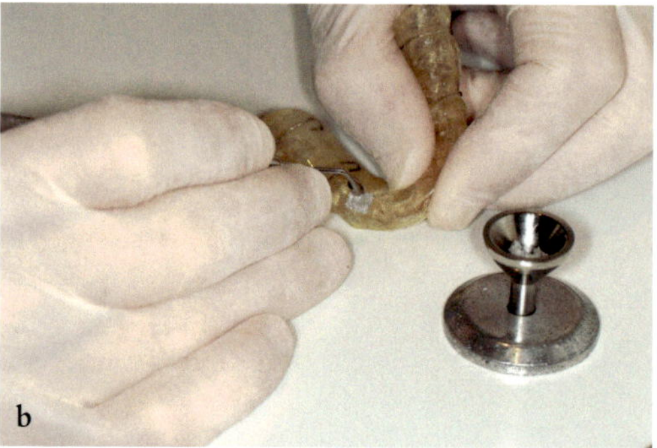

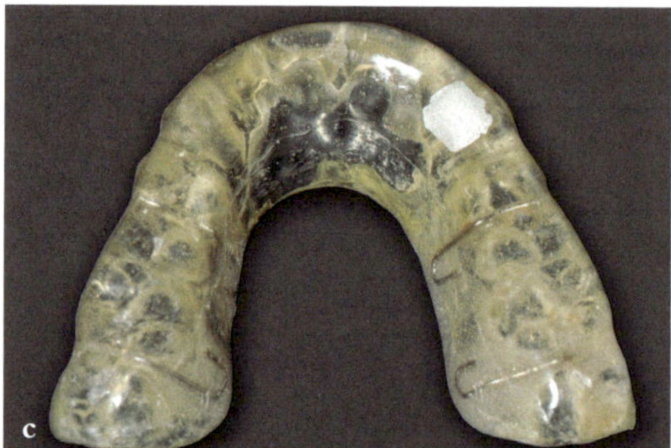

Fig 25-51 **(a–c)** Silver-amalgam canine guidance fabrication. A retaining cavity is carved and amalgam is condensed into it. It is advisable to use an excess of amalgam and then wait at least 2 hours to perform the adjustment in the mouth.

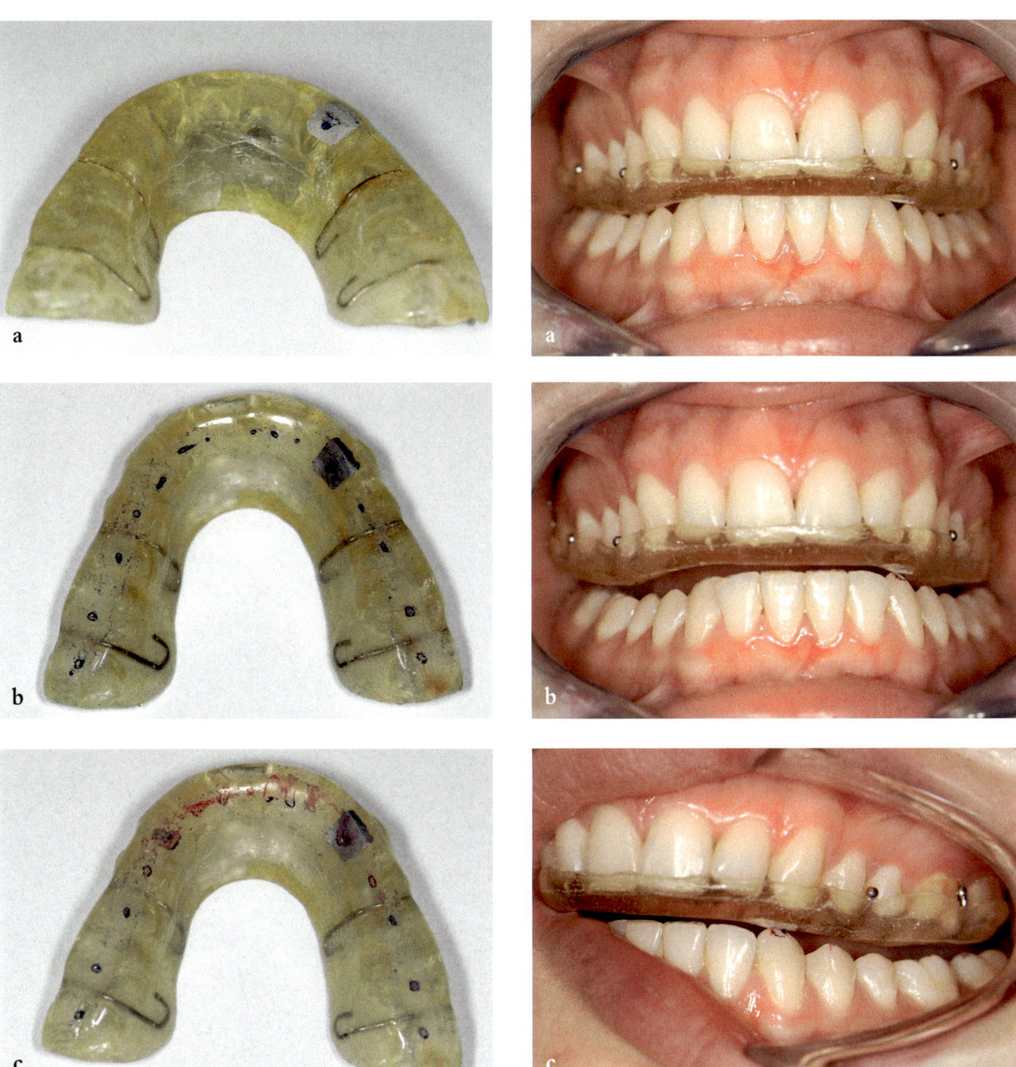

Fig 25-52 **(a–c)** Adjustment in the mouth. A single contact on the amalgam guide is observed, resulting from excessive obturation. The premature contact is adjusted on the guide by using abrasive rubber, until all the antagonists occlude simultaneously.

Fig 25-53 **(a–c)** Using paper of a different color, final adjustments are made to the anterior guidance during protrusion and lateral movements.

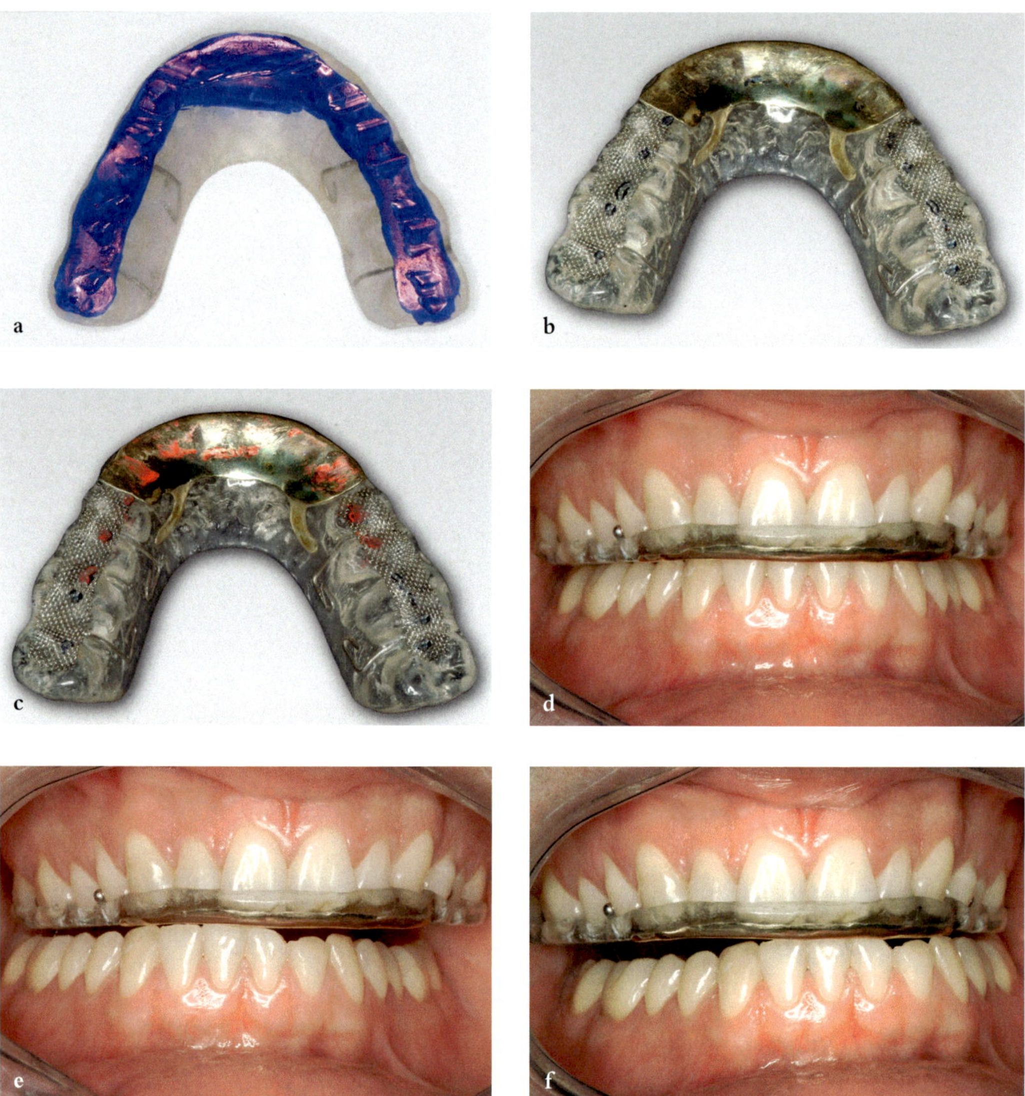

Fig 25-54 **(a)** Bruxism splint for sleep wear that was "devoured" within 30 days. **(b)** A new splint with gold anterior guidance was fabricated; closure stops are shown in blue. **(c)** Anterior guidance functioning is shown in red. **(d–f)** The splint during closure and lateral movements.

## Bruxism Splint Maintenance

The dental practitioner's services do not end with the delivery of the splint to the patient. It is advisable to present the patient with printed instructions on splint wear and maintenance. Since bruxism splints are made of the same material used for fabricating removable prostheses and are thus subject to similar deterioration, the instructions given for maintenance are not different from the traditional tips usually given to removable prosthesis wearers.

The splint should be washed immediately after use to prevent the saliva that impregnates it from fermenting. A toothbrush should not be used for washing the splint; ideally, a prosthesis brush should be used, or, if not available, a common nail brush will serve the purpose, since nail brushes are harder than toothbrushes. Dentifrice should not be used either, since its abrasive contents will affect the surface of the splint and boost the appearance of unpleasant pigmentations. Gel with no abrasive content can be used, or the splint can simply be washed with neutral soap. Once a week, it is advisable to submerge the splint for some hours in water to which a dental cleanser has been added (e.g., Corega Tab).

The splint should not be allowed to dry up, since this will cause it to undergo unpleasant appearance changes and to aquire a nasty odor. The best thing is to keep the splint inside one of the special cases designed for storing splints and mouthguards. It is also advisable to include a piece of foam rubber in the box and moisten it with oral deodorant every day; this way, the splint will be kept in a damp, antiseptic environment, and the deodorant will cause it to have a nice taste (Fig 25-55). The case containing the splint should be kept in a safe place and away from domestic pets, since they may nibble on the splint and destroy it (Fig 25-56).

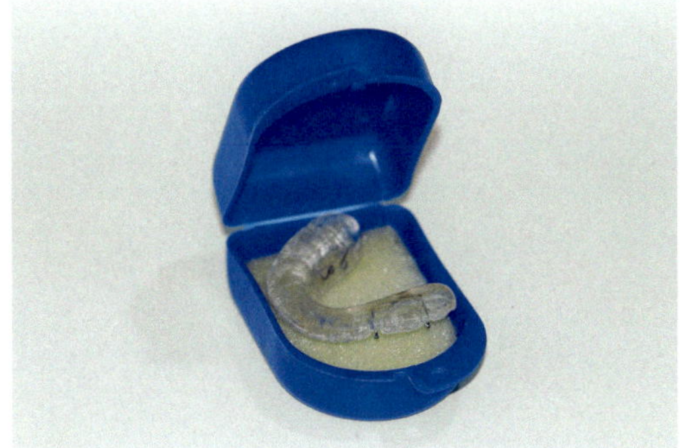

Fig 25-55 The splint should be stored in its case. It is advisable to include a piece of foam rubber moistened with antiseptic to keep the splint moistened and well-scented.

The patient should be informed that wearing the splint in an intermittent way or interrupting its use for a long time may cause the device to become maladjusted with respect to the dental arch.

The patient should be asked to attend control visits regularly, so that the splint can be monitored. Apart from monitoring and maintaining the occlusal aspect of the device, retainers will be adjusted and the splint will be intensively polished to smooth it and improve its appearance. The interval between control visits should not exceed 1 year, though in fact it will depend on the degree of bruxism developed by the patient.

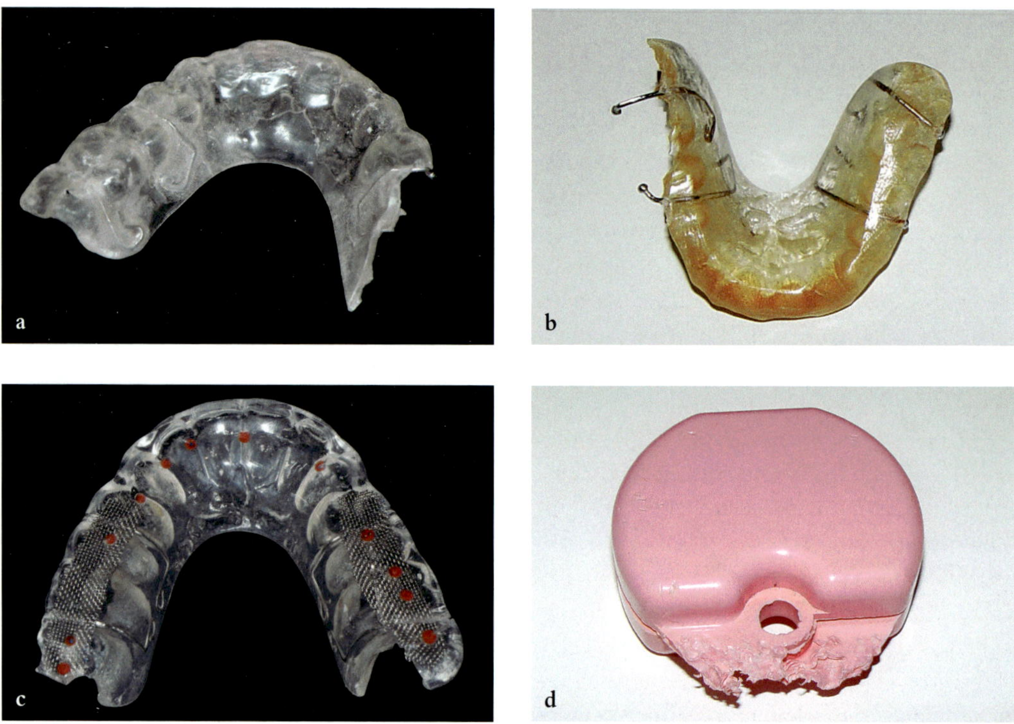

Fig 25-56 **(a–c)** Splints destroyed by pets. **(d)** This case was nibbled by a dog, but the splint inside was not touched by the animal.

## Treatments with Botulinum Toxin

Chapter 24 of this volume is devoted to the use of botulinum toxin in dentistry. Its author presents a historical review of the use of this toxin and deals with its action mechanism, indications, contraindications, and use as treatment for several pathologies. Here we will discuss the use of the toxin as a treatment for bruxism sequelae from a practical clinical point of view.

### *Overview*

Awake bruxism is characterized mainly by sustained tooth clenching. The muscle power exerted during bruxism episodes is highest during maximum dental intercuspation; that is, when stability between dental arches is greater.[28,29] Bruxism is an automated habit consisting of a repeated, contractile activity of the levator muscles of the jaw based on an isometric-type exercise that is deemed to be the cause of the progressive bulging of the masseter muscles.[30]

The so-called masseter "bulging" is cause of discussion. The term "hypertrophy" has lately been called into question as a result of a study in which biopsies were performed showing that there were twice as many muscle fibers as in a normal muscle; thus, the designation "masseter hyperplasia" has been proposed instead.[31] However, in a similar study, Guggenheim and Cohen[30] found muscle fiber size to be significantly greater than in normal muscles. Anabolic steroid use (which is widespread nowadays) has been reported to be an aggravating factor in patients with unilateral mastication.[32]

The use of splints as treatment for awake tooth clenching bruxism does not seem to be the most advisable, for several reasons. First, the patient will have to wear the splint at work, and on social occasions. Even if this were not a problem for the patient, splints have also been shown to cause increased interjaw stability in healthy individuals, which results in such a maximum voluntary contraction (MVC) that masseter EMG values are greater than the ones registered before, in the intercuspal position and with the patient not wearing the splint. Wood and Tobias[33] recorded 17% more masseter activity during tooth clenching on the splint, and Fitins and Sheikholeslam[34] recorded 13%. Others were not able to record any differences.[35–37] Christensen[38] found decreased masseter activity during maximum tooth clenching on the splint, though the decrease in EMG activity was insignificant. Although splints protect teeth, distribute stress over the dental arch, and cause levator muscle activity to be harmonious, they fail to inhibit masseter activity, and the masseter muscles will continue to develop an intensive isometric activity. It is also possible that splints act as an aide-memoire thus causing the number of bruxism episodes to decrease. However, this has not been documented.

Masseter muscle hypertrophy is a common presenting complaint. Sometimes, patients are only interested in finding out whether it represents any risk for health. Other patients are concerned with esthetics and request hypertrophy elimination. One possibility is to surgically remove a portion of the masseter muscles. This treatment is irreversible, and no recurrence has been reported. As in any surgical procedure, there are risks. Besides, many people are reluctant to accept surgical treatments. A technique based on radio-frequency-induced coagulation tissue necrosis has recently been presented in the reconstructive surgery field. Postsurgical follow-up 6 months later showed a 27% average masseter reduction, with a reduction range of 10–60%.[39]

The use of botulinum toxin to reduce masseter hypertrophy volume has lately become widespread. The results, as reported by most publications, are very good; however, the changes achieved are not permanent. Significant improvement of pain variables, mouth opening, function, and tenderness on palpation was reported, and the MVC returned to the original values within 4 weeks;[40] in contrast, others report that MVC decrease will only return to normal 3 months after injection of the toxin.[41,42] One study reports that the greatest muscle mass reduction was of 7.5 mm – the measurement was performed by means of cranial teleradiography – and it occurred 3 months after injection; from that moment onwards, the muscle started to slowly recover its original shape, which eventually fully materialized 12 months after toxin injection.[43]

### *Drug Preparation and Injection*

Several registered trademarks for botulinum toxin exist, and they vary according to country. The most widespread brands are Botox (Allergan, USA), available in 100 U vials, and Dysport (Ipsen, UK), available in 500 U vials. The drug is marketed in lyophilized dust form, and sterile saline solution must be added. The recommended diluent is a sodium chloride solution at 0.9% concentration; the number of toxin units per milliliter obtained will depend on the amount of diluent added.

Allergan Laboratory, the manufacturer of Botox, recommends a dosage of up to 25 U per muscle. Although the effects of 25 U and 35 U doses per masseter muscle have been compared, no significant differences were found regarding effectiveness.[44] If Botox is used, it is advisable to dilute it by adding 2 mL of sodium chloride at 0.9% concentration (Fig 25-57), and this amount will be enough for four muscles. The manufacturer states that the drug should be kept in a freezer at a temperature of –5°C or lower until preparation time. In fact, the drug is transported to the clinic in thermal containers with dry ice; once in the clinic, it should be kept in a refrigerator until preparation time. As specified by the manufacturer, once pre-

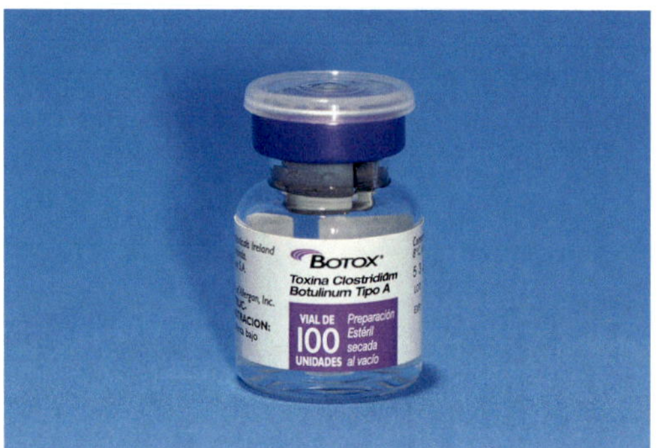


**Fig 25-57** Botox vial.

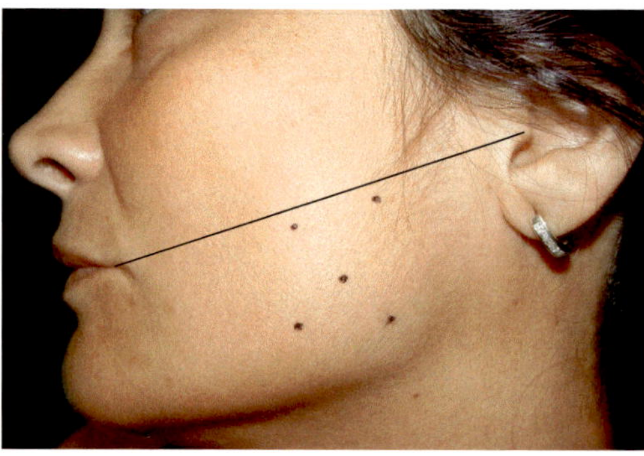

**Fig 25-58** The toxin is injected in five masseter prominent areas, below the level of an imaginary line drawn from the auricular tragus to the commissure of the lips.

pared, the drug lasts only 4 hours and must be kept in the refrigerator at a temperature between 2°C and 8°C; after that period of time has elapsed, the toxin loses its effectiveness completely.

The fact that the lifespan of botulinum toxin is so short causes some problems. Usually, 25 U per masseter muscle is needed for each patient, since temporalis muscles will hardly need treatment; in other words, each 100 U vial is enough for two patients (four muscles). It is a very expensive drug, so it is advisable to place the first patient on a waiting list until a second patient requires the same treatment; then both patients are called back simultaneously. If another brand is chosen, such as Dysport which comes in vials with five times as many drug units, the situation is more complicated – except when the patients scheduled for this treatment are many.

As for unilateral masseter hypertrophy, injection of 25 U on the affected side and also of 10 U in the contralateral muscle has been recommended in order to prevent marked hyperfunction on the latter side.[45]

The treatment can be repeated as many times as desired, provided it continues to be effective. Risk of antibody formation has been reported, though it can be prevented by allowing at least 12 weeks between applications.[46]

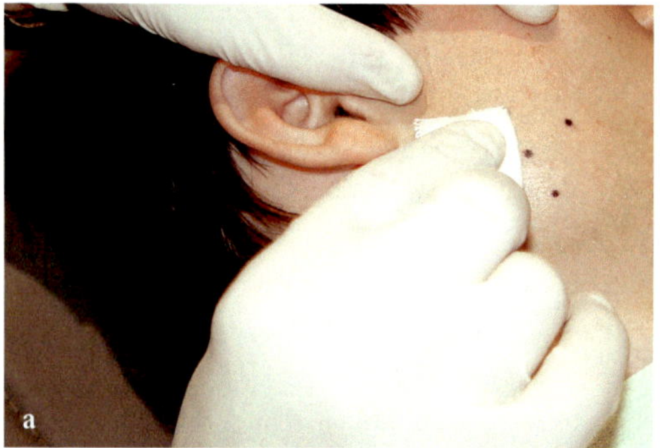


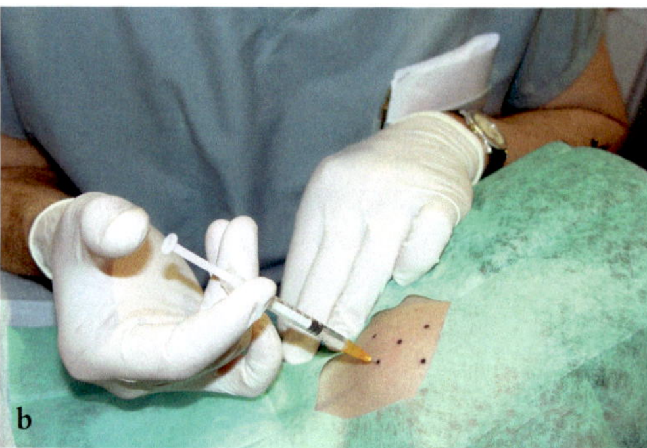


**Fig 25-59 (a and b)** Before injecting the drug, the area is disinfected and covered with a sterile surgical field.

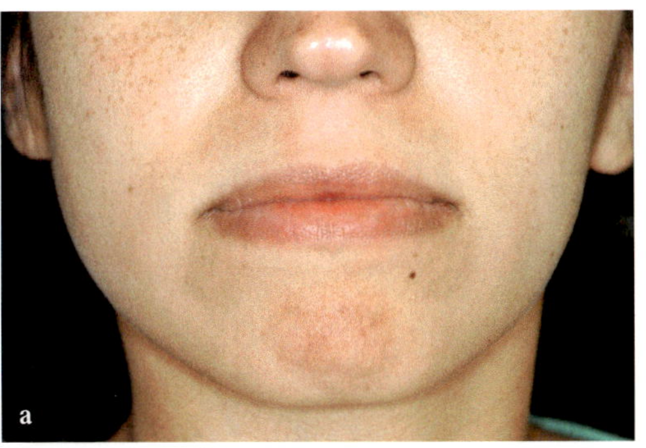

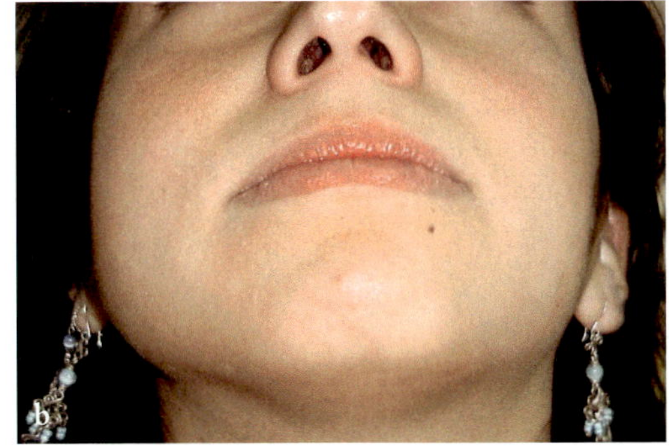

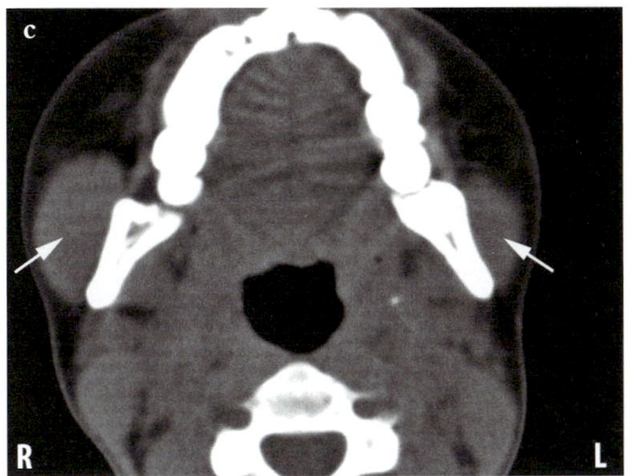


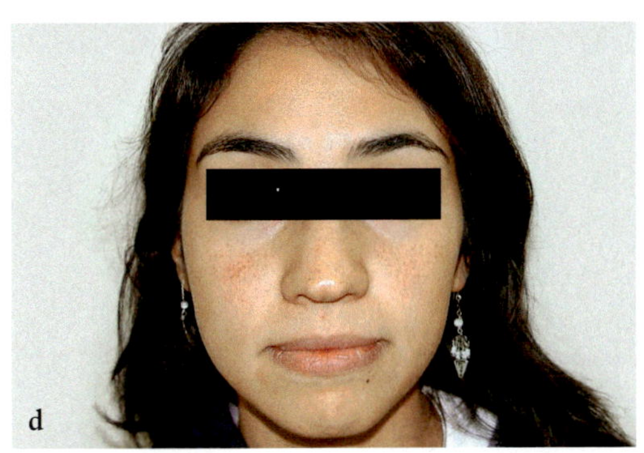

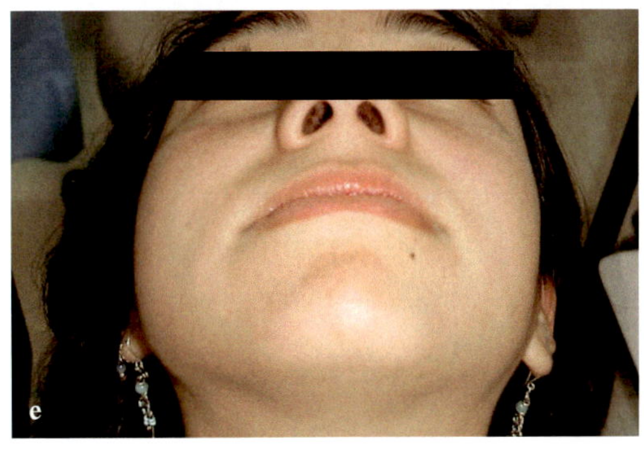

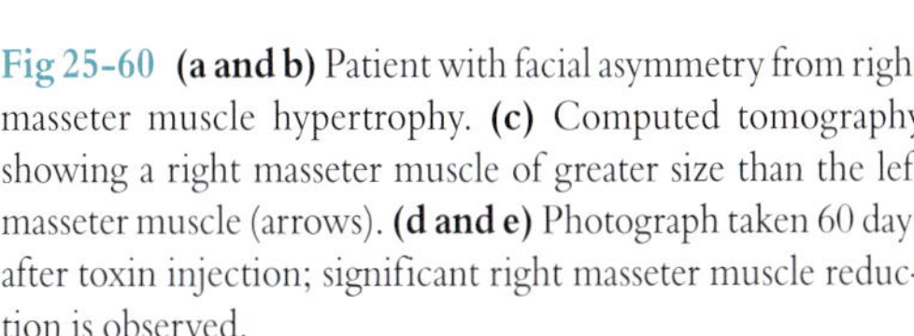

Fig 25-60 **(a and b)** Patient with facial asymmetry from right masseter muscle hypertrophy. **(c)** Computed tomography showing a right masseter muscle of greater size than the left masseter muscle (arrows). **(d and e)** Photograph taken 60 days after toxin injection; significant right masseter muscle reduction is observed.

### *Application Technique*

The patient is placed supine and requested to perform sustained tooth clenching in order to properly identify the whole muscle volume. Five punctures will be made in each masseter muscle, in those muscle areas that are more prominent and harder on palpation. Then, a small mark is made with an indelible marker pen. It has been suggested that injections be always given below the level of an imaginary line drawn from the auricular tragus to the corner of the mouth (Fig 25-58). The whole area is disinfected with antiseptic; it is advisable to have a small sterile surgical field (Fig 25-59). This treatment is absolutely contraindicated in patients with skin lesions, even if such lesions are simply acne.

The toxin is extracted from the vial using a 1 mL tuberculin-type syringe, and the solution is

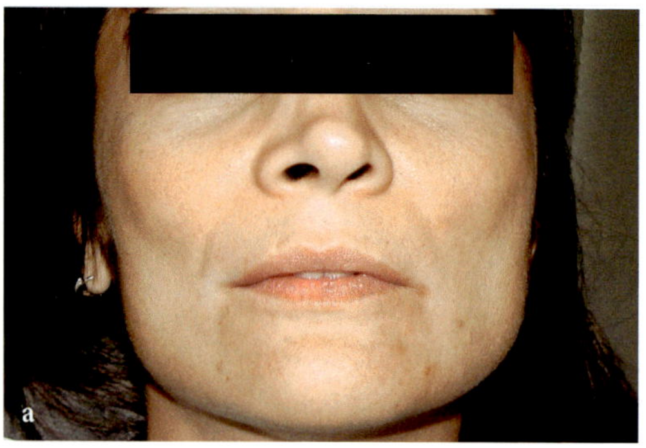


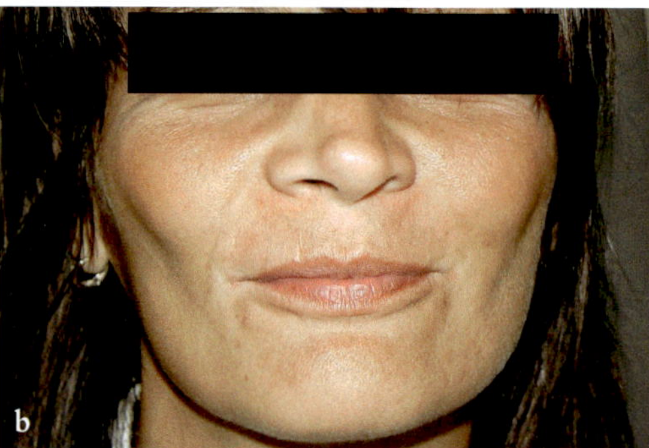


Fig 25-61 **(a and b)** Hypertrophy of both masseter muscles before and after toxin injection.

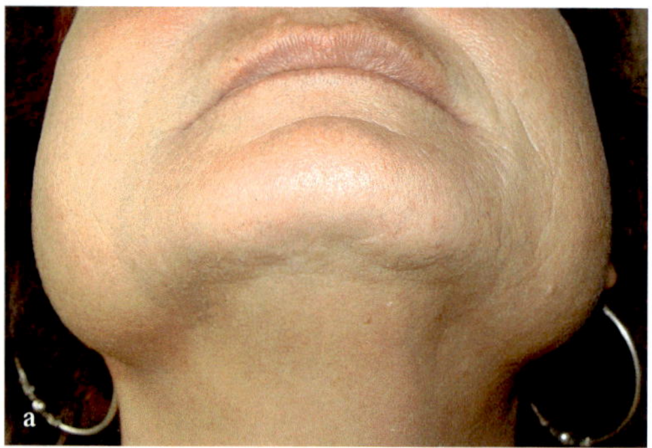


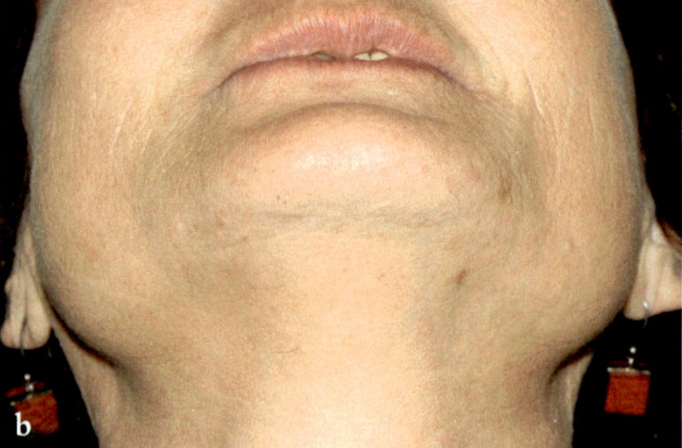


Fig 25-62 **(a)** Significantly developed masseter muscles in a female tooth clencher. **(b)** Picture taken after toxin injection shows significant reduction of both muscles.

added to fill the syringe; this amount is enough for both masseter muscles. The needle should be discarded after withdrawal of the vial content, since the needle bevel will be spoiled during the process of puncturing the vial's rubber cap. The thinnest needles available on the market should be used; we suggest using 0.5-inch 30G needles. Also, it is advisable to change needles every two punctures, so that the procedure is painless and imperceptible to the patient. The toxin is injected at the location of the previously drawn marks, while having the patient relax their muscles completely; the needle should penetrate in full. With each puncture, 0.1 mL of toxin (equivalent to 5 units) will be injected inside the muscle, and the five punctures performed will add up to 25 U (0.5 mL), which is the dosage recommended for each muscle. Once the five punctures have been performed, the procedure is repeated on the opposite side.

Figures 25-60 to 25-65 show some clinical cases treated with the technique which has just been described.

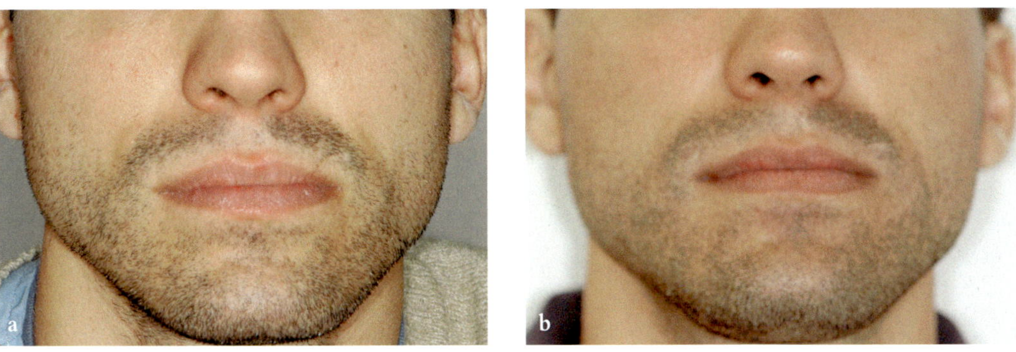

Fig 25-63 **(a and b)** Toxin injection "before" and "after" pictures.

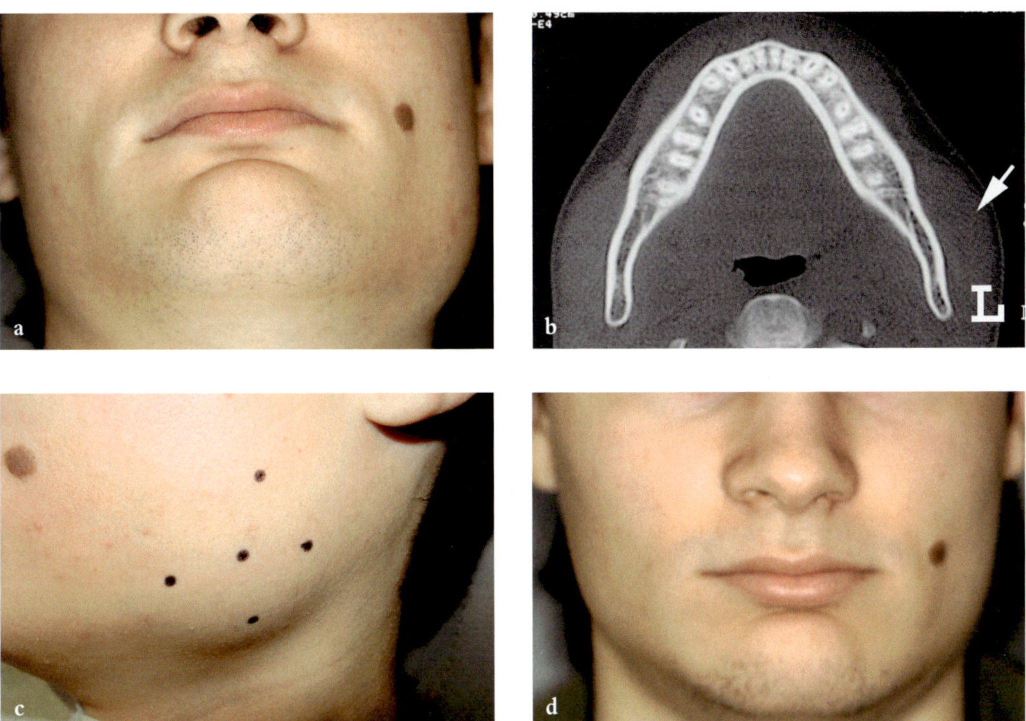

Fig 25-64 **(a)** Patient with facial asymmetry from left masseter muscle hypertrophy. **(b)** Computed tomography was performed: potential osseous etiology was excluded and the left masseter muscle (arrow) was found to be bigger than the right masseter muscle. **(c)** The five areas to be punctured are marked on the skin. **(d)** Toxin application has corrected the asymmetry.

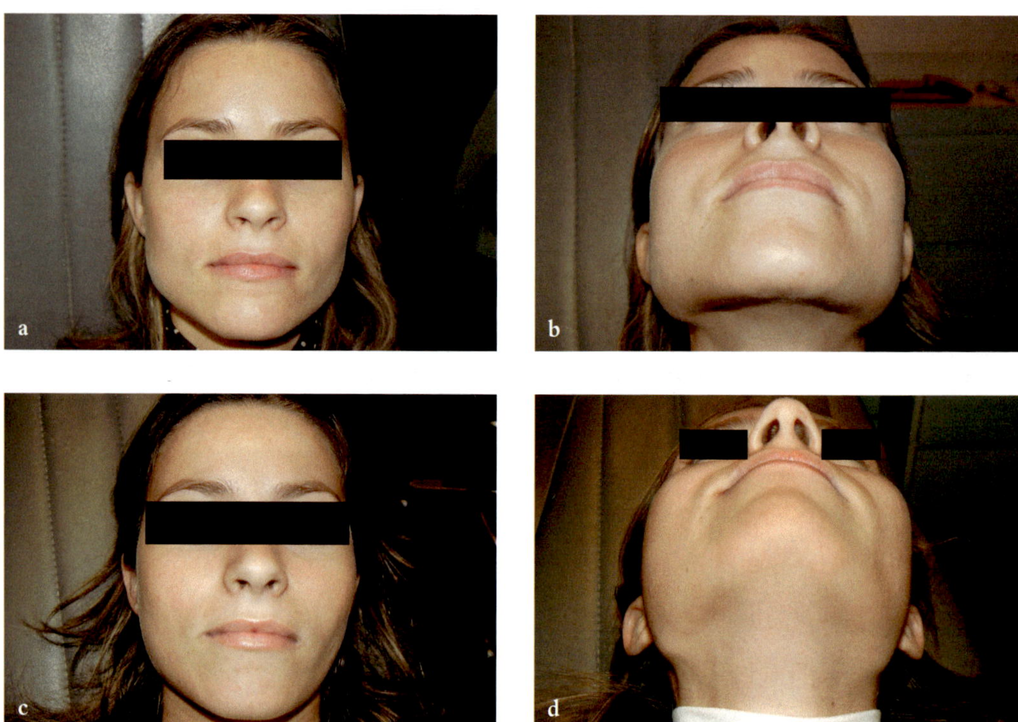

Fig 25-65 **(a and b)** Female bruxer with hypertrophy of both masseter muscles. **(c and d)** Toxin injection has resulted in hypertrophy regression.

## References


1. Glossary of prosthodontic terms. J Prosthet Dent 2005; 94:10–92.
2. McLean DW. Physiologic vs. pathologic occlusion. J Am Dent Assoc 1938;25:1583–1594.
3. Schuyler CH. Fundamental principles in the correction of occlusal disharmony, natural and artificial. J Am Dent Assoc 1935;22:1193–1202.
4. Alexander PC. The periodontium and the canine function theory. J Prosthet Dent 1967;18:571–578.
5. O'Leary TJ, Shanley DB, Drake RB. Tooth mobility in cuspid protected and group function occlusions. J Prosthet Dent 1972;27:21–25.
6. Beyron H. Occlusion: point of significance in planning restorative procedures. J Prosthet Dent 1973;30:641–652.
7. Weinberg LA. Temporomandibular joint function and its effect on concepts of occlusion. J Prosthet Dent 1976;35: 553–566.
8. D'Amico A. The canine teeth. Normal functional relation of the natural teeth of man. J South Calif Dent Assoc 1958; 26:194–208.
9. Stuart CE, Stallard H. Diagnosis and treatment of occlusal relations of the teeth. In: Stuart CE, Stallard H (eds). A Syllabus on Oral Rehabilitation and Occlusion. San Francisco: University of California, 1959.
10. Bonaguro JG, Dusza GR, Bowman DC. Ability of human subjects to discriminate forces applied to certain teeth. J Dent Res 1969;48:236–241.
11. Arpád T. Distribution of the last 1–4 teeth in the mouth. Fogorv Sz 1970;63:180–186.
12. Huffman RW, Regenos JW. Principles of occlusion. Laboratory and clinical teaching manual, ed 6. Columbus: Ohio State University, 1977.
13. Scaife RR. Natural occurrence of cuspid guidance. J Prosthet Dent 1969;22:225–229.
14. Woda A, Vigneron P, Kav D. Nonfunctional and functional occlusal contacts: a review of the literature. J Prosthet Dent 1979;42:335–341.

15. Belser UC, Hannam AG. The influence of altered working-side occlusal guidance on masticatory muscles and related jaw movement. J Prosthet Dent 1985;53:406–413.
16. Baba K, Ai M, Mizutani H, Enosawa S. Influence of experimental oclusal discrepancy on masticatory muscle activity during clenching. J Oral Rehabil 1996;23:55–60.
17. Akören AC, Karaağçlioğlu L. Comparison of the electromyographic activity of individuals with canine guidance and group function occlusion. J Oral Rehabil 1995; 22:73–77.
18. Carlsson GE, Johansson A, Lundqvist S. Occlusal wear: a follow-up study of 18 subjects with extensively worn dentitions. Acta Odontol Scand 1985;43:83–90.
19. Hasegawa K, Okamoto M, Nishigawa G, Oki K, Minagi S. The design of non-occlusal intraoral appliances on hard palate and their effect on masseter muscle activity during sleep. Cranio 2007;25:8–15.
20. Minagi S, Shimamura M, Sato T, Natsuaki N, Ohta M. Effect of a thick palatal appliance on muscular symptoms in craniomandibular disorders: a preliminary study. J Craniomandibular Pract 2001;19:42–47.
21. Manns A, Miralles R, Guerrero F. The changes in electrical activity of the postural muscles of the mandible upon varying the vertical dimension. J Prosthet Dent 1981;45:438–445.
22. Dao TTT, Lavigne GJ. Oral splints: the crutches for temporomandibular disorders and bruxism? Crit Rev Oral Biol Med 1998;9:345–361.
23. Dos Santos J, De Rijk WG. Vectorial analysis of the equilibrium of forces transmitted to TMJ and occlusal biteplane splints. J Oral Rehabil 1995;22:301–310.
24. Dahl BL, Krogstad O, Karlsen K. An alternative treatment in cases with advanced localized attrition. J Oral Rehabil 1975;2:209–214.
25. Yustin D, Neff P, Rieger MR, Hurst T. Characterization of 86 bruxing patients and long-term study of their management with occlusal devices and other forms of therapy. J Orofac Pain 1993;7:54–60.
26. Lucia VO. A technique for recording centric relation. J Prosthet Dent 1964;14:493–505.
27. Davis CR. Maintaining immediate posterior disclusion on an occlusal splint for patient with severe bruxism habit. J Prosthet Dent 1996;75:338–339.
28. Møller E, Bakke M. Occlusal harmony and disharmony: frauds in clinical dentistry? Int Dent J 1988;38:7–18.
29. Wood WW. A review of masticatory muscle function. J Prosthet Dent 1987;57:222–232.
30. Guggenheim P, Cohen L. The nature of maseteric hypertrophy. Arch Otolaryngol 1961;73:15–28.
31. Newton JP, Cowpe JG, McClure IJ, Delday MI, Maltin CA. Masseteric hypertrophy? Preliminary report. Br J Oral Maxillofac Surg 1999;37:405–408.
32. Skoura C, Mourouzis C, Saranteas T, Chatzigianni E, Tesseromatis C. Masseteric hypertrophy associated with administration of anabolic steroids and unilateral mastication: a case report. Oral Surg Oral Med Oral Pathol Oral Radiol Endod 2001;92:51–58.
33. Wood WW, Tobias DL. EMG response to alteration of tooth contacts on occlusal splints during maximal clenching. J Prosthet Dent 1984;51:394–396.
34. Fitins D, Sheikholeslam A. Effect of canine guidance of maxillary occlusal splint on level of activation of masticatory muscles. Swed Dent J 1993;17:235–241.
35. Dahlström L, Haraldson T. Immediate electromyographic response in masseter and temporal muscles to bite plates and stabilization splints. Scand J Dent Res 1989;97: 533–538.
36. Roark AL, Glaros AG, O'Mahony AM. Effects of interocclusal appliances on EMG activity during parafunctional tooth contact. J Oral Rehabil 2003;30:573–577.
37. Lobbezoo F, Van der Glas HW, Van Kampen FMC, Bosman F. The effect of an occlusal stabilization splint and the mode of visual feedback on the activity balance between jaw-elevator muscles during isometric contraction. J Dent Res 1993;72:876–882.
38. Christensen LV. Effects of an occlusal splint on integrated electromyography of masseter muscle in experimental tooth clenching in man. J Oral Rehabil 1980;7:281–288.
39. Jin Park Y, Woo Jo Y, Bang SI et al. Radiofrequency volumetric reduction for masseteric hypertrophy. Aesthetic Plast Surg 2007;31:42–52.
40. Freund B, Schwartz M, Symington J. Botulinum toxin: new treatment for temporomandibular disorders. Br J Oral Maxillofac Surg 2000;38:466–471.
41. Yu CC, Chen PK, Chen YR. Botulinum toxin A for lower facial contouring: a prospective study. Aesthetic Plast Surg 2007;31:445–451.
42. Ahn KY, Kim ST. The change of maximum bite force after botulinum toxin type A injection for treating masseteric hypertrophy. Plast Reconstr Surg 2007;120:1662–1666.
43. Lee CJ, Kim SG, Kim YJ et al. Electrophysiologic change and facial contour following botulinum toxin A injection in square faces. Plast Reconstr Surg 2007;120:769–778.
44. Kim JH, Shin JH, Kim ST, Kim CY. Effects of two different units of botulinum toxin type A evaluated by computed tomography and electromyographic measurements of human masseter muscle. Plast Reconstr Surg 2007;119: 711–717.
45. Bentsianov B, Aren F, Blitzer A. Botulinum toxin treatment of temporomandibular disorders, masseteric hypertrophy, and cosmetic masseter reduction. Oper Tech Otolaryngol Head Neck Surg 2004;15:110–113.
46. Clark GT. The management of oromandibular motor disorders and facial spasm with injections of botulinum toxin. Phys Med Rehabil Clin N Am 2003;14:727–748.

## A

## B

## E

## I



## J

## K



## L



## M

## Q



## R

## S

T